Handbook of
Psychopharmacology

Volume 19

New Directions in Behavioral Pharmacology

Handbook of
Psychopharmacology

SECTION I: BASIC NEUROPHARMACOLOGY
Volume 1   Biochemical Principles and Techniques in Neuropharmacology
Volume 2   Principles of Receptor Research
Volume 3   Biochemistry of Biogenic Amines
Volume 4   Amino Acid Neurotransmitters
Volume 5   Synaptic Modulators
Volume 6   Biogenic Amine Receptors

SECTION II: BEHAVIORAL PHARMACOLOGY IN ANIMALS
Volume 7   Principles of Behavioral Pharmacology
Volume 8   Drugs, Neurotransmitters, and Behavior
Volume 9   Chemical Pathways in the Brain

SECTION III: HUMAN PSYCHOPHARMACOLOGY
Volume 10   Neuroleptics and Schizophrenia
Volume 11   Stimulants
Volume 12   Drugs of Abuse
Volume 13   Biology of Mood and Antianxiety Drugs
Volume 14   Affective Disorders: Drug Actions in Animals and Man

SECTION IV: BASIC NEUROPHARMACOLOGY: AN UPDATE
Volume 15   New Techniques in Psychopharmacology
Volume 16   Neuropeptides
Volume 17   Biochemical Studies of CNS Receptors

SECTION V: BEHAVIORAL PHARMACOLOGY: AN UPDATE
Volume 18   Drugs, Neurotransmitters, and Behavior
Volume 19   New Directions in Behavioral Pharmacology

Volume 19

New Directions in Behavioral Pharmacology

Edited by

Leslie L. Iversen
Department of Pharmacology
University of Cambridge

Susan D. Iversen
Department of Psychology
University of Cambridge

and

Solomon H. Snyder
Departments of Neuroscience, Pharmacology, and Psychiatry
The Johns Hopkins University
School of Medicine

PLENUM PRESS • NEW YORK AND LONDON

Library of Congress Cataloging in Publication Data

New directions in behavioral pharmacology.

(Handbook of psychopharmacology; v. 19)
Includes bibliographies and index.
1. Neuropsychopharmacology. I. Iversen, Leslie L. II. Iversen, Susan D., 1940–
III. Snyder, Solomon H., 1938–   . IV. Series. [DNLM: 1. Behavior—drug effects. 2.
Neuropharmacology. 3. Psychopharmacology. QV 77 H236 sect.5 v.19]
RM315.H345 1975 vol. 19   615'.78 s   87-2551
ISBN 0-306-42447-9   [615'.78]

© 1987 Plenum Press, New York
A Division of Plenum Publishing Corporation
233 Spring Street, New York, N.Y. 10013

All rights reserved

No part of this book may be reproduced, stored in a retrieval system, or transmitted
in any form or by any means, electronic, mechanical, photocopying, microfilming,
recording, or otherwise, without written permission from the Publisher

Printed in the United States of America

CONTRIBUTORS

MICHAEL J. BANNON, *Departments of Psychiatry and Pharmacology, Yale University School of Medicine and the Abraham Ribicoff Research Facilities, Connecticut Mental Health Center, New Haven, Connecticut 06508; present address: Center for Cell Biology, Sinai Hospital of Detroit, Detroit, Michigan 48235*

JOHN E. BLUNDELL, *BioPsychology Laboratories, Psychology Department, University of Leeds, Leeds LS2 9JT, United Kingdom*

BENJAMIN S. BUNNEY, *Departments of Psychiatry and Pharmacology, Yale University School of Medicine and the Abraham Ribicoff Research Facilities, Connecticut Mental Health Center, New Haven, Connecticut 06508*

LOUIS A. CHIODO, *Departments of Psychiatry and Pharmacology, Yale University School of Medicine and the Abraham Ribicoff Research Facilities, Connecticut Mental Health Center, New Haven, Connecticut 06508; present address: Center for Cell Biology, Sinai Hospital of Detroit, Detroit, Michigan 48235*

DONALD J. COHEN, *Departments of Pediatrics, Psychiatry, and Psychology, Yale University School of Medicine and the Child Study Center, New Haven, Connecticut 06510*

ROELOF EIKELBOOM, *Department of Psychology, Queen's University, Kingston, Ontario, Canada K7L 3N6*

MICHAEL S. EISON, *Central Nervous System Research, Pharmaceutical Research and Development Division, Bristol-Myers Company, Wallingford, Connecticut 06429*

S. J. ENNA, *Nova Pharmaceutical Corporation, Baltimore, Maryland 21224*

ARTHUR S. FREEMAN, *Departments of Psychiatry and Pharmacology, Yale University School of Medicine and the Abraham Ribicoff Research Facilities, Connecticut Mental Health Center, New Haven, Connecticut 06508; present address:* Center for Cell Biology, Sinai Hospital of Detroit, Detroit, Michigan 48235

A. RICHARD GREEN, *MRC Clinical Pharmacology Unit, Radcliffe Infirmary, Oxford OX2 6HE, England; present address: Astra Neuroscience Research Unit, 1 Wakefield Street, London WC1N 1PJ, England*

JEFFREY M. HALPERIN, *Division of Child and Adolescent Psychiatry, Mount Sinai School of Medicine of the City University of New York, New York, New York 10029*

GEORGE F. KOOB, *Division of Preclinical Neuroscience and Endocrinology, Scripps Clinic and Research Foundation, La Jolla, California 92037*

LEONARD I. LEVEN, *Division of Child and Adolescent Psychiatry, Mount Sinai School of Medicine of the City University of New York, New York, New York 10029*

DAVID J. MAYER, *Department of Physiology and Biophysics, Medical College of Virginia, Virginia Commonwealth University, Richmond, Virginia 23298*

KLAUS A. MICZEK, *Department of Psychology, Tufts University, Medford, Massachusetts 02155*

DAVID J. NUTT, *Department of Psychiatry, Research Unit, Littlemore Hospital, Oxford OX4 4NX, England; present address: National Institute for Alcohol Abuse and Alcoholism, Bethesda, Maryland 20205*

ROBERT H. ROTH, *Departments of Psychiatry and Pharmacology, Yale University School of Medicine and the Abraham Ribicoff Research Facilities, Connecticut Mental Health Center, New Haven, Connecticut 06508*

JOHN D. SALAMONE, *Department of Behavioral Neuroscience, University of Pittsburgh, Pittsburgh, Pennsylvania 15260*

BENNETT A. SHAYWITZ, *Departments of Pediatrics and Neurology, Yale University School of Medicine, New Haven, Connecticut 06510*

JANE STEWART, *Department of Psychology, Center for Studies in Behavioral Neurobiology, Concordia University, Montreal, Quebec, Canada H3G 1M8*

I. P. STOLERMAN, *Departments of Pharmacology and Psychiatry, Institute of Psychiatry, London SE5 8AF, England*

J. GERALD YOUNG, *Division of Child and Adolescent Psychiatry, Mount Sinai School of Medicine of the City University of New York, New York, New York 10029*

PREFACE

Volumes 7 and 8 of the *Handbook* were published in 1977. In Volume 7 methods for studying unconditioned and conditioned behavior were reviewed. Attention was given to both ethological methods and operant conditioning techniques as applied to some selected aspects of behavior. Genetic, developmental, and environmental factors influencing behavior were also discussed. In Volume 8, neurotransmitter systems, and in particular brain circuits, were discussed in relation to behavior and to the effects of psychoactive drugs on behavior. The coverage was not exhaustive because of space limitations. The topics selected for review were, at the time, the focus of considerable experimental effort; they included homeostasis-motivated behaviors: sleep, locomotion, feeding, drinking, and sexual behavior. Brain dopamine systems were therefore discussed in depth, since they were already known to be centrally involved in motivated behaviors. Learning mechanisms and emotion were reviewed in the remaining chapters.

In 1984 we initiated an update of behavioral pharmacology to review areas of progress within the same scope as the earlier volumes. This update continues in Volume 19. Among the contributions are several that represent important advances in analyzing behavior and the use of more sophisticated methods to define the effect of drugs on particular aspects of behavior. The chapters by Blundell on feeding and Miczek on aggression illustrate the sophistication of modern ethopharmacology. Conceptual advances have also been made, but it is important to realize that computer analysis of patterns and sequences of responses has opened up a new era in ethology.

The effects of drugs on behavior depend not only on their neuropharmacological properties but also on the age and state of development of the animal (see the chapter by Young), and are influenced by the ongoing behavior and drug history of that animal. The latter topic has become an extremely important one, since it is now clear that animals learn about drug experiences in much the same way that they learn about other stimuli in their environment (see the chapter by Stewart and Eikelboom).

The last decade has seen the identification of a large number of neuropeptides as CNS chemical messengers. In this area, work on the opiates and the issue of peptide involvement in memory were selected for review, since it is in these two areas that substantial progress has been made in understanding the modulatory role of peptides for integrative CNS activity. The future will, it is hoped, bring novel drugs to influence peptide function in CNS.

Finally, the behavioral effects of some of the classical psychotropics, such as nicotine, antidepressants, neuroleptics, and anticonvulsants, are receiving renewed attention as more is discovered about their neuropharmacological sites and modes of action in the CNS. Novel drugs to treat the major neurological and psychoactive conditions continue to be sought, since many of the existing ones have unwanted side effects.

L. L. I.
S. D. I.
S. H. S.

CONTENTS

CHAPTER 1

Conditioned Drug Effects

JANE STEWART AND ROELOF EIKELBOOM

 1. Introduction 1
   1.1. Terminology 2
   1.2. Basic Procedures and Designs 2
   1.3. Tests for Conditioning 3
   1.4. Optimal Conditions for Conditioning 5
   1.5. Confounding Factors 6
 2. Conditioned Drug Effects: Evidence and Explanations 9
   2.1. Conditioning of Drug-Induced Physiological Responses 9
   2.2. Conditioning Factors in the Changing Effectiveness of Drugs 18
   2.3. Conditioning of Affective Changes 26
 3. Implications 36
   3.1. Drug Self-Administration 37
   3.2. Treatment of Addictions 40
 4. References 41

CHAPTER 2

Developmental Neuropharmacology: Clinical and Neurochemical Perspectives on the Regulation of Attention, Learning, and Movement

J. GERALD YOUNG, JEFFREY M. HALPERIN, LEONARD I. LEVEN, BENNETT A. SHAYWITZ, AND DONALD J. COHEN

 1. Clinical Phenomena and Research Design 59
   1.1. Developmental Influences 59

		1.2.	Methodological Issues in Pediatric Psychopharmacological Research	63
	2.	Attention Deficit Disorder with Hyperactivity		68
		2.1.	Component Symptoms	68
		2.2.	Clinical Effects of Stimulants	70
		2.3.	Cellular and Molecular Effects of Stimulants	74
		2.4.	Neurochemistry: Animal Studies	75
		2.5.	Neurochemistry: Clinical Studies	79
	3.	Learning Disorders		84
		3.1.	General Considerations	84
		3.2.	Stimulants	86
		3.3.	Piracetam	92
	4.	Tourette's Syndrome of Chronic, Multiple Tics		93
		4.1.	Clinical Features	93
		4.2.	Neurobiological and Genetic Basis	94
		4.3.	Clinical Neurochemical Research	95
		4.4.	Treatment	98
	5.	Overview		106
	6.	References		107

CHAPTER 3

Structure, Process, and Mechanism: Case Studies in the Psychopharmacology of Feeding

JOHN E. BLUNDELL

1.	Introduction		123
2.	Control of Feeding: A First Look		125
3.	Drugs and Food Intake		126
	3.1.	Suppression of Food Intake	128
	3.2.	Enhancement of Food Intake	132
4.	Interpretation of Pharmacological Action		136
5.	Contextual and Temporal Dimensions of Behavior		137
6.	Structure, Process, and Mechanism		138
7.	Methodological Developments		140
	7.1.	Free-Feeding Animals	141
	7.2.	Microanalysis of the Structure of Feeding Behavior	141
	7.3.	Macroanalysis of Feeding Patterns	142
	7.4.	Variety and Palatability of Food	143
	7.5.	Motivation Measured by Instrumental Performance	143
	7.6.	Nutritional Aspects of Eating	144

8. Case Studies in the Pharmacological Analysis of
   Feeding 145
   8.1. Serotonin Manipulations and the Structure of
        Feeding Behavior 145
   8.2. Behavioral Analysis of the Effects of Opioid
        Antagonists on Feeding 155
   8.3. Behavioral Calibration of Natural and
        Abnormal Anorexia 161
9. Control of Feeding: A Second Look 168
   9.1. Impact of Pharmacological Studies 168
   9.2. A Paradox: The Orexic and Anorexic Effects
        of Amphetamine 169
   9.3. Models of Feeding Control 171
10. References 173

Chapter 4

The Psychopharmacology of Aggression

Klaus A. Miczek

1. Recent History of Psychopharmacological Aggression
   Research 183
   1.1. Psychiatric Research Questions 183
   1.2. Origins of Behavioral Methodology 185
   1.3. Emerging Neuroscientific Objectives 186
2. Framework for the Behavioral Analysis of Aggression 187
   2.1. Experimental–Psychological Approach 187
   2.2. Neurological Approach 193
   2.3. Ethological Approach 199
3. Preclinical and Clinical Aggression Research 204
   3.1. Antiaggressive Drug Treatments 204
   3.2. Drugs of Abuse and Aggression 235
4. References 277

Chapter 5

The Electrophysiological and Biochemical Pharmacology of the Mesolimbic and Mesocortical Dopamine Neurons

Michael J. Bannon, Arthur S. Freeman, Louis A. Chiodo, Benjamin S. Bunney, and Robert H. Roth

1. Introduction 329

2.	Anatomy of Midbrain Dopamine Systems	330
	2.1. The Nigrostriatal DA System	330
	2.2. Mesolimbic and Mesocortical DA Systems	330
3.	Distinguishing between A9 and A10 Dopamine Systems	332
	3.1. Behavioral Studies	332
	3.2. Anatomical Considerations	333
4.	Identification and Characterization	334
5.	Dopamine Neuron Function Regulation	337
	5.1. Effects of DA Agonists on A10 DA Neuron Activity	338
	5.2. DA Receptor Antagonist Actions	348
6.	Effects of Neurotransmitters on A10 Dopamine Neuron Activity	355
	6.1. The Influence of GABA on A10 DA Neurons	355
	6.2. The Effects of Serotonin on A10 DA Neurons	358
	6.3. The Effects of Noradrenergic Agonists and Antagonists on A10 DA Neurons	359
	6.4. The Effects of Substance P on A10 DA Neurons	360
7.	Summary	362
8.	References	363

CHAPTER 6

Psychopharmacology of Repeated Seizures: Possible Relevance to the Mechanism of Action of Electroconvulsive Therapy

A. RICHARD GREEN AND DAVID J. NUTT

1.	Introduction	375
2.	Functional Changes after Seizures	377
	2.1. 5-Hydroxytryptamine	377
	2.2. Dopamine	380
	2.3. Noradrenaline	382
	2.4. GABA	383
	2.5. Acetylcholine	386
	2.6. Opioids	386
	2.7. Histamine	387
3.	Biochemical Consequences of Seizures	387
	3.1. 5-Hydroxytryptamine	387
	3.2. Dopamine	390
	3.3. Noradrenaline	390

	3.4.	GABA	393
	3.5.	Opioid Peptides	397
	3.6.	Acetylcholine	398
	3.7.	Adenosine and Cyclic Nucleotides	399
	3.8.	Peptides	400
	3.9.	Calcium	400
4.	Neuroendocrine Markers of Neurotransmitter Changes Following Electroconvulsive Shock		401
5.	Are Any Biochemical and Functional Changes Associated?		402
	5.1.	5-Hydroxytryptamine	402
	5.2.	Dopamine	402
	5.3.	Noradrenaline	403
	5.4.	GABA	403
	5.5.	Acetylcholine	406
	5.6.	Opioid Peptides	406
6.	Can Biochemical or Behavioral Changes Be Associated with Antidepressant Action of Electroconvulsive Shock?		406
7.	References		408

Chapter 7

Psychopharmacology of Nicotine: Stimulus Effects and Receptor Mechanisms

I. P. Stolerman

1.	Introduction		421
	1.1.	Historical Background	421
	1.2.	Behavioral Background	423
	1.3.	Neurochemical Background	424
2.	Nicotine as a Positive Reinforcer		429
	2.1.	Introduction	429
	2.2.	Studies in Animals	429
	2.3.	Studies in Human Subjects	432
	2.4.	Conclusions	433
3.	Nicotine as an Aversive Stimulus		434
	3.1.	Introduction	434
	3.2.	Nicotine as a Punisher	434
	3.3.	Nicotine as a Negative Reinforcer	435
	3.4.	Conditioned Taste Aversions	435
	3.5.	Conclusions	436

4. Discriminative Stimulus of Nicotine 437
   4.1. Introduction 437
   4.2. Generalization Tests: Nicotinic Agonists 438
   4.3. Generalization Tests: Nonnicotinic Drugs 442
   4.4. Pretreatment Experiments............... 444
   4.5. Conclusions 447
5. Nicotine and Brain Mechanisms of Reward 448
   5.1. Introduction 448
   5.2. Studies of Intracranial Self-Stimulation...... 448
   5.3. Intake of Palatable Substances 450
   5.4. Conditioned Place Preferences 450
   5.5. Neuropharmacological Observations 450
   5.6. Evidence from Nicotine Self-Administration .. 452
6. General Conclusions 452
   6.1. Integration of Different Approaches 452
   6.2. Models of the CNS Nicotinic Receptor 454
7. References 458

Chapter 8

The Behavioral Effects of Opiates

David J. Mayer

1. Introduction 467
   1.1. Historical Perspective 467
   1.2. Methodological Considerations 468
2. The Effects of Opiates on Pain 469
   2.1. The Neurobiology of Afferent Pain
        Transmission 470
   2.2. The Effects of Opiates on Pain Transmission .. 478
   2.3. Environmental Activation of Endogenous
        Analgesia Systems 485
3. The Effects of Opiates on Reward 495
   3.1. The Neural Substrate of Opiate Reward 495
   3.2. The Opiate Reward and Other Forms of
        Reward 496
4. The Effects of Opiates on Cardiovascular
   Function 499
   4.1. The Cardiovascular Effects of Exogenously
        Administered Opiates 499
   4.2. Endogenous Opioids and Environmentally
        Produced Cardiovascular Effects 501
5. Other Effects of Opiates on Behavior 502
6. References 511

Chapter 9

Neuropeptides and Memory

George F. Koob

1.	Neuropeptides	531
2.	Conceptual and Methodological Considerations	533
	2.1. Conceptual Model	533
	2.2. Animal Tests	534
3.	Hypophyseal Peptides and Memory	535
	3.1. Vasopressin	535
	3.2. Oxytocin	542
	3.3. Adrenocorticotropic Hormone	543
	3.4. Endorphins	546
	3.5. Somatostatin	548
4.	Nonhypophyseal Peptides and Memory	549
	4.1. Neurotensin	549
	4.2. Angiotensin	550
	4.3. Cholecystokinin	550
	4.4. Substance P	551
5.	Synthesis	553
	5.1. Hypophyseal Peptides—Summary	553
	5.2. Nonhypophyseal Peptides—Summary	554
	5.3. Site and Mechanism of Action	554
	5.4. U-Shaped Dose–Effect Functions	555
	5.5. Blood–Brain Barrier	556
	5.6. Is It Memory?	557
	5.7. James–Lange Theory of Memory	559
	5.8. State Dependency	560
	5.9. Homology of Function	561
6.	References	561

Chapter 10

The Actions of Neuroleptic Drugs on Appetitive Instrumental Behaviors

John D. Salamone

1.	Introduction	575
2.	Hypotheses on the Behavioral Actions of Neuroleptics	576
	2.1. Behavioral Profile of Neuroleptic Effects	576
	2.2. Early Motor Hypotheses	578
	2.3. Anhedonia and the Link between Dopamine and Reinforcement	579

3. Evaluation of Experiments on Dopaminergic
   Involvement in Reinforcement 581
   3.1. On the Proposed Similarity between
        Neuroleptics and Extinction 581
   3.2. The Response Capacity Argument........... 583
   3.3. The Use of Paradigms Purported to Dissociate
        Reinforcement from Performance........... 584
   3.4. Conclusions 592
4. Incentive Explanation of Neuroleptic Actions 594
5. An Alternative Explanation of Dopamine Antagonist
   Effects on Operant Behavior..................... 597
   5.1. A Multiprocess Model for Describing Control
        of Operant Response Output 598
   5.2. On the Role of Brain Dopamine Systems in
        Appetitive Instrumental Behavior 600
6. References 602

Chapter 11

Second-Generation Antidepressants

S. J. Enna and Michael S. Eison

1. Introduction 609
2. General Properties of Second-Generation
   Antidepressants................................ 612
3. Methodological Approaches 616
   3.1. Neurochemical Assays 616
   3.2. Behavioral Assays........................ 619
4. Summary and Conclusions 625
5. References 626

Index 633

CONDITIONED DRUG EFFECTS

Jane Stewart and Roelof Eikelboom

1. INTRODUCTION

The repeated administration of a drug or hormone in the presence of a common set of environmental stimuli leads to conditions under which the organism can learn the contingent relation between the environmental stimulus and the drug-produced stimulus. In the terminology of Pavlovian conditioning, the stimulus that signals the occurrence of drug-produced stimuli is the *conditioned stimulus* (CS) and the drug-produced stimulus is the *unconditioned stimulus* (US). Evidence that the relation between the CS and the US is learned comes from the change in the way the organism responds to the originally neutral CS. If the CS reliably predicts the occurrence of the US, the CS becomes capable of eliciting responses in anticipation of the US that were originally elicited, unconditionally, by the US; that is, the CS becomes a substitute for the US. Although conditioning experiments in which the USs are drug produced have been carried out for over 75 years (see Lynch *et al.*, 1976; Wikler, 1973), only in the last 10 years has the study of conditioned drug effects become of major interest in psychopharmacology (see Baker and Tiffany, 1985; Eikelboom and Stewart, 1982; Goudie and Demellweek, 1985; Grabowski and O'Brien, 1981; Hinson, 1985; Poulos *et al.*, 1981a; Siegel, 1977b, 1983, 1985; Solomon, 1977; Stewart *et al.*, 1984). No doubt, the possible relevance of conditioned effects for understanding drug tolerance, sensitization, and

---

Jane Stewart • Department of Psychology, Center for Studies in Behavioral Neurobiology, Concordia University, Montreal, Quebec, Canada H3G 1M8.   *Roelof Eikelboom* • Department of Psychology, Queen's University, Kingston, Ontario, Canada K7L 3N6.

compulsive drug use has sparked the large increase in the number of studies. In this chapter, we review the evidence for conditioned drug effects and discuss its implications.

1.1. Terminology

In the study of conditioned drug effects, a set of stimuli, previously relatively neutral to the animal, is paired with an injection of a drug known or thought to bring about some observable, measurable change either in a physiological variable (e.g., heart rate or body temperature) or in overt behavior (e.g., increased activity, analgesia). These changes we shall call *observed drug effects*. In the terminology of Pavlovian conditioning, the neutral stimuli are the CSs, and the drug-produced stimuli are the USs. Drug-produced stimuli elicit *unconditioned responses* (URs) via their effect on the central nervous system (CNS). Effects elicited by the drug via the CNS have the potential to become elicitable by the CS and thus to become *conditioned responses* (CRs) or *conditioned drug effects*.

Note that, according to this terminology, the ritual surrounding the injection of the drug as well as other environmental events associated with the drug action have the potential to act as CSs. It is the drug-produced stimuli that act as the USs and that, in turn, elicit URs via the CNS. It is inaccurate and misleading, therefore, to refer casually to the drug injection as the US and to the observed drug effect as the UR. The observed drug effect may indeed be the UR elicited by the action of drug on the CNS, but it may not be; the initially observed drug effect may result from direct actions on effectors and thus act as an indirect stimulus for the elicitation of a CNS-mediated response that opposes or compensates for the observed drug effect. In this way, therefore, we see that it is possible for conditioned drug effects to mimic or to oppose the initially observed drug effect (see Eikelboom and Stewart, 1982).

1.2. Basic Procedures and Designs

The procedures and designs required for the unequivocal demonstration of Pavlovian CRs have been the concern of many workers in the field and continue to be discussed (see Mackintosh, 1974; Rescorla, 1967). In essence, these procedures have been established to demonstrate that the changes in behavior observed in the presence of the CS after explicit pairings of the CS and US result from learning the contingent relation between the CS and the US and not from changes in responding to the CS brought about by repeated presentations of the CS alone, of the US alone (so-called pseudoconditioning), or from random (noncontingent) presentations of both sets of stimuli.

It has become standard to include at least three groups of animals in studies of conditioned drug effects: a group that receives the drug in the presence of a distinctive set of stimuli (the CS) and receives a saline or drug vehicle in the absence of these distinctive stimuli (an explicitly paired group), a group that receives saline in the presence of the distinctive stimuli and the drug injection in their absence (an explicitly unpaired group), and a group that receives saline under both conditions.

A note of caution about the use of this design: In many instances, distinctive environments or places are used as CS in drug experiments. Animals are brought to the CS environment where they are given the appropriate injection (drug or saline) and remain for a fixed time. The second set of injections are given in the home cage. In many experiments, the second set of injections is given immediately upon return to the home cage. Under these conditions, it is possible that the time spent in the distinctive CS environment will come to serve as a cue, predictive of drug administration for animals that receive the injection when taken back to the home cage. Therefore, such regular spatial–temporal contiguities should be avoided.

Another problem with this design is that the distinctive CS environment, being negatively correlated with drug injections, may come to serve as an inhibitory stimulus for animals that receive saline there and drug in the home cage or second environment. For this reason, it may be preferable to include a group that receives random presentations of the CS and the drug. Additional groups, of course, may be added to control for other variables that might affect the results of particular experiments. This phase of the conditioning experiment is usually referred to as the *training* or *conditioning phase*. The training phase may be interrupted by occasional *tests* for conditioning.

1.3. Tests for Conditioning

In a standard test for conditioning, all groups are presented with the CS without drug administration and their responses are compared. Tests given during the training phase allow one to follow the course of conditioning. In many instances, however, tests for conditioning may be made only upon the completion of the conditioning phase. Repeated tests without resumption of conditioning trials constitute an *extinction phase* during which differences among groups should diminish. These are the simplest and most fundamental procedures used in studies of conditioning. For a more complete description of the various training and test procedures used to study the range of conditioning phenomena, see Mackintosh (1974) and Rescorla and Solomon (1967).

Evidence for conditioning is best assessed, as described earlier, using a between-groups design in which the responses of various treatment groups are compared to the presentation of the CS in the absence of drug. In some experiments, however, subjects are given the CS before the conditioning phase and the responses elicited by the CS on these tests are compared to those elicited after conditioning. In other experiments, the change in response to the CS is assessed by taking measurements in the same animal immediately before and after the CS. These variations in tests for conditioned drug effects constitute within-subjects designs and can lead to results that differ from those obtained with between-group designs. They have, in addition, revealed the operation of confounding variables that preclude simple interpretation of results and often have led to contradictory conclusions.

In most studies, tests for conditioning are done immediately after the end of the conditioning phase, that is, when the drug would normally be administered. Termination of drug administration, however, can have physiological consequences that may confound tests for conditioning or mask the CR. A conditioning test given after a drug-free period may thus reveal a different conditioned drug effect than a test given immediately after conditioning (Eikelboom and Stewart, 1979).

The assessment of conditioned drug effects has, in recent years, often been done in the context of the study of tolerance and sensitization of specific drug effects. In many instances, tolerance, and in some cases sensitization, has been shown to be specific to the contextual stimuli repeatedly associated with drug administration. These findings have led to the view that context-specific tolerance could arise from the conditioning of drug-opposite responses to the context, whereas context-specific sensitization might arise from the conditioning of drug-similar responses (Siegel, 1975*b*, 1977*a*). In these cases, evidence of conditioned drug effects is sometimes inferred from the differential response to drug observed in the presence and absence of drug-related stimuli (CSs). These indirect tests for "conditioning" are made by giving subjects in all treatment groups injections of the drug in the presence of the CS, in its absence, or in both. It should be pointed out, however, that although these tests may indicate context- or stimulus-specific tolerance or sensitization, they do not provide direct evidence for the operation of conditioned drug-induced responses. There are many reports of context-specific tolerance, for example, when no evidence for the operation of drug-opposite responses was found. Alternative explanations for these effects have been proposed and will be discussed in a later section.

1.4. Optimal Conditions for Conditioning

In this section, we will mention a few of the conditions that have been found to facilitate conditioning in animals and that may be particularly important for the understanding of results in conditioning studies using drugs. Animals are most likely to learn the relation between the CS and the US when the CS predicts the occurrence of the US reliably and uniquely. Thus, not only must there be a reliable contingent relation between the CS and the US for conditioning to develop, but, in addition, the intended CS will be more effective if it alone reliably predicts the occurrence of the US, that is, if it is not a redundant cue. One way to ensure that predictive relations between paired events are perceived is to give discrete, widely spaced presentations of the CS–US pairings. Separation in time of conditioning trials when drugs are used to produce the US may be particularly important, for although the injection of the drug is a relatively short-duration event, drug actions are not. If a drug were injected too frequently, its effects might continue until the time of the next injection, thus masking its contingent relation to the CS. Furthermore, drug-produced stimuli of long duration would lose their salience and effectiveness as USs if injections were closely spaced in time. Frequent injections of long-acting drugs would also affect the uniqueness of the CS as a predictive cue for the drug effect, inasmuch as other intervening stimuli might equally predict the drug effects. Because drugs in higher doses have longer duration of action, it may be that under some circumstances stronger evidence for conditioning will be obtained with lower doses of drugs. This may be so when conditioning trials are frequent or when animals are removed from the presence of the CS before the effects of the drug have subsided (see also Baker and Tiffany, 1985).

Post (1981) made the interesting point that the interval between drug doses is an important variable in determining sensitization or tolerance to the drug. In some instances, for example, continuous exposure to a drug may lead to tolerance, whereas intermittent exposure may lead to sensitization (see also Giknis and Damjanov, 1984). The extent to which such observed differences can be attributed to conditioning factors, which would more likely be operative under intermittent exposure, needs to be explored in more detail.

Salience of the CS is another important factor in the development of conditioning. Animals will show greater evidence for conditioning when the CS is relatively novel and distinct from the background. Preexposure to the CS will reduce its effectiveness as a CS event (for a more complete discussion of these issues, see Mackintosh, 1974). There now is considerable evidence that these factors operate in studies of drug conditioning and that contradictory findings are obtained in certain instances.

In conclusion, it seems reasonable to state that more evidence for conditioned drug effects and context-specific effects will be obtained when the CS is a reliable and unique predictor of the drug effect, when individual pairings of CS and drug are widely spaced in time, and when the CS is a highly salient and discriminable event in the animal's daily routine. See Section 1.5.4 for further discussion of the choice of the CS.

1.5. Confounding Factors

1.5.1. Multiple Drug Effects

Most drugs used in studies of conditioning affect several different response systems through the CNS as well as peripheral tissues. Sometimes the same drug produces opposing changes in some measure being used to monitor the response of the system. A high dose of morphine, for example, may cause an initial drop in body temperature, followed by a rise in temperature to above normal. These biphasic effects of certain drugs may reflect, on the one hand, the output of two independent response systems that are activated simultaneously, with one initially masking the other, perhaps by different doses of the drug. On the other hand, the second response may be elicited to compensate for the initial response. For example, the drop in body temperature could occur because of passive loss of heat, for example, as the result of some direct peripheral action of the drug on blood vessels, not of CNS-mediated cooling responses. In this case, the compensatory activation of heat mechanisms would be the only response elicited unconditionally. One must be aware that, depending on how the responses are elicited, one or both of them could become conditioned. The problem for the experimenter is that a particular physiological indicator reflects only the net effect of these conditioned changes and, under some circumstances, may indicate that little or no conditioning occurred, whereas in fact, conditioning did occur and may be perceived later under different circumstances.

As outlined earlier, some conditioned drug effects may arise because of the direct or indirect action of the drug on a particular regulatory system. Other conditioned drug effects, however, may reflect consequences secondary to direct actions of the drug. For example, CSs that predict the injection of a highly preferred euphoria-producing drug could elicit general anticipatory excitement, increasing activity levels and indirectly increasing body temperature. The conditioned changes in activity and body temperature observed under these circumstances would not necessarily reflect specific conditioning of drug-produced changes in activity or thermoregulatory responses. An awareness of this possibility is particularly important for an understanding of the behavioral significance of conditioned physiological changes in the mediation of drug taking and, perhaps, of placebo effects.

1.5.2. Stress Responses

Probably the most significant confounding variable that has come to light as a source of contradictory results in studies of conditioned drug effects is the response to stressors. Experimental procedures, including handling, injection, testing, response measurement, associated pain, and even exposure to a novel stimulus condition, have all been shown to act as stressors and to affect physiological and behavioral measurements. This is particularly true in studies with opiates; many of the effects of opiates are mimicked by stressors; and thus stress can augment the effects of opiate drugs. Furthermore, stress responses in themselves can become conditioned to stimuli associated with stressors; these conditioned stress responses can, in turn, lead to misinterpretation of experimental results.

Bardo and Hughes (1979) first explored in detail the role that exposure to novel stimuli plays in the assessment of the analgesic effects of morphine. Animals exposed to apparatus cues for the first time had augmental analgesic responses to morphine, compared to animals preexposed to the testing environment. Similar effects of the stress of handling and novel stimuli have been shown to interact with the temperature effects of morphine to potentiate the hyperthermic effect of low doses and the hypothermic effect of high doses (Benedek *et al.*, 1983; Stewart and Eikelboom, 1981) and to interact with the assessment of conditioned temperature responses to morphine (Sherman, 1979). Colpaert *et al.* (1980) have demonstrated that repeatedly testing for analgesia (every 5 min) under the influence of the narcotic Fentanyl increases the degree of analgesia induced by a single dose, and that antecedent exposure to pain augments the analgesic response to Fentanyl. Sherman *et al.* (1982) and Sherman *et al.* (1984) have shown that morphine analgesia is enhanced in the presence of stress-associated environmental stimuli, which suggests that conditioned stress-induced analgesia interacts with drug-induced analgesia and could, therefore, affect the assessment of drug-induced conditioned effects.

These conditioned stress-induced analgesic effects appear to be mediated, at least in part, by endogenous opioids (Fanselow and Baackes, 1982). Naloxone can attenuate the conditioned stress-induced analgesia (Fanselow and Bolles, 1979) and plasma β-endorphin levels are elevated in an environment in which pain had previously been experienced (Scallet, 1982).

Studies with stimulant drugs also point to the importance of stress responses in the assessment of unconditioned and conditioned drug effects. Preexposure to a stressor appears to sensitize responses elicited by a dose of amphetamine much in the way that prior exposure to the drug does (Antelman *et al.*, 1980). This finding suggests that both effects are mediated through the dopamine systems of the brain. The role such effects might play in the development and assessment of conditioned effects obtained with stimulants is yet to be determined.

Such examples of the interaction between stress responses and drug effects make it appear that the operation of stress factors may account for many of the contradictory findings in the drug-conditioning literature. We are well aware that it is all too easy to call upon the operation of stress factors to "explain" these contradictions. Quite clearly, it will take some time to sort out whether and how stress is having an effect in each instance.

1.5.3. Circadian and Ultradian Rhythms

Another potential source of discrepant findings in the literature on conditioned drug effects is in the changing effectiveness of drugs as a function of changes in physiological systems over the day (for examples see Fredrickson *et al.*, 1977; Glimcher *et al.*, 1984; Nakano *et al.*, 1980; Walker *et al.*, 1982). Changes in receptor number, in endogenously released pituitary peptides, and in neurotransmitters and enzymes could change the degree of a given drug effect and thereby affect the magnitude, and even the direction, of the unconditioned drug effect. Although little attention has been paid to these effects in studies of drug conditioning, drug injections are often given in such studies at the same time each day. This practice, in itself, may lead to problems of interpretation. It appears that regular daily injections may act to entrain physiological responses and to bring certain conditioned drug effects under temporal control (see, for example, Eikelboom and Stewart, 1981*a*). These temporally conditioned effects may, in turn, modify the development of CRs to other stimuli in the environment. Such observations highlight another confounding factor, the choice of the CS, in the study of conditioned drug effects.

1.5.4. Choice of Conditional Stimuli

Evidence has been accumulating for some time that the relative effectiveness of stimuli to act as CSs varies as a function of the US (Garcia and Koelling, 1966; Garcia *et al.*, 1966). Garcia and his colleagues showed that, in rats, aversion based on x-ray or drug-induced illness could be conditioned to taste stimuli but not to sights and sounds. Subsequent work with a variety of drugs has shown that the different effects produced by a drug are more easily conditioned to some environmental stimuli than to others (e.g., Lett, 1985). This evidence will be discussed in subsequent sections. As has been stated before, drugs have multiple effects that elicit responding in different systems, both simultaneously and over time. It is important to note, then, that these different responses may be selectively conditioned to different features of the environment. The choice of the CS used in a drug-conditioning experiment may determine not only the magnitude of the conditioned effect observed but also its direction and quality.

2. CONDITIONED DRUG EFFECTS: EVIDENCE AND EXPLANATIONS

Early studies of conditioned drug effects were largely concerned with the conditioning of drug-elicited physiological responses. These studies were conceptualized within the stimulus-substitution theory of conditioning first suggested by Pavlov (see Bykov, 1957), in which the CS, through pairing with the US, comes to elicit responses that mimic those originally elicited by the US. Among the early findings, however, were examples of so-called *paradoxical conditioning*. Paradoxical conditioning was said to occur when the observed drug effect and the CRs were in opposite directions. We have argued that cases of paradoxical conditioning are entirely consistent with stimulus substitution theory and that their paradoxical nature arises from failure to determine the relation between the observed drug effect and the drug produced US and UR (Eikelboom and Stewart, 1982). The conditioning of responses that oppose the observed drug effect occurs, in our view, when the observed drug effect acts as a stimulus to elicit a compensatory physiological response. In this section, we will review studies from four physiological systems in which conditioning studies with drugs have been continuing: the thermoregulatory system, the blood glucose regulation system, the cardiovascular system, and the immune system.

2.1. Conditioning of Drug-Induced Physiological Responses

2.1.1. Conditioning of Changes in Body Temperature

Many drugs have profound effects on the thermoregulatory system and, consequently, on body temperature. In several instances, the explicit pairing of environmental stimuli with a drug-induced temperature change has been shown to result in changes in body temperature that are elicited by CSs in the absence of the drug. Two drugs, morphine and ethanol, have been used in the majority of studies and serve well to illustrate the complexity of the nature of conditioned temperature effects.

Morphine has complex effects on body temperature that vary across species, strain, dose, route of administration, degree of restraint, ambient temperature, sex, and housing. In rats, the species used in these conditioning studies, morphine produces hyperthermia at lower doses and hypothermia followed by hyperthermia at higher doses. The hyperthermia appears to involve recruitment of centrally elicited heat production mechanisms. Morphine can be thought of as elevating the thermoregulatory set point, in that animals will actively defend the hyperthermia (Cox *et al.*, 1976*b*). Microinjections of morphine at temperature-sensitive sites in the medial preoptic area of the brain cause a directly elicited hyperthermia (Martin and Morrison, 1978). In contrast, the initial hypothermia following high systemic injections of morphine appears to be caused by the animal's inability to thermoregulate; in hot environments, the animal becomes hyperthermic, whereas at normal room temperature or in cold environments, the animal becomes hypothermic (Cochin *et al.*, 1978; Paolina and Bernard, 1968). The mechanisms underlying these two temperature effects are obviously very different, a view that is consistent with the suggestion that they are mediated by different opiate receptors (Geller *et al.*, 1983). Usually after one or two injections, the hypothermic effect of morphine disappears (Gunne, 1960), but the hyperthermia, which occurs earlier in time after the injection, (Gunne, 1960; Mucha *et al.*, 1979; Sherman, 1979). If, after long-term administration, morphine injections are terminated, or if an opiate antagonist is injected, one of the symptoms of withdrawal is severe hypothermia. There is evidence that this withdrawal hypothermia is mediated by mechanisms that are unrelated to the hypothermia initially seen following high doses of morphine (Cox *et al.*, 1976*a*).

In one series of experiments on conditioned temperature effects of morphine, the high doses of morphine that produced hyperthermia were given several times a day accompanied by the presentation of a tone. When morphine injections were terminated, it was found that presentation of the tone (the CS) prevented the hypothermia of withdrawal (Drawbaugh and Lal, 1974, 1976; Roffman *et al.*, 1973). Several subsequent studies in which much lower doses of morphine were used showed that environmental stimuli paired with morphine injections elicit conditioned hyperthermia, both when tests are given 1 day following the last injection of morphine (Lal *et al.*, 1976; Miksic *et al.*, 1975; Sherman, 1979) and following a drug-free period of several days (Eikelboom and Stewart, 1979, 1981*a*). Thus, there is considerable evidence that the conditioned temperature response to morphine mimics the hyperthermia that is elicited by the drug acting directly on the CNS.* It should be noted that when high doses of morphine are given at room temperature, the resulting initial hypothermia could elicit compensatory heating responses. These heating responses could, in turn, become conditioned to the injection environment. To date, the possible contribution of such compensatory responses to the conditioned hyperthermia that results when high doses of morphine are used has not been investigated. In any case, both the drug-elicited heat production and the indirectly recruited compensatory responses should produce conditioned hyperthermic effects.

In a related set of experiments, we have shown that hyperthermia-producing doses of amphetamine also lead to conditioned hyperthermic responses, but the mechanisms that mediate this conditioned hyperthermic effect have not been investigated (Eikelboom and Stewart, 1981b).

Ethanol is the other drug for which conditioning of temperature responses has been studied in some detail. Ethanol induces hypothermia in rats, an effect that shows tolerance with repeated ethanol exposure. As in the case of morphine hypothermia, ethanol hypothermia is thought to reflect a disruption of the thermoregulatory system (Myers, 1981). The animal is unable to maintain body temperature, and as a consequence, the body temperature approaches the environmental temperature. Several studies have shown that the tolerance to ethanol hypothermia is context-specific (Crowell et al., 1981; Lê et al., 1979; Mansfield and Cunningham, 1980). Only in the presence of environmental stimuli associated with ethanol injections does the animal show tolerance to this effect. Furthermore, conditioned hyperthermia has been observed when animals receive saline in an environment previously paired with ethanol (Crowell et al., 1981; Lê et al., 1979; Mansfield and Cunningham, 1980). In this case, the observed drug effect and the CR are opposite in direction. As suggested previously, this should occur when the observed drug effect acts as an US to elicit a response to counteract or to compensate for the drug effect. We predicted that if, in such a situation, the observed drug effect (hypothermia) were passively prevented, for example, by heating up the environment, conditioned compensatory responses would not be observed because the thermoregulatory mechanisms would not be recruited.

---

* There is one study reported by Siegel (1978) in which conditioned hypothermia was found when a low, hyperthermia-inducing dose of morphine was used. In that study it was reported as well that the hyperthermic effects of morphine showed tolerance with repeated administration, an almost unique finding (see Eikelboom and Stewart, 1982). Sherman (1979) was unable to replicate these findings. He and, more recently, Zelman et al. (1985) have suggested that the excessive stress known to interact with the temperature effects of morphine (Stewart and Eikelboom, 1981) possibly accounts for this anomalous result.

Alkana et al. (1983) have reported that tolerance to the hypothermic effect of ethanol did not develop in mice that were prevented from becoming hypothermic following ethanol injections. This finding suggests that tolerance to ethanol hypothermia is normally due to the recruitment of heat production mechanisms that come to be elicited by the drug-associated environment.

Context-specific tolerance of pentobarbital-induced hypothermia has been reported by Cappell et al. (1981). They also found that animals that displayed tolerance to pentobarbital hypothermia in the injection environment also showed tolerance to ethanol in that environment. This finding suggests that the heat production mechanisms recruited by the loss of heat under pentobarbital, which were presumably elicited by the conditioned stimuli of the injection environment, were able to compensate for the effects of the ethanol. Such mechanisms could help account for the instances of cross-tolerance (and presumably cross-sensitization) observed between drugs having very different mechanisms of action.

2.1.2. Conditioning of Changes in Insulin Secretion and Blood Glucose Levels

Most investigations of conditioned changes in blood glucose have involved the repeated pairing of a CS with insulin injection. When low physiological doses of insulin, which decrease blood glucose levels, are paired with CS, a conditioned increase in blood glucose level is observed (Siegel, 1972), although, unlike Siegel, Woods and Shogren (1972) have attributed this effect to pseudoconditioning. This increase is presumably brought about by a compensatory release of glucose in response to insulin. When high doses of insulin are used, the most frequently reported CR is hypoglycemia (see Woods, 1983). This conditioned hypoglycemia is a consequence of the association between the CS and the insulin, and is not due to pseudoconditioning (Hutton et al., 1970). The strength of the CR varies with the number of pairings (Woods et al., 1969), the dose of insulin (Woods and Shogren, 1972), and the nature of the CS; and the decrease in strength with unreinforced trials (Woods et al., 1969). The conditioned hypoglycemia can be elicited by using tolbutamide (a compound that causes the pancreas to release insulin) (Woods et al., 1972); it is blocked by atropine (Woods, 1972; Flaherty et al., 1980) or vagotomy (Woods, 1972), and it does not depend on an insulin-induced change in blood glucose levels (Woods, 1976). The phenomenon has been seen in dogs (Alvarez-Buylla and Carrasco-Zanini, 1960), in rats (Alvarez-Buylla and Alvarez-Buylla, 1975; Flaherty et al., 1980; Matysiak and Green, 1984; Woods, 1976), and in humans (Lichko, 1959).

Since in these studies the doses of insulin are usually large, the finding that the CS also elicits a hypoglycemia, and potentially augments the insulin effect seems maladaptive. Woods (1976, 1983), however, has suggested a mechanism that could account for the direction of the CR in terms of normal blood glucose regulations. Small doses of insulin (which would be without effect if injected peripherally) when injected into the brain produce a fall in blood glucose. This is true whether the insulin is injected directly into the ventromedial hypothalamus (Weider and Waldbilling, 1982), into the cerebrospinal fluid (Chen et al., 1975; Chowers et al., 1961, 1966; Woods and Porte, 1975), or into the carotid artery (Szabo and Szabo, 1983, but see Davidson and Organ, 1982). This centrally mediated fall in blood glucose is blocked by atropine administration or by vagotomy (Szabo and Szabo, 1975; Woods and Porte, 1975) and does not appear to be the result of insulin leaking into the general circulation (Szabo and Szabo, 1972; Weider and Waldbilling, 1982; Woods and Porte, 1975, but see Margolis and Altszuler, 1968). Thus, one of the consequences of an increased insulin level appears to be a neurally mediated fall in blood glucose level. It is not clear whether this effect is brought about by changes in the liver (Szabo and Szabo, 1983) or the pancreas (Chen et al., 1975) or both. The discovery of insulin receptors in the arcuate nucleus and the median eminence area (a region with no blood–brain barrier) provides a site of action and a possible mechanism for the mediation of this neural effect on insulin (Van Houten and Posner, 1983). This effect of insulin may seem unexpected, but it should be noted that, under normal circumstances, insulin levels are elevated only when blood glucose levels are high. Woods (1976, 1983) argues that it is this action of insulin on the CNS that elicits the UR in these conditioning studies and thus determines the direction of the CR.

As stated earlier, in most studies in which high doses of insulin are utilized, conditioned hypoglycemia occurs. Siegal (1972, 1975a), however, has found conditioned hyperglycemia using both high and low doses. The results of some recent studies by Flaherty and co-workers may partially explain this contradictory finding. They found originally (Flaherty et al., 1980) that an insulin injection paired with one set of environmental stimuli led to conditioned hypoglycemia, whereas pairing of the same injection with a second set of environmental stimuli led to conditioned hyperglycemia. The hypoglycemia found in the first environment was similar to that found by Woods (1972), in that it was blocked by atropine. But why would the same dose lead to conditioned hyperglycemia in a different environment? One answer might involve an uncontrolled stressor that is responsible for the conditioned hyperglycemia found in this and in Siegel's experiment with high doses of insulin. Stress is known to bring about the release of epinephrine, a response that can be conditioned to stimuli associated with stress (Woods and Burchfield, 1980). Epinephrine leads to increased blood glucose and to decreased insulin release. The hypoglycemia induced by an injection of insulin given in a stressful environment could, in turn, cause further release of epinephrine (see Axelrod and Reisine, 1984) and lead to increased mobilization of glucose stores. Thus, it is interesting to note that in the Flaherty *et al.* (1980) study, and again in a study by Flaherty and Becker (1984), the conditioned hyperglycemia was obtained in the group exposed to the more novel (and thus more stressful?) set of conditioning stimuli. Subsequently, Flaherty *et al.* (1984) have shown that chlordiazepoxide attenuated the hyperglycemia induced by the stress of a novel environment. And finally, insulin injections led to conditioned hypoglycemia in a novel environment when animals were pretreated with chlordiazepoxide. It is possible, therefore, that the anomalous results of Woods and Siegel could be explained by differential amounts of stress induced in their experiments; it should be noted, however, that the procedures used by them seem similar in most major aspects.

When CSs are paired with elevations in blood glucose produced by intravenous injections of glucose in dogs (Mitiushov, 1954; Russek and Pina, 1962) and in humans (Mitiushov, 1954) and by intragastric (Deutsch, 1974) or intraperitoneal injections (Matysiak and Green, 1984) in rats, the CR observed is a fall in blood glucose level. The results obtained with glucagon and epinephrine, both of which increase blood glucose levels, have been inconsistent. Balagura (1968) reported conditioned hyperglycemia with glucagon, but his study lacked appropriate control groups (see Woods *et al.*, 1969) and the dose of glucagon used was high enough to induce a conditioned taste aversion (see Revusky, 1967). Woods and Kulkosky (1976) have reported that they found conditioned hypoglycemia after multiple injections of glucagon in rats. When epinephrine was used to produce hyperglycemia, Gantt *et al.* (1937) found no evidence for conditioning; Russek and Pina (1962) reported a small conditioned hypoglycemic effect, but the study lacked an appropriate control group for pseudoconditioning. Thus, it seems that only with large doses of glucose is there consistent evidence for conditioned hypoglycemia. This effect is presumably the result of the neurally mediated release of insulin brought about by the sudden increase in blood glucose levels. It is interesting to note, in this regard, that sensory contact with foodstuff can trigger insulin secretion. This so-called cephalic phase response can be elicited during sham feeding (Berthoud and Jeanrenaud, 1982; Hommel *et al.*, 1972) and by saccharin (Berthoud *et al.*, 1980) or carbohydrate-free diets (Strubbe and Steffens, 1975), suggesting that actual rises in blood glucose are not required for its elicitation, at least in experienced animals. The sight as well as the smell of food (Johnson and Wildman, 1983; Parra-Covarrubias *et al.*, 1971) also leads to insulin release which suggests that it is a CR that mimics the response to meals. Cephalic-phase insulin secretion can be blocked by vagotomy (Louis-Sylvestre, 1976) or by atropine administration (Berthoud and Jeanrenaud, 1982) and does not occur in animals with transplanted pancreatic islets (Berthoud et al., 1980; Louis-Sylvestre, 1978). Odors or the time of day that reliably predict food can elicit a release of insulin that is mediated by the same vagal pathway as the conditioned insulin secretion produced by glucose injections (Woods et al., 1977). These naturally occurring CRs could contribute to the control of food intake, meal initiation, and meal size (Powley, 1977; Woods, 1977).

2.1.3. Conditioning of Changes in the Cardiovascular System

The study of conditioned drug effects on cardiovascular functioning has been hindered by our lack of understanding of how the drugs used induce the observed changes in the cardiovascular system. Often researchers have failed to recognize that a drug can affect the system by several different actions (both central and peripheral) and that direct effects on one part of the system can indirectly elicit effects in another part of the system. Bulbocapnine, a drug that is thought to act centrally to increase heart rate and T-wave amplitude, has been reported to lead to conditioned increased in heart rate and T-wave amplitude (Perez-Cruet and Gantt, 1964). Similarly, small doses of morphine that act centrally to increase heart rate lead to conditioned increases in heart rate that mimic those elicited by the drug itself (Rush et al., 1970). High doses of morphine also lead to conditioned increases in heart rate despite the fact that these doses decreased the heart rate initially (Rush et al., 1970). High doses of morphine have nonspecific depressant effects (see Section 2.1.1) and may act, therefore, to depress effector mechanisms. Such an effect could cause the recruitment of compensatory cardiovascular changes. In support of this argument, Rush et al. (1970) found that at the higher dose of morphine dogs became sedated and hung limply in their support straps. This suggests that at the higher dose morphine could act both directly to stimulate heart rate increases centrally and indirectly to recruit compensatory cardiovascular changes via its depressant actions on effector mechanisms.

Studies with the drug epinephrine have led to conditioned decreases in heart rate (Russek and Pina, 1962; Subkov and Zilov, 1937). Epinephrine is known to act directly on heart muscle to increase heart rate. This increases the blood pressure, as the result of epinephrine's vasoconstrictor activity. The increase in blood pressure could, in turn, result in a CNS-elicited heart rate deceleration. This deceleration would, in fact, be the UR elicited by the actions of epinephrine on the heart and vasculature, and thus the response to be conditioned.

Both Rush et al. (1970) and Mackenzie and Gantt (1950) reported that a dose of atropine that produced tachycardia (presumably via blockade of muscarinic receptors in the heart) did not support conditioning.

Examination of the results of these studies indicates, however, that small decreases in heart rate did occur in response to CS presentation, suggesting that with different parameters conditioning might have been more evident.

In a recent study, Dafters and Anderson (1982) found evidence for context-specific tolerance to the tachycardia effect of ethanol in humans. Using a carefully counterbalanced design, they found tolerance to the effects of ethanol on heart rate only in the environment in which ethanol had been administered previously. Although they did not test directly for conditioned changes in heart rate by presenting the CS alone, they argued that conditioned compensatory slowing of heart rate could account for the context-specific tolerance.

Although no drugs were used in their study, Furedy and Poulos (1976) report a conditioned heart rate effect in humans that bears directly on the issue of how to predict the nature and direction of conditioned cardiovascular responses. They induced an unconditioned heart rate deceleration directly by rapidly (1.7 sec) tilting the subject backward on a table from a 45° head-up position through 90° to a head-down position. This led to a drop in heart rate of about 30 beats/min in 6–7 sec. The change was probably brought about, at least in part, by the increased arterial pressure in the head and upper body, which reflexively elicited vagus activation. In this case, the US (apparent high blood pressure) activated the CNS directly to bring about the UR (heart rate deceleration). The CR observed was heart rate deceleration, a response that mimicked the UR.

These studies generally support the conclusion that when a drug or other manipulation affects the heart directly or peripherally, to elicit a neurally mediated compensatory change in heart rate, it is this compensatory change that will become conditioned. Drugs that act centrally to elicit a cardiovascular response will lead to CRs that mimic the direction of the drug-elicited change.

2.1.4. Conditioning of Immune Responses

There are indications that activation of the immune system can be influenced by conditioning factors. In early studies by Russian researchers (reviewed by Ader, 1981), a CS was paired several times with injection of an antigen. Subsequent presentation of the CS resulted in an increased antibody titer, that is, increased immunoreactivity in the conditioning group relative to that shown by groups receiving only the antigen. Jenkins *et al.* (1983) replicated these findings using a more salient CS and only one CS–US pairing. Although the earlier studies lacked many of the controls and procedural details that today would be considered necessary in a study of conditioning, the results are consistent with the principles of classical conditioning. The question of how the conditioned immune responses might be mediated was not addressed in these studies, however, and the question of the mechanisms mediating conditioned changes in the immune system is still unanswered.

In recent years, Ader and his associates have studied learned changes in immunoreactivity, using the taste aversion paradigm. In their studies, a novel taste (saccharin) is paired with an immunosuppressive drug, cyclophosphamide. The animals are then given an antigen (sheep red blood cells), and several days later antibody titers are measured. Animals reexposed to saccharin in the interval showed a lower antibody titer than animals not reexposed (Ader and Cohen, 1975); that is, relative immunosuppression occurred. These results have been replicated several times, and although the effects are not large, they are consistent (Rogers et al., 1976; Wayner et al., 1978). Ader has attempted to determine whether an elevation in adrenocortical steroids could mediate this conditioned immunosuppression. Other drugs, however, that are not immunosuppressive, but do produce a change in corticosterone levels, do not support a conditioned immunosuppressive response (Ader, 1976). Furthermore, injections of corticosterone given at the time of antigen injection do not lower antibody titers significantly (Ader et al., 1979). Ader concludes, therefore, that the conditioned immunosuppressive effect is not mediated by adrenocortical steroids, but to date there is no explanation of the phenomenon.

Similar conditioned effects have been seen in investigations of the other main class of immune reactions—the cellular response. Bovbjerg et al. (1982) demonstrated that the graft-versus-host reaction could be suppressed by the presentation of a distinctive taste previously paired with the immunosuppressive drug cyclophosphamide. Again, these effects are small, suggesting either that the role of conditioned effects is minimal or that the conditioning procedures themselves are less than ideal.

Ader and Cohen (1982) studied the effects of conditioning on the development of an autoimmune disease in female New Zealand hybrid mice. In these mice, weekly administrations of cyclophosphamide delayed the mortality rate. Each week animals were allowed to drink a saccharin solution, the CS, which every second week was followed by the drug administration (50% pairing). The rate of development of proteinuria and the occurrence mortality in these animals was slower in animals with an equivalent cyclophosphamide exposure that was not paired with the CS exposure. It appears that exposure to the CS further retards the development of this autoimmune disease through its immunosuppressive action. The results of these studies, as a whole, suggest that although the nature of the learned responses remains unknown, learning can modulate the functioning of the immune system, a finding consistent with other studies showing CNS effects on immune responses (Fauman, 1982).

2.2. Conditioning Factors in the Changing Effectiveness of Drugs

As mentioned in the introduction, conditioned drug effects are frequently assessed in the context of the study of tolerance and sensitization. Tolerance and sensitization to the effects of drugs is often context-specific. This finding has led to the view that context-specific tolerance and sensitization arise from the conditioning of drug-opposite and drug-similar responses, respectively. In this section, we will explore the evidence for this view from studies of the effects of drugs on general activity, on eating and drinking, on responsivity to pain, and on convulsions.

2.2.1. Conditioning of Changes in General Activity

Most studies of conditioning of changes in activity have been done with the stimulants amphetamine and cocaine, and with morphine. It was observed early that with repeated injections of these drugs, animals would become increasingly excited or active, displaying sensitization or "reverse tolerance" (Seevers and Deneau, 1963) to the activity-enhancing effects. The question arose whether conditioning factors could account for these changes in activity. In some studies, direct tests for conditioned increases in activity were made by comparing in activity in the drug-associated environment of experimental and control groups treated with saline. In other studies, only context-specific sensitization was tested, by measuring activity in the drug-associated environment when all animals were treated with the drug. In few studies have animals been tested under both drug and saline conditions. In nearly all these studies, the distinctive cues of the activity measuring environment served as the CSs. It must also be noted that in most studies, activity measures appeared to include all movements; in other studies, locomotor activity and rearing were differentiated from stereotyped movements.

Conditioned increases in activity have been reported in studies with methamphetamine and d-amphetamine (Beninger and Hahn, 1983; Irwin and Armstrong, 1961; Pickens and Crowder, 1967; Pickens and Dougherty, 1971; Schiff, 1982; Tilson and Rech, 1973) and with cocaine (Barr et al., 1983; Tatum and Seevers, 1929). Context-specific sensitization of activity has been found with d-amphetamine (Tilson and Rech, 1973) and with cocaine (Post and Rose, 1976; Post et al., 1981; Hinson and Poulos, 1981). One cannot conclude from these studies, however, that conditioning accounts for all instances of sensitization seen with these drugs. For example, Post et al. (1981) found large context-specific increases in cocaine-induced activity with little evidence of conditioned increases in activity. The conclusion of Post (1983) that conditioning cannot account for these sensitization effects is based on the finding that the size of the sensitization effect is much greater than the sum of the initial drug effect plus the conditioned effect. There is no reason, however, to expect these to be additive; rather, it seems more probable that these would be multiplicative. In some instances, the effect of the drug in the absence of CSs is negligible; the drug, however, appears to potentiate the behavioral effectiveness of the CSs. What is obviously needed here are dose × context studies of context-specific sensitization.

In other instances, it is difficult to draw any conclusions about the relation between conditioning and sensitization from the available data. Barr *et al.* (1983), for example, who found strong evidence for conditioning cocaine-induced activity, did not test for context-specific sensitization. Furthermore, despite repeated demonstrations of conditioned activity using *d*-amphetamine, little or no evidence for context-specific sensitization of amphetamine-induced behaviors has been found (Post, 1981; Robinson *et al.*, 1982; Robinson, 1984; Segal, 1975). In cases in which one group of workers found conditioned or context-specific effects and another group did not, one might reasonably conclude that details of the experimental situation could explain the discrepancies. In other cases, however, differences in the behaviors measured might better account for the differing results. In a study designed to examine possible neurochemical changes underlying the sensitization of amphetamine-induced stereotypes, Robinson and Becker (1982) found that amphetamine-stimulated release of endogenous dopamine *in vitro* was enhanced in striatal tissue taken from rats repeatedly injected with amphetamine compared to that taken from saline-treated animals. Although there is nothing in the design of their experiment to suggest that conditioning could account for these results, it should be noted that CSs associated with amphetamine injections have been found to elicit conditioned changes in dopamine turnover (Schiff, 1982). Finally, it needs to be emphasized that although repeated exposure to a drug may bring about long-term neurochemical changes, the behavioral expression of these changes may be made manifest, that is, facilitated (or sensitized), only by environmental stimuli previously associated with the elicitation and expression of these behaviors.

The analysis of the conditioning of morphine-induced changes in activity raises a different set of issues. Acute systemic injections of morphine have both depressant and excitatory actions on locomotor activity. In rats, medium to high doses produce an initial decrease in activity followed by an increase above base line; low doses produce only an increase in activity. With repeated injections of higher doses, the decrease in activity shows tolerance and the increase in activity becomes stronger (shows sensitization) and occurs earlier (Babbini and Davis, 1972; Babbini *et al.*, 1979; Fog, 1970; Martin *et al.*, 1963; Vasko and Domino, 1978). Similar results have been found in hamsters (Schnur, 1985; Schnur *et al.*, 1983).

Studies aimed at conditioning the changes in general activity induced by systemic injections of morphine showed only increases in activity in the drug-associated environment (Hinson and Siegel, 1983; Kamat *et al.*, 1974; Mucha *et al.*, 1981; Perez-Cruet, 1976). One explanation of this finding has been that the excitatory effect of morphine is a compensatory response to the initial depressant effect of the drug and that this compensatory response becomes conditioned to stimuli associated with the morphine injection and is ultimately responsible for the development of tolerance (Hinson and Siegel, 1983; Mucha *et al.*, 1981). Another explanation for the finding is suggested by the observation that low doses of morphine elicit only an increase in activity, which is blocked by the opiate receptor antagonist naloxone (Oka and Hosoya, 1976). Morphine appears, therefore, to act directly on opiate receptors to increase activity independently of its depressant actions (Schnur, 1985). Joyce and Iversen (1979) found that morphine injected into the ventral tegmental area of the brain, the site of the cell bodies of the mesolimbic dopamine system, produced only an increase in activity, and that this increase was enhanced with repeated injection. Vezina and Stewart (1984) have shown that this increase in activity becomes conditioned to the environment in which morphine is administered and furthermore that the sensitization produced by repeated injections is situation-specific. Such results may provide an explanation for the conditioned increases in activity seen following repeated systemic injections of morphine. These researchers suggest that the conditioned increases reflect the independent conditioning of the excitatory effects of morphine on general activity, and not the conditioning of a response compensatory to the depressant effects. A similar conclusion has been reached by Tabakoff and Kiianmaa (1982) in their studies of the development of tolerance to the depressant effects of ethanol. Although not concerned with conditioning in these studies, they point out that the depressant effects show tolerance, whereas the excitatory effects do not. Furthermore, they argue that the excitatory actions of ethanol are independent from the depressant actions and are not compensatory reactions to the initial depression.

In a variety of operant tasks, tolerance to the depressant effects of ethanol on performance has been found to occur. It occurs, however, only if there is practice of the task under the influence of ethanol; it does not occur if ethanol is given after performance of the operant task (Chen, 1968). There is, however, disagreement about the importance of this practice under the influence of ethanol on the development of tolerance. LeBlanc and his associates (LeBlanc *et al.*, 1973, 1975, 1976) have argued that this behavioral tolerance reflects only a more rapid acquisition of tolerance, rather than the existence of a specific learned tolerance. This suggestion has been criticized because, in their studies, animals in the control groups received multiple tests for tolerance that involved practice while under the influence of ethanol. This may have resulted in the acquisition of behavioral tolerance in these control group animals. Experiments avoiding or controlling for this confounding factor have generally found evidence for the existence of behavioral tolerance to the depressive effects of ethanol (Mansfield et al., 1983; Wenger et al., 1980, 1981). For a more extensive discussion of this problem, see Goudie and Demellweek (1985).

2.2.2. Conditioning Factors in Tolerance to Drug-Produced Anorexia and Adipsia

In 1971, Carlton and Wolgin reported that rats on a restricted feeding schedule developed tolerance to the anorexic effect of amphetamine only when it was given before the daily meal. Animals with the same schedule, injected after the daily meal, did not show tolerance to amphetamine anorexia in a test session in which both groups received amphetamine before the meal. Carlton and Wolgin labeled the phenomenon *contingent tolerance*, inasmuch as development of tolerance was contingent on the animal being exposed to food at the time of drug injection. Because the drug history of the two groups of animals was identical, this form of tolerance could not be accounted for easily by traditional pharmacological explanations. Carlton and Wolgin (1971) suggested that associative learning factors might be responsible for this differential tolerance.

Contingent tolerance to the anorexic effects of amphetamine and related drugs has been demonstrated in a number of later studies (Demellweek and Goudie, 1982, 1983a; Pearl and Seiden, 1979; Poulos et al., 1981b; Rowland and Carlton, 1983; Woolverton et al., 1978), and several other explanations for the phenomenon have been suggested. The degree of amphetamine-induced anorexia is known to be a function of the deprivation state of the animal; the more severe the food deprivation, the less effect the amphetamine has (Cole, 1980). In the contingent tolerance procedure, the group of animals that receives amphetamine before food eats less than the group that receives amphetamine after the meal, and thus, over days, experiences greater deprivation. This has led some researchers to suggest that contingent tolerance is the result of increased deprivation and subsequent weight loss in the group receiving amphetamine before feeding (Levitsky et al., 1981; Wolgin, 1983). Stunkard (1982) has gone so far as to suggest that tolerance to amphetamine anorexia is an artifact of the weight change induced by the drug. He argues that amphetamine lowers the point at which the body regulates its weight and the animal simply reduces its food consumption until it reaches this new set point. Explicit tests of this explanation for contingent tolerance have been carried out using manipulations that affect body weight, either by restricting food intake (Demellweek and Goudie, 1983a) or by pair-feeding of animals in amphetamine before and after groups (Demellweek and Goudie, 1982). These studies demonstrate that although deprivation plays a role in the strength of the amphetamine anorexia, it cannot explain contingent tolerance.

A second explanation put forward to account for the apparent lack of tolerance in animals repeatedly given amphetamine after eating is the possible development of a conditioned taste aversion to food. Several studies have reported decreases in food consumption in animals given amphetamine after eating (Carey, 1978; Cawthorne, 1981; Milloy and Glick, 1976). Explicit tests for a taste aversion made in the context of a contingent tolerance experiment have found no evidence for food aversion in either amphetamine group (Demellweek and Goudie, 1983a; Emmett-Oglesby and Taylor, 1981).

The explanation for contingent tolerance that has received the most attention is the loss-of-reinforcement hypothesis first suggested by Schuster et al. (1966). According to this hypothesis, there is behavioral adaptation to those effects of the drug that disrupt rewarded behavior. If no food is present, no reward is lost, and no behavioral adaptation occurs (see Demellweek and Goudie, 1983b). Recently, however, Poulos et al. (1981b) have presented data that suggest that a more complete explanation of contingent tolerance phenomena can be made within a classical conditioning model. They found, as have others, that tolerance to amphetamine anorexia only develops in animals exposed to food while drugged. They also found, however, that the development of contingent tolerance was context-specific. Animals displayed tolerance to the anorexic effect of amphetamine only in the environment where they had experienced the drug in the presence of food. They argue that tolerance develops as a result of conditioning of an opponent, compensatory mechanism to amphetamine's anorexic effect. Furthermore, this response is recruited only in the presence of food in food-deprived animals and, therefore, only conditioned to drug-associated stimuli in the presence of food. More recently, Poulos and Hinson (1984) have reported a similar set of data in studies of tolerance to the adipsic effects of scopolamine. Although their studies have been criticized (see Demellweek and Goudie, 1983a), we feel that their analysis may be applicable to a broader range of contingent phenomena than the "loss-of-reinforcement" hypothesis.

Finally, we have found one example of what might be considered to be "contingent sensitization" of feeding. Siegel and Nettleton (1970) reported an experiment in which animals were repeatedly injected with insulin either in the presence or in the absence of food. They found that animals injected with insulin in the presence of food showed marked increases in food-getting behavior over trials. On a saline test trial, these animals had high rates of responding for food compared to animals that had received similar injections of insulin in the same environment, but in the absence of food. At the time, these data were considered to reflect an instrumental contingency, and tests for context-specific effects were not made. They do, however, raise the interesting possibility that classical conditioning may operate in contingent sensitization as well as in tolerance.

2.2.3. Conditioning Factors in Pain Sensitivity

The study of conditioning factors in the development of tolerance to morphine analgesia began with a series of experiments by Mitchell and his colleagues (Adams *et al.*, 1969; Ferguson *et al.*, 1969; Kayan and Mitchell, 1972; Kayan *et al.*, 1969). They showed that tolerance to the analgesic effects of morphine was specific to the environment in which morphine was injected. Subsequently, Siegel (1975b, 1976, 1977a) conducted a series of experiments from which he concluded that tolerance to morphine analgesia resulted from the conditioning of a compensatory hyperalgesic response elicited by the environmental stimuli (CSs) associated with the morphine injections. This explanation of context-specific tolerance to the analgesic effects of morphine has come under close scrutiny in recent years and has sparked considerable controversy. In this chapter, we briefly outline some of the contentious issues and try to point to areas in which further research is needed.

First, it is increasingly apparent that stress-induced analgesia operates in many of these studies as a confounding factor. It may be possible, for example, that stress-induced analgesia contributes to the initial high levels of analgesia seen in the pain tests used in these experiments and that the gradual loss of stress-induced analgesia contributes to the apparent tolerance to morphine analgesia that occurs over test trials. Second, in many experiments, tests for context specificity of tolerance are made by comparing analgesia in animals that were repeatedly exposed to the test environment to analgesia in animals exposed to that environment for the first time. Although it is true that efforts have been made to control for such stress effects in some experiments, it is difficult to compare results across experiments when they have not been controlled for. For a further discussion of this issue, see Baker and Tiffany (1985) and Goudie and Demellweek (1985).

While the role of conditioning factors in tolerance to the analgesic effects of morphine was being studied, endogenous pain control mechanisms were being studied extensively. It is now thought that multiple opioid and nonopioid mechanisms involved in endogenous pain control which operate at several levels in the CNS and pituitary gland (Basbaum and Fields, 1978, 1984; Chance, 1980; Gebhart, 1982; Watkins and Mayer, 1982). These systems are activated by stressful situations and by painful stimuli and can come under control of stimuli that are predictive of pain (Bolles and Fanselow, 1980; Fanselow, 1984; Fanselow and

Baackes, 1982; Watkins *et al.*, 1982, 1983, 1984). Clearly, conditions exist for conditioning of such autoanalgesia in most experiments on tolerance to morphine. Control group animals that repeatedly undergo experimental procedures and that are then given pain tests following saline injections would be expected to develop some degree of conditioned autoanalgesia. Animals pretreated with morphine presumably would not; because pain is suppressed, endogenous pain suppression mechanisms would not be recruited. To date, the operation of endogenous pain control mechanisms in studies of morphine analgesia has been given little attention (but see Rochford and Stewart, 1985).

Although numerous studies provide evidence for context-specific tolerance to morphine analgesia (Adams *et al.*, 1969; Advokat, 1980; Carder, 1978; Dafters *et al.*, 1983; Morris *et al.*, 1981; Sherman, 1979; Tiffany and Baker, 1981; Tiffany *et al.*, 1983a,b), little direct evidence for conditioned compensatory hyperalgesia was found. When direct tests for hyperalgesia were performed, only Krank *et al.* (1981) and Siegel (1975b) found evidence of such hyperalgesia; others did not (Hughes and Bardo, 1978; LaHoste *et al.*, 1980; Morris *et al.*, 1981; Sherman, 1979; Tiffany *et al.*, 1983a). This failure led Kesner and Baker (1981) and Kesner and Cook (1983) to propose a two-process model of opiate tolerance involving a habituation process. More recently, Baker and Tiffany (1985) have developed the habituation model more fully.

2.2.4. Conditioning Factors in Tolerance to Anticonvulsant Drugs

Mention should be made of an interesting phenomenon reported by Pinel *et al.* (1983). They studied the anticonvulsant effects of ethanol in "kindled" rats in which electrical stimulation normally elicited seizures. They found tolerance to this anticonvulsant effect only when the rats were stimulated during the periods of ethanol intoxication. Animals given similar daily injections of ethanol, but after the seizure episodes, developed no tolerance to the anticonvulsant effect. This finding resembles that found for the effects of amphetamine on feeding. It is an example of contingent tolerance, which depends on the animal being exposed to the stimulation while drugged, just as the development of tolerance to the anorexic effect of amphetamine depended on the hungry animal being exposed to food while drugged. Pinel *et al.* point out, however, that it is unlikely that their findings can be explained in terms of loss of reinforcement. It would seem rather that tolerance develops when some response, recruited under the drug, antagonizes the drug-induced inhibition of the afterdischarge necessary for seizures. What is not clear from their experiment, however, is whether that antagonistic response is conditioned to the environmental stimuli associated with recruitment under ethanol. They did not test for the context specificity of the tolerance or for conditioned facilitation of kindling in the absence of drug. It does appear, however, although it is not stated explicitly, that, in their experiment, animals in the contingent group experienced the drug in the seizure-test apparatus, whereas animals in the noncontingent group were given the seizure test and then injected with ethanol and returned to the home cage. It would be interesting to explore the parallels between this phenomenon and those involved in tolerance to anorexia- and adipsia-producing drugs.

Let us consider some of the common features of the studies reviewed in this section. We saw, for example, that tolerance to the anorexic, adipsic, analgesic, and anticonvulsant properties of a drug is assessed by its changing effects on a behavior that is elicited by a stimulus in the context, e.g., food-elicited eating, water-elicited drinking, heat-elicited withdrawal, and electrical stimulation-elicited seizure. What seems to happen in these studies is that tolerance develops when some response, recruited while the animal is drugged, antagonizes the drug-induced inhibition or disruption of the behavior. In the language of instrumental learning, tolerance to the disruptive effect of a drug on performance occurs when the disruption of behavior results in reinforcement loss. Tolerance results from the acquisition over trials of adaptive responses or coping strategies that compensate for the drug-induced disruption and consequent reinforcement loss (Corfield-Sumner and Stolerman, 1978; Schuster *et al.*, 1966; Wenger *et al.*, 1980). This idea requires that the compensatory responses be "practiced" while the animal is drugged. A similar analysis in terms of reinforcement loss has been applied to studies on such consummatory behaviors as feeding; here, tolerance development is contingent on a hungry animal being exposed to food while drugged (Demellweek and Goudie, 1983*b*). In this theoretical framework, tolerance development should be specific to the behavioral effects that were disrupted by the drug. In our view, the essential requirement for tolerance development in these experiments is not reinforcement loss, but rather the recruitment of a response that counteracts the effect of the drug. This idea could account for such effects as tolerance to the anticonvulsant effects of ethanol, as described by Pinel *et al.* (1983). In our analysis of the conditioning of drug-induced physiological responses, we argued that CRs that opposed the observed drug effect would be observed only when the drug effect acted as a stimulus to recruit a regulatory response (Eikelboom and Stewart, 1982). The conditioned activation of this compensatory response would contribute to context-specific tolerance (Siegel, 1975*b*). Poulos *et al.* (1981*b*) and Poulos and Hinson (1984) have applied these ideas to results from studies of contingent tolerance of the anorexic and adipsic effects of drugs. They suggest that feeding and drinking behaviors are regulated in a homeostatic manner by some mechanism that compares actual consumption with a level of consumption that is appropriate to the animal's needs at the time. Without the incentive stimulus of food or water, this mechanism is not activated. The drug-induced disruptions result in the recruitment of unconditioned adaptive responses, and these URs become conditioned to the environmental stimuli and result in context-specific tolerance. Thus, their analysis parallels ours in that the disturbance induced by the drug is the stimulus to which the system (through homeostatic or feedback mechanisms) responds.

Clearly, not all studies of context-specific tolerance can be easily accounted for within this general kind of theorizing. There are, for example, cases of context-specific tolerance of the analgesic effects of morphine occurring when morphine is given repeatedly in a specific environment in the absence of tests for analgesia (e.g., Krank *et al.*, 1981). It would seem here that the elicitation of pain is not necessary for the recruitment of hyperalgesia. More difficult than this, however, is the fact that context-specific tolerance often occurs in the absence of evidence for conditioned compensatory responses (see, e.g., Sherman, 1979; Shapiro *et al.*, 1983; Tiffany *et al.*, 1983*a*). This failure to find conditioned compensatory responses has occurred primarily in studies of context-specific tolerance to the analgesic effects of morphine and has led to an alternative explanation in terms of habituation (Baker and Tiffany, 1985). It should also be noted, however, that the operation of compensatory responses in tolerance to amphetamine anorexia or in other examples of contingent tolerance have rarely been tested for. Until more direct evidence is obtained for the operation of these opponent processes, all of our explanations must remain tentative.

2.3. Conditioning of Affective Changes

The affective states associated with traditionally used incentive stimuli, such as food, sexual partner, and electric shock, are intuitively inferred from our observations of the effects of these stimuli on ourselves and other animals. Such stimuli induce approach or withdrawal, and often little attention is given to the physiological bases of their positive and negative affective properties. In the study of conditioning using such incentive events, we often assume their affective value and go on to study the nature of the physiological responses that CSs associated with them elicit. In studies of the affective states produced by drugs, however, response to the CS has been used to infer the affective nature of the drug-induced effects. Approach responses made to a CS are said to reflect the positive incentive properties of a drug, and avoidance responses elicited by CSs are said to reflect the aversive properties. For example, if a rat presses a lever that results in drug administration, the drug is said to have positive affective properties, and, conversely, if the animal avoids stimuli paired with the drug administration, the drug is assumed to have aversive properties. The fact that for large classes of drugs the human experience is consistent with the animal results adds some validity to this approach. What makes this area of study of special interest is that drugs often elicit both approach and avoidance. In the sections that follow we will discuss studies concerned with the conditioning of affective consequences of drug presentations and the related issue of the affective consequences of drug termination (the withdrawal problem).

2.3.1. Conditioning of the Aversive Properties of Drugs

Most of the evidence which suggests that drugs can have aversive properties comes from studies of conditioned taste aversion (CTA). In their initial exploration of this phenomenon, Garcia et al. (1966, 1967) demonstrated that if a drug known to produce illness and gastric distress were paired with a distinctive taste, animals would subsequently avoid ingestion of a similar-tasting substance. Their observations have sparked hundreds of studies aimed at uncovering the conditions for such learning. In addition, the experimental paradigm has been used to investigate possible aversive properties of a wide variety of psychoactive drugs. No attempt will be made to review this large literature here (see Barker et al., 1977; Goudie, 1979, 1987; Milgram et al., 1977 for recent reviews). Instead, in this section we will deal only with some of the questions that CTA studies raise about the nature of the aversive properties elicited by different drugs, and about the relation between various unconditioned and conditioned drug effects.

The measure used to estimate the aversive properties of drugs in most studies of CTA is an indirect one. As Goudie (1979, 1987) has noted, the fact that an animal consumes less of a flavored substance tells us little about the CR elicited by the taste CS or about the particular action of the drug on which the aversion is based. CTA has been found using drugs with a wide variety of pharmacological actions, but because the early studies were done using drugs such as lithium that were known to produce illness and malaise, nausea and vomiting, it was assumed that the taste CS was avoided because it acquired the ability to elicit conditioned physiological symptoms of illness (Garcia et al., 1974). This view has received considerable support from studies reporting that lesions of the area postrema (a medullary area sensitive to chemical irritants that can activate the emetic system) and sectioning of the vagus nerve (which can carry messages from the stomach to the emetic system) attenuate in expected ways CTAs based on blood-borne chemical toxins or gastrointestinal irritants known to elicit nausea and vomiting (Coil et al., 1978a,b; Coil and Nogren, 1981). These manipulations, which should attenuate the severity of the drug effect, were thought to reduce the reactions to the CS. Studies with antiemetic drugs, administered just before the test and after the establishment of the CTA, however, have provided mixed results. For example, whereas Coil *et al.* (1978a) found that pretreatment with such drugs would block a previously acquired CTA to lithium chloride, Goudie *et al.* (1982) and Rabin and Hunt (1983) did not. It is interesting to note in this regard that anticipatory nausea and vomiting that often occurs in response to smells and tastes associated with chemotherapy in cancer patients is also resistent to treatment with antiemetic drugs (Redd and Andrykowski, 1982).

Although these studies do point to the unconditioned stimulus effects responsible for the CTA produced by drugs that act on the emetic system, they do not provide direct measures of the conditioned responses elicited by the taste CSs. No measures are made, for example, of conditioned gagging or vomiting. Most studies have been carried out in rats, however, and rats do not vomit. As mentioned earlier, however, conditioned nausea, gagging, and vomiting are seen in human subjects subjected to chemotherapy or radiation treatments that elicit nausea and vomiting (Redd and Andrykowski, 1982). Evidence for conditioning of related oral–gastric–intestinal distress response when lithium is used in studies with rats has been found. Conditioned defecation (Krane, 1980), conditioned pica (Mitchell *et al.*, 1977), and conditioned orofacial rejection responses (Berridge *et al.*, 1981; Pelchat *et al.*, 1983) have all been reported to be elicited by taste CS previously paired with lithium. The food rejection responses are particularly interesting because they suggest that the taste CS has truly acquired aversive affective properties. Whether it is the pairing of the taste CS with the nausea-inducing properties of lithium that is responsible for the change in palatability is not clear. It is interesting, however, that Parker (1982) has reported that although both lithium and amphetamine produced strong CTA, only the stimuli paired with lithium elicited the stereotyped rejection movements, suggesting that different mechanism mediate the CTA produced by these drugs (see also Parker, 1982, 1984; Parker *et al.*, 1984).

The idea that CTA produced by nausea-producing drugs and toxins is mediated by mechanisms different from those mediating the CTA produced by a number of other psychoactive drugs is not new (Amit *et al.*, 1977; Berger, 1972; Berger *et al.*, 1973; Goudie, 1979; Riley *et al.*, 1978). Of particular interest are the drugs of abuse. Most, if not all, drugs that are self-administered by animals are capable of producing CTA. Furthermore, it has been found in a series of recent studies that many of these same drugs "paradoxically" produce both aversive effects as measured by a CTA and reinforcing effects as measured by self-administration and conditioned place preference (CPP) at the same doses (Cappell and LeBlanc, 1971; Mucha *et al.*, 1982, Reicher and Holman, 1977; Sherman *et al.*,

1980*a,b*; Switzman *et al.*, 1978; Vander Kooy *et al.*, 1983*a;* White *et al.*, 1977; Wise *et al.*, 1976).

Numerous attempts have been made to specify the actions of self-administered drugs that are responsible for their aversive properties as revealed in CTA studies. One approach has been to suggest that the aversions are based on some negative reaction to the novelty of the drug experience (Amit and Baum, 1970) and not to some independent actions of the drugs. The fact that preexposure to these drugs prior to their pairing with taste stimuli weakens or eliminates the development of the CTA but does not reduce the reinforcing properties of drugs such as morphine and amphetamine lends support to such a view (Cappell *et al.*, 1975; Goudie *et al.*, 1975, 1976). Studies showing that in the case of stimulants, for example, lesions of the ascending dopamine pathways known to attenuate the reinforcing properties of these drugs also eliminate CTA based on them (Robert and Fibiger, 1975; Wagner *et al.*, 1981) can be similarly interpreted. On the other hand, data from preexposure studies (Bardo *et al.*, 1984*a;* Domjan and Siegel, 1983; Stewart and Eikelboom, 1978) and from lesion studies (Blair and Amit, 1981; Van der Kooy *et al.*, 1983*a*) suggest that, at least in some instances, the aversive properties of a drug can be differentiated from other actions of the same drug. In conclusion, it can be said that, although the data from CTA studies strongly support the view that the aversive properties of psychoactive self-administered drugs are different from those of drugs such as lithium chloride, neither a general nor a specific mechanism mediating the effects has been identified. In an excellent recent review of CTA studies, Goudie (1987) has made the point that the CTA-inducing potency of drugs does not correlate with their other known pharmacological actions. Clearly, the question of identifying the basis of the aversive actions calls for new and different approaches. Perhaps the application of drugs to specific central nervous system sites (e.g., Amit *et al.*, 1977), a technique that is proving effective in the identification of the positive incentive properties of drugs (see Section 2.3.3), will provide some of the answers (see White *et al.*, 1987, for additional studies).

Finally, it should be mentioned that there are a few reported instances of conditioned place aversion in rats due to the pairing of a drug with a distinctive compartment of a two-choice apparatus. Ethanol, for example, has been found to induce an aversion to a place (Cunningham, 1979; Van der Kooy *et al.*, 1983*b*), as have naloxone (Mucha and Iversen, 1984; Mucha *et al.*, 1982), methamphetamine (Martin and Ellinwood, 1974), and drugs known to produce gastrointestinal distress such as lithium chloride (Krane, 1980). We shall see later, however, that both amphetamine and ethanol have also been reported to produce place preferences. No systematic studies of the pharmacological basis of these place aversions has been carried out.

2.3.2. Conditioning of Withdrawal Symptoms and Aversion Based on Withdrawal

Numerous studies have been carried out which demonstrate that abstinence symptoms accompanying withdrawal from morphine can become conditioned to stimuli associated with their occurrence. Rats repeatedly placed in a distinctive environment during the period of withdrawal from daily dependence-producing doses of morphine show a higher incidence of withdrawal symptoms in that environment than they do in a home-cage environment (Trost, 1973; Wikler and Pescor, 1967). Goldberg and Schuster (1967) showed that presentation of a tone paired with an injection of the opiate antagonist nalorphine to morphine-dependent monkeys elicited withdrawal symptoms and suppressed responding for food reinforcement, mimicking the effect of nalorphine. Similarly, in humans, an environment paired with small doses of naloxone has been shown to produce withdrawal symptoms in heroin addicts maintained on methadone (O'Brien *et al.*, 1977). Inasmuch as abstinence symptoms resemble illness and include nausea, vomiting, tearing, and excessive salivation, it is somewhat surprising that even abstinent animals do not display an aversion to a place that was previously paired with drug withdrawal (Kuman, 1972). Furthermore, although abstinent animals show an increased preference for an opiate solution, the same animals do not drink more of an opiate solution than a control group when placed in a distinctive environment previously associated with the experience of withdrawal (Wikler and Pescor, 1967).

It should perhaps be noted Mucha *et al.* (1982) and Mucha and Iversen (1984) have reported a dose-related conditioned aversion to a place paired with naloxone given either intravenously or subcutaneously in drug-naive animals, although no such effect was found with naloxone given intraperitoneally (Bozarth and Wise, 1982). Similarly, Holtzman (1979) found that naloxone suppressed eating and drinking in rats to the same degree whether they were dependent on morphine or drug-naive. It has been speculated that opiate antagonists might produce mild withdrawallike effects by blocking endogenous opiate systems. Whether these conditioned aversions that are seen in drug-naive animals are based on mechanisms similar to those seen in opiate-dependent animals in not at all clear.

Evidence that withdrawal effects have aversive properties comes from studies of CTA. Morphine-dependent rats have been shown to avoid a taste stimulus paired with naloxone-precipitated withdrawal (Pilcher and Stolerman, 1976; Ternes, 1975), but not to avoid an audiovisual stimulus (Frumkin, 1976). Rats avoid a usually preferred saccharin solution during opiate withdrawal (Parker and Radow, 1974), another finding that may be indicative of the ease of association between gastrointestinal malaise and taste stimuli. It may be that, at least in the rat, this constellation of withdrawal symptoms is selectively associated with taste stimuli and provides the basis for the taste aversion. Again it should be mentioned here that CTA has been found with naloxone in drug-naive animals (LeBlanc and Cappell, 1975). Again, whether the basis of this aversion is the same as that seen in opiate-dependent animals is not known.

In the studies discussed earlier, conditioning stimuli that were explicitly paired with the onset of withdrawal from drug were found to elicit withdrawallike symptoms. Siegel (1977b, 1983) has pointed out, however, that drug-opposite compensatory responses that resemble the symptoms of withdrawal are often elicited by stimuli repeatedly paired with drug administration. He has argued that these conditioned compensatory responses can account for context-specific tolerance to drugs such as morphine and ethanol and that, when elicited by the contextual stimuli in the absence of drug, they are responsible for withdrawal symptoms and signs of dependence. In a recent experiment, Zellner *et al.* (1984) attempted to assess whether the aversive symptoms of withdrawal that are assessed by taste aversion would manifest themselves specifically in the context in which morphine had been repeatedly administered. They argued that if the conditioned compensatory responses are the basis of withdrawal symptoms, then one should see evidence for greater taste aversion following drug withdrawal in the drug-associated environment. Their findings were negative; all animals showed a taste aversion to saccharin during withdrawal whether tested in the presence of morphine-related stimuli or not. These results raise the question whether the constellation of withdrawal symptoms that is conditionable to taste stimuli is the same as the constellation of compensatory responses that is elicited by the morphine-associated contextual stimuli. If we look at the full range of data on compensatory responses, it appears probable that they are not. Drug-contextual cues elicit a variety of different responses. For example, morphine-contextual cues elicit a number of morphine-mimicking responses, such as hyperthermia, increased activity, and appetitive motivational effects, as well as compensatory responses. Even some of the conditioned compensatory effects, such as those that are thought to be responsible for tolerance to lethal actions of morphine or heroin (Siegel *et al.*, 1979, 1982), might not contribute to withdrawal malaise. It is interesting to note in this regard that Melchior and Tabakoff (1981, personal communication) have found that contextual stimuli previously paired with ethanol injections elicit alterations in ethanol distribution; mice given ethanol in an environment previously paired with ethanol injections had lower brain levels of ethanol accompanied by a larger "volume of distribution" than animals given ethanol in a neutral environment. One wonders what mechanisms mediate these effects and what symptoms would be produced by them in animal returned to the ethanol environment in the absence of ethanol.

Finally, it should be mentioned here that drugs themselves can be used as stimuli to condition what appear to be *antisickness* responses. Revusky *et al.* (1979) reported that when pentobarbital was paired with lithium chloride, making pentobarbital a CS for the lithium injection, instead of gaining effectiveness as an aversive agent, pentobarbital lost its capacity to produce taste aversion. Similar effects have been found when other drugs such as morphine, amphetamine, and chlordiazepoxide are substituted for pentobarbital. Lett (1983) has attributed this so-called aversion failure (Avfail) to the conditioning of an "antisickness" response to the CS drug. To date no mechanism has been found that could account for the "antisickness" effect. It appears, however, that the phenomenon cannot be explained in terms of some unique pharmacological effect of the CS drug.

2.3.3. Conditioning of the Positive Incentive Properties of Drugs

When discrete stimuli are repeatedly paired with the presentation of an opiate or a stimulant in a self-administration paradigm, such stimuli will maintain behavior for some time when they are presented alone following responding (Davis and Smith, 1976; Levine, 1974; O'Brien, 1976; O'Brien *et al.*, 1974; Schuster and Woods, 1968; Wikler *et al.*, 1971). Because these stimuli maintain the behavior upon which they are contingent, they can be said to act as reinforcers and have been called conditioned reinforcers. These stimuli may maintain responding because being paired with the drug, as in a standard Pavlovian conditioning procedure, they should acquire the ability to elicit some of the same druglike effects as were elicited by the drugs themselves.

Evidence that such stimuli can acquire positive incentive properties through their association with the positive affective properties of drugs comes mainly from studies of CCP. In these studies, following repeated experience with a drug in one compartment of a two-compartment box, animals show a shift in preference for the compartment previously paired with drug. Such effects have been found with systemic injections of amphetamine (Reicher and Holman, 1977; Sherman *et al.*, 1980), cocaine (Mucha *et al.*, 1982; Spyraki *et al.*, 1982*b*), morphine (Beach, 1957; Blander *et al.*, 1984; Katz and Gormezano, 1978; Mucha *et al.*, 1982; Rossi and Reid, 1976; Sherman *et al.*, 1980*a*; White *et al.*, 1977), and heroin (Bozarth and Wise, 1981*b*). Evidence that the shift in preference is related to the positive incentive properties of these drugs comes from studies showing that central administration of such drugs to sites known to support self-administration in other paradigms will serve as an adequate incentive stimulus for CPP (Bozarth, 1983). For example, Carr and White (1983) have shown that rats developed a significant preference for a place associated with intraaccumbens, but not intracaudate amphetamine injections, the dopamine terminal region also found to support amphetamine self-administration (Monaco et al., 1981). Similarly, Bozarth and Wise (1982) and Phillips and LePiane (1980, 1982) found a preference shift for a place associated with injections of opiates into the ventral tegmental area, the dopamine cell body region found to support morphine self-administration (Bozarth and Wise, 1981a). In addition, there is evidence that sites supporting the development of CPP can be clearly dissociated from sites responsible for other actions of these same drugs (Bozarth and Wise, 1982, 1984; Van der Kooy et al., 1982; White et al., 1987). In general, lesion studies also provide support for the view that the drug actions responsible for CPP established with stimulants and opiates are similar to those underlying their self-administration (Spyraki et al., 1982a, 1983). An exception is the cocaine-induced place preference. Spyraki et al. (1982b) found that nucleus accumbens lesions that are known to disrupt cocaine self-administration (Roberts et al., 1980) did not affect cocaine-induced place preference. Whether this finding should be interpreted to mean that the CPP is based on some other property of cocaine, e.g., its anesthetic action, is not clear.

In general, these studies support the view that the positive incentive properties of both opiates and stimulants are mediated by their actions on the mesolimbic and/or mesocortical dopamine pathway. However, studies attempting to block CPP based on stimulants and opiates by prior administration of dopamine receptor blockers have produced mixed results. For example, Spyraki et al. (1982a, 1982b) found haloperidol blocked the development of amphetamine-induced CPP, but neither haloperidol nor pimozide blocked cocaine-induced CPP. In other studies Bozarth and Wise (1981b) found that pimozide blocked heroin-induced CPP, but Mackey and Van der Kooy (1983) found no effect of pimozide. Obviously, considerable work is required to work out these discrepancies.

Several features of the results from CPP studies have been of concern to a number of investigators (for recent reviews of some of these issues see Bardo et al., 1984a; Blander et al., 1984; Bozarth, 1987; Van der Kooy, 1987). The principal concern has been the magnitude of the effect. Animals given conditioning trials in one part of a two-compartment box rarely spend close to 100% of the time on the drug-paired side when given a free choice. This may be due in part to the way in which these studies are conducted. In most, animals are initially placed in the apparatus for a fixed period of time and allowed to move freely between the compartments. The amount of time spent in each compartment is recorded. Often animals show a distinct preference for one side, spending more than half the time there. In order to demonstrate that conditioning trials lead to a clear preference shift, drug is usually paired with the nonpreferred side. On the test trial, animals are again free to move between the two sides, and the amount of time spent in the compartment previously paired with drug is recorded. If the animals show a net increase in time on this side, a preference shift is said to have occurred. Sometimes, however, animals do not show an absolute preference for the drug-paired side, but only an increase in total time spent. Van der Kooy (1987) has argued that this lack of absolute preference is due to the unbalanced initial valence of the two compartments, and that if care is taken to make them equally attractive initially, absolute preferences will be demonstrated. It is interesting that White et al. (1987) have found, using a three-compartment box (a box with a start compartment that opens out on to two choice compartments), that animals rarely divide the total time between the two choice compartments. Instead they spend a significant amount of time in the start compartment. In their experiments, however, the animals demonstrate an absolute preference for the drug-paired side over the unpaired side following conditioning trials. The fact that under the conditions of these experiments animals often fail to spend the large majority of their time on the drug-preferred side might be explained in part by the fact that animals do not actually have to enter the drug-paired side to be fully in view of the drug-paired stimuli. In the two-compartment box, animals can usually be in close proximity to the drug-paired stimuli while standing on the often initially preferred floor of the unpaired side. A similar situation exists in the three-compartment box, where the animals continue to spend a considerable amount of time in the start compartment. Vezina and Stewart (1985) have recently found evidence for a strong absolute CPP when morphine is paired exclusively with tactile stimuli on the floor of an open field. These observations are reminiscent of the early failures to observe autoshaping or "sign tracking" (see Hearst and Jenkins, 1974) in rats when the arbitrary response requirement was physical contact with a stimulus. When approaches and visual surveillance were included as evidence for sign tracking, stimuli paired with reinforcers could clearly be seen to have changed in valence as a function of the conditioning procedures. Some recent observations of Bardo et al. (1984a) bear on this question. In a CPP study using morphine, they recorded, in addition to total time spent on the morphine-paired side, the number of entries to that side and the duration per entry. They found that in the test trial given after conditioning, the number of entries was not different from a saline control group, but that the time spent per entry was significantly longer. Following a period of extinction trials, previously conditioned animals showed a significant reduction in the time spent per entry, as did a saline control group, but, interestingly, they significantly increased the number of entries made into the compartment previously paired with drug. This analysis bears directly on another aspect of the results from CPP studies that have been puzzling. Some workers have found that extinction trials often do not lead to a significant decrease in total time spent on the drug-paired side (Bozarth, 1987). Clearly, the results of Bardo and colleagues suggest that the animals are sensitive to the extinction procedures, but the measure of total time spent is not.

Other puzzling aspects of CPP studies may also be interpretable within the analysis offered here. Most researchers have found, for instance, that the relation between dose and the magnitude of CPP is evident within a very small range of doses and reaches an asymptote at relatively low doses. We suggest that the ceiling found on the magnitude of preference may be explained by the same factors discussed earlier. It may be that the very aspect of the CPP paradigm that has made it so attractive as a research tool, the simplicity of the response requirement, is also the source of its apparent limitations. If the animal does not actually have to go some place or make some specific response in order to get "in touch" with the drug-related stimuli, its response may appear to lack vigor or strength. It is interesting, however, that when a more traditional runway is used, with a start box, an alley, and an enclosed goal box, animals quickly learn to run to the goal box where drug has been experienced previously (Beach, 1957; White *et al.*, 1977). It appears, as in the case of CTA, that in order to better assess the affective responses associated with drug-related stimuli, a closer observation of the animal's behavior in the presence of these stimuli will be required. One such study has been done by Berridge *et al.* (1984). They studied the orofacial ingestion sequences of rats to a morphine solution. Animals responded initially by passive rejection and stereotyped movements typically seen toward quinine solutions, but following experience with oral self-administration of morphine, they responded with positive orofacial ingestion sequences.

One of the questions that has relevance for understanding compulsive drug use is whether positive incentive properties of drugs change with repeated exposure. Although the CPP paradigm is one in which this question could be studied, in most studies of CPP with stimulants and opiate drugs, tests for preference shift have been made after three of four pairings in previously drug-naive animals. As has been stated already, the magnitude of the preference has usually been modest. Recently Blander *et al.* (1984) reported a study using morphine in which animals were given three series of conditioning trials interspersed with drug-free test trials. In each series of four trials, the dose of morphine was doubled. It is interesting to note that in this experiment the absolute magnitude of the preference attained was greater than that normally seen; in some groups over 80% of the time was spent in the morphine-paired side. This finding suggests that repeated exposure to morphine increases its positive reinforcing properties possibly by decreasing either its aversive properties (see Section 2.3.1), its depressant actions (see Section 2.1.1), or both. A related set of findings comes from conditioning studies using ethanol. As mentioned earlier, conditioned place aversion has typically been found when place cues are paired with ethanol injections. There is, however, at least one report in the literature of a preference for cues associated with ethanol (Black *et al.*, 1973), and recently Reid *et al.*, (1985) have reported a CPP to emerge after only a few conditioning trials in animals habituated to drinking ethanol. In both these studies animals were placed in the conditioning apparatus for brief periods of time; in the earlier study, for 15 min, 5 min after injection, and in the Reid *et al.* study, for 4 min, 4 min after the injection, during a period when ethanol has transient excitatory effects (Shippenberg *et al.*, 1984). Reid *et al.* argue that, in other CPP studies with ethanol, animals are usually placed in the conditioning apparatus for longer periods of time following the ethanol injection, creating the opportunity for both excitatory and depressant actions of alcohol to become associated with the environment. It is interesting to note here that others have proposed that it is the excitatory actions of ethanol which may be associated with its positive reinforcing properties (Ahlenius *et al.*, 1973; Carlsson *et al.*, 1972) and that while the depressant actions show tolerance with repeated administration, the excitatory actions do not (Masur and Boerngen, 1980; Tabakoff and Kiianmaa, 1982). Similar findings have been reported for the opiate drugs (see Stewart *et al.*, 1984). These findings suggest that, in general, experience with the effects of self-administered drugs may alter the magnitude of the positive and negative affective components associated with them. This would seem to be especially true for drugs with biphasic effects on behavior such as morphine and ethanol, but the same could apply to drugs such as amphetamine and might account for the effects of preexposure to these drugs on CTA as well as on CPP.

3. IMPLICATIONS

The fact that repeated administration of a drug or hormone in the presence of a common set of environmental stimuli often results in the conditioning of drug-induced responses has both practical and theoretical implications. The observation that conditioned drug effects can alter the pharmacological response to drugs should be a major concern of the experimental pharmacologist as well as the physician. A role for conditioned drug effects in tolerance and sensitization of the responses to drugs has been proposed and discussed in a number of major papers by Siegel (1977*b*, 1979, 1983, 1985), and the evidence has been reviewed recently by Goudie and Demellweek (1985). We will not, therefore, deal with the issues again in this section.

The practical use of conditioned taste aversions based on drugs for the control of predators has been studied and reviewed by Gustavson (1977). Conditioned taste aversions arising during the course of chemotherapy in the treatment of cancer have also become the subject of recent studies (Bernstein, 1978; Bernstein and Webster, 1980). It has been considered, for example, that the anorexia that occurs during cancer treatment may be due in part to the development of food aversions. Recent studies by Lett (1983) and Revusky *et al.* (1979) suggest that it may be possible to ameliorate these aversions by drug–drug conditioning procedures that counteract the development of conditioned food aversions.

The practical role for conditioned changes in the immune response, though of great interest, is just beginning to be considered. Early studies have been concerned with demonstrating the effects and with attempting to determine the physiological bases of the effects. The recent rise in interest in CNS involvement in immunoresponsivity will no doubt bring greater attention to the potential involvement of conditioned factors in disease and treatment (see Ader, 1981, 1983; Fauman, 1982).

In our review of the conditioning of changes in blood glucose and insulin, we touched on the role of conditioned endocrine changes in the control of food intake. Woods and Burchfield (1980) have discussed the field of conditioned endocrine changes more broadly in their recent review.

Many of the issues discussed under the heading conditioned drug effects or drug-anticipatory responses are those discussed under the heading placebo effects. See a recent book edited by White *et al.* (1987) for a fuller discussion of conditioning factors in placebo effects.

Finally, to conclude this chapter, we will deal with two phenomena in which conditioned drug effects have been implicated and which have been topics of wide interest in recent years: drug self-administration and treatment of addiction.

3.1. Drug Self-Administration

One of the most interesting questions in the area of conditioned drug effects is what role, if any, conditioned drug effects play in drug self-administration. We have recently reviewed this question in some depth (Stewart *et al.*, 1984) and will therefore contain our remarks to a summary and updating of that review. Two types of conditioned drug effects have assumed importance in theories of drug self-administration, conditioned incentive or appetitive effects and conditioned withdrawal effects. It has been proposed, for example, that conditioned withdrawal effects could account for relapse to drug taking in drug-free individuals (Siegel, 1977b; Wikler, 1948). This idea is consistent with the view that it is escape or avoidance of withdrawal that maintains drug, or at least opiate, use.

As discussed in Section, 2.3.2, there is considerable evidence that stimuli previously paired with withdrawal from opiates do elicit withdrawallike symptoms. We find no evidence to suggest that animals resume or increase drug taking in environments paired exclusively with opiate withdrawal. It should be noted, however, that in most instances, whether in the laboratory or in life, the positive affective properties of drugs are experienced in the same settings where withdrawal effects are experienced. It becomes difficult, therefore, to determine whether conditioned appetitive effects or conditioned withdrawal effects underlie the resumption of drug taking when it is observed in such an environment. An experiment by Thompson and Ostlund (1965) throws some light on the issue and suggests that experiencing withdrawal in an environment does not increase the likelihood of drug taking in that environment. They reported that animals that had experienced withdrawal in the same environment in which they initially learned to drink morphine had a lesser preference for morphine during readdiction than did animals that had experienced withdrawal in a different environment.

Morphine-dependent animals self-administer orally larger amounts of opiates when in a state of natural withdrawal (see, for example, Wikler and Pescor, 1967) and learn to prefer a flavored substance that has been paired with morphine injections that alleviate withdrawal symptoms (Parker *et al.*, 1973). Similarly, Goldberg *et al.* (1969) have shown that monkeys will self-administer morphine more frequently following intravenous nalorphine injections. After several days of this experience, a saline injection also yielded higher rates of self-administration on at least the first occasion when it was substituted, but interestingly, a tone paired with the nalorphine injections did not. These data have been interpreted to mean that conditioned withdrawal symptoms increase drug self-administration, but an alternative explanation seems more probable. Animals increase their rate of intravenous self-administration when the dose is decreased, or in the early stages of extinction conditions. Nalorphine blocks opiate receptors and probably acts to effectively reduce the dose. The higher rates may reflect this dose change. The fact that saline injections also caused a slight, though significant increase in rate on the first trial might reflect conditioning, but it is not obvious that this behavioral effect was due to the elicitation of conditioned withdrawal symptoms.

Stimuli paired with morphine injections have been found to prevent (Roffman *et al.*, 1973) and to reverse (Tye and Iversen, 1975) morphine withdrawal symptoms in dependent animals. As discussed previously, stimuli paired with injections of opiates and stimulants elicit many effects that mimic those elicited by the drugs themselves. We have argued that it is the elicitation of conditioned druglike effects, and especially of conditioned appetitive motivational effects, that underlies the maintenance and resumption of drug-taking behavior; conditioned stimuli associated with self-administered drugs, we suggest, arouse central states that mimic features of those produced by the drugs themselves and, thereby, serve to increase the attractiveness of other drug-related stimuli in the environment and to increase the probability of drug-related thoughts and actions. These ideas arise from findings on the effectiveness of "priming" injections in reinstating drug taking in animals experienced in drug taking (de Wit and Stewart, 1981, 1983; Gerber and Stretch, 1975; Stewart, 1983, 1984; Stewart and de Wit, 1987). More direct evidence that priming injections increase the attractiveness of drug-related stimuli comes from studies carried out within the CPP paradigm. Bozarth (1987) has found that the magnitude of the preference for heroin-associated place cues is considerably increased when animals are given the test trial following an injection of heroin. A somewhat similar finding has been reported by Chew (1984), who studied the effects of priming injections on place preferences based on morphine and amphetamine. He found that in animals given 10 mg/kg morphine injections paired with one set of place cues and 1.5 mg/kg amphetamine with the other showed an initial preference for the morphine-associated side when tested under saline. Following an injection of amphetamine, the preference shifted to the less preferred, amphetamine-associated side. After a series of extinction trials during which animals were enclosed in the morphine-associated side after saline injections, a clear preference for the amphetamine side emerged. Following a morphine priming injection, however, the preference for the morphine-associated side was reinstated at a magnitude even greater than that originally seen.

The idea that conditioned changes associated with the mesolimbic dopamine systems might underlie the excitatory and positive affective properties of stimulants and opiates has been discussed in previous sections (see also Perez-Cruet, 1976; Schiff, 1982). Activation of such conditioned changes by drug-paired stimuli might act similarly to the priming injection of the drug to reinstate drug-taking behavior. A recent study (Friedman and Coons, 1983) suggests that a similar mechanism might underlie conditioned feeding responses. They found that intracranial dopamine injections into basal forebrain dopamine-containing areas potentiated food intake in deprived animals. Furthermore, feeding was potentiated in the environment associated with the injections on recurrent tests and was specific to that situation. They suggest "that brain DA activity normally may modulate the hedonic responsiveness of the rat to consummatory stimuli" (see also Carr and Simon, 1984; Jenck, et al., 1985).

In a study of conditioned factors in ethanol intake, Krank (1984) found that rats increased free-choice ethanol consumption in an environment that had been previously paired with ethanol injections. Such findings, as well as the many earlier reports that discrete stimuli repeatedly paired with drugs in a self-administration paradigm can maintain drug-taking behavior when they are presented alone following responding in both laboratory animals and human drug users (Davis and Smith, 1976; Levine, 1974; O'Brien *et al.*, 1974; Schuster and Woods, 1968; Wikler *et al.*, 1971), all support the view that conditioned stimuli associated with the positive affective and reinforcing properties of drugs play an important role in drug-taking behavior.

3.2. Treatment of Addictions

Findings such as those discussed in the previous section have led to some new approaches to treatment of addictions. If it is the case that drug-paired stimuli arouse central states and physiological effects that increase and maintain interest in drugs and other drug-related stimuli, that is, create drug "craving" (see, for example, Meyer and Mirin, 1979), then one direct approach to treatment would be to try to extinguish the conditioned drug responses elicited by these stimuli. Several researchers have tried this approach. Hodgson and Rankin (1976) repeatedly exposed an excessive drinker to a single drink of ethanol (a treatment that immediately created a strong desire for ethanol) and then prevented any further consumption of ethanol. Over a course of six sessions, rating of desire for ethanol, taken 4 hr after the priming dose, was reduced to a scale value of 1 from a high of 10 on the first session. Similarly, Blakey and Baker (1980) repeatedly exposed alcoholics to stimulus situations previously determined to create a strong desire to drink and to set off drinking behavior, but without allowing them to drink. Stimuli included drinking companions, drinking environments, and sights and smells of preferred alcoholic drinks. Rating of desire to drink in the presence of these stimuli was reduced to zero over the course of therapy. In some instances individuals found that the smell of liquor actually became aversive as the extinction treatments progressed. Interestingly, the smell of tobacco smoke often is reported to change from being very positive to aversive by ex-smokers who are inevitably repeatedly exposed to tobacco smoke throughout the period following the decision to stop smoking.

A finding reported by O'Brien *et al.* (1974) may be related. They found that detoxified former heroin addicts initially reported opiatelike effects and showed druglike physiological responses when self-injecting saline under conditions where drug was expected. After repeated injections of saline, the opiatelike effects extinguished and subjects showed withdrawallike effects and dysphoria. In a similar study, Sideroff and Jarvik (1980) exposed heroin addicts who had just finished a 14-day detoxification program to videotapes of heroin-related stimuli. Subjects experienced anxiety and craving and increases in heart rate and galvanic skin responses in the presence of these stimuli. In these subjects, the conditioned drug effects appeared to be primarily aversive, a finding that might be related to the recency of detoxification. But as the authors point out, because the addict often experiences abstinence just prior to his next heroin injection, one might expect the same stimuli to be conditioned to withdrawal and to the "high" resulting from the injection. Such an explanation might account for the fact that both druglike and withdrawallike effects seem often to be elicited by opiate-related stimuli. Because both types of effects are repeatedly paired with drug taking they could acquire positive affective properties through repeated association with those of the drug. During extinction, however, when these effects are elicited in the absence of drug, they should lose any positive properties, perhaps revealing aversive ones. It would seem important, whatever the case, that extinction trials be continued until all these conditioned effects are extinguished.

ACKNOWLEDGMENTS

Preparation of this paper was supported by a grant from the Medical Research Council of Canada to Jane Stewart (MT 6678) and from the Natural Sciences and Engineering Research Council of Canada to Roelof Eikelboom (A 2575). Roelof Eikelboom holds a Career Scientist Award from the Ontario Ministry of Health. We gratefully acknowledge the work of Elizabeth Chau in typing and preparing the manuscript.

4. REFERENCES

ADAMS, W. J., YEH, S. Y., WOODS, L. A., and MITCHELL, C. L., 1969, Drug-test interaction as a factor in the development of tolerance to the analgesic effect of morphine, *J. Pharmacol. Exp. Ther.* **168**:251–257.
ADER, R., 1976, Conditioned adrenocortical steroid elevations in the rat, *J. Comp. Physiol. Psychol.* **90**:1156–1163.
ADER, R., 1981, A historical account of conditioned immunobiologic responses, in: *Psychoneuroimmunology* (R. Ader, ed.), Academic Press, New York.
ADER, R., 1983, Developmental psychoneuroimmunology, *Dev. Psychobiol.* **16**:251–267.
ADER, R., and COHEN, N. 1975, Behaviorally conditioned immunosuppression, *Psychosom. Med.* **37**:333–340.
ADER, R., and COHEN, N., 1982, Behaviorally conditioned immunosuppression and murine systemic lupus erythematosus, *Science* **215**:1534–1536.
ADER, R., COHEN, N., and GROTA, L. J., 1979, Adrenal involvement in conditioned immunosuppression, *Int. J. Immunopharmacol.* **1**:141–145.
ADVOKAT, C., 1980, Evidence for conditioned tolerance of the tail flick reflex, *Behav. Neural Biol.* **29**:385–389.
AHLENIUS, S., CARLSSON, A., ENGEL, J., SVENSSON, H., and SODERSTEN, P., 1973, Antagonism by alphamethyltyrosine of the ethanol-induced stimulation and euphoria in man, *Clin. Pharmacol. Ther.* **14**:586–591.
ALKANA, R. L., FINN, D. A., and MALCOLM, R. D., 1983, The importance of experience in the development of tolerance to ethanol hypothermia, *Life Sci.* **32**:2685–2692.

ALVAREZ-BUYLLA R., and ALVEREZ-BUYLLA, E., 1975, Hypoglycemic conditioned reflex in rats: Preliminary study of its mechanism, *J. Comp. Physiol. Psychol.* **88**(1):155–160.

ALVAREZ-BUYLLA, R., and CARRASCO-ZANINI, J., 1960, A conditioned reflex which reproduces the hypoglycemic effect of insulin, *Acta Physiol. Latinoam.* **10**:153–158.

AMIT, Z., and BAUM, M., 1970, Comment on the increased resistance-to-extinction of an avoidance response induced by certain drugs, *Psychol. Rep.* **27**:310.

AMIT, Z., LEVITAN, D. E., BROWN, Z. W., and ROGAN, F., 1977, Possible involvement of central factors in the mediation of conditioned taste aversion, *Neuropharmacology* **16**:121–124.

ANTELMAN, S. M., EICHLER, A. J., BLACK, C. A., and KOCAN, D., 1980, Interchangeability of stress and amphetamine in sensitization, *Science* **207**:329–331.

AXELROD, J., and REISINE, T. D., 1984, Stress hormones: Their interaction and regulation, *Science* **224**:452–459.

BABBINI, M., and DAVIS, W. M., 1972, Time-dose relationships for locomotor activity effects of morphine after acute or repeated treatment, *Br. J. Pharmacol.* **46**:213–224.

BABBINI, M., GAIARDI, M., and BARTOLETTI, M., 1979, Dose-time motility effects of morphine and methadone in naive and morphinized rats, *Pharmacol. Res. Commun.* **11**:809–816.

BAKER, T. B., and TIFFANY, S. T., 1985, Morphine tolerance as habituation, *Psychol. Rev.* **92**:78–108.

BALAGURA, S., 1968, Conditioned glycemic responses in the control of food intake, *J. Comp. Physiol. Psychol.* **65**:30–32.

BARDO, M. T., and HUGHES, R. A., 1979, Exposure to a nonfunctional hot plate as a factor in the assessment of morphine-induced analgesia and analgesic tolerance in rats, *Pharmacol. Biochem. Behav.* **10**:481–485.

BARDO, M. T., MILLER, J. S., and NEISEWANDER, J. L., 1984a, Conditioned place preference with morphine: The effect of extinction training on the reinforcing CR, *Pharmacol. Biochem. Behav.* **21**:545–550.

BARDO, M. T., MILLER, J. S., and RISNER, M. E., 1984b, Opiate receptor supersensitivity produced by chronic naloxone treatment: Dissociation of morphine-induced antinociception and conditioned taste aversion, *Pharmacol. Biochem. Behav.* **21**:591–597.

BARKER, L. M., BEST, M. R., and DOMJAN, M. (eds.), 1977, *Learning Mechanisms in Food Selection*, Baylor University Press, Waco, TX.

BARR, G. A., SHARPLESS, N. S., COOPER, S, SCHIFF, S. R., PAREDES, W., and BRIDGER, W. H., 1983, Classical conditioning, decay and extinction of cocaine-induced hyperactivity and stereotypy, *Life Sci.* **33**:1341–1351.

BASBAUM, A. I., and FIELDS, H. L., 1978, Endogenous pain control mechanisms: Review and hypothesis, *Ann. Neurol.* **4**:451–462.

BASBAUM, A. I., and FIELDS, H. L., 1984, Endogenous pain control systems: Brain-stem spinal pathways and endorphin circuitry, *Ann. Rev. Neurosci.* **7**:309–338.

BEACH, H. D., 1957, Morphine addiction in rats, *Can. J. Psychol.* **11**: 104–112.

BENEDEK, G., SZIKSZAY, M., and OBAL, F., 1983, Stress-related changes of opiate sensitivity in thermoregulation, *Life Sci.* **33**(Suppl. I):591–593.

BENINGER, R. J., and HAHN, B. L., 1983, Pimozide blocks establishment but not expression of amphetamine-produced environment-specific conditioning, *Science* **220**:1304–1306.

BERGER, B. D., 1972, Conditioning of food aversions by injections of psychoactive drugs, *J. Comp. Physiol. Psychol.* **81**:21–26.

BERGER, B. D., WISE, C. D., and STEIN, L., 1973, Area postrema damage and bait shyness, *J. Comp. Physiol. Psychol.* **82**:475–479.

BERNSTEIN, I. L., 1978, Learned taste aversion in children receiving chemotherapy, *Science* **200**: 1302–1303.

BERNSTEIN, I. L., and WEBSTER, M. M., 1980, Learned taste aversions in humans, *Physiol. Behav.* **25**:363–366.

BERRIDGE, K., GRILL, H. J., and NORGREN, R., 1981, Relation of consummatory responses and preabsorptive insulin release to palatability and learned taste aversions, *J. Comp. Physiol. Psychol.* **95**:363–382.

BERRIDGE, K. C., ZELLNER, D. A., GRILL, H. J., and TERNES, J. W., 1984, Increases in palatability of bitter morphine in morphine drinking rats, paper presented at the Eastern Psychological Association, Philadelphia.

BERTHOUD, H. R., and JEANRENAUD, B., 1982, Sham feeding-induced cephalic phase insulin release in the rat, *Am. J. Physiol.* **242**:E280–E285.

BERTHOUD, H. R., TRIMBLE, E. R., SIEGEL, E. G. BEREITER, D. A., and JEANRENAUD, B., 1980, Cephalic-phase insulin secretion in normal and pancreatic islet-transplanted rats, *Am. J. Physiol.* **238**:E336–E340.

BLACK, R. W., ALBINIAK, T., DAVIS, M., and SCHUMPERT, J., 1973, A preference in rats for cues associated with intoxication, *Bull. Psychonom. Soc.* **2**:423–424.

BLAIR, R., and AMIT, Z., 1981, Morphine conditioned taste aversion reversed by periaqueductal gray lesions, *Pharmacol. Biochem. Behav.* **15**(4):651–653.

BLAKEY, R., and BAKER, R., 1980, An exposure approach to alcohol abuse, *Behav. Res. Ther.* **18**:319–325.

BLANDER, A., HUNT, T., BLAIR, R., and AMIT, Z., 1984, Conditioned place preference: An evaluation of morphine's positive reinforcing properties, *Psychopharmacology* **84**:124–127.

BOLLES, R. C,. and FANSELOW, M. S., 1980, A perceptual-defensive-recuperative model of fear and pain, *Behav. Brain Sci.* **3**:291–323.

BOVBJERG, D., ADER, R., and COHEN, N., 1982, Behaviorally conditioned suppression of a graft-versus-host response, *Proc. Natl. Acad. Sci. USA* **79**:583–585.

BOZARTH, M. A., 1983, Opiate reward mechanisms mapped by intracranial self-administration, in: *The Neurobiology of Opiate Reward Processes* (J. E. Smith and J. D. Lane, eds.), Elsevier Biomedical Press, Amsterdam, pp. 331–359.

BOZARTH, M. A., 1987, Conditioned place preference: A parametric analysis using systemic heroin injections, in: *Methods of Assessing the Reinforcing Properties of Abused Drugs* (M. A. Bozarth, ed.), Springer-Verlag, New York.

BOZARTH, M. A., and WISE, R. A., 1981*a*, Intracranial self-administration of morphine into the ventral tegmental area in rats, *Life Sci.* **28**:551–555.

BOZARTH, M. A., and WISE, R. A., 1981*b*, Heroin reward is dependent on a dopaminergic substrate, *Life Sci.* **29**:1881–1886.

BOZARTH, M. A., and WISE, R. A., 1982, Localization of the reward-relevant opiate receptors, in: *Problems of Drug Dependence 1981* (L. S. Harris, ed.), National Institute of Drug Abuse, Rockville, MD, pp. 158–164.

BOZARTH, M. A., and WISE, R. A., 1984, Anatomically distinct-opiate receptor fields mediate reward and physical dependence, *Science* **224**:516–517.

BYKOV, K. M., 1957, *The Cerebral Cortex and the Internal Organs* (W. H. Gantt, ed. and trans.), Chemical Publishing Co'., New York.

CAPPELL, H. D., and LEBLANC, A. E., 1971, Conditioned aversion to saccharin by single administrations of mescaline and *d*-amphetamine, *Psychopharmacologia* **22**:352–356.

CAPPELL, H., LEBLANC, A. E., and Herling, S., 1975, Modification of the punishing effects of psychoactive drugs in rats by previous drug experience, *J. Comp. Physiol. Psychol.* **89**:347–356.

CAPPELL, H., ROACH, C., and POULOS, C. X., 1981, Pavlovian control of cross-tolerance between pentobarbital and ethanol, *Psychopharmacology* **74**:54–58.

CARDER, B., 1978, Environmental influences on morphine tolerance, in *Behavioral Toler-*

ance: *Research and Treatment Implications* (N. A. KRASNEGOR, ed.), NIDA Res. Mono. 18, U.S. Government Printing Office, Washington, DC.

CAREY, R. J., 1978, A comparison of the food intake suppression produced by giving amphetamine as an aversion treatment versus as an anorexic treatment, *Psychopharmacology* **56**:45–48.

CARLSSON, A., ENGEL, J., and SVENSSON, T. H., 1972, Inhibition of ethanol-induced excitation in mice and rats by α-methyl-p-tyrosine, *Psychopharmacologia* **26**:307–312.

CARLTON, P. L., and WOLGIN, D. L., 1971, Contingent tolerance to the anorexigenic effects of amphetamine, *Physiol. Behav.* **7**:221–223.

CARR, G. D., and WHITE, N. M., 1983, Conditioned place preference from intraaccumbens but not intra-caudate amphetamine injections, *Life Sci.* **33**:2551–2557.

CARR, K. D., and SIMON, E. J., 1984, Potentiation of reward by hunger is opiate mediated, *Brain Res.* **297**:369–373.

CAWTHORNE, M. A., 1981, Is tolerance to anorectic drugs a real phenomenon or an experimental artifact? in: *Anorectic Agents: Mechanisms of Action and Tolerance* (S. Garattini and R. Samanin, eds.), Raven Press, New York, pp. 1–17.

CHANCE, W. T., 1980, Autoanalgesia: Opiate and non-opiate mechanisms, *Neurosci. Biobehav. Rev.* **4**:55–67.

CHEN, C. S., 1968, A study of the alcohol-tolerance effect and an introduction of a new behavioral technique, *Psychopharmacologia* **12**:443–440.

CHEN, M., WOODS, S. C., and PORTE, D. Jr., 1975, Effect of cerebral intraventricular insulin on pancreatic insulin secretion in the dog, *Diabetes* **24**:910–914.

CHEW, H. Y. J., 1984, The effects of priming on place preference using morphine and amphetamine, B. S. Honours thesis, University of Western Ontario.

CHOWERS, I., LAVY, S., and HALPERN, L., 1961, Effect of insulin administered intracisternally in dogs on the glucose level of the blood and cerebrospinal fluid, *Exp. Neurol.* **3**:197–205.

CHOWERS, I., LAVY, S., and HALPERN, L., 1966, Effect of insulin administered intracisternally on the glucose level of the blood and the cerebrospinal fluid in vagotomized dogs, *Exp. Neurol.* **14**:383–389.

COCHIN, J., ROSOW, C., and MILLER, J., 1978, Ambient temperature and morphine action, in: *Factors Affecting the Action of Narcotics* (M. L. Adler, L. Manara, and R. Samanin, eds.), Raven Press, New York, pp. 631–641.

COIL, J. D., and NOGREN, R., 1981, Taste aversions conditioned with intravenous copper sulphate: Attenuation by ablation of the area postrema, *Brain Res.* **212**:425–433.

COIL, J. D., HANKINS, W. D., JENDEN, D. J., and GARCIA, J., 1978a, The attenuation of a specific cue-to-consequence association by antiemetic agents, *Psychopharmacology* **56**:21–25.

COIL, J. D., ROGERS, R. C., GARCIA, J., and NOVIA, D., 1978b, Conditioned taste aversions: Vagal and circulatory mediation of the toxic unconditioned stimulus, *Behav. Biol.* **24**:509–519.

COLE, S. O., 1980, Deprivation-dependent effects of amphetamine on concurrent measures of feeding and activity, *Pharmacol. Biochem. Behav.* **12**:723–727.

COLPAERT, F. C., NIEMEGEERS, C. J. E., JANSSEN, P. A. J., and MAROLI, A. N., 1980, The effects of prior fentanyl administration and of pain on fentanyl analgesia: Tolerance to and enhancement of narcotic analgesia, *J. Pharmacol. Exp. Ther.* **213**:418–424.

CORFIELD-SUMNER, P. K., and STOLERMAN, I. P., 1978, Behavioral tolerance, in: *Contemporary Research in Behavioural Pharmacology* (D. E. Blackman and D. J. Sanger, eds.), Plenum Press, New York, pp. 391–448.

COX, B., ARY, M., and LOMAX, P., 1976a, Dopaminergic involvement in withdrawal hypothermia and thermoregulatory behavior in morphine dependent rats, *Pharmacol. Biochem. Behav.* **4**:259–262.

Cox, B., Ary, M., Chesarek, W., and Lomax, P., 1976b, Morphine hyperthermia in the rat: An action on the central thermostats, *Eur. J. Pharmacol.* **36**:33–39.

Crowell, C. R., Hinson, R. E., and Siegel, S., 1981, The role of conditional drug responses in tolerance to the hypothermic effects of ethanol, *Psychopharmacology* **73**:51–54.

Cunningham, C. L., 1979, Flavor and location aversions produced by ethanol, *Behav. Neural Biol.* **27**:362–367.

Dafters, R., and Anderson, G., 1982, Conditional tolerance to the tachycardia effect of ethanol in humans, *Psychopharmacology* **78**:365–367.

Dafters, R., Hetherington, M., and McCartney, H., 1983, Blocking and sensory preconditioning effects in morphine analgesic tolerance: Support for a Pavlovian conditioning model of drug tolerance, *Q. J. Exp. Psychol.* **35B**:1–11.

Davidson, M. B., and Organ, G., 1982, Small doses of intracarotid insulin do not lower plasma glucose in rats, *Peptides* **3**:721–725.

Davis, W. M., and Smith, S. G., 1976, Role of conditioned reinforcers in the initiation, maintenance and extinction of drug-seeking behavior, *Pavlov. J. Biol. Sci.* **11**:222–236.

Demellweek, C., and Goudie, A. J., 1982, The role of reinforcement loss in the development of tolerance to amphetamine anorexia, *IRCS Med. Sci.* **10**:903–904.

Demellweek, C., and Goudie, A. J., 1983a, An analysis of behavioural mechanisms involved in the acquisition of amphetamine anorectic tolerance, *Psychopharmacology* **79**:58–66.

Demellweek, C., and Goudie, A. J., 1983b, Behavioural tolerance to amphetamine and other psychostimulants: The case for considering behavioural mechanisms, *Psychopharmacology* **80**:287–307.

Deutsch, R., 1974, Conditioned hypoglycemia: A mechanism for saccharin-induced sensitivity to insulin in the rat, *J. Comp. Physiol. Psychol.* **86**:350–358.

de Wit, H., and Stewart, J., 1981, Reinstatement of cocaine-reinforced responding in the rat, *Psychopharmacology* **75**:134–143.

de Wit, H., and Stewart, J., 1983, Drug reinstatement of heroin-reinforced responding in the rat, *Psychopharmacology* **79**:29–31.

Domjan, M., and Siegel, S., 1983, Attenuation of the aversive and analgesic effects of morphine by repeated administration: Different mechanisms, *Physiol. Psychol.* **11**:155–158.

Drawbaugh, R., and Lal, H., 1974, Reversal by narcotic antagonist of a narcotic action elicited by a conditional stimulus, *Nature* **247**:65–67.

Drawbaugh, R. B., and Lal, H., 1976, Effect of pharmacological interference with various neuropathways on blockage of morphine-withdrawal hypothermia by morphine and by conditional stimulus, *Neuropharmacology* **15**:375–378.

Eikelboom, R., and Stewart, J., 1979, Conditioned temperature effects using morphine as the unconditioned stimulus, *Psychopharmacology* **61**:31–38.

Eikelboom, R., and Stewart, J., 1981a, Temporal and environmental cues in conditioned hypothermia and hyperthermia associated with morphine, *Psychopharmacology* **72**:147–153.

Eikelboom, R., and Stewart, J., 1981b, Conditioned temperature effects using amphetamine as the unconditioned stimulus, *Psychopharmacology* **75**:96–97.

Eikelboom, R., and Stewart, J., 1982, The conditioning of drug-induced physiological responses, *Psychol. Rev.* **89**:507–528.

Emmett-Oglesby, M. W., and Taylor, K. E., 1981, Role of dose interval in the acquisition of tolerance to methylphenidate, *Neuropharmacology* **20**:995–1002.

Fanselow, M. S., 1984, Shock-induced analgesia on the formalin test: Effects of shock severity, naloxone, hypophysectomy, and associative variables, *Behav. Neurosci.* **98**:79–95.

Fanselow, M. S., and Baackes, M. P., 1982, Conditioned fear-induced opiate analgesia on the formalin test: Evidence for two aversive motivational systems, *Learn. Motiv.* **13**:200–221.

FANSELOW, M. S., and BOLLES, R. C., 1979, Triggering of the endorphin analgesic reaction by a cue previously associated with shock: Reversal by naloxone, *Bull. Psychonom. Soc.* **14:**88–90.

FAUMAN, M. A., 1982, The central nervous system and the immune system, *Biol. Psychiatry* **17:**1459–1482.

FERGUSON, R. K., ADAMS, W. J., and MITCHELL, C. L., 1969, Studies of tolerance development to morphine analgesia in rats tested on the hot plate, *Eur. J.Pharmacol.* **8:**83–92.

FLAHERTY, C. F., and BECKER, H. C., 1984, Influence of conditioned stimulus context on hyperglycemic conditioned responses, *Physiol. Behav.* **33:**587–593.

FLAHERTY, C. F., UZWIAK, A. J., LEVINE, J., SMITH, M., HALL, P., and SCHULER, R., 1980, Apparent hyperglycemic and hypoglycemic conditioned responses with exogenous insulin as the unconditioned stimulus, *Anim. Learn. Behav.* **8:**382–386.

FLAHERTY, C. F., BECKER, H. C., ROWAN, G. A., and VOELKER, S., 1984, Effects of chlordiazepoxide on novelty-induced hyperglycemia and conditioned hyperglycemia, *Physiol. Behav.* **33:**595–599.

FOG, R., 1970, Behavioral effects in rats of morphine and amphetamine and of a combination of the two drugs, *Pharmacologia (Berlin)* **16:**305–312.

FREDERICKSON, R. C. A., BURGIS, V., and EDWARDS, J. D., 1977, Hyperalgesia induced by naloxone follows diurnal rhythm in responsivity to painful stimuli, *Science* **198:**756–758.

FRIEDMAN, H. R., and COONS, E. E., 1983, Dopaminergic modulation of consummatory behavior in hungry and sated rats, *Abst. Soc. Neurosci.* **9:**468.

FRUMKIN, K., 1976, Differential potency of taste and audiovisual stimuli in the conditioning of morphine withdrawal in rats, *Psychopharmacologia* **46:**245–248.

FUREDY, J. J., and POULOS, C. X., 1976, Heart-rate decelerative Pavlovian conditioning with tilt as UCS: Towards behavioral control of cardiac dysfunction, *Biol. Psychol.* **4:**93–106.

GANTT W. H., KATZENELEBOGEN, S., and LOUCKS, R. B., 1937, An attempt to condition adrenalin hyperglycemia, *Bull. John Hopkins Hosp.* **60:**400–411.

GARCIA, J., and KOELLING, R. A., 1966, Relation of cue to consequence in avoidance learning, *Psychonom. Sci.* **4:**123–124.

GARCIA, J., McGOWAN, B. K., ERVIN, F. R., and KOELLING, R. A., 1966, Cues: Their relative effectiveness as a function of the reinforcer, *Science* **160:**794–795.

GARCIA, J., ERVIN, F. R., and KOELLING, R. A., 1967, Bait-shyness: A test for toxicity with $N = 2$, *Psychonom. Sci.* **7:**245–246.

GARCIA, J., HANKINS, W. G., and RUSINIAK, K. W., 1974, Behavioral regulation of the milieu interne in man and rat, *Science* **18:**824–831.

GEBHART, G. F., 1982, Opiate and opioid peptide effects on brain stem neurons: Relevance to nociception and antinociceptive mechanisms, *Pain* **12:**93–140.

GEBHART, G. F., SHERMAN, A. D., and MITCHELL, C. L., 1972, The influence of stress on tolerance development to morphine in rats tested on the hot plate, *Arch. Int. Pharmacodyn. Ther.* **197:**328–337.

GELLER, E. B., HAWK, C., KEINATH, S. H., TALLARIDA, R. J., and ADLER, M. W., 1983, Subclasses of opioids based on body temperature change in rats: Acute subcutaneous administration, *J. Pharmacol. Exp. Ther.* **225:**391–399.

GERBER, G. J., and STRETCH, R., 1975, Drug-induced reinstatement of extinguished self-administration behavior in monkeys, *Pharmacol. Biochem. Behav.* **3:**1055–1061.

GIKNIS, M. L. A., and DAMJANOV, I., 1984, Time interval between sequential exposures to ethanol is critical for the development of neural tolerance and sensitivity, *Psychopharmacology* **82:**229–232.

GLIMCHER, P. W., GIOVINO, A. A., MARGOLIN, D. H., and HOEBEL, B. G., 1984, Endogenous opiate reward induced by an enkephalinase inhibitor, Thiorphan, injected into the ventral midbrain, *Behav. Neurosci.* **98:**262–268.

GOLDBERG, S. R., and SCHUSTER, C. R., 1967, Conditioned suppression by a stimulus associated with nalorphine in morphine-dependent monkeys, *J. Exp. Anal. Behav.* **10**:235–242.
GOLDBERG, S. R., WOODS, J. H., and SCHUSTER, C. R., 1969, Morphine: Conditioned increases in self-administration in rhesus monkeys, *Science* **166**:1306–1307.
GOUDIE, A. J., 1979, Aversive stimulus properties of drugs, *Neuropharmacology* **18**:971–979.
GOUDIE, A. J., 1987, Aversive stimulus properties of drugs: The conditioned taste aversion paradigm, in: *Experimental Approach in Psychopharmacology* (A. J. Greenshaw and C. T. Dourish, eds.), Humana Press Inc., Crescent Manor, NJ.
GOUDIE, A. J., and DEMELLWEEK, C., 1987, Conditioning factors in drug tolerance, in: *Behavioural Analysis of Drug Dependence* (S. R. Goldberg and I. P. Stolerman, eds.), Academic Press, New York.
GOUDIE, A. J., TAYLOR, M., and ATHERTON, H., 1975, Effects of prior drug experience on the establishment of taste aversions in rats, *Pharmacol. Biochem. Behav.* **3**:947–952.
GOUDIE, A. J., THORNTON, E. W., and WHEELER, T. J., 1976, Drug pretreatment effects in drug induced taste aversions: Effects of dose and duration of pretreatment, *Pharmacol. Biochem. Behav.* **4**:629–633.
GOUDIE, A. J., STOLERMAN, I. P., DEMELLWEEK, C., and D'MELLO, G. D., 1982, Does conditioned nausea mediate drug-induced conditioned taste aversion? *Psychopharmacology* **78**:277–281.
GRABOWSKI, J., and O'BRIEN, C. P., 1981, Conditioning factors in opiate use, in: *Advances in Substance Abuse*, Vol. 2 (N. K. Mello, ed.), Jai Press, Greenwich, CT.
GUNNE, L. M., 1960, The temperature response in rats during acute and chronic morphine administration a study of morphine tolerance, *Arch. Int. Pharmacodyn. Ther.* **129**:416–428.
GUSTAVSON, C. R., 1977, Comparative and field aspects of learned food aversions, in: *Learning Mechanisms in Food Selection* (L. M. Barker, M. R. Best, and M. Domjan, eds.), Baylor University Press, Waco, TX, pp. 23–43.
HEARST, E., and JENKINS, H. M., 1974, *Sign-Tracking: The Stimulus-Reinforcer Relation and Directed Action*, The Psychonomic Society, Austin, TX.
HINSON, R., 1985, Individual differences in tolerance and relapse: A Pavlovian conditioning perspective, in: *Determinants of Substance Abuse: Biological, Psychological and Environmental Factors* (M. Galizio and S. A. Maisto, eds.), Plenum Press, New York.
HINSON, R. E., and POULOS, C. X., 1981, Sensitization to the behavioral effects of cocaine: Modification by Pavlovian conditioning, *Pharmacol. Biochem. Behav.* **15**:559–562.
HINSON, R. E., and SIEGEL, S., 1983, Anticipatory hyperexcitability and tolerance to the narcotizing effect of morphine in the rat, *Behav. Neurosci.* **97**:759–767.
HODGSON, R. J., and RANKIN, H. J., 1976, Modification of excessive drinking by cue exposure, *Behav. Res. Ther.* **14**:305–307.
HOLTZMAN, S. G,. 1979, Suppression of appetitive behavior in the rat by naloxone: Lack of effect of prior morphine dependence, *Life Sci.* **24**:219–226.
HOMMEL, H., FISCHER, U,. RETZLAFF, K., and KNOFLER, H., 1972, The mechanism of insulin secretion after oral glucose administration. II. Reflex insulin secretion in conscious dogs bearing fistulas of the digestive tract by sham-feeding of glucose or tap water, *Diabetologia* **8**:111–116
HUGHES, R. A., and BARDO, M. T., 1978, Morphine analgesic tolerance in rats: A search for hyperalgesia, Paper presented at the Psychonomic Society meeting, San Antonio, TX.
HUTTON, R. A., WOODS, S. C., and MAKOUS, W. L., 1970, Conditioned hypoglycemia: Pseudoconditioning controls, *J. Comp. Physiol. Psychol.* **71**:198–201.
IRWIN, S., and ARMSTRONG, P., 1961, Conditioned locomotor response with drug as the unconditioned stimulus: Individual differences, in: *Neuropsychopharmacology* (E. Rothlin, ed.), Elsevier, Amsterdam, pp. 151–157.

JENCK, F., QUIRION, R., and WISE, R. A., 1985, Microinjected opioids into VTA or PAG induce opposite effects on LH stimulation-induced feeding, *Soc. Neurosci. Abstr.* **11**:61.

JENKINS, P. E., CHADWICK, R. A., and NEVIN, J. A., 1983, Classically conditioned enhancement of antibody production, *Bull. Psychonom. Soc.* **21**:485–487.

JOHNSON, W. G., and WILDMAN, H. E., 1983, Influence of external and covert food stimuli on insulin secretion in obese and normal persons, *Behav. Neurosci.* **97**:1025–1028.

JOYCE, E. M., and IVERSEN, S. D., 1979, The effect of morphine applied locally to mesencephalic dopamine cell bodies on spontaneous motor activity in the rat, *Neurosci. Lett.* **14**:207–212.

KAMAT, K. A., DUTTA, S. N., and PRADHAM, S. N., 1974, Conditioning of morphine-induced enhancement of motor activity, *Res. Comm. Chem. Pathol. Pharmacol.* **7**:367–373.

KATZ, R. J., and GORMEZANO, G., 1978, A rapid and inexpensive technique for assessing the reinforcing effects of opiate drugs, *Pharmacol. Biochem. Behav.* **11**:231–233.

KAYAN, S,. and MITCHELL, C. L., 1972, Studies on tolerance development to morphine: Effect of the dose-interval on the development of single dose tolerance, *Arch. Int. Pharmacodyn. Ther.* **199**:407–414.

KAYAN, S., WOODS, L. A., and MITCHELL, C. L., 1969, Experience as a factor in the development of tolerance to the analgesic effect of morphine, *Eur. J. Pharmacol.* **6**:333–339.

KESNER, R. P., and BAKER, T. B., 1981, A two-process model of opiate tolerance, in: *Endogenous Peptides and Learning and Memory Processes* (J. L. Martinez, R. A. Jensen, R. B. Messing, H. Rigter, and J. L. McGaugh, eds.), Academic Press, New York, pp. 479–518.

KESNER, R. P., and COOK, D. G., 1983, Role of habituation and classical conditioning in the development of morphine tolerance, *Behav. Neurosci.* **97**:4–12.

KRANE, R. V., 1980, Toxicophobia conditioning with exteroceptive cues, *Anim. Learn. Behav.* **8**:513–523.

KRANK, M. D., 1984, Environmental signals for ethanol enhance free-choice ethanol consumption. *Can. Psychol.: Abstr.* **25**:262.

KRANK, M. D., HINSON, R. E., and SIEGEL, S., 1981, Conditioned hyperalgesia is elicited by environmental signals of morphine, *Behav. Neural Biol.* **32**:148–157.

KUMAR, R., 1972, Morphine dependence in rats: Secondary reinforcement from environmental stimuli, *Psychopharmacologia* **25**:332–338.

LaHOSTE, G. A., OLSON, R. A., OLSON, G. A., and KASTIN, A. J., 1980, Effects of Pavlovian conditioning and MIF-1 on the development of morphine tolerance in rats, *Pharmacol. Biochem. Behav.* **13**:799–804.

LAL, H., MIKSIC, S., and SMITH, N., 1976, Naloxone antagonism of conditioned hyperthermia: An evidence for release of endogenous opioid, *Life Sci.* **18**:971–975.

LÊ, A. D., POULOS, C. X., and CAPPELL, H., 1979, Conditioned tolerance to the hypothermic effect of ethyl alcohol, *Science* **206**:1109–1110.

LEBLANC, A. E., and CAPPELL, H., 1975, Antagonism of morphine-induced aversive conditioning by naloxone, *Pharmacol. Biochem. Behav.* **3**:185–188.

LEBLANC, A. E., GIBBINS, R. J., and KALANT, H., 1973, Behavioral augmentation of tolerance to ethanol in the rat, *Psychopharmacologia* **30**:117–122.

LEBLANC, A. E., GIBBINS, R. J., and KALANT, H., 1975, Generalization of behaviorally augmented tolerance to ethanol and its relation to physical dependence, *Psychopharmacologia* **44**:241–246.

LEBLANC, A. E., KALANT, H,. and GIBBINS, R. J., 1976, Acquisition and loss of behaviorally augmented tolerance to ethanol in the rat, *Psychopharmacologia* **48**:153–158.

LETT, B. T., 1983, Pavlovian drug-sickness pairings result in the conditioning of an antisickness response, *Behav. Neurosci.* **97**:779–784.

LETT, B. T., 1985, The painlike effect of gallamine and naloxone differs from sickness induced by lithium chloride, *Behav. Neurosci.* **99**:145–150.

LEVINE, D. G., 1974, "Needle freaks": Compulsive self-injections by drug users, *Am. J. Psychiatry* **131**:297–300.
LEVITSKY, D. A., STRUPP, B. J., and LUPOLI, J., 1981, Tolerance to anorectic drugs: Pharmacological or artifactual, *Pharmacol. Biochem. Behav.* **14**:661–667.
LICHKO, A. E., 1959, Conditioned reflex hypoglycemia in man, *Zh. Vyssh. Nervn. Deiatel.* **9**:823–829. (Also in *Pavlov. J. Higher Nervous Act.* **9**:731–737.)
LOUIS-SYLVESTRE, J., 1976, Preabsorptive insulin release and hypoglycemia in rats, *Am. J. Physiol.* **230**:56–60.
LOUIS-SYLVESTRE, J., 1978, Relationship between two stages of prandial insulin release in rats, *Am. J. Physiol.* **235**:E103–E111.
LYNCH, J. J., STEIN, E. A., and FERTZIGER, A. P., 1976, An analysis of 70 years of morphine classical conditioning: Implications for clinical treatment of narcotic addiction, *J. Nerv. Ment. Dis.* **163**:47–58.
MACKENZIE, T. M., and GANTT, W. H., 1950, Cardiac acceleration to atropine cannot be conditioned, *Fed. Proc.* **9**:83–84.
MACKEY, W. B., and VAN DER KOOY, D., 1983, Neuroleptics do not block the reinforcing effects of opiates in the conditioned place preference paradigm, *Neurosci. Abstr.* **9**:981.
MACKINTOSH, N. J., 1974, *The Psychology of Animal Learning*, Academic Press, London.
MANSFIELD, J. G., and CUNNINGHAM, C. L., 1980, Conditioning and extinction of tolerance to the hypothermic effect of ethanol in rats, *J. Comp. Physiol. Psychol.* **94**:962–969.
MANSFIELD, J. G., BENEDICT, R. S., and WOODS, S. C., 1983, Response specificity of behaviorally augmented tolerance to ethanol supports a learning interpretation, *Psychopharmacology* **79**:94–98.
MARGOLIS, R. U., and ALTSZULER, N., 1968, Effect of intracisternally administered insulin-^{131}I in normal and vagotomized dogs, *Proc. Soc. Exp. Biol. Med.* **127**:1122–1125.
MARTIN, G. E., and MORRISON, J. E., 1978, Hyperthermia evoked by the intracerebral injection of morphine sulphate in the rat: The effect of restraint, *Brain Res.* **145**:127–140.
MARTIN, J. C., and ELLINWOOD, E. H., 1974, Conditioned aversion in spatial paradigms following methamphetamine injection, *Psychopharmacologia* **36**:323–335.
MARTIN, W. R,. WIKLER, A., EADES, C. G., and PESCOR, F. T., 1963, Tolerance to and physical dependence on morphine in rats, *Psychopharmacologia* **4**:247–260.
MASUR, J., and BOERNGEN, R., 1980, The excitatory component of ethanol in mice: A chronic study, *Pharmacol. Biochem. Behav.* **13**:777–780.
MATYSIAK, J., and GREEN, L., 1984, On the directionality of classically-conditioned glycemic responses, *Physiol. Behav.* **32**:5–9.
MELCHIOR, C. L., and TABAKOFF, B., 1981, Conditioned tolerance: Cued alterations in ethanol distribution, *Alcohol.: Clin. Exp. Res.* **5**:161.
MEYER, R. E., and MIRIN, S. M., 1979, *The Heroin Stimulus: Implications for a Theory of Addiction*, Plenum Press, New York.
MIKSIC, S., SMITH, N., NUMAN, R., and LAL, H., 1975, Acquisition and extinction of a conditioned hyperthermic response to a tone paired with morphine administration, *Neuropsychobiology* **1**:277–283.
MILGRAM, N. W., KRAMES, L., and ALLOWAY, T., 1977, *Food Aversion Learning*, Plenum Press, New York.
MILLOY, S., and GLICK, S. D., 1976, Factors affecting tolerance to d-amphetamine-induced anorexia in rats, *Arch. Int. Pharmacodyn. Ther.* **221**:87–95.
MITCHELL, D., WINTER, W., and MORISAKI, C. M., 1977, Conditioned taste aversions accompanied by geophagia: Evidence for the occurrence of "psychological" factors in the etiology of pica, *Psychosom. Med.* **39**:402–412.
MITIUSHOV, M. I., 1954, The conditional reflex incretion of insulin, *Pavlov. J. Higher Nerv. Act.* **4**:206–212.
MONACO, A. P., HERNANDEZ, L., and HOEBEL, B. G., 1981, Nucleus accumbens: Site of

amphetamine self-injection; comparison with the lateral ventricle, in: *The Neurobiology of Nucleus Accumbens* (R. B. Chronister and J. F. de France, eds.), Haer Institute, Brunswick, ME.

MORRIS, R. G. M., JONZEN, R. A. I., WELSH, B., and CAHUSAC, P. M. B., 1981, Environmentally specific opiate tolerance: Is it due to compensatory conditioning? Paper presented at meeting of Experimental Psychology Society, Liverpool, U.K.

MUCHA, R. F., and IVERSEN, S. D., 1984, Reinforcing properties of morphine and naloxone revealed by conditioned place preferences: A procedural examination, *Psychopharmacology* **82**:241–247.

MUCHA, R. F., KALANT, H., and LINSEMAN, M. A., 1979, Quantitative relationships among measures of morphine tolerance and physical dependence in the rat, *Pharmacol. Biochem. Behav.* **10**:397–405.

MUCHA, R. F., VOLKOVSKIS, C., and KALANT, H., 1981, Conditioned increases in locomotor activity produced with morphine as an unconditioned stimulus, and the relation of conditioning to acute morphine effect and tolerance, *J. Comp. Physiol. Psychol.* **95**:351–362.

MUCHA, R. F., VAN DER KOOY, D., O'SHAUGHNESSY, M., and BUCENIEKS, P., 1982, Drug reinforcement studied by the use of place conditioning in rat, *Brain Res.* **243**:91–105.

MYERS, R. D., 1981, Alcohol's effect on body temperature: Hypothermia, hyperthermia or poikilothermia? *Brain Res. Bull.* **7**:209–220.

NAKANO, S., HARA, C., and OGAWA, N., 1980, Circadian rhythm of apomorphine-induced stereotypy in rats, *Pharmacol. Biochem. Behav.* **12**:459–461.

O'BRIEN, C. P., 1976, Experimental analysis of conditioning factors in human narcotic addiction, *Pharmacol. Rev.* **27**:533–543.

O'BRIEN, C. P., CHADDOCK, B., WOODY, G., and GREENSTEIN, R., 1974, Systematic extinction of addiction-associated rituals using narcotic antagonists, *Psychosom. Med.* **36**:458.

O'BRIEN, C. P., TESTA, T., O'BRIEN, T. J., BRADY, J. P., and WELLS, B., 1977, Conditioned narcotic withdrawal in humans, *Science* **195**:1000–1002.

OKA, T., and HOSOYA, E., 1976, Effects of humoral modulators and naloxone on morphine-induced changes in the spontaneous locomotor activity of the rat, *Psychopharmacology* **47**:243–248.

PAOLINO, R. M., and BERNARD, B. K., 1968, Environmental temperature effects on the thermoregulatory response to systemic and hypothalamic administration of morphine, *Life Sci.* **7**(1):857–863.

PARKER, L. A., 1982, Nonconsummatory and consummatory behavioral CRs elicited by lithium- and amphetamine-paired flavors, *Learn. Motiv.* **13**:281–303.

PARKER, L. A., 1984, Behavioral conditioned responses across multiple conditioning/testing trials elicited by lithium- and amphetamine-paired flavors, *Behav. Neural Biol.* **41**:190–199.

PARKER, L., FAILOR, A., and WEIDMAN, K., 1973, Conditioned preferences in the rat with an unnatural need state: Morphine withdrawal, *J. Comp. Physiol. Psychol.* **82**:294–300.

PARKER, L. A., HILLS, K., and JENSEN, K., 1984, Behavioral CRs elicited by a lithium- or an amphetamine-paired contextual test chamber, *Anim. Learning Behav.* **12**:307–315.

PARKER, L. F., and RADOW, B. L., 1974, Morphine-like physical dependence: A pharmacologic method for drug assessment using the rat, *Pharmacol. Biochem. Behav.* **2**:613–618.

PARRA-COVARRUBIAS, A., RIVERA-RODRIGUEZ, I., and ALMARAZ-UGALDE, A., 1971, Cephalic phase of insulin secretion in obese adolescents, *Diabetes* **20**:800–802.

PEARL, R. G., and SEIDEN, L. S., 1979, D-amphetamine-induced increase in catecholamine synthesis in the corpus striatum of the rat: Persistence of the effect after tolerance, *J. Neural Transm.* **44**:21–38.

PELCHAT, M. L., GRILL, H. J., ROZIN, P., and JACOBS, J., 1983, Quality of acquired responses to tastes by *Rattus norvegicus* depends on type of associated discomfort, *J. Comp. Psychol.* **97**:140–153.

PEREZ-CRUET, J., 1976, Conditioning of striatal dopamine metabolism with methadone, morphine or bulbocapnine as an unconditioned stimulus, *Pavlov. J. Biol. Sci.* **11**:237–250.

PEREZ-CRUET, J., and GANTT, W. H., 1964, Conditioned reflex electrocardiogram of bulbocapnine: Conditioning of the T wave, *Am. Heart J.* **67**:61–72.

PHILLIPS, A. G., and LEPIANE, F. G., 1980, Reinforcing effects of morphine microinjection into the ventral tegmental area, *Pharmacol. Biochem. Behav.* **12**:965–968.

PHILLIPS, A. G., and LEPIANE, F. G., 1982, Reward produced by microinjection of (D-Ala^2), Met^5-enkephalinamide into the ventral tegmental area, *Behav. Brain Res.* **5**:225–229.

PICKENS, R. W., and CROWDER, W. F., 1967, Effects of CS–US interval on conditioning of drug response, with assessment of speed of conditioning, *Psychopharmacologia* **11**:88–94.

PICKENS, R., and DOUGHERTY, J. A., 1971, Conditioning of the activity effects of drugs, in: *Stimulus Properties of Drugs* (T. Thompson and R. Pickens, eds.) Appleton-Century-Crofts, New York, pp. 39–50.

PILCHER, C. W. T., and STOLERMAN I. P., 1976, Conditioned flavor aversions for assessing precipitated morphine abstinence in rats, *Pharmacol. Biochem. Behav.* **4**:159–163.

PINEL, J. P. J., COLBORNE, B., SIGALET, J. P., and RENFREY, G., 1983, Learned tolerance to the anticonvulsant effects of alcohol in rats, *Pharmacol. Biochem. Behav.* **18**(Suppl 1):507–510.

POST, R. M., 1981, Central stimulants: Clinical and experimental evidence on tolerance and sensitization, in: *Research Advances in Alcohol and Drug Problems*, Vol. 6 (Y. Israel, F. B. Glaser, H. Kalant, R. E. Popham, W. Schmidt, and R. G. Smart, eds.), Plenum Press, New York, pp. 1–65.

POST, R. M., and ROSE, H., 1976, Increasing effects of repetitive cocaine administration in the rat, *Nature* **260**:731–732.

POST, R. M., LOCKFELD, A., SQUILLACE, K. M., and CONTEL, N. R., 1981, Drug-environment interaction: Context dependency of cocaine-induced sensitization, *Life Sci.* **28**:755–760.

POULOS, C. X., and HINSON, R. E., 1984, A homeostatic model of Pavlovian conditioning: Tolerance to scopolamine-induced adipsia, *J. Exp. Psychol.: Anim. Behav. Proc.* **10**:75–89.

POULOS, C. X., HINSON, R. E., and SIEGEL, S., 1981a, The role of Pavlovian processes in drug tolerance and dependence: Implications for treatment, *Addict. Behav.* **6**:205–211.

POULOS, C. X., WILKINSON, D. A., and CAPPELL, H., 1981b, Homeostatic regulation and Pavlovian conditioning in tolerance to amphetamine-induced anorexia, *J. Comp. Physiol. Psychol.* **95**:735–746.

POWLEY, T. L., 1977, The ventromedial hypothalamic syndrome, satiety, and a cephalic phase hypothesis, *Psychol. Rev.* **84**:89–126.

RABIN, B. M., and HUNT, N. A., 1983, Effects of antiemetics on the acquisition and recall of radiation- and lithium chloride-induced conditioned taste aversions, *Pharmacol. Biochem. Behav.* **18**:629–635.

REDD, W. H., and ANDRYKOWSKI, M. A., 1982, Behavioral intervention in cancer treatment: Controlling aversion to chemotherapy, *J. Consult. Clin. Psychol.* **50**:1018–1029.

REICHER, M. A., and HOLMAN, E. W., 1977, Location preference and flavor aversion reinforced by amphetamine in rats, *Anim. Learn. Behav.* **5**:343–346.

REID, L. D., HUNTER, G. A., BEAMAN, C. M., and HUBBELL, C. L., 1985, Toward understanding ethanol's capacity to be reinforcing: A conditioned place preference following injections of ethanol, *Pharmacol. Biochem. Behav.* **22**:483–488.

RESCORLA, R. A., 1967, Pavlovian conditioning and its proper control procedures, *Psychol. Rev.* **74**:71–80.

RESCORLA, R. A., and SOLOMON, R. L., 1967, Two-process learning theory: Relationships between Pavlovian conditioning and instrumental learning, *Psychol. Rev.* **74:**151–182.

REVUSKY, S. H., 1967, Aversiveness of glucagon injection to hungry rats, US Army Medical Research Laboratory Report No. 723.

REVUSKY, S., TAUKULIS, H. K., PARKER, L. A., and COOMBES, S., 1979, Chemical aversion therapy: Rat data suggest it may be countertherapeutic to pair an addictive drug state with sickness, *Behav. Res. Ther.* **17:**177–188.

RILEY, A. L., JACOBS, W. J., and LOLORDO, V. M., 1978, Morphine-induced taste aversions: A consideration of parameters, *Physiol. Psychol.* **6:**96–100.

ROBERTS, D. C. S., and FIBIGER, H. C., 1975, Attenuation of amphetamine-induced conditioned taste aversion following intraventricular 6-hydroxydopamine, *Neurosci. Lett.* **1:**343–347.

ROBERTS, D. C. S., KOOB, G. F., KLONOFF, P., and FIBIGER, H. C., 1980, Extinction and recovery of cocaine self-administration following 6-hydroxydopamine lesions of the nucleus accumbens, *Pharmacol. Biochem. Behav.* **12:**781–787.

ROBINSON, T. E., Behavioral sensitization: Characterization of enduring changes in rotational behavior produced by intermittent injections of amphetamine in male and female rats, *Psychopharmacology* **84:**466–475.

ROBINSON, T. E., and BECKER, J. B., 1982, Behavioral sensitization is accompanied by an enhancement in amphetamine-stimulated dopamine release from striatal tissue *in vitro,* *Eur. J. Pharmacol.* **85:**253–254.

ROBINSON, T. E., BECKER, J. B., and PRESTY, S. K., 1982, Long-term facilitation of amphetamine-induced rotational behavior and striatal dopamine release produced by a single exposure to amphetamine: Sex differences, *Brain Res.* **253:**231–241.

ROCHFORD, J., and STEWART, J., 1985, Morphine attenuation of conditioned autoanalgesia: Implications for environment-specific morphine analgesic tolerance, *Soc. Neurosci. Abstr.* **11:**132.

ROFFMAN, M., REDDY, C., and LAL, H., 1973, Control of morphine-withdrawal hypothermia by conditional stimuli, *Psychopharmacologia* **29:**197–201.

ROGERS, M. P., REICH, P., STROM, T. B., and CARPENTER, C. B., 1976, Behaviorally conditioned immunosuppression: Replication of a recent study, *Psychosom. Med.* **38:**447–451.

ROSSI, N. A., and REID, L. D., 1976, Affective states associated with morphine injections, *Physiol. Psychol.* **4:**269–274.

ROWLAND, N., and CARLTON, J., 1983, Different behavioral mechanisms underlie tolerance to the anorectic effects of fenfluramine and quipazine, *Psychopharmacology* **81:**155–157.

RUSH, M. L., PEARSON, L., and LANG, W. J., 1970, Conditional autonomic responses induced in dogs by atropine and morphine, *Eur. J. Pharmacol.* **11:**22–28.

RUSSEK, M., and PINA, S., 1962, Conditioning of adrenalin anorexia, *Nature* **193:**1296–1297.

SCALLET, A. C., 1982, Effects of conditioned fear and environmental novelty on plasma β-endorphin in the rat, *Peptides* **3:**203–206.

SCHIFF, S. R., 1982, Conditioned dopaminergic activity, *Biol. Psychiatry* **17:**135–154.

SCHNUR, P., 1985, Morphine tolerance and sensitization in the hamster, *Pharmacol. Biochem. Behav.* **22:**157–158.

SCHNUR, P., 1985, Effects of naloxone and naltrexone on morphine-elicited changes in hamster locomotor activity, *Physiol. Psychol.* **13:**26–32.

SCHNUR, P., BRAVO, F., and TRUJILLO, M., 1983, Tolerance and sensitization to the biphasic effects of low doses of morphine in the hamster, *Pharmacol. Biochem. Behav.* **19:**435–439.

SCHUSTER, C. R., and WOODS, J. H., 1968, The conditioned reinforcing effects of stimuli associated with morphine reinforcement, *Int. J. Addict.* **3:**223–230.

SCHUSTER, C. R., DOCKENS, W. S., and WOODS, J. H., 1966, Behavioural variables affecting the development of amphetamine tolerance, *Psychopharmacologia* **9:**170–182.

SEEVERS, M. H., and DENEAU, G. A., 1963, Physiological aspects of tolerance and physical dependence, in: *Physiological Pharmacology*, Vol. 1 (W. S. Root and F. G. Hofmann, eds.), Academic Press, New York.

SEGAL, D. S., 1975, Behavioral and neurochemical correlates of repeated *d*-amphetamine administration, *Adv. Biochem. Psychopharmacol.* **13:**247–262.

SHAPIRO, N. R., DUDEK, B. C., and ROSELLINI, R. A., 1983, The role of associative factors in tolerance to the hypothermic effects of morphine in mice, *Pharmacol. Biochem. Behav.* **19:**327–333.

SHERMAN, J. E., 1979, The effects of conditioning and novelty on the rat's analgesic and pyretic responses to morphine, *Learn. Motiv.* **10:**383–418.

SHERMAN, J. E., PICKMAN, C., RICE, A., LIEBESKIND, J. C., and HOLMAN, E. W., 1980a, Rewarding and aversive effects of morphine: Temporal and pharmacological properties, *Pharmacol. Biochem. Behav.* **13:**501–505.

SHERMAN, J. E., ROBERTS, T., ROSKAM, S. E., and HOLMAN, E. W., 1980b, Temporal properties of the rewarding and aversive effects of amphetamine in rats, *Pharmacol. Biochem. Behav.* **13:**597–599.

SHERMAN, J. E., PROCTOR, C., and STRUB, H., 1982, Prior hot plate exposure enhances morphine analgesia in tolerant and drug-naive rats, *Pharmacol. Biochem. Behav.* **17:**229–232.

SHERMAN, J. E., STRUB, H., and LEWIS, J. W., 1984, Morphine analgesia: Enhancement by shock-associated cues, *Behav. Neurosci.* **98:**293–309.

SHIPPENBERG, T. S., KNAPPENBERGER, E., and ALTSCHULER, H. L., 1984, Drug discrimination analysis of the dual behavioral effects of ethanol, *Soc. Neurosci. Abstr.* **9:**1240.

SIDEROFF, S. I., and JARVIK, M. E,. 1980, Conditioned responses to a videotape showing heroin-related stimuli, *Int. J. Addict.* **15:**529–536.

SIEGEL, S., 1972, Conditioning of insulin-induced glycemia, *J. Comp. Physiol. Psychol.* **78:**233–241.

SIEGEL, S., 1975a, Conditioning insulin effects, *J. Comp. Physiol. Psychol.* **89:**189–199.

SIEGEL, S,. 1975b, Evidence from rats that morphine tolerance is a learned response, *J. Comp. Physiol. Psychol.* **89:**498–506.

SIEGEL, S., 1976, Morphine analgesic tolerance: Its situation specificity supports a Pavlovian conditioning model, *Science* **193:**323–325.

SIEGEL, S., 1977a, Morphine tolerance acquisition as an associative process, *J. Exp. Psychol.: Anim. Behav. Proc.* **3:**1–13.

SIEGEL, S., 1977b, Learning and psychopharmacology, in: *Psychopharmacology in the Practice of Medicine* (M. E. JARVIK, ed.), Appleton-Century-Crofts, New York.

SIEGEL, S., 1978, Tolerance to the hyperthermic effect of morphine in the rat is a learned response, *J. Comp. Physiol. Psychol.* **92:**1137–1149.

SIEGEL, S., 1979, The role of conditioning in drug tolerance and addiction, in: *Psychopathology in Animals: Research and Treatment Implications* (J. D. Keehn, ed.), Academic Press, New York.

SIEGEL, S., 1983, Classical conditioning, drug tolerance, and drug dependence, in: *Research Advances in Alcohol and Drug Problems*, Vol. 7 (R. G. Smart, F. B. Glaser, Y. Israel, H. Kalant, R. E. Popham, and W. Schmidt, eds.), Plenum Press, New York, pp. 207–245.

SIEGEL, S., 1985, Drug-anticipatory responses in animals, in: *Placebo: Theory, Research, and Mechanisms* (L. White, B. Tursky, and B. Schwartz, eds.), Guilford Press, New York, pp. 288–305.

SIEGEL, S., and NETTLETON, N., 1970, Conditioning of insulin-induced hyperphagia, *J. Comp. Physiol. Psychol.* **72:**390–393.

SIEGEL, S., HINSON, R. E., and KRANK, M. D., 1979, Modulation of tolerance to the lethal effect of morphine by extinction, *Behav. Neural Biol.* **25**:257–262.

SIEGEL, S., HINSON, R. E., KRANK, M. D., and McCULLY, J., 1982, Heroin "overdose" death: Contribution of drug-associated environmental cues, *Science* **216**:436–437.

SOLOMON, R. L., 1977, An opponent-process theory of acquired motivation: IV. The affective dynamics of addiction, in: *Psychopathology: Experimental Models* (J. D. Maser and M. E. P. Seligman, eds.), Freeman, San Francisco, pp. 66–103.

SPYRAKI, C., FIBIGER, H. C., and PHILLIPS, A. G., 1982a, Dopaminergic substrates of amphetamine-induced place preference conditioning, *Brain Res.* **253**:185–193.

SPYRAKI, C., FIBIGER, H. C., and PHILLIPS, A. G., 1982b, Cocaine-induced place preference conditioning: Lack of effects of neuroleptics and 6-hydroxydopamine lesions, *Brain Res.* **253**:195–203.

SPYRAKI, C., FIBIGER, H. C., and PHILLIPS, A. G., 1983, Attenuation of heroin reward in rats by disruption of the mesolimbic dopamine system, *Psychopharmacology* **79**:278–283.

STEWART, J., 1983, Conditioned and unconditioned drug effects in relapse to opiate and stimulant drug self-administration, *Prog. Neuro-Psychopharmacol. Biol. Psychiat.* **7**:591–597.

STEWART, J., 1984, Reinstatement of heroin and cocaine self-administration behavior in the rat by intracerebral application of morphine in the ventral tegmental area, *Pharmacol. Biochem. Behav.* **20**:917–923.

STEWART, J., and DE WIT, H., 1987, Reinstatement of drug-taking behavior as a method of assessing incentive motivational properties of drugs, in: *Methods of Assessing the Reinforcing Properties of Abused Drugs* (M. A. Bozarth, ed.), Springer-Verlag, New York.

STEWART, J., and EIKELBOOM, R., 1978, Pre-exposure to morphine and the attenuation of conditioned taste aversion in rats, *Pharmacol. Biochem. Behav.* **9**:639–645.

STEWART, J., and EIKELBOOM, R., 1981, Interaction between the effects of stress and morphine on body temperature in rats, *Life Sci.* **28**:1041–1045.

STEWART, J., DE WIT, H., and EIKELBOOM, R., 1984, The role of unconditioned and conditioned drug effects in the self-administration of opiates and stimulants, *Psychol. Rev.* **91**:251–268.

STRUBBE, J. H., and STEFFENS, A. B., 1975, Rapid insulin release after ingestion of a meal in the unanesthetized rat, *Am. J. Physiol.* **229**:1019–1022.

STUNKARD, A. J., 1982, Anorectic agents lower a body weight set point, *Life Sci.* **30**:2043–2055.

SUBKOV, A. A., and ZILOV, G. N., 1937, The role of conditioned reflex adaptation in the origin of hyperergic reactions, *Byull. Eksp. Biol. Med.* **4**:294–296.

SWITZMAN, L., AMIT, Z., WHITE, N., and FISHMAN, B., 1978, Novel tasting food enhances morphine discriminability in rats, in: *Stimulus Properties of Drugs: Ten Years of Progress* (F. C. Colpaert and J. A. Rosecrans, eds.), Elsevier North Holland Biomedical Press, Amsterdam.

SZABO, A. J., and SZABO, O., 1975, Influence of the insulin sensitive central nervous system glucoregulator receptor on hepatic glucose metabolism, *J. Physiol.* **253**:121–133.

SZABO, A. J., and SZABO, O., 1983, Insulin injected into CNS structures or into the carotid artery: Effect on carbohydrate homeostasis of the intact animal, *Adv. Metabol. Disorders* **10**:385–400.

SZABO, O., and SZABO, A. J., 1972, Evidence for an insulin-sensitive receptor in the central nervus system, *Am. J. Physiol.* **223**:1349–1353.

TABAKOFF, B., and KIIANMAA, K., 1982, Does tolerance develop to the activating, as well as the depressant, effects of ethanol? *Pharmacol. Biochem. Behav.* **17**:1073–1076.

TATUM, A. L., and SEEVERS, M. H., 1929, Experimental cocaine addiction, *J. Pharmacol. Exp. Ther.* **36**:401–410.

TERNES, J. W., 1975, Conditioned aversion to morphine with naloxone, *Bull. Psychonom. Soc.* **5**:292–294.
THOMPSON, T., and OSTLUND, W., Jr., 1965, Susceptibility to readdiction as a function of the addiction and withdrawal environments, *J. Comp. Physiol. Psychol.* **60**:388–392.
TIFFANY, S. T., and BAKER, T. B., 1981, Morphine tolerance in rats: Congruence with a Pavlovian paradigm, *J. Comp. Physiol. Psychol.* **95**:747–762.
TIFFANY, S. T., PETRIE, E. C., BAKER, T. B., and DAHL, J. L., 1983a, Conditioned morphine tolerance in the rat: Absence of a compensatory response and cross-tolerance with stress, *Behav. Neurosci.* **97**:335–353.
TIFFANY, S. T., PETRIE, E. C., MARTIN, E. M., and BAKER, T. B., 1983b, Drug signals enhance morphine tolerance development in hypophysectomized rats, *Psychopharmacology* **79**:84–85.
TILSON, H. A., and RECH, R. H., 1973, Conditioned drug effects and absence of tolerance to *d*-amphetamine-induced motor activity, *Pharmacol. Biochem. Behav.* **1**:149–153.
TROST, R. C., 1973, Differential classical conditioning of abstinence syndrome in morphine-dependent rats, *Psychopharmacologia* **30**:153–161.
TYE, N. C., and IVERSEN, S. D., 1975, Some behavioral signs of morphine withdrawal blocked by conditional stimuli, *Nature* **255**:416–418.
VAN DER KOOY, D., 1987, Place conditioning: A simple and effective method for assessing the motivational properties of drugs, in: *Methods of Assessing the Reinforcing Properties of Abused Drugs* (M. A. Bozarth, ed.), Springer-Verlag, New York.
VAN DER KOOY, D., MUCHA, R. F., O'SHAUGHNESSY, M., and BUCENIEKS, P., 1982, Reinforcing effects of brain microinjections of morphine revealed by conditioned place preference, *Brain Res.* **243**:107–117.
VAN DER KOOY, D., SWERDLOW, N. R., and KOOB, G. F., 1983a, Paradoxical reinforcing properties of apomorphine: Effects of nucleus accumbens and area postrema lesions, *Brain Res.* **259**:111–118.
VAN DER KOOY, D., O'SHAUGHNESSY, M., MUCHA, R. F., and KALANT, H., 1983b, Motivational properties of ethanol in naive rats as studied by place conditioning, *Pharmacol. Biochem. Behav.* **19**:441–445.
VAN HOUTEN, M., and POSNER, B. I., 1983, Circumventricular organs: Receptors and mediators of direct peptide hormone action on brain, *Adv. Metabol. Disorders* **10**:269–289.
VASKO, M. R., and DOMINO, E. F., 1978, Tolerance development to the biphasic effects of morphine on locomotor activity and brain acetylcholine in the rat, *J. Pharmacol. Exp. Ther.* **207**:848–858.
VEZINA, P., and STEWART, J., 1984, Conditioning and place-specific sensitization of increases in activity induced by morphine in the VTA, *Pharmacol. Biochem. Behav.* **20**:925–934.
VEZINA, P., and STEWART, J., 1985, Strong absolute conditioned place preference is obtained when morphine is paired exclusively with tactile stimuli in an open field, *Soc. Neurosci. Abstr.* **11**:1278.
WAGNER, G. C., FOLTIN, R. W., SEIDEN, L. S., and SCHUSTER, C. R., 1981, Dopamine depletion by 6-hydroxydopamine prevents conditioned taste aversion induced by methylamphetamine but not lithium chloride, *Pharmacol. Biochem. Behav.* **14**:85–88.
WALKER, P. Y., SOLIMAN, K. F. A., and WALKER, C. A., 1982, Diurnal rhythm of ethanol hypothermic action in mice, *Res. Commun. Subst. Abuse* **3**:503–506.
WATKINS, L. R., and MAYER, D. J., 1982, The neural organization of endogenous opiate and non-opiate pain control systems, *Science* **216**:1185–1192.
WATKINS, L. R., COBELLI, D. A., and MAYER, D. J., 1982, Classical conditioning of front paw and hind paw footshock-induced analgesia (FSIA): Naloxone reversibility and descending pathways, *Brain Res.* **243**:119–132.
WATKINS, L. R., YOUNG, E. G., KINSCHECK, I. B., and MAYER, D. J., 1983, The neural basis

of footshock analgesia: The role of specific ventral medullary nuclei, *Brain Res.* **276**:305–315.

WATKINS, L. R., JOHANNESSEN, J. W., KINSCHECK, I. B., and MAYER, D. J., 1984, The neurochemical basis of footshock analgesia: The role of spinal cord serotonin and norepinephrine, *Brain Res.* **290**:107–117.

WAYNER, E. A., FLANNERY, G. R., and SINGER, G., 1978, Effects of taste aversion conditioning on the primary antibody response to sheep red blood cell and *Brucella abortus* in the albino rat, *Physiol. Behav.* **21**:995–1000.

WEIDER, G. E., and WALDBILLING, R. J., 1982, Evidence for an insulin-sensitive hypothalamic circuit controlling hepatic glucose production, *Soc. Neurosci. Abstr.* **8**:144.

WENGER, J. R., BERLIN, V., and WOODS, S. C., 1980, Learned tolerance to the behaviorally disruptive effects of ethanol, *Behav. Neur. Biol.* **28**:418–430.

WENGER, J. R., TIFFANY, T. M., BOMBARDIER, C., NICHOLLS, K., and WOODS, S. C., 1981, Ethanol tolerance in the rat is learned, *Science* **213**:575–577.

WHITE, L., TURSKY, B., and SCHWARTZ, B. (eds.), 1985, *Placebo: Theory, Research, and Mechanisms,* Guilford Press, NY.

WHITE, N., SKLAR, L., and AMIT, Z., 1977, The reinforcing action of morphine and its paradoxical side effect, *Psychopharmacology* **52**:63–66.

WHITE, N. M., MESSIER, C., and CARR, G. D., 1987, Operationalizing and measuring the organizing influence of drugs on behavior, in: *Methods of Assessing the Reinforcing Properties of Abused Drugs* (M. A. Bozarth, ed.), Springer-Verlag, New York.

WIKLER, A., 1948, Recent progress in research on the neurophysiologic basis of morphine addiction, *Am. J. Psychiatry* **105**:329–338.

WIKLER, A., 1973, Conditioning of successive adaptive responses to the initial effects of drugs, *Cond. Reflex* **8**:193–210.

WIKLER, A., and PESCOR, F. T., 1967, Classical conditioning of a morphine abstinence phenomenon, reinforcement of opioid-drinking behavior and "relapse" in morphine-addicted rats, *Psychopharmacologia* **10**:255–284.

WIKLER, A., PESCOR, F. T., MILLER, D., and NORELL, H., 1971, Persistent potency of a secondary (conditioned) reinforcer following withdrawal of morphine from physically dependent rats, *Psychopharmacologia* **20**:103–117.

WISE, R. A., YOKEL, R. A., and DE WIT, H., 1976, Both positive reinforcement and conditioned aversion from amphetamine and from apomorphine in rats, *Science* **191**:1273–1275.

WOLGIN, D. L., 1983, Tolerance to amphetamine anorexia: Role of learning versus body weight settling point, *Behav. Neurosci.* **4**:549–562.

WOODS, S. C., 1972, Conditioned hypoglycemia: Effect of vagotomy and pharmacological blockade, *Am. J. Physiol.* **223**:1424–1427.

WOODS, S. C., 1976, Conditioned hypoglycemia, *J. Comp. Physiol. Psychol.* **90**:1164–1168.

WOODS, S. C., 1977, Conditioned insulin secretion, in: *Food Intake and the Chemical Senses* (Y. Katsuki, M. Sato, S. F. Takagi, and Y. Oomura, eds.), University of Tokyo Press, Tokyo, pp. 357–365.

WOODS, S. C., 1983, Conditioned hypoglycemia and conditioned insulin secretion, *Advan. Metabol. Disorders* **10**:485–495.

WOODS, S. D., and BURCHFIELD, S. R., 1980, Conditioned endocrine responses, in: *The Comprehensive Handbook of Behavioral Medicine,* Vol. 1 (J. M. Ferguson and C. B. Taylor, eds.), Spectrum Publications Inc., New York, pp. 239–254.

WOODS, S. C., and KULKOSKY, P. J., 1976, Classically conditioned changes of blood glucose level, *Psychosom. Med.* **38**:201–219.

WOODS, S. C., and PORTE, D., Jr., 1975, Effect of intracisternal insulin on plasma glucose and insulin in the dog, *Diabetes* **24**:905–909.

WOODS, S. C., and SHOGREN, R. E., 1972, Glycemic responses following conditioning with different doses of insulin in rats, *J. Comp. Physiol. Psychol.* **81**:220–225.

WOODS, W. C., MAKOUS, W., and HUTTON, R. A., 1969, Temporal parameters of conditioned hypoglycemia, *J. Comp. Physiol. Psychol.* **69**:301–307.

WOODS, S. C., ALEXANDER, K. R., and PORTE, D., Jr., 1972, Conditioned insulin secretion and hypoglycemia following repeated injections of tolbutamide in rats, *Endocrinology* **90**:227–231.

WOODS, S. C., VASSELLI, J. R., KAESTNER, E., SZAKMARY, G. A., MILBURN, P., and VITIELLO, M. V., 1977, Conditioned insulin secretion and meal feeding in rats, *J. Comp. Physiol. Psychol.* **91**:128–133.

WOOLVERTON, W. L., KANDEL, D., and SCHUSTER, C. R., 1978, Tolerance and cross-tolerance to cocaine and *d*-amphetamine, *J. Pharmacol. Exp. Ther.* **205**:525–535.

ZELLNER, D. A., DACANAY, R. J., and RILEY, A. L., 1984, Opiate withdrawal: The result of conditioning or physiological mechanism? *Pharmacol. Biochem. Behav.* **20**:175–180.

ZELMAN, D. C., TIFFANY, S. T., and BAKER, T. B., 1985, Influence of stress on morphine-induced pyrexia: Relevance to a Pavlovian model of tolerance development, *Behav. Neurosci.* **99**:122–144.

2

DEVELOPMENTAL NEUROPHARMACOLOGY: CLINICAL AND NEUROCHEMICAL PERSPECTIVES ON THE REGULATION OF ATTENTION, LEARNING, AND MOVEMENT

J. Gerald Young, Jeffrey M. Halperin, Leonard I. Leven, Bennett A. Shaywitz, and Donald J. Cohen

1. CLINICAL PHENOMENA AND RESEARCH DESIGN

1.1. Developmental Influences

Pharmacological agents are typically grouped according to their target diseases, chemical structures, or molecular mechanisms of action. Categorization of drugs according to their use in the treatment of specific diseases is most common in clinical practice, but a disease-oriented classifi-

---

J. Gerald Young, Jeffrey M. Halperin, and Leonard I. Leven • Division of Child and Adolescent Psychiatry, Mount Sinai School of Medicine of the City University of New York, New York, New York 10029.   *Bennett A. Shaywitz* • Departments of Pediatrics and Neurology, Yale University School of Medicine, New Haven, Connecticut 06510. *Donald J. Cohen* • Departments of Pediatrics, Psychiatry, and Psychology, Yale University School of Medicine and the Child Study Center, New Haven, Connecticut 06510.

cation requires thoughtful consideration during childhood. Development compromises the nomenclature for childhood psychiatric disorders. The features of an illness are continuous variables which are the result of the timing and nature of an insult, subsequent maturational processes, and environmental molding. The clinician makes his observations at relatively few cross-sectional points and is unable to reliably estimate the relative contributions of these factors. These diagnostic problems crucially affect our understanding of drugs acting on the central nervous system, so the examination of developmental influences on drug effects has become a major topic for pediatric psychopharmacology.

The impact of development on the clinical presentation of an illness can be illustrated by three commonly observed effects. The first is that severe insults at an early age can lead to pervasive developmental impairments; although subject to later improvement, there is a ceiling on the amount of mending that can be anticipated. There is substantial evidence that mild or moderate pathogenic conditions during the perinatal period or early infancy will be responsive to treatment when the child is favored by the optimal socioeconomic conditions which facilitate development. Nevertheless, when the injury to brain tissue is severe, there is substantial lasting damage and a deficit that impairs a range of functions. This widespread involvement of central nervous system (CNS) function interferes with the healing potential of development and the child is unable to adapt to even the most harmonious environment. This leaves the child with an odd appearance and maladaptive behaviors which can actually increase the distance between his intact competencies and the normal abilities of a similar-aged child. This convergence of pathogenic factors makes diagnosis difficult, as the clinician attempts to fit the child's symptoms and strengths into a standard nosological framework. Progress in development of these children is difficult to assess; the likelihood that children with different etiological agents, anatomical involvement, and/or compensatory adaptations will be lumped together diagnostically often makes assessment of progress on an individual dimension confusing. There is a tendency, in the face of this confusion, to impose on these syndromes an adult model which is sometimes ill-fitting, if at other times useful.

A second example of developmental influences on the form of childhood neuropsychiatric illness is that motoric behavior, language, and attentional functioning are primary areas of expression for the lesion. Motor learning is a central childhood activity, and a child's relatively limited repertoire of responses to stress means that modulation of the rate or form of activity will be a frequently employed adaptive or maladaptive response. Even when there is no physical insult to tissue, if the environmental stress exceeds the child's coping, it is likely that the child's first line of defense will include a motor component that is vulnerable to extension to a symptomatic form. A child is less likely to assemble a complex psychological defense if this more immediate motoric display of his overwhelmed defenses is still available to him. There is also accumulating evidence to suggest that there are biological factors that promote greater activity levels in childhood, making children more vulnerable to manifestations of motor dysregulation during illness. Boys show a much higher prevalence of certain childhood illnesses with major motor components, and clinical neurochemical research suggests a basis for this sex difference.

A child's vulnerability to language disorders may have somewhat different determinants. Here the vulnerability may be derived from the complexity of the biological and psychological processes involved, requiring optimal environmental conditions for full development. Language is an instrument that exquisitely expresses the state of the organism, and this applies to the effects of diseases, stress, or their sequelae. The measurement of a language impairment can be more open to error or misinterpretation than the comparatively concrete manifestations of a motor abnormality.

The frequency of attentional dysfunction in childhood disorders may not indicate a greater prevalence than during adulthood; instead it may more often be discriminated from other symptoms in children (Buchsbaum et al., 1985). Similarly, there is no particular reason to think that attentional processes are necessarily more important in childhood, since the complexity of tasks in adult work and everyday life suggests a need for optimal attentional functioning. Two other features of attention suggest why it assumes such a central position in childhood psychopathology. First, children must learn to utilize attentional mechanisms as their potential capacities mature. This requires environmental incentives that will induce motivation within the child. This environmental–child interaction can be finely tuned, and the presence of interfering factors (such as structural deficits in the child) or the absence of necessary provisions (such as adequate stimulation for the child) may lead to deficiencies in his attentional performance. In contrast, there may be less emphasis on learning in the life of an adult afflicted with an attentional deficit. Second, the lack of satisfaction with a nosology for the childhood disorders has led to a particular openness to new observations and organization of clinical phenomena. An attentional deficit can be a relatively subtle component of a hyperactive child's chaotic presentation, until clinicians are alerted to look for it and have the proper assessment techniques to identify it.

Similarly, children spend most of their public day in school, so the presence of an attentional disorder has a better chance of being detected. This might not be the case for adults. If they adapt to such a chronic handicap, it is likely that they will have elaborated psychological defenses and found a niche in their work and social lives that accommodates their limitations. This process is gauged to reduce the likelihood that they will be stressed and, therefore, that their attentional deficit will be identified. Other symptoms will be more prominent and become the basis for the diagnoses assigned to them.

A third illustration of the impact of development on the clinical features of psychiatric disorders in childhood concerns the pattern and rate of development. Daily observation by a parent or teacher gives the impression of a gradual, imperceptible, steady process of maturation. Yet, there is substantial evidence to show that this is deceptive. Examination of old photos or filmstrips indicates intermittent periods of rapid change in a child's development. A favorite example for a clinical child psychiatrist is the evidence marshalled to show the discontinuity of development at about the age of 7 years. Data from biological studies, cognitive testing, and behavioral assessment indicate a marked alteration in the child's capacities and accomplishments at this age (Shapiro and Perry, 1976). The coincidence of these advances in separate domains suggests that they reflect a decisive transition to a higher level when the neural matrix reaches a critical ripeness. Of course, it is not as if there had never been a cultural recognition of this new capacity: nevertheless, it was too easily assumed that the basis for the child's expanding knowledge and abilities was the initiation of formal education at this time. The alternative view is that this age was chosen by multiple cultures for the initiation of education of their young because they observed a readiness in their children that was supplied by maturation.

Clinicians commonly emphasize the importance of these changes at about 7 years of age, whatever their roots. Symptoms that have gone unnoticed in the privacy of the family and neighborhood can be striking when a child comes under public scrutiny at the time of school entry. Beyond that is the fact that children of this age are capable of the requisite formal rules for rudimentary functioning in a technological society. The absence of certain capacities by this age becomes much more clearly discriminated as pathology, in contrast to the situation 2 or 3 years before. For example, a reading or arithmetic lag, or a visuomotor abnormality on formal testing, will be diagnosed as a disorder and treatment recommended. Even in profound pathological states this discontinuity in development is recognized by clinical practice. Clinicians do not feel confidence in their ability to predict the future development of severely disturbed preschool children with great precision, yet they commonly estimate that if a child with autism or a related condition does not have language by the age of 7 or 8 years, he is unlikely to acquire much language in the future and his overall level of function will tend to be congruent with that limited language development.

The application of neurochemical methods to clinical studies of childhood neuropsychiatric disorders has been initiated in the past decade as a method to unravel underlying mechanisms which are the determinants of these clinical phenomena. They promise to aid in the clarification of developmental patterns and change, and to be an important guide for the use of psychopharmacological agents. In the years ahead, clinical neurochemical methods will assume the status of a standard assessment tool for child psychiatrists, as they are linked to systematic clinical evaluation protocols. This chapter will first consider the influence of research design on the development of new knowledge concerning childhood disorders. This will be followed by an examination of the major clinical, neurochemical, and psychopharmacological research that has investigated impairments in three major sectors of childhood development: attention, learning, and movement.

1.2. Methodological Issues in Pediatric Psychopharmacological Research

The methodology utilized in clinical developmental psychopharmacology is subject to numerous errors related to experimental design. Excellent reviews outline the major questions concerning research methods in preclinical and adult clinical psychopharmacology, yet few reports examine the difficulties specific to psychopharmacological research with children (Conners, 1985; Shapiro, 1985; Young *et al.*, 1982). Numerous clinical, diagnostic, pharmacological and ethical issues arise in pediatric research, and a few will be mentioned here.

1.2.1. Diagnostic Specificity

Any treatment study employing a pharmacological agent that acts selectively on specific neurophysiological systems is vulnerable to confounded results because of etiological and genetic heterogeneity. When investigating a childhood disorder that has multiple causes and several underlying neurophysiological dysfunctions, careful application of diagnostic criteria will enhance the likelihood that specific drug effects will be observed. This can reduce the variance, so that eventual replication by other investigators might indicate that an underlying mechanism for a drug effect has been determined. Difficulties encountered in the establishment of reliable classification systems for childhood disorders, mentioned earlier, have impeded progress in these efforts. Additional troublesome factors accounting for these difficulties in classification, which are especially important for psychopharmacological research, include the following. First, symptoms in childhood tend to be multiple, fluid, and less specific than in adults. Therefore, as the diagnostic criteria are currently specified, it is common for children to receive multiple diagnoses. Second, unlike with adults, diagnostic decisions regarding children are based on the observations of parents, teachers, and relatives, in addition to information obtained through examination of the child.

The difficulties caused by the multisymptomatic nature of childhood psychiatric disorders have been apparent for years. Some progress has been made by more clearly delineating specific symptoms associated with each disorder. For example, as recently as the 1970s, a large proportion of research was conducted on undifferentiated groups of children referred to as minimal brain dysfunction (MBD), hyperkinetic, or learning disabled. There was likely to be little difference among the groups of children classified by these diagnostic labels, and a child could be placed in any of these groups for different reasons, including the presence of a learning problem, a behavioral problem, neurological soft signs, or a discrepancy between his verbal and performance IQ. Thus, this research must be carefully scrutinized before conclusions can be drawn.

More recently, the tendency has been to examine symptom clusters as discrete groups. Although this has many advantages, when compared to earlier methods, the degree of overlap among "different" diagnostic groups is considerable. For example, it is estimated that 30–70% of children diagnosed as having attention deficit disorder with hyperactivity (ADDH) also meet criteria for conduct disorder; approximately 10–50% of ADDH children are likely to meet criteria for a specific developmental disorder, and a large number of them may be anxious and depressed. Some of these children also have a suggestion of neurological dysfunction by EEG or clinical neurological examination. Therefore, unlike the past, when our nomenclature resulted in the assignment of the same diagnosis to very different children (e.g., MBD), the current tendency is to assign several diagnoses to the same child. The same child could conceivably be a subject for studies examining ADDH, conduct disorders, learning disabilities, and depression in childhood.

Clinical investigators have attempted to achieve clarity in their research, in spite of diagnostic heterogeneity, by clearly defining subgroups within a given diagnostic category; in other words, they examine and quantify specific clinical dimensions while retaining diagnostic categories. For example, one may study conduct-disordered children with and without a learning disability, attentional dysfunction, or hyperactivity. Obviously, numerous small, highly differentiated subgroups can be generated by varying the combinations of symptoms. An alternative approach is to select a unitary dimension such as hyperactivity, but include in the sample description the number of hyperactive subjects in each of the diagnostic categories represented in the sample. Regardless of the approach, it is essential that all subjects be evaluated across a broad spectrum of potential diagnoses and not limited to those disorders under study.

The selection of categories of information for assessment (e.g., behavioral observation, neurological examination, continuous performance task, etc.), and their sources, is a crucial consideration when assessing a child's symptoms in relation to diagnostic criteria and will also be discussed in terms of effects on outcome criteria.

The child is usually neither the primary informant nor the one who decides that treatment is necessary, so diagnosis is commonly based more upon how others perceive the child's problem than on the child's subjective experience. Typically, clinical information comes from one of four sources: the child, the parents (or other close relative), the teacher, or the observing clinician. Unfortunately, this can be confusing because they frequently disagree. Information gathered from all four sources is optimal, but, although diagnostic criteria and rating-scale items are specific and often operationally defined, observers are variably objective, and the results may differ according to the subjective tolerance of the parents, teachers, or clinicians. On the other hand, a child may be unwilling to acknowledge difficulties or aberrant behaviors. Therefore, the difficult task of the clinician is to sort out the child's difficulties from variations in parental and teacher observational skills and tolerance levels. Fortunately, numerous parent, teacher, and child rating scales can be objectively scored to assist in this difficult procedure. Despite this, concordance among the various reporters may be limited. Therefore, for the purpose of research, subjects should be selected who meet inclusion criteria according to two or three different informants, preferably in at least two separate settings (e.g., home and school). Although this stringent procedure may result in greater difficulty gathering subjects, it will optimize the likelihood that the sample is homogeneous. Children selected on the basis of a single informant, when others fail to observe the symptoms, should be separately classified as a situation-specific subgroup of the disorder.

1.2.2. Dosage

Four methodological strategies guide the evaluation of drug dosage in clinical investigation:

1. The use of relative rather than absolute doses
2. The determination of a dose–response curve
3. The estimation of side effects relative to drug efficacy
4. The use of blood levels of drugs

Most clinical psychopharmacological research is designed to vary dosage and report findings in terms of absolute drug level administered. This practice may be acceptable for studies with adults because intersubject weight differences may be small relative to the absolute weight of the subject, and the mg/kg dose level remains relatively constant. However, this is rarely the case with children. It is not uncommon for studies with children to include subjects ranging from age 6 through early adolescence.

The average body weight of a 12-year-old is nearly twice that of a 6-year-old, and administering a predetermined absolute drug dosage is usually an error. Unless the dosage is carefully regulated relative to body weight, it is difficult to determine whether a poor response by a subject group is due to a lack of action of the drug on the target symptoms or whether the *actual* dose (mg/kg) was outside of the therapeutic range.

The use of multiple dose levels is essential in all clinical psychopharmacological research. The absence of therapeutic effects at a single dose provides little clinical information about the medication. On the other hand, a behavioral response after a single dose may have clinical utility but fails to clarify the optimal dose or illuminate possible pharmacological actions of the drug. At high doses many medications can reduce symptoms such as hyperactivity or aggression. However, determination of a dose–response curve might indicate the absence of specific links among the clinical findings, dosage, and the neuropharmacological actions of the drug.

A sequential fixed/flexible dosage procedure is often a practical plan for clinical investigation. This schedule is composed of an initial series of predetermined dose increments for a brief period of time, followed by a flexible, response-dependent variation in dosage. The flexible schedule is altered until either an optimal dose or a predetermined maximum dose is attained.

As the dose of medication is increased, the probability of eliciting side effects increases. Individuals vary in their sensitivity to drugs, and it is not uncommon for subjects to be removed from drug studies because they develop side effects. A question then arises concerning a subject who is terminated from a study, without symptom relief, because of side effects: if this occurs prior to the time that he reached the maximum dose, should he be considered a treatment failure? Some investigators argue that these subjects should be considered untestable, rather than treatment failures, and should be eliminated from the data analysis because a fair test of the drug's efficacy is not possible. However, this may create a bias in favor of finding drug efficacy, because those for whom the drug is ineffective, and who develop side effects at higher doses, are not counted as treatment failures; on the other hand, those who have positive drug effects at low doses and, therefore, are not tested at higher doses (where they may encounter side effects) are counted as treatment successes. Thus, when the maximum dose is not substantially above a typically effective dose, many treatment failures are selectively removed from the analysis. Regardless of the statistical manner in which this is handled, the side effects for all subjects should be clearly reported with the dosages at which they occurred.

A final method for determining proper dosages is measurement of blood levels of the drug and/or its active metabolites. After oral ingestion of a drug, numerous factors (including gender, age, body composition, and metabolism) affect the distribution of the drug and the amount actually active at CNS neuronal sites. Lipid-soluble drugs have greater potency in women and water-soluble drugs are more active in men; this is due to the presence of more fat tissue in women and more muscle in men. The body composition of children changes markedly, and the fat and muscle content at about age 10 or 11 years is particularly variable. Therefore, even careful control of dose relative to body weight may be inadequate, as the amount of drug becoming available in the CNS is likely to be inconstant. For this reason, monitoring blood levels of a medication can improve our understanding of variability in individual drug response and be used to regulate dosage. The determination of blood levels can also ensure parental and child medication compliance.

1.2.3. Controls in Clinical Research Design

An optimal medication trial is designed so that the clinician and the patient (as well as the parents, if a child) are blind to the content of the pill ingested, knowing only that it may be a placebo or an active agent. However, this "double-blind" design is often difficult to carry out successfully and deserves a brief comment. Similarly, there are advantages and disadvantages to using a "within-subject" design in which the subject becomes "his own control" through comparison of responses to sequentially altered drug conditions.

Most psychoactive drugs have readily observable side effects or clearly affect the subjective state of the patient, making it possible for clinician and patient to distinguish active compound from placebo. It is essential that side effects be carefully monitored, and these differences become all too apparent. Although the physician and patient are sometimes wrong, these nontarget responses suggest which subjects are on active medication and which are on placebo. This "guessing" affects outcome judgments and can add to error variance. This difficulty can be minimized by employing active control medications and/or independent judges.

Active control medications are drugs that may or may not be effective for treatment of the target disorder; they are psychoactive and likely to yield side effects, thus camouflaging the trial drug under examination. However, the ethical difficulties involved in giving a child a noneffective substance can be complex; the severity of side effects and length of time on the active control drug must be carefully weighed. A variation on this design which is easier to apply in pediatric medication studies is simultaneous evaluation of two different drugs for the same disorder. These active controls should be used in addition to, and not replace, placebo controls.

Another strategy for overcoming these design limitations is to designate a clinician other than the treating physician to evaluate outcome. This enhances the likelihood that the final evaluation of drug efficacy will focus on differential effects on target symptoms, rather than guessing by observation of side effects. Of course, this does not control for the possibility that the patient recognizes that he is receiving an active agent.

1.2.4. Outcome Criteria

Determination of outcome criteria in psychopharmacological treatment studies for children is complicated by the need to specify who determines improvement. Is a child considered to be successfully treated when he says he feels better, when his teacher rates his behavior as improved, or when his parents state that his symptoms are no longer present? Unfortunately, the disparity among the ratings of these different informants can be disconcerting. There is not a single best informant, and the integration of multiple informant ratings into the research design has substantial advantages until these differences are better understood.

Several behavioral rating scales are currently available to quantify changes in the child's behavior. They are designed to evaluate the child's behavior on a variety of dimensions, including hyperactivity, aggression, depression, and anxiety. The reliability and validity of these scales have been assessed in varying degrees, and each is designed for specific use by teachers, parents, or children. While further research is required to determine which reporter is most useful for specified purposes, the use of these scales during pre- and posttreatment conditions can produce meaningful and replicable data that are understood by others in the field. Despite the fact that it is advantageous to generate global improvement scores, based on the summation of specific individual ratings, these global scores are less replicable and should only be utilized as an addition to individual rating scores.

2. ATTENTION DEFICIT DISORDER WITH HYPERACTIVITY

2.1. Component Symptoms

Hyperactivity is routinely described as the most common pediatric behavioral disorder. Nevertheless, a wide range of prevalence rates have been reported (Huessy and Gendron, 1970; Satin *et al.*, 1985; Shekim *et al.*, 1985), reflecting the difficulties encountered when defining criteria for the sample (Lambert *et al.*, 1978; Sandberg *et al.*, 1980). Many symptoms are encompassed within the diagnosis of "hyperactivity," and clinicians continue their analysis of which symptoms ought to be designated as primary. Child psychiatrists currently assign the attentional deficit as the primary symptom and indicate the presence or absence of additional features such as hyperactivity (the "attention deficit disorder with hyperactivity" syndrome, or ADDH). Multiple overlapping functions may be impaired in these children (hyperactivity, inattention, impulsivity, learning disorders, "soft" neurological signs, clumsiness, perceptual deficits, visuomotor abnormalities, aggression, conduct disorder, and antisocial personality disorder), and this extensive symptom list was the basis for the earlier broad designation of these children as suffering from "minimal brain dysfunction." This is reflected in the general agreement that efforts to formally define a distinctive syndrome have failed to achieve adequate validation through well-designed empirical research (Shaffer and Greenhill, 1979; Rutter, 1983; Ferguson and Rapoport, 1983). Nevertheless, clinical investigators must proceed with mutually agreed upon syndrome constructs, such as ADDH or conduct disorder.

Controversy concerning the differential significance of hyperactivity, inattention, and impulsivity has led to increasing clarification of their relations. There is new evidence that increased motor activity, after relinquishing its place as a preeminent symptom defining a childhood disorder, is a fundamental sign of disturbance that can reliably distinguish hyperactive from normal boys. Hyperactive boys demonstrate greater levels of motor activity in all their usual home and school situations, across all days of the week and all hours of the day. Hyperactivity is an independent symptom dimension, separate from attentional dysfunction, and a motor activity measure is equal or superior to an attention measure as a discriminator among this broad group of children. These data indicate that there is not yet sufficient information to define either hyperactivity or inattention as "the" core symptom in these children (Porrino *et al.*, 1983*a*).

The simultaneous occurrence of these related symptoms has stimulated more sophisticated nosological research. While separate factors (e.g., hyperactivity, inattention, or conduct disorder) may be derived, the component symptoms for the factors show substantial association with one another. Thus, the attempt to distinguish separate syndromes founders on the ambiguity of symptom constructs that do not easily yield to operationalization and the interrelatedness of component symptoms across syndromes. For example, attentional dysfunction has obvious detrimental effects on learning, so that clinicians commonly labor to differentiate ADDH and learning disorders, or to establish that both are present in an individual child. However, the elusiveness of this goal is inherent in the problem of adequately isolating such phenomena as impulsivity, arousal level, hyperactivity, inattention, selective attention, distractibility, sustained attention, vigilance, impulsivity, inhibitory control, motivation, response to reward, task and treatment conditions, perceptual discrimination, and aspects of memory (Douglas, 1983). While clinical measures of these functions are continually improved, their limitations affect all studies of biological markers or treatment efficacy.

In spite of so many factors complicating the design and interpretation of research, recent empirical studies have increased confidence that groups defined according to current clinical criteria are validly distinguished as specific diagnostic groups and subgroups. For example, children with attention deficit disorder (ADD) appear to exhibit a particular pattern of behaviors and symptoms that are characterized by inattention, and they are not simply a group of children with a greater frequency and severity of problems. These children have poor work habits, poor self-concept, behave inappropriately, and their tendency to learn less is reflected in poor school performance. The determination of ADD subgroups on the basis of the presence or absence of hyperactivity has also begun to have empirical support. Hyperactive ADD boys demonstrate greater motor activity and nervousness on teacher ratings and tend to be characterized by more aggressive and self-destructive behavior without guilt and less popularity among their peers; conduct disorders are common in this group. On the other hand, the "pure" ADD group is much less common, and these boys are less aggressive and more anxious, shy, and withdrawn (Maurer and Stewart, 1980; Edelbrock *et al.*, 1984; Lahey *et al.*, 1984). Other behavioral dimensions have also been supported by empirical studies as the basis for subgrouping children in ways that may have important implications for treatment and prediction of outcome, particularly aggression (Goyette *et al.*, 1978; Loney *et al.*, 1978; Stewart *et al.*, 1981) and learning disabilities (Cantwell and Satterfield, 1978; Lambert and Sandoval, 1980; Silver, 1981; Halperin *et al.*, 1984).

2.2. Clinical Effects of Stimulants

Stimulant medications are the optimal drugs for treatment of hyperactivity and are prescribed in the context of other treatment methods specifically selected for the individual child. Increased knowledge concerning stimulant treatment has important public health ramifications, because stimulants may be the most frequently prescribed medication for children (Krager *et al.*, 1979; Gadow, 1981). The term "stimulants" refers primarily to two drugs, methylphenidate (MPH) and *d*-amphetamine. They differ slightly in their mechanism of action at the nerve terminal (MPH acting on storage pools of catecholamines, and amphetamine acting on newly synthesized, free catecholamines in the nerve terminal), but for clinical purposes they are interchangeable (Moore, 1978; Kuczenski, 1983). Pemoline will not be discussed here (Conners and Taylor, 1980).

Stimulants elicit behavioral effects within the few hours immediately following administration whether the subject is a hyperactive child, normal child, or normal adult. Amphetamine reduces the motor activity of both groups of children, as well as adult males. There is an age effect on the mood change subsequent to an oral dose of the drug, with a typical euphoria experienced by adults not characteristic in children; the children feel "funny" or "tired" after the medication, but this could be a result of a child's limited ability to differentiate and verbally describe mood states. Both hyperactive and normal children perform better on reaction time or vigilance (continuous performance) tests after stimulant administration, but the response of adults is more variable and dose-dependent. A clinically intriguing difference is that normal children improve by having fewer omission errors while receiving stimulants, but hyperactive children reduce their commission errors. Scores on verbal learning and memory tasks also improve and there is increased speech production (Rapoport et al., 1980). In short, the observations of clinicians and teachers that stimulants have immediate salutary effects for hyperactive children are crystallized in these experimental findings. Yet, it is now evident that these nonspecific stimulant effects pertain to normal subjects also (Rapoport et al., 1978a, 1980). Other studies indicate that stimulants administered to ADDH children reduce aggressive behavior (Winsberg et al., 1972; Amery et al., 1984), facilitate fine motor activity (Knights and Hinton, 1969), and improve classroom social behavior (Sprague et al., 1970; Pelham et al., 1985). Do these benefits of stimulants lead to short-term acceleration of academic achievement? Research findings are encouraging, documenting improved short-term (Sprague and Sleator, 1977) and long-term memory (Weingartner et al., 1980), enhanced learning (Swanson and Kinsbourne, 1979; Gan and Cantwell, 1982; Stephens et al., 1984), and better classroom academic performance (Pelham et al., 1985) (see Table 1).

TABLE 1
Short-Term Effects of Stimulant Medications

	Hyperactive boys	Normal boys	Normal adult males
1. Motor activity	Reduced	Reduced	Reduced
2. Performance on reaction time and vigilance tests	Improved	Improved	Variably improved
3. Mood	Unclear	Unclear	Euphoria
4. Memory	Improved	Improved	Improved
5. Learning	Improved	Improved	Improved
6. Speech production	Increased	Increased	Increased
7. Aggressive behavior	Reduced	??	??
8. Fine motor activity	Improved	??	??
9. Classroom behavior	Improved	??	??
10. Classroom academic performance	Improved	??	??

Stimulants reduce motor activity levels in hyperactive boys in the classroom or during sedentary activities. However, the effects of the setting and type of activity and the time of medication administration require consideration when assessing stimulant effects. Hyperactive boys engaged in physical education and sports activities actually show greater motor activity following dextroamphetamine than during off-drug periods. This does not lead to a deterioration in performance, and apparently indicates greater on-task, directed physical activity in the sports events (Porrino et al., 1983b).

Another confounding factor in research concerning stimulants has been parental dissatisfaction with medication effects in the face of improved behavior on teacher reports. A "rebound" effect has been demonstrated, in which an increase in activity levels occurs in the early evening, 6–8 hr after dextroamphetamine administration. Activity levels of the hyperactive boys during sleep were greater also, when compared to off-medication weeks, giving further evidence of a rebound effect following a therapeutic response earlier in the day. This suggests that one cause of "situational" hyperactivity might be a combination of therapeutic and rebound effects in children evaluated after a prior clinician prescribed a stimulant (Porrino et al., 1983b).

The long-term effects of administering a stimulant to a hyperactive child are beginning to be clarified by detailed follow-up studies. In order to judge their effects, an appraisal of the natural history (the usual outcome for hyperactive children not given treatment) is required. Although follow-up studies are plagued by innumerable methodological pitfalls (Cantwell, 1985), and those targeted on hyperactivity are not in perfect agreement, a general outline of the natural history has begun to emerge. Hyperactive children, when they reach adolescence, will be more likely to be characterized by a persistence of the ADDH syndrome; poor academic performance or failure; conduct disorders and delinquent behavior; substance use disorders; poor social skills and more aggressive behavior; depression and low self-esteem; and continued hyperactivity, attentional dysfunction, or impulsivity when the full ADDH syndrome is absent (Mendelson et al., 1971; Minde et al., 1972; Hoy et al., 1978; Satterfield et al., 1981; Loney et al., 1981; Gittelman et al., 1985). Preliminary findings describing outcome in young adulthood paint a similarly gloomy picture for many of them when they reach adulthood: continuing restlessness and impulsivity; more personality disorders, particularly of the impulsive and immature-dependent types; poor academic achievement; low self-esteem; poor social skills and more aggressive behavior; more nonmedical drug use; and more car accidents. The rate of antisocial personality disorder reaches 25–50% of the sample in young adulthood (Table 2) (Weiss et al., 1985; Satterfield et al., 1982; Weiss, 1983).

Administration of stimulants during childhood may modify this outcome, but the fundamental natural history of the disorder remains

TABLE 2
Survey of Outcome Studies of Hyperactive Boys during Adolescence and Young Adulthood: Types of Impairment Accounting for Poor Outcome Relative to Normal Controls

Adolescence	Young adulthood
1. No increase in rate of psychosis	1. No increase in rate of psychosis
2. Restless, hyperactive, impulsive, and distractible; persistent ADDH syndrome	2. Restless and impulsive
3. Emotionally immature and impulsive	3. More personality disorders: impulsive and immature-dependent
4. Poor academic achievement	4. Poor academic achievement
5. Low self-esteem	5. Low self-esteem
6. Poor social skills	6. Poor social skills
7. Delinquent behavior (25%)	7. Increased antisocial personality disorder (25–50%)
8. More nonmedical drug use	8. More nonmedical drug use
9. More aggressive	9. More aggressive
10. Poor motor skills	10. More car accidents
11. More alcohol use	11. No increase in rate of alcoholism

unchanged. A few studies have attempted to examine the outcome in adolescence and young adulthood. In general, they suggest that, while medication may continue to improve the child's behavior at home and school, the long-term outcome is not altered in the areas of poor academic performance, antisocial behavior, work record, and poor emotional adjustment. On the other hand, hyperactive children treated with stimulants appear to have better self-esteem and social skills at follow-up (Hechtman et al., 1984). These results emphasize that we must treat short-term and long-term outcomes as separate, although possibly related, phenomena when considering stimulant effects on hyperactive children. Whatever immediate performance benefits may accrue from their use, there appears to be minimal carryover in lasting amelioration of the child's impaired functioning. Children receiving other therapies in addition to medication, according to their individual needs, appear to have a better prognosis (Satterfield et al., 1981, 1982).

Two fundamental considerations weave through all clinical research on the nature of ADD and the efficacy of stimulant treatment that require clarification in the next generation of research. First, the clinical characteristics of the smaller number of girls with ADD or ADDH have received little attention by investigators. Preliminary research suggests that there may be sex differences: girls with ADDH have more severe cognitive and language deficits, show fewer disruptive behaviors, are younger at the time of referral, and their families have a lower socioeconomic status when compared with boys. Girls with ADD, but lacking symptoms of hyperactivity, are older and have poorer self-esteem when compared with boys with ADD without hyperactivity. These diagnostic differences, especially a relative emphasis on cognitive and language impairment in girls in contrast to disruptive behavior in boys, may lead to an underestimate of the prevalence of ADDH among girls (Berry *et al.*, 1985). Second, inadequate understanding of dose effects continues to confound research on stimulants. The possibility that there are differential drug effects on separate target symptoms, improved symptom response as dosage increases, and/or an optimal dose (with subsequent decline in efficacy at higher doses) characteristic for each child leads to alternative interpretations of research on the clinical effects of stimulants (Sprague and Sleator, 1977; Pelham *et al.*, 1985; Rapoport *et al.*, 1985). Examination of these alternative clinical response profiles for stimulants may clarify their molecular mechanisms of action (Young, 1981; Solanto, 1986).

The minimal ameliorative effect of stimulants on long-term outcome has initiated a closer look at nonpharmacological therapies (Abikoff and Gittelman, 1985) and a renewed emphasis on multiple therapies tailored to the requirements of each child. However, clinical investigators have also examined alternative medications. Clonidine, a partial α_2-adrenergic agonist, may be useful in the treatment of a subgroup of ADDH children (Hunt *et al.*, 1985). Monoamine oxidase inhibitors have beneficial clinical effects comparable to those of dextroamphetamine, with an immediate therapeutic response. They also might be a useful alternative medication in a subgroup of hyperactive children (Zametkin *et al.*, 1985*a*). Caffeine has been suggested as a substitute for conventional stimulants in the treatment of hyperactive children for many years. Research has not shown caffeine to be efficacious (Elkins *et al.*, 1981), but this may reflect individual physiological differences in the children that determine their dietary caffeine preferences (Rapoport *et al.*, 1984). Similarly, although various antidepressant medications have not been shown to be superior to stimulants, some specific advantages (such as a longer duration of action that reduces behavioral problems in the evening) may recommend their use in certain children (Rapoport *et al.*, 1974; Garfinkel *et al.*, 1983; Langer *et al.*, 1985).

2.3. Cellular and Molecular Effects of Stimulants

Amphetamine exerts its effects on brain function through multiple mechanisms. While it acts on several neurotransmitter-related neuronal systems, the profound behavioral effects characteristic of stimulants are secondary to actions at the dopaminergic system. In single-cell studies, amphetamine has been shown to depress the firing rate of dopamine-containing neurons in the substantia nigra through striatonigral feedback inhibition and through activation of dopamine (DA) autoreceptors by locally released DA. Autoreceptors are distributed at nerve terminals and soma of dopaminergic neurons and are more sensitive to DA and DA agonists than are postsynaptic receptors (Bunney and Aghajanian, 1978; Aghajanian, 1978; Skirboll *et al.*, 1979). New information concerning the neuroanatomy of dopamine and related neuronal systems, the sequential interactions of several neuronal systems (e.g., dopamine, acetylcholine, GABA, substance P) in the striatum, the coexistence of peptide and classical neurotransmitters in the same neuron, and the development of new drugs acting on dopamine systems promises to build a more complex description of dopamine function (Glowinski *et al.*, 1984; Selemon and Goldman-Rakic, 1985; Groves and Tepper, 1983; Creese, 1983; Bunney, 1984).

The molecular effects of amphetamine at DA nerve terminals appear to include three major actions: (1) release of presynaptic DA; (2) interference with reuptake of DA by the presynaptic neuron; and (3) inhibition of monoamine oxidase (MAO) activity. Amphetamine has similar effects on neurons containing norepinephrine (NE); blockade of NE uptake is particularly important (Moore, 1978; Kuczenski, 1983). The structure of amphetamine and MPH is closely related to phenylethylamine, the molecular structure basic to catecholamines, and accounts for the actions of stimulants at catecholaminergic neurons (Biel and Bopp, 1978).

Amphetamine also has effects on the serotonergic neuronal system, especially at high dosages. Dopaminergic neurons are known to facilitate the activity of serotonin containing neurons, and serotonergic input inhibits DA neurons. When amphetamine is chronically administered to cats, it leads to a reduction in serotonin and 5-hydroxyindoleacetic acid (5-HIAA), the major serotonin metabolite (Sloviter *et al.*, 1978; Lloyd, 1978; Lees *et al.*, 1979; Trulson and Jacobs, 1979).

2.4. Neurochemistry: Animal Studies

Dopamine, norepinephrine, and serotonin have been demonstrated to play important roles in the production or mediation of behaviors involved in ADDH: motor activity, rate and coordination of movements, aggression, attention, cognition, and emotional responsivity. There is ample evidence that the DA neuronal system modulates activity levels and learning and may be a source of pathological influences in ADDH.

The motor behaviors elicited by amphetamine administered to the rat are dose related and consist of a replicable sequence initiated by coordinated locomotor activity. Increasing doses cause augmented locomotor activity that is accompanied by sniffing and subsequent evidence of disruption of motor coordination into repetitive isolated motor acts (stereotypies). At high doses, the behavioral sequence culminates in a final phase in which motor behavior deteriorates into intense stereotypies and tremor and an inability to carry out integrated, purposive behavior (Lyon and Robbins, 1975; Iversen, 1977; Kelly, 1977; Groves and Tepper, 1983). Research examining the function of the four dopamine systems in the brain (nigrostriatal, mesolimbic, mesocortical, and tuberoinfundibular) has ascribed a predominant influence of the mesolimbic system on locomotor activity and the nigrostriatal system on stereotypic behaviors. However, this apparent anatomical localization is less clear as information is accumulated about mesocortical and corticostriatal influences on motor behavior, as well as the contributions of nondopamine neuronal systems. For example, dopaminergic systems may not act directly on motor systems in the brain, but may mediate the outflow of other neuronal systems (e.g., GABA and substance P) on motor centers in the brain (Iversen and Koob, 1977; Koob et al., 1977; van Rossum et al., 1977; Fink and Smith, 1980a,b; Groves, 1983; Goldman-Rakic, 1984; Selemon and Goldman-Rakic, 1985).

There are significant clinical phenomena related to this continuum of dose effects on motor behaviors. While stimulants are administered, in part, to reduce hyperactivity in children, chronic administration occasionally leads to the development of fragmented motor acts, such as tics or choreic movements (Denckla et al., 1976; Lowe et al., 1982; Goetz and Klawans, 1983). Similarly, an alternative type of motor disorganization, tardive dyskinesia, can appear following chronic neuroleptic use (Klawans et al., 1980).

Dose-related effects of stimulants on cognition and emotional aspects of behavior are well known. Low doses of a stimulant produce enhanced attention, euphoria, and improved performance on cognitive tests, but increasing doses and chronic administration lead to anxiety, obsessive thoughts, paranoia, and eventual decay into stimulant-induced psychosis characterized by delusions and hallucinations (Angrist and Sudilovsky, 1978; Young, 1981; Angrist, 1983).

Animal models of stimulant-induced psychosis have confirmed this progression of symptoms (Nielsen et al., 1983; Segal and Schukit, 1983). When treating children with stimulants, a pragmatic problem is encountered in that the dosage threshold for eliciting perseverative and disorganized thinking or frank hallucinations varies widely. Even apparent low doses of a stimulant may precipitate mildly disturbed cognition that is sometimes difficult to discern as a drug effect (Young, 1981).

Several animal models have been suggested for hyperactivity. One described in 1976, and subsequently confirmed by many investigators, closely parallels the clinical disorder (Shaywitz et al., 1976a,b). Hyperactivity is produced in the developing rat pup by intracisternal administration of desmethylimipramine (DMI) and the neurotoxin 6-hydroxydopamine (6-OHDA); these procedures selectively ablate central DA systems. There is a rapid, permanent reduction of brain DA to concentrations of 10–25% of that in controls, while brain NE and serotonin levels remain unaffected. Dopamine-depleted rat pups develop in ways that are similar to the clinical disorder observed in children (Sorenson et al., 1977; Eastgate et al., 1978; Stoof et al., 1978; Erinoff et al., 1979). For example, DMI/6-OHDA-treated animals are significantly more active than their littermate controls during a period of behavioral arousal that occurs at 2–3 weeks of age. However, the hyperactivity disappears with maturity, a finding that corresponds to the clinical syndrome for those children in whom hyperactivity is pronounced until adolescence, but then diminishes. Furthermore, pups treated with DMI/6-OHDA remain active throughout the entire experimental observation period: i.e., they fail to habituate. This is similar to the inability of the child with attentional difficulties to adjust easily to a change in his environment (Shaywitz et al., 1977a; Stoof et al., 1978). Impaired cognitive performance is commonly a significant clinical problem in the child with attentional disorders. Deficits in learning have been demonstrated in appetitive, escape, and avoidance tasks in the DMI/6-OHDA-treated rat pups as well as in the acquisition of an operant response. The learning deficits persist in the DA-depleted rat pups, approximating the continuing cognitive difficulties occurring in hyperactive adolescents (Shaywitz et al., 1976b; Heffner and Seiden, 1983).

Another counterpart to the clinical syndrome is the response of DMI/6-OHDA-treated rat pups to pharmacological agents used in the management of children with attentional difficulties. Administration of stimulants produces an ameliorative effect on both the hyperactivity and attentional deficits in affected children. Administration of either amphetamine or methylphenidate reduces activity in DMI/6-OHDA animals while phenobarbital aggravates the hyperactivity (Shaywitz et al., 1976a, 1978; Shaywitz and Pearson, 1978).

The DMI/6-OHDA model has been a useful tool for examining the interaction between biological factors (depletion of brain DA) and environmental influences (alterations in litter composition) as they affect locomotor activity and avoidance performance. DMI/6-OHDA pups were reared from 5 days of age through weaning with other comparably treated animals or with littermates who were sham-treated. Both the hyperactivity and avoidance-learning deficits observed in the DMI/6-OHDA pups were significantly improved by rearing the DA-depleted pups with normal littermates, rather than solely with other damaged animals; the degree of improvement was comparable to that achieved with drugs. These findings may be related to clinical reports which suggest that modifications of the environment may be therapeutic for children with attentional difficulties (Pearson *et al.*, 1980). A further intriguing finding is that gastric infusion of food dyes causes increased activity and impaired avoidance performance in both dopamine-depleted and sham-treated rat pups (Goldenring *et al.*, 1980).

Interruption of the dorsal noradrenergic pathways ascending to the forebrain in an adult animal (by lesions of the dorsal NE bundle) has little effect on motor activity or acquisition of avoidance learning; however, it does interfere with the ability of the damaged animal to extinguish previously learned responses. This has been termed the dorsal bundle extinction effect (DBEE) and is a partial model for attentional processes. Therefore it appears that lesions affecting noradrenergic pathways influence attentional functions (Robbins, 1984). Selective damage to the noradrenergic system in the developing rat pup (leaving the dopaminergic system intact) has little effect on activity, although such treatment does affect cognitive performance. Further research will examine the hypothesis that the dopaminergic system mediates hyperactivity and some cognitive deficits, while noradrenergic pathways predominantly influence attentional processes (Shaywitz *et al.*, 1984).

A "dose–response" relationship in the dopamine depletion model of hyperactivity further enhances its application in research. Four different doses of 6-OHDA have been shown to generate a progression in symptom severity: the amount of hyperactivity during neonatal life is related to the extent of destruction of brain dopamine neurons. In addition, the duration of locomotor activity is greater in those rat pups with more complete brain dopamine depletion (Miller *et al.*, 1981). In sum, dopamine depletion leads to hyperactivity and learning deficits in rat pups. The severity and duration of impairment are related to the extent of damage, the effects on activity level are age-related (Erinoff *et al.*, 1979), and the symptoms are responsive to treatment, either with stimulants or through alteration of the environment.

A genetic model that would partially account for behavioral differences among hyperactive and normal children has been described. This model represents a natural paradigm for the development of reduced brain dopaminergic activity and behavioral hyperactivity in the absence of environmental insult. A series of studies has demonstrated differences in the activity of a critical enzyme in two inbred mice strains. The enzyme, tyrosine hydroxylase (TH), is the rate-limiting enzyme in the synthesis of dopamine and NE (Ciaranello *et al.*, 1972). The difference in enzyme activity is due to genetic differences in the number of midbrain dopamine neurons in these two strains; one strain has 20–25% more dopamine neurons in the substantia nigra (A9) and ventral midbrain (A10) neuronal groups than the other strain (Ross *et al.*, 1976; Reis *et al.*, 1982, 1983).

The variation in the number of A9 dopamine neurons (substantia nigra) is associated with differences in the morphology and biochemistry of its principal terminal field, the caudate. The caudate of the BALB/cJ strain is larger, has more neurons (probably cholinergic), and has more dopaminergic receptors which bind 3H-spiroperidol than CBA/J mice (Fink et al., 1979; Baker et al., 1980). At the same time, the number of NE neurons, which also contain tyrosine hydroxylase, does not differ in the two strains. These differences in the number of dopamine neurons and the density of innervation of their terminal fields alter the animal's behavior in a recognizable fashion. Amphetamine, which acts by releasing DA, produces a greater locomotor and stereotype response in BALB/cJ mice over a wide dose range; this greater response is not explainable on a pharmacokinetic basis. In addition, BALB/cJ mice exhibit more spontaneous activity and rear more in a test cage before and after saline injection than CBA/J mice. In other words, naturalistic behavior differs across the two strains in a way that reflects the difference in the number of DA neurons in the midbrain. This activity appears to represent greater locomotor exploration of a novel environment, as the locomotion habituates during the trial (Fink and Smith, 1979, 1980a,c; Fink and Reis, 1981; Reis et al., 1983). Other research has indicated that genetic control of both dopamine and serotonin receptor density is specific for each brain region (Boehme and Ciaranello, 1982).

Animal models suggest that we should anticipate overlapping symptom clusters (e.g., hyperactivity, attention deficit, conduct disorder). While specific neuronal systems innervate discrete functional areas, some neuronal systems act through widespread modulation of multiple neuronal systems, so that many behaviors may be affected through one modulatory system (e.g., the noradrenergic system). Biology most often exerts its observable effects through altered behavioral dimensions, not discrete, reproducible syndromes. These dimensions are embedded in different symptom constellations according to the functional brain areas involved. In short, from a biological viewpoint symptom overlap across syndromes is to be expected.

2.5. Neurochemistry: Clinical Studies

The breadth of functional capacities for which there is evidence of minor dysfunction in ADDH individuals, coupled with animal models which give surface credibility to the hypothesis of "minor" brain damage, has generated a continuing stream of attempts to document brain impairment in these individuals. Unfortunately, the variable findings in individuals are not easily integrated into coherent, reliable classification procedures. The multiple studies of classical neurological signs, "soft" neurological signs, and developmental stigmata have left us on unsteady footing (Shaffer *et al.*, 1983, 1985). Computed tomographic scans have failed to differentiate a specific abnormality in ADDH children. A variety of electrophysiological studies (spectral analysis and event-related potentials) have begun to produce intriguing findings, but methodological problems (e.g., differing protocols at each research site, failure to take account of developmental changes in variables) prevent agreement or definitive findings at this time. All these factors continue to press the clinical investigator toward specification of a biological indicator of the developmental delay in ADDH children. In this context, a range of clinical neurochemical studies have been carried out.

There have been few clinical studies of dopaminergic function in ADDH because of several methodological difficulties. The major metabolite of dopamine is homovanillic acid (HVA), and urinary HVA levels primarily reflect the peripheral dopaminergic contribution; thus, urinary HVA levels do not produce a reliable estimate of brain dopaminergic activity.

There is evidence that plasma HVA concentrations may be a useful index of brain dopaminergic function, but further research is required and this measure has required assay by mass spectrometry; this expensive instrumentation is not available in all clinical centers. Finally, children with ADDH do not have symptoms of sufficient severity to justify a lumbar puncture to obtain spinal fluid. Those few ADDH children for whom cerebrospinal fluid (CSF) HVA levels are available had spinal taps as a component of a workup for a concurrent condition (e.g., persistent headache). Investigation of CSF HVA levels in these small ADDH groups failed to show differences between these patients and contrast groups. However, CSF HVA levels following probenecid loading or amphetamine treatment are significantly reduced (Shetty and Chase, 1978; Shaywitz *et al.*, 1977*b*).

Relatively few studies of serotonergic function have been completed. Examination of CSF 5-hydroxyindoleacetic acid (5-HIAA) levels has shown no difference from contrast groups either before or after probenecid loading (Shaywitz *et al.*, 1977*b*). Investigation of blood and urinary indoleamines has not yet defined a clear utility for these measures in children with ADDH (Irwin *et al.*, 1981; Zametkin *et al.*, 1985*a*). The interaction of dopaminergic and serotonergic systems may be a particularly fruitful area of future clinical research with ADDH children.

The preferential metabolism of brain NE to 3-methoxy-4-hydroxyphenylethylene glycol (MHPG), in contrast to the peripheral conversion of NE to vanillylmandelic acid (VMA), makes urinary studies of central noradrenergic metabolism feasible. A large portion of urinary MHPG, estimated to be in the range of 30–60%, is derived from brain NE metabolism (Mass *et al.*, 1979; Blomberg *et al.*, 1980; Maas and Leckman, 1983). Consequently extensive studies of urinary MHPG in hyperactive children have been completed.

While hyperactive boys appear to have lower mean 24-hr urinary MHPG levels than normal boys, the distributions of the hyperactive and control groups overlap broadly (Shekim *et al.*, 1977, 1979a,b; Yu-Cun and Wang, 1984), and there are dissenting studies (Khan and Dekirmenjian, 1981; Rapoport *et al.*, 1978b; Wender *et al.*, 1971). A number of studies have attempted further discrimination of characteristics of the hyperactive boys in relation to MHPG excretion levels. These have included (1) investigation of the response to drugs acting on catecholamine neuronal systems (*d*-amphetamine, levodopa/carbidopa, and piribedil); (2) comparison of subgroups with normal to high pretreatment urinary MHPG levels to those with low MHPG levels, including their drug response and their association with clinical variables; (3) the relationship of drug response to the presence or absence of soft neurological signs; and (4) simultaneous measurement of levels of other urinary metabolites. MHPG excretion is also decreased in nonhyperactive, learning-disabled children when compared to controls (Shekim and Dekirmenjian, 1978). A reduction in 24-hr urinary MHPG level in hyperactive or learning-disabled boys is not specific to these diagnostic groups, and its meaning requires further study.

When *d*-amphetamine is administered to hyperactive boys, MHPG excretion decreases (Brown *et al.*, 1981; Shekim *et al.*, 1977, 1979a,b), an effect observed in some adult patient groups (Fawcett *et al.*, 1972). Other investigators describe a decrease that fails to reach statistical significance in normal and hyperactive subjects (Rapoport *et al.*, 1978b; Wender *et al.*, 1971). The time at which the urinary MHPG response to amphetamine is measured may be a critical factor in that one study suggests that there may be a progressive decline in urinary MHPG levels for a week or more.

Those findings indicate that *d*-amphetamine simultaneously reduces symptoms, but aggravates the metabolic abnormality suggested to be a marker for the illness (low urinary MHPG level). There is no simple clinical–biological relationship to explain the possible reduction in urinary MHPG levels in hyperactive boys. Studies of the effects of carbidopa/levodopa and piribedil in hyperactive boys make this point again. According to the hypothesis that some children with hyperactivity might have a relative dopamine deficiency, L-dopa should be a beneficial medication. Although L-dopa does lead to a reduction in hyperactivity and some improvement in a vigilance measure, the overall effects are much less substantial than those achieved with *d*-amphetamine (Langer *et al.*, 1982). The partial clinical improvement is accompanied by the expected increase in urinary MHPG levels (due to administration of large amounts of precursor), in contrast to the decrease observed with amphetamine-induced clinical improvement. An attempt to augment dopaminergic function in these children by administering piribedil (a dopamine agonist) failed to elicit clinical improvement (Brown *et al.*, 1979). Thus, three drugs administered in order to achieve a similar effect on catecholamine systems led to a good clinical response, a partial clinical response, and a lack of response, along with inconsistent effects on urinary MHPG levels.

Division of hyperactive boys into those with normal to high MHPG excretion levels and those with low urinary MHPG levels does not lead to any association between high or low MHPG excretion levels and clinical variables. In fact, in both the normal/high and low MHPG groups, the clinical responders to *d*-amphetamine show a reduction in MHPG excretion levels, whereas the nonresponders do not, regardless of their baseline MHPG level (Shekim *et al.*, 1979*b*; Yu-Cun and Wang, 1984). This is consistent with another study in which clinical responders to *d*-amphetamine had a decrease in urinary MHPG levels whereas one nonresponder showed an increased MHPG excretion level (Brown *et al.*, 1981). The responder group, which shows a decrease in urinary MHPG level following *d*-amphetamine, also has more soft neurological signs (Shekim *et al.*, 1979*a*); the presence of soft neurological signs has previously been suggested as a predictor for favorable clinical response to stimulants (Satterfield *et al.*, 1973).

Reduction in urinary MHPG during a single-dose trial with *d*-amphetamine might serve as a metabolic marker for the subgroup of hyperactive children most likely to benefit; it also might begin to clarify the underlying molecular mechanism for symptom reduction. Among the 21 hyperactive boys studied before and after *d*-amphetamine treatment by Shekim and his colleagues, there were 15 responders and six nonresponders. The responders showed a reduction in urinary MHPG levels after stimulant treatment, whereas nonresponders did not. In addition, pretreatment urinary MHPG levels were higher in responders than nonresponders. The percentage change on conduct problems and activity (measured by Factors I and IV on the Conners Teacher Questionnaire) after treatment was correlated with the percentage change in urinary MHPG levels (Shekim *et al.*, 1979*b*). Although further studies of noradrenergic metabolism in hyperactive children could lead to discrimination of a subgroup amenable to treatment with stimulants, the molecular basis for differences in metabolic response in responder and nonresponder groups is a much more complicated problem. Also, because responders have higher urinary MHPG levels than nonresponders, the reduced mean urinary MHPG level for the entire hyperactive group might be due to the inclusion of the nonresponder group. Decreased urinary MHPG levels might be a nonspecific finding unrelated to this diagnostic group or indicative of a poor prognosis.

Another method for establishing the meaning of MHPG levels in childhood disorders is simultaneous measurement of levels of other urinary metabolites [e.g., urinary normetanephrine (NM), metanephrine (MN), and homovanillic acid (HVA)]. Homovanillic acid, the major metabolite of dopamine (DA), may be an index of concurrent central and peripheral dopaminergic effects of the stimulants; the methylated urinary catecholamine metabolites, NM and MN, derive predominantly from peripheral metabolic pools. Urinary HVA does not differentiate hyperactive and control groups or responders from nonresponders nor is it altered following d-amphetamine administration (Brown et al., 1981; Rapoport et al., 1978b; Wender et al., 1971). Similarly, urinary MN levels are not a consistent discriminator of these clinical groups (Wender et al., 1971; Shekim et al., 1979b). On the other hand, urinary NM levels are increased in both hyperactive and learning-disabled boys as compared to normal controls (Shekim et al., 1979b; Shekim and Dekirmenjian, 1978; Wender et al., 1971). Urinary NM levels are not significantly altered by d-amphetamine and are similar in responder and nonresponder groups. The MHPG:NM ratio, suggested to reflect central versus peripheral noradrenergic activity, is sharply reduced in hyperactive and learning-disabled groups, but is not altered by d-amphetamine (Shekim et al., 1979b).

Levels of vanillylmandelic acid (VMA), a product of peripheral NE metabolism, are increased by administration of carbidopa–levodopa to hyperactive boys, as are MHPG levels (Langer et al., 1982). This parallel change may reflect increased NE synthesis, both centrally and peripherally, subsequent to precursor administration. However, plasma NE levels do not increase, just as they show no increase after d-amphetamine administration in most studies (Langer et al., 1982; Mikkelsen et al., 1981; Rapoport et al., 1978b; Wender et al., 1971).

A recent study of other urinary metabolites produced intriguing results. Phenylethylamine (PEA) is an endogenous amine with molecular structure and pharmacological properties similar to those of amphetamine. Twenty-four-hour excretion of PEA was reduced in ADDH children compared to age-matched controls, although it was not different when expressed as a ratio to creatinine excretion. The excretion of tyrosine, phenylalanine, and phenylacetic acid (PAA, the major metabolite of phenylalanine) did not differ between the groups, suggesting specificity of the group differences in PEA (Zametkin et al., 1984b).

Although methylphenidate and dextroamphetamine are similar in their clinical actions, the two stimulants have marked differences in their effects on catecholamine metabolism in ADDH children. Dextroamphetamine administration causes reduced MHPG excretion and stable or reduced NE and NMN levels, but methylphenidate elicits an increase in urinary MHPG, NE, and NMN. Levels of urinary dopamine and its metabolites were not altered by either stimulant. Dextroamphetamine treatment produced a 1600% increase in urinary PEA, but methylphenidate failed to change PEA excretion (Zametkin et al., 1984b, 1985a,b). These findings could be the basis for establishing biological indices that correspond to differential clinical effects of stimulants in hyperactive children.

Plasma NE and MHPG levels are not markedly altered following dextroamphetamine administration, but further research may demonstrate their utility. Changes in monoamine metabolites also occur following treatment with monoamine oxidase inhibitors, but are not consistently associated with clinical response. Rapid clinical relapse after discontinuation of these drugs is dissociated from the sluggish return of NE metabolites to baseline levels (Zametkin et al., 1985c).

3. LEARNING DISORDERS

Bradley's (1937) report that Benzedrine had a favorable effect on a child's performance on schoolwork initiated the evaluation of psychopharmacological interventions for the treatment of learning disorders. Despite this, until recently, relatively few empirical studies assessed the effects of drugs on learning in childhood, and these have been plagued by methodological and conceptual difficulties. It is imperative that research examining pharmacological effects on learning include the determination of each child's attentional capacities. Obviously, attentional dysfunction will impair learning abilities, and these two capacities will be confounded if investigators fail to distinguish them. Regrettably, the difficulties encountered when attempting to dissociate attention and learning are formidable, so that the distinctions are ignored or blurred by most investigators. In spite of the acknowledged problems in this realm of research, it is worthwhile to consider the findings in clinical studies of learning disorders separately from the research on ADDH just described. This will clarify the questions that will be the basis for further examination.

Very little clinical research concerning the neurobiological basis of learning in childhood has been attempted (Young, 1985) and little information is available concerning clinical indices of the brain development that makes learning possible in childhood (Young et al., 1984).

3.1. General Considerations

3.1.1. Definition and Diagnostic Criteria

Learning disorders in childhood have different forms and numerous etiologies. Most research has examined reading disabilities, although other types of specific disorders occur (e.g., arithmetic or spelling disabilities). A variety of specific reading impairments have been identified, so that the unelaborated diagnosis of reading disability is inadequate. Historically, children were considered to be "disabled" if their reading score was 2 years below grade level, and this evaluative system characterizes some of the educational research on this topic. The shortcomings of this definition for a reading disability (Cone and Wilson, 1981; Reynolds, 1981; Rutter and Yule, 1975) include the problem that a child with a low-average IQ can be reading at the expected level for his IQ and still be classified as learning disabled. Therefore, it is essential that reading ability be carefully considered in relation to age and IQ.

It is also preferable to utilize either percentiles or standard scores for the determination of reading level in research. Grade-level scores vary considerably according to the reading test used. Thus, for example, grade-level scores on the Gray Oral Reading Test are consistently lower than those generated by the Wide Range Achievement Test (WRAT) on the same sample. Although differences in results between tests apparently measuring the same abilities are not uncommon, tying the score to an everyday classification system (i.e., grade level) can be quite deceptive; the percentage of children designated as learning disabled can vary by as much as 20%.

Despite clear warnings from test designers not to use grade level ratings for comparisons of either individuals or groups, this practice persists. As stated by Jastak and Jastak (1978), "Months and years are suitable measures for time, but their relationship to performance is not arithmetical. The often-heard statement that there has been a 3-month growth is *not* an accurate representation of how learning takes place." In fact, a 7-year-old who is reading 2 years below grade level on the WRAT is performing at the 1st percentile relative to his age; a 12-year-old reading 2 years below grade level is at the 14th percentile for his age; and a 15-year-old reading 2 years below grade level is at the 47th percentile for his age.

Thus, any studies that define a learning-disabled sample without regard to IQ should be considered inadequate; those that use grade level criteria should be regarded with skepticism and the age of the sample carefully considered.

Another consideration not taken into account in research examining drug effects on learning disabilities is that reading disabilities are due to multiple cognitive and neurophysiological deficits and will not respond identically to medication. For example, several investigators have reported independent neuropsychological syndromes associated with dyslexia in children (Mattis *et al.,* 1975; Mattis, 1978; Denckla, 1979). Children presenting with these disparate cognitive disorders would all meet stringent criteria for reading disabilities, but it is unlikely that they would respond in the same way to medication; if only one subgroup responded, significant group effects would not emerge. Therefore, drug effects on learning-disabled children should be assessed by examining separate patient groups (defined *a priori*) representing the spectrum of impairments associated with these disorders.

3.1.2. Outcome Measures

The selection of outcome measures for research with learning-disabled children is a persistent difficulty. Target symptoms, such as reading or arithmetic disabilities, are generally assessed in a rudimentary, unrefined manner by standardized achievement tests. While these tests are useful for demonstrating large performance decrements for diagnostic purposes, they are relatively insensitive to small changes in academic achievement over brief periods of time. Despite this, most studies have used the WRAT or other similarly insensitive achievement tests not designed for this purpose.

Another approach to evaluating the effects of drugs on learning disabilities has been to apply laboratory measures of learning. These include tasks of specific memory, perception, and linguistic abilities and are more likely to show small changes than tests of academic achievement, but are also more likely to be improved by the attention-focusing properties of the drugs. Furthermore, there is little evidence indicating that improvements on these measures are related to improvements in academic performance.

A final approach used to examine the effects of drugs on learning disorders is to determine changes in scores on tests of academic achievement in children treated with drugs over many years. This approach has limited applicability (e.g., only hyperactive children who are treated with stimulants for years can be subjects). However, if the drug has a facilitatory effect on learning, it may be most apparent in these children, and improved academic performance is commonly a primary result sought by parents and physician.

3.2. Stimulants

Most research examining drug effects in learning-disabled children has focused on the psychostimulants. The first person to note the possible facilitating effects of stimulants on learning was Bradley (1937), who administered Benzedrine to 30 children with a broad array of problems ranging from educational difficulties to aggressive behavior. Among his many findings in this uncontrolled trial was an improvement due to enhanced cognitive processing. He concluded that these results were due to "altering the emotional attitude of the individual toward his task" (Bradley and Green, 1940). Since then, numerous studies have examined the effects of stimulants on learning-disabled children. Minimal evidence supports the position that different stimulants have differential effects on learning (Dykman *et al.*, 1980); the various stimulant drugs will not be reviewed separately here.

Research examining the effects of stimulants on learning-disabled children has produced complex results; some investigators conclude that little evidence currently supports the efficacy of stimulants (Aman, 1980; Barkley and Cunningham, 1978; Gadow, 1983; Aman and Werry, 1982), while others (Kavale, 1982; Pelham, 1983; Pelham et al., 1985) are more optimistic. Only minimal evidence exists demonstrating that psychostimulants facilitate learning in learning-disabled children; methodological and conceptual difficulties, and a lack of sensitive measures of learning, leave the question unanswered. Improved methods for examining specific stages of information processing may bring new information.

3.2.1. Effects of Dosage and Administration Schedules

Dosage differences have been a source of controversy among investigators. Virtually all studies that have examined the effects of stimulants on learning have titrated the dose on the basis of the child's behavior (Gadow, 1981). Yet, using a short-term memory task and classroom behavior ratings, Sprague and Sleator (1977) demonstrated that methylphenidate has differential dose–response effects for cognitive and behavioral improvement. Although others have failed to replicate these findings (Charles et al., 1981), they suggest that the optimal dose for producing cognitive improvement is 0.3 mg/kg, while behavioral improvement is greatest at 1.0 mg/kg. Furthermore, high doses of stimulants that improve behavior have disruptive effects on cognitive performance (Robbins and Sahakian, 1979). Despite this, the majority of studies examining methylphenidate effects on learning have used dosages well above 0.3 mg/kg.

Stimulant medications are short-acting, and the schedule of administration must be considered. Orally ingested methylphenidate has a behavioral and biological half-life of 2–4 hr (Shaywitz et al., 1982; Swanson et al., 1978). Therefore, medication administered in the morning, prior to school, is no longer active by the afternoon. Assessment of long-term effects on learning and academic achievement requires that the medication regimen be structured so that it is active throughout the child's school day.

In addition to ensuring adequate medication levels during learning, test protocols to determine outcome measures should be administered during times of peak drug action. State-dependent learning may be characteristic of hyperactive children learning while medicated with a stimulant, but not normal controls (Swanson and Kinsbourne, 1976). Therefore, facilitatory learning effects would be apparent only if the child was medicated during testing. However, others have been unable to detect evidence indicating state-dependent learning in stimulant-treated children (Gan and Cantwell, 1982; Weingartner et al., 1982; Becker-Mattes et al., 1985).

3.2.2. Learning versus Performance

Further research on stimulants must clarify the distinction between improved *performance* and enhanced *learning*. Stimulants help children focus their attention, contain impulsivity, and reduce hyperactivity. Some have argued (Gittelman *et al.*, 1983; Rie and Rie, 1977) that stimulants may enhance learning performance by reducing inattention. This is particularly salient because most research examining the effects of stimulants on learning has used hyperactive children as subjects; hyperactive children with and without learning disabilities do not differ on many measures that distinguish learning-disabled children from normals (Ackerman *et al.*, 1982; Halperin *et al.*, 1984). Therefore, it is difficult to say whether improvement is due to better attention and cooperation during testing, or to enhanced learning.

One method suggested for controlling for improved performance (versus learning) in trials of medication effects on learning is to obtain baseline (unmedicated) measures, after 1–3 days of medication, and long-term assessment when chronically medicated. For example, one study indicated that medication, relative to placebo, significantly improved reading scores after 2 days. The investigators concluded that it is unlikely that true learning took place in such a brief period of time, so that the improvement was secondary to enhanced performance (Rie and Rie, 1977). However, this conclusion is controversial.

3.2.3. Reviews of Research on Short-Term Effects of Stimulants

Reviews summarizing research on the effects of short-term stimulant treatment on learning provide an interesting perspective. In a review of 10 studies, 40 of 196 perceptual–cognitive measures were significantly improved following stimulant treatment, while only 2 of 26 reading measures improved (Aman, 1982). Similarly, another review indicated that only 6 of 17 studies showed significant improvement on any measures examined (Barkley and Cunningham, 1978). The large number of dependent variables used in these studies suggests that this is not much above chance levels of occurrence.

On the other hand, Kavale (1982) conducted a meta-analysis of the literature evaluating stimulant effects on learning-disabled children and found that stimulants have moderate positive effects on achievement. He estimated an average 15% increase in performance level for drug-treated subjects when compared to nontreated subjects. Pelham's (1983) review suggests that the research studies indicating weak or absent effects of stimulants on learning disabilities were poorly designed and concludes that a lack of positive effects has not been proven. However, the burden of proof is conventionally on those claiming medication effects.

3.2.4. Short-Term Stimulant Effects on Learning-Disabled Children Who Are Not Hyperactive

Among 20 studies examining the short-term effects of psychostimulants on academic achievement in children, only six (Aman and Werry, 1982; Conners *et al.*, 1969; Gittelman *et al.*, 1983; Gittelman-Klein and Klein, 1976; Rie and Rie, 1977; Rie *et al.*, 1976) selected children primarily on the basis of learning problems. Three of these studies (Aman and Werry, 1982; Gittelman *et al.*, 1983; Gittelman-Klein and Klein, 1976) clearly met stringent diagnostic criteria for defining their sample as learning disabled. Two studies (Gittelman *et al.*, 1983; Gittelman-Klein and Klein, 1976) gave clear evidence that their sample was *not* hyperactive.

A group of 61 carefully diagnosed nonhyperactive reading-disabled children were treated with either methylphenidate (average dose, 52 mg/day) or placebo for 12 weeks and assessed on a variety of cognitive, behavioral and academic achievement measures before and after treatment. Methylphenidate significantly improved performance on several psychological and cognitive tasks, but did not affect performance on standardized achievement tests (Gittelman-Klein and Klein, 1976). The same data were later reanalyzed to identify predictors of academic improvement in the children; none were found (Gittelman, 1980).

If stimulant drugs enhance cognitive functioning, the lack of effect on academic achievement may be due to a lack of remediation in conjunction with the medication. Therefore, a sample of 65 reading-disabled children was divided into three treatment groups; (1) reading remediation and placebo, (2) generalized tutoring (no reading instruction) and placebo, and (3) reading remediation and methylphenidate. Following 18 weeks of intervention, it was concluded that the drug enhanced cognitive test performance, but it did not add much to the improvement due to remediation on academic achievement tests (the WRAT and the Gray Oral Reading Test) (Gittelman and Feingold, 1983; Gittelman *et al.*, 1983).

The negative findings might be due to the fact that the dependent achievement measures were relatively insensitive grade scores, or that the drug dose was above the optimal range (Sprague and Sleator, 1977). However, these data suggest that nonhyperactive reading-disabled children receive minimal benefit to academic performance (over a few months) from stimulant drug treatment regardless of the presence or absence of additional tutoring.

3.2.5. Short-Term Stimulant Effects on Mixed Groups of Learning-Disabled Children

Fifteen children with severe reading retardation were examined in a crossover, double-blind, placebo-controlled procedure which compared methylphenidate (0.35 mg/kg) to diazepam (0.1 mg/kg). No behavioral exclusion criteria were used in the selection of subjects, and their behavior was not well described, but the children were *not* selected primarily for hyperactivity. The results again indicated that these drugs had little or no effect on reading achievement measures or cognitive tests believed to be associated with academic performance. However, drugs were given for only 6 days, which may be too brief a period to elicit effects on learning (Aman and Werry, 1982).

The effects of methylphenidate treatment (at doses ranging from 5 to 40 mg daily) using a double-blind crossover procedure were evaluated in two studies (Rie and Rie, 1977; Rie *et al.*, 1976). The children had relatively mild reading impairments and concomitant behavior problems. Assessment scores on the Iowa Test of Basic Skills after either 12 or 15 weeks of treatment showed significant drug improvements on one of six achievement measures. However, the improved measure differed between the studies and the authors concluded that methylphenidate treatment has minimal, if any, effects on learning.

Eight additional studies with hyperactive subjects (Blacklidge and Ekblad, 1971; Conners, 1972; Conrad *et al.*, 1971; Finnerty *et al.*, 1971; Hoffman *et al.*, 1974; Rapoport *et al.*, 1974; Werry and Sprague, 1974; Wolrich *et al.*, 1978) reported no significant drug effects on achievement tests. The duration of treatment in these studies ranged from 2 weeks to 6 months, and the outcome measures were scores on the WRAT in six of the eight studies.

Another seven studies demonstrated some positive effects of stimulants on learning or academic achievement. A non-double-blind, placebo-controlled study showed dextroamphetamine (5.25 mg), over an 8-week period, to significantly improve arithmetic, but not reading or spelling scores (Conners *et al.*, 1969). A later, double-blind, placebo-controlled study reported significant improvement in WRAT spelling and Gray Oral Reading but not in WRAT reading and arithmetic or the Gates Diagnostic Reading Test (Conners *et al.*, 1972). Following 4–6 weeks of methylphenidate, improvement was also shown on tests of oral reading, silent memory, and spelling (Weiss *et al.*, 1971); the researchers attributed these findings to enhancement of attention.

Two recent studies examined methylphenidate effects at multiple doses (0.15 mg/kg, 0.3 mg/kg, and 0.6 mg/kg) in a placebo-controlled crossover study with hyperactive children. A dose-dependent increase was found in the proportion of reading questions answered correctly by the children. In addition, the children, while medicated, attempted a greater number of arithmetic problems, but there was no increase in the proportion answered correctly. These subjects were selected primarily for hyperactivity rather than a learning disability (Pelham, 1983; Pelham *et al.*, 1985).

A single-subject design was used to compare interactional effects of behavior therapy and several doses of methylphenidate on academic productivity and accuracy in two underachieving hyperactive boys. The drug enhanced productivity without compromising accuracy. At the highest dose (0.92 mg/kg) productivity was disrupted and deteriorated to levels below baseline (Rapoport et al., 1982).

Overall, research examining the effect of short-term stimulant treatment on academic achievement yields minimal support for the notion that these drugs are significant learning enhancers. However, it should be noted that, despite the dearth of significant findings, numerous trends have been reported in the direction of a positive drug effect. Furthermore, no study has adequately assessed drug effects on well-defined, nonhyperactive, learning-disabled children using appropriate drug doses, duration of treatment, and sensitive outcome measures.

3.2.6. Long-Term Effects of Stimulants on Learning

Relatively few follow-up studies have evaluated the long-term effects of stimulant medication on learning. Published research describes subjects selected for hyperactivity, rather than learning disabilities, and frequently the findings are expressed in terms of school success, rather than achievement test scores.

A 2- to 5-year follow-up of 83 hyperactive children included a majority who had been treated with stimulants. Despite behavioral improvement in many children, 58% had failed at least one grade in school, 57% had reading difficulties, and 44% had arithmetic difficulties (Mendelson et al., 1971). Although no untreated control data were presented for comparison, these numbers are higher than percentages of unmedicated hyperactive children with learning disabilities reported by others (Cantwell and Satterfield, 1978; Halperin et al., 1984; Keogh, 1971; Lambert and Sandoval, 1980).

Hyperactive boys treated with methylphenidate, imipramine, or placebo were followed after 1 year. Despite teacher-reported behavioral improvements, academic performance (as measured by WRAT reading, spelling, and arithmetic scores) showed no drug-related improvements (Quinn and Rapoport, 1975). More than half of these boys received stimulant medication for an additional year and no drug-related improvements in academic achievement were evident (Riddle and Rapoport, 1976).

Other follow-up studies of stimulant-treated hyperactive children (Huessy et al., 1974; Minde et al., 1972; Weiss et al., 1975) ranging in duration from 5 to 10 years, also failed to document any medication-related effects on subsequent academic performance. Overall, these studies indicate that long-term stimulant treatment has minimal, if any, effect on long-term academic performance in hyperactive children. However, none of these studies examined children who were selected for the presence of learning disabilities; it is not clear whether the school difficulties described for these children were due to behavioral or cognitive problems. Therefore, little can be said regarding the long-term effects of chronic stimulant treatment of learning-disabled children.

3.3. Piracetam

Psychopharmacological research on childhood learning disabilities has begun to evaluate a new class of pharmacological agents, the nootropic drugs (*noos* = mind, *tropein* = toward). The most extensively studied of these is piracetam (2-pyrrolidone acetamide). This compound, structurally related to γ-aminobutyric acid (GABA), putatively acts on telencephalic structures and facilitates the integrative actions of the brain.

Piracetam's clinical effects were initially evaluated in patients suffering from senile dementia and other degenerative disorders; it was suggested to have a positive effect on learning and memory (Stegnick, 1972). Two groups of normal volunteers, given either piracetam (400 mg/day) or placebo for 14 days, were compared on a verbal memory test and a nonverbal pursuit motor task. No significant differences emerged at 7 days posttreatment; the drug-treated group did better on the verbal, but not on the nonverbal, task, after 14 days of treatment. The group difference was quite small, and reached statistical significance only after data from several trials were collapsed, but the authors interpret the findings to be indicative of a selective enhancement of mental action (Dimond and Brouwers, 1976).

Piracetam was first evaluated in dyslexics by comparing it to placebo in dyslexic adults and normal college students (Wilsher *et al.*, 1979). This study utilized several laboratory measures of learning and an initial double-blind, crossover design. However, for reasons not specified, only data from the initial treatment period were published. The drug significantly improved several measures of memory from predrug trials, while improvements with placebo did not reach significance. However, drug effects were never actually compared to placebo.

Two additional studies (Simeon *et al.*, 1979, 1980) examined the effects of piracetam and placebo in dyslexic children; no significant differences were demonstrated on a battery of neuropsychological tests (unspecified) for verbal, nonverbal, sensory, and motor tasks. However, they suggest that piracetam is likely to be psychoactive because it did cause significant reductions in delta EEG.

In a 12-week, placebo-controlled trial with 60 dyslexic boys, it was found that 3.3 g/day of piracetam generated a significant improvement in WISC-R similarities subtest scores, but not in vocabulary (Wilsher and Milewski, 1983). However, a subsequent study by the same investigators (Wilsher *et al.*, 1984) found no significant differences on several reading measures between groups of dyslexic children treated for 8 weeks with piracetam or placebo.

Using a well-defined group of 55 reading-disabled boys, performance on a variety of perceptual, linguistic, memory, and achievement measures (using standardized instruments) was compared after treatment with 3.3 g/day of piracetam or placebo. Boys treated with piracetam for 12 weeks showed significant improvements in reading accuracy, comprehension, speed, and writing accuracy when compared to the placebo group (Chase *et al.*, 1984). These results, which are more promising than others reported, require replication; only 4 of 29 statistical comparisons were significant.

Two additional double-blind studies (Helfgott *et al.*, 1984; Rudel, 1984) compared the effects of 12 weeks of piracetam treatment to placebo treatment in well-defined groups of dyslexic children. The first study (Helfgott *et al.*, 1984) indicated that individual word reading (on the WRAT), but not oral reading, was significantly improved by the drug relative to placebo. However, one-tailed tests of significance were utilized in the statistical analysis. The second study (Rudel and Helfgott, 1984) employed the Neimarck Memory Test (Neimarck *et al.*, 1971) to evaluate memory and verbal retrieval strategies in the two groups. Again, the data indicated significant (one-tailed) pre-post changes in the group treated with piracetam, but not the placebo-treated group; the two groups were not directly compared.

Overall, little evidence supports the concept that piracetam facilitates learning in learning-disabled children. The research is difficult and has been burdened with methodological (primarily statistical) difficulties; only weak positive findings have emerged. However, piracetam appears to be safe and free of side effects, so it may be fruitful to pursue further research on the properties and efficacy of piracetam and similar compounds for the treatment of learning disorders.

4. TOURETTE'S SYNDROME OF CHRONIC, MULTIPLE TICS

4.1. Clinical Features

Tourette's syndrome (TS) is a constellation of symptoms that are quite unusual and disabling when severe. The classical features of the illness are vocal and phonic tics, which are designated as chronic (lasting more than 1 year) and multiple (several types of tics are evident). A childhood onset and intermittently remitting and recurring course is typical of the symptoms; tics diminish over a period of time only to reappear later in more severe form (the phenomenon known as "waxing and waning"). While tics can be voluntarily suppressed for seconds to minutes, they ultimately exhibit their involuntary nature by breaking through in a sudden rush. Eye blinking, lip pursing, grimacing, arm thrusting, head bobbing, leg jerking, mumbling, throat clearing, snorting, barking, cursing, and other motor and phonic tics have been emphasized as the central symptoms of TS for many years (Shapiro *et al.*, 1978). While they can be embarrassing, seriously interfere with social and vocational activities, and sometimes reach a debilitating level of severity, it is often true that other associated behavioral features of TS are the greatest impediment to enjoying usual life activities. For example, complex motor tics involve multiple muscle groups and assume a more purposeful appearance. At some point, these more elaborate tics take on the character of recognizable actions which are repetitively carried out and are designated as compulsions. These complex behaviors can occupy a major share of a patient's time and energy, or be dangerous or socially inappropriate in a dramatic way. The resulting profound interference in a patient's life often makes compulsions the major target symptoms for medication. Other associated behavioral disorders may have a similarly serious impact on a TS patient's life. Attentional impairment, hyperactivity, and impulsivity may make it especially difficult for a child to undertake and master the challenges confronting him at school, on the athletic field, or in peer groups. Cursing or ethnic slurs may provoke attacks by adults. Poorly modulated behavior may leave him outside his old group of friends, his self-esteem may plummet, and depression may become a complicating addition to his symptoms (Young *et al.*, 1985; Comings and Comings, 1985*a*).

4.2. Neurobiogical and Genetic Basis

There is strong evidence that molecular pathology underlies the impaired regulation of behavior in TS. The syndrome has occurred in association with known biological causes, such as carbon monoxide poisoning, head trauma, encephalitis lethargica, and prolonged neuroleptic use. Most series of TS patients report that on neurological examination about half these children have nonlocalizing, "soft" neurological signs involving mild disturbances of motor coordination and body schema maturation (Shapiro *et al.*, 1973*a*). A similarly large number of TS patients have an EEG abnormality (Bergen *et al.*, 1982; Volkmar *et al.*, 1984). In both instances—the "soft" signs and the EEG abnormalities—the findings are nonspecific and fail to illuminate either etiological questions or the proper treatment for an individual child. Computed tomographic scans have not demonstrated specific brain abnormalities in TS patients (Caparulo *et al.,* 1981). Clinicians have been aware of a familial aggregation of TS for many years, but the systematic investigation of a genetic basis for TS began in the late 1970s. Boys are more often afflicted than girls, who require a stronger genetic predisposition for expression of the disorder; therefore, girls must have more afflicted individuals in their family to be likely to be symptomatic themselves. The sons of mothers with TS have the highest risk for developing symptoms, possibly as high as 30–50%. Clarification of the genetic endowment for TS patients requires examination of pedigrees both for the full expression of TS and for chronic, multiple tics (CMT). The actual mode of genetic transmission has not yet been determined for TS, and several models are under consideration. Some pedigrees suggest a dominant autosomal gene, while other data fit polygenic models with sex thresholds of expression affecting the trait (Eldridge *et al.,* 1977; Kidd *et al.,* 1980; Pauls *et al.,* 1981; Comings *et al.,* 1984). Environmental factors are important, and there are many sporadic cases of TS which lack a family history of tics or TS. There is also increasing evidence of an association between TS and other neuropsychiatric disorders, particularly ADDH and obsessive–compulsive disorder (Cohen *et al.,* 1980, 1982; Comings and Comings, 1984). The prevalence of TS among adults (0.5 per 10,000) is substantially lower than the prevalence in school-age children (5.2 per 10,000), emphasizing developmental influences on the expression and form of the disorder (Burd *et al.,* 1986).

4.3. Clinical Neurochemical Research

The mechanisms mediating the influence of these genetic factors are not known. Neurochemical research, utilizing several strategies, has identified specific brain neuronal systems whose function has been altered, but the etiology and the locus of primary involvement remain elusive. The strong genetic contribution and distinctive motor and behavioral symptoms make TS an especially useful model for the investigation of neurochemical alterations in childhood neuropsychiatric disorders.

The compelling evidence indicating dopaminergic involvement in TS rests primarily on symptom response to drugs. Haloperidol, a dopamine-receptor blocking agent, has been the principal medication used in the treatment of TS. Approximately 80% of TS patients have a good initial response to haloperidol, suggesting that an excess of dopaminergic activity contributes to symptom formation. Other neuroleptics that block dopamine receptors (e.g., phenothiazines or pimozide) have a similar effect. Congruent with this theory is the possible role of stimulant medications, which release dopamine, in symptom genesis. Amphetamine, methylphenidate (MPH), and pemoline aggravate existing TS symptoms, and there is evidence suggesting that stimulants may trigger an earlier appearance of tics in vulnerable children (Golden, 1974; Lowe et al., 1982). While this remains a controversial issue in clinical practice (Shapiro and Shapiro, 1981; Caine et al., 1984), there are enough data to warrant caution when considering the administration of stimulants to children with a family history of TS. Stimulant medications are known to produce complex stereotypies in animals which may be amplified by stress, adding further credence to this model (Knott and Hutson, 1982).

Clinical neurochemical studies have been undertaken to examine these questions in TS patients undergoing treatment. Several laboratories have now reported reduced levels of homovanillic acid (HVA, the principal dopamine metabolite) in the cerebrospinal fluid (CSF) of TS patients (Cohen et al., 1978; Butler et al., 1979; Singer et al., 1982; Koslow and Cross, 1982). These findings have been interpreted to indicate a supersensitivity of postsynaptic dopamine receptors, leading to a reduction in presynaptic dopamine release. In agreement with this hypothesis, CSF HVA was further reduced following administration of d-amphetamine to an individual TS patient (Cohen et al., 1978).

There is less direct evidence supporting a serotonergic contribution to TS symptoms. CSF levels of 5-hydroxyindoleacetic acid (5-HIAA, the major serotonin metabolite) also have been reported to be reduced. Serotonergic activity may have a balancing, modulatory relation to dopaminergic control of motor function (Cohen et al., 1978; Butler et al., 1979; Singer et al., 1982; Koslow and Cross, 1982; Jacobs et al., 1982).

On this basis, the reduced CSF 5-HIAA in TS has been hypothesized to reflect an inadequate modulation of dopaminergic activity by serotonergic neurons. The response of CSF 5-HIAA to d-amphetamine in an individual TS patient was in agreement with this hypothesis, as it increased after the stimulant induced activation of dopaminergic receptors. When group means were examined, the CSF 5-HIAA/HVA ratio was correlated with the degree of clinical impairment in the patients; inadequate serotonergic compensatory balance is postulated to contribute to the dysregulation of motor and impulse control (Cohen et al., 1978). Other strategies for elucidating a serotonergic role in the pathophysiology of TS have left the picture clouded. Peripheral serotonin measures in TS (i.e., plasma tryptophan and blood serotonin) have not been useful, and medications acting on the serotonergic system have had a range of indeterminate effects. A precursor of serotonin (5-hydroxytryptophan), a serotonin receptor blocker (methysergide), and a serotonin reuptake blocker (chlorimipramine) all failed to demonstrate useful effects (Van Woert et al., 1977a, 1982).

A recent study cautions the investigator to meticulously examine individual patients when considering these theories. Employing a design using challenge doses of a drug and simultaneous behavioral observations, the mean results for a group of six TS patients indicated predictable behavioral responses to stimulants and haloperidol. Nevertheless, examination of the isolated behaviors of individual patients showed a surprising diversity of responses. They did *not* always improve with haloperidol or worsen with stimulants. The biological heterogeneity of disorders, and individual differences among patients, make predictions concerning single patients hazardous (Caine et al., 1984).

Clinicians have come to this conclusion through a number of observations. Not all patients respond to haloperidol; there is a wide therapeutic dose range among those who do. Some clinicians have observed beneficial effects of stimulants in TS patients, particularly through improving attentional function. A transient beneficial effect has been reported for apomorphine, a potent dopamine agonist; the effect has been suggested, however, to reflect a presynaptic inhibitory influence on dopaminergic turnover through stimulation of a dopamine autoreceptor (Feinberg and Carroll, 1979).

The role of the noradrenergic system has been an intriguing question since the introduction of clonidine for treatment of TS. Clonidine was initially considered as a potential medication when a child with TS was found to have elevated CSF MHPG levels (Cohen et al., 1979a). The effects of clonidine on the locus ceruleus (the principal nucleus of noradrenergic cell bodies in the brain stem) were the subject of animal studies, and clonidine's capacity to reduce noradrenergic activity made it a candidate for a trial for boys afflicted with severe TS symptoms. Clonidine is an imidazoline derivative used widely as an antihypertensive agent. It presumably stimulates α-2-presynaptic adrenergic inhibitory receptors, reducing spontaneous firing in the locus ceruleus, although effects at α-1-adrenergic receptors must also be considered (Bunney and DeRiemer, 1982; Kehne et al., 1985). Approximately 30–60% of patients show improvement in their symptoms following clonidine (Cohen et al., 1979b, 1980; Bruun, 1982b; Leckman et al., 1982; Shapiro and Shapiro, 1982a).

Further clinical research indicated that most TS patients have normal CSF and plasma MHPG levels; occasional patients have elevated CSF MHPG. While urinary total MHPG is reduced, there is not a clear, significant decrease in plasma MHPG levels following acute clonidine challenge. However, challenge with clonidine after a 12-week course of clonidine treatment does elicit a significant reduction in plasma MHPG. This research has also suggested that the therapeutic effects of clonidine might, in part, be exerted through indirect effects on dopaminergic function. Following a 12-week course of clonidine, baseline plasma HVA levels are increased (Young *et al.*, 1981a,b; Leckman *et al.*, 1983). This finding is similar to the rise in plasma HVA that occurs after chronic administration of haloperidol. Elucidation of the neurochemical basis of clonidine's therapeutic effects may require determination of the nature of noradrenergic–dopaminergic interactions in these subjects (Bunney and DeRiemer, 1982).

Attempts to specify the role of the cholinergic system in TS have produced contradictory reports. Elevated levels of red blood cell choline have been observed in a group of TS patients and their relatives, but no clear relation to brain cholinergic function has yet been established (Hanin *et al.*, 1979; Comings *et al.*, 1982). A report of symptom reduction following the administration of intravenous physostigmine (an acetylcholinesterase inhibitor that increases cholinergic activity) was a hopeful step, but intramuscular physostigmine caused an aggravation of symptoms. Blockage of cholinergic receptors led to mixed responses, leaving the overall status of the cholinergic system in TS unclear (Stahl and Berger, 1980, 1981, 1982; Rosenberg and Davis, 1982).

Individual patients have treated themselves with opiates and noted improvement in their symptoms. Enkephalin-containing neurons have been identified in the basal ganglia, establishing a neuroanatomical basis for further study of opioid peptide systems in TS (Buck and Yamamura, 1982). Clonidine is an effective agent for treating withdrawal symptoms after narcotic abuse, presumably through its inhibition of the adrenergic overactivity characteristic of the withdrawal state; this is further encouragement for careful study of opioid peptide neuronal systems in TS.

Close attention to associated behavioral disorders may be a basis for subgrouping TS patients in the future. Determination of associated neurochemical and behavioral changes in TS patients will be an enlightening strategy for investigation of attentional impairment, hyperactivity, and compulsive symptoms; it is possible that these symptom dimensions may have different neurochemical correlates in TS patients, as contrasted to those patients with disorders in which the symptoms are primary. In addition, these associated disorders are often present in particularly severe form in TS patients, and associated neurochemical alterations may be of greater magnitude.

4.4. Treatment

The choice of treatment evolves from the diagnosis and the degree to which symptoms interfere with the child's development. The primary goal should be to help the child manage normal developmental tasks—for the school-age child, to feel competent in school, develop friendships, experience trust in his parents, and enjoy life's adventures. Many children with multiple tics and TS progress satisfactorily, and pharmacological treatment is not required. Anxiety and confusion about the symptoms require calm discussion and education about available treatments. If treatment is agreed upon by the child, family, and physician, developmental issues must be continually reassessed (Cohen and Leckman, 1984; Bruun, 1984; Van Woert *et al.*, 1982).

4.4.1. Monitoring and Reassurance

It is best if the clinician can follow a patient for several months before initiating a specific treatment plan. The goals of this first stage of treatment are to establish a baseline of symptoms; define associated difficulties in school, family, and peer relations; obtain necessary medical tests; monitor, through check lists and interviews, the range and fluctuation of symptoms; determine aggravating and alleviating factors; and establish a relationship.

The child's tics may be of minimal functional significance. He may satisfy the criteria for TS, yet have good peer relations, school achievement, and sense of himself, and no treatment may be needed. Parents may be worried about the child's future. In general, the severity of TS is apparent within a short period after its appearance; by the time a child has had TS for 2 or 3 years, one can guess with reasonable accuracy how severe the disorder ultimately will be. For transient single tics, reassurance is fully appropriate. Families should also be informed about emerging knowledge concerning genetic factors.

4.4.2. Pharmacological Treatment

The only effective treatment for simple and complex motor and phonic tics is pharmacological. Psychotherapy may help children with TS understand the effects of the illness on their personality and on the response of peers, the nature of their own adjustment, and the usual conflicts accompanying development. While psychotherapy may reduce the severity of tics slightly in individual children as a result of relief of general stress and anxiety, tics are generally not responsive to psychotherapy. Behavior modification, hypnotherapy, and relaxation methods have been tried with TS with little success; they may act synergistically with pharmacotherapy, but no firm evidence supports this. Some patients are able to learn methods of self-control, particularly as they grow older.

Three medications have broad use in the treatment of TS today.

4.4.2a. Haloperidol. Haloperidol has been the most common treatment for TS since the 1960s. During the first years of its use, dosage was rapidly increased to very high levels (up to 300 mg/day), followed by gradual reduction. However, it is now accepted that haloperidol is most effective at quite low doses. Patients are given an initial dose of 0.5 mg/day and slowly increased up to 3–4 mg/day, usually in twice-daily dosage. Impressive benefits are seen at these low doses, and patients may have almost complete remission with few side effects (Shapiro et al., 1973b, 1978, 1982b). Patients for whom low doses of haloperidol are ineffective may find that higher doses (10–15 mg) are useful, but improvement is often limited and side effects troubling. While there has been a suggestion that patients with a family history of TS may respond better to haloperidol than those without, other studies do not indicate that family history of tics or the presence of EEG abnormalities is specifically associated with a favorable response.

As many as 80% of patients with TS initially benefit from haloperidol, sometimes dramatically. However, long-term follow-up suggests that only a smaller number, perhaps 20–30%, continue haloperidol for an extended period of time. Haloperidol is discontinued because of the emergence of side effects, including lethargy, weight gain, dysphoria, pseudoparkinsonian symptoms, intellectual dulling, personality changes, feeling like a "zombie," and akathisia (Cohen et al., 1980; Shapiro et al., 1978; Bruun, 1982a; Bogomolny et al., 1982). Pseudoparkinsonian and acute dystonic reactions can be controlled with antiparkinsonian agents (1–2 mg/day of benztropine). Akathisia is less responsive to anticholinergic agents. A school phobia occasionally appears during the first weeks of treatment with low doses of haloperidol, while tics are improving. Social phobias in adults involve acute anxiety about going to work or performing at work; like school phobia, they can be extremely disabling. When these phobias are not recognized as drug side effects, they continue for months; they remit within weeks of haloperidol discontinuation. Intellectual dulling can lead to a marked deterioration of school and work performance. Children who are excellent students and enjoy many friendships may become poor students, unhappy, and isolated after beginning haloperidol for tics. Some clinicians prescribe methylphenidate in combination with haloperidol in order to counter the attentional impairment caused by haloperidol. While good results have been described, the aggravation of tics by stimulant medications suggests that adding a stimulant to haloperidol should be considered experimental and performed only with informed consent and careful monitoring until long-term effects can be assessed.

Haloperidol has been incriminated in the onset of tardive dyskinesia (TD). The appearance of new facial or hand movements may be difficult to assess in a patient with a preexisting movement disorder. Tics must be distinguished from the first signs of TD. Orofacial movements suspected to be TD sometimes disappear several weeks after discontinuation of haloperidol (Shapiro and Shapiro, 1982b; Klawans et al., 1982; Fog et al.,

1982). Some animal studies suggest TD may be more likely to appear after multiple discontinuations and reintroductions of neuroleptics, so it is probably wise not to attempt frequent drug holidays with haloperidol. Withdrawal exacerbations seldom make this feasible, in any case.

Anticholinergic agents need not be prescribed until required to combat specific side effects (parkinsonian tremor or rigidity, dystonia, oculogyric crisis, or akathisia). However, some clinicians prefer to begin low doses of these agents once the haloperidol is above a certain threshold, perhaps 2 mg/day, because of fear of the occurrence of these frightening side effects in school. Antiparkinsonian agents have their own side effects, so prophylactic use may be unwise. Patients should be instructed about haloperidol's potential side effects and have an antiparkinsonian drug at home and with them on trips in the event that they develop extrapyramidal symptoms. They should also be informed that, in an emergency, acute dystonic reactions can be treated with other drugs, such as Valium, Librium, or Benadryl.

4.4.2b. Clonidine. The first description of the use of clonidine for treatment of TS appeared in 1979 (Cohen *et al.*, 1979b) and was followed by other open and controlled trials indicating that from 30 to 70% of TS patients benefit from its use (Cohen *et al.*, 1979b, 1980; Shapiro and Shapiro, 1982a; Bruun, 1982b; Leckman *et al.*, 1982, 1983, 1984). Clonidine has been approved by the Federal Drug Administration (FDA) only for use in hypertension, but clinicians can prescribe it for TS without special government approval as long as they understand its indications and describe the basis for their decision to the family and child. Formal FDA approval for the use of clonidine in TS is anticipated. Clonidine primarily inhibits noradrenergic functions, while haloperidol alters dopaminergic functioning. Interactions between central dopaminergic and noradrenergic systems may be involved in the pathophysiology of TS, and there is evidence that clonidine indirectly affects central dopaminergic systems (Leckman *et al.*, 1983; Antelman and Caggiula, 1977). Clonidine reduces simple motor and phonic tics, and is particularly useful in improving attentional problems and ameliorating complex motor and phonic symptoms. Clonidine treatment should be initiated at low doses of 0.05 mg/day and slowly titrated over several weeks to 0.15–0.30 mg/day (or approximately 3 µg/kg per day). Doses of 0.4 mg/day are not infrequent, but doses above 0.5 mg/day are more likely to lead to side effects. When medication is working effectively, patients may experience the need for their next dose by sensing increasing anxiety, frequency of symptoms, or irritability. Haloperidol may bring a clear improvement within a few days, but clonidine has a slower onset of action. This can make the evaluation of its therapeutic effects treacherous with an expectant and anxious family. When larger doses are used earlier, improvement may occur sooner, but there may be more sedation.

Using a slower titration to therapeutic levels, clonidine may take 3 weeks or longer to show a beneficial effect. The patient may experience a reduction in tension, a sense of being calm, or have a "longer fuse" before tics are reduced. A gradual decrease in complex motor tics and compulsions also may precede clear improvement in simple tics. Evaluation of the medication's effectiveness may not be possible before 3–4 months. When there is a positive response, improvement may progress for up to a year or more. Patients gain confidence in themselves, adjust better to school, feel less irritable, and have fewer tic symptoms. Clonidine has only recently been used in TS, so the longest individual period of treatment is 7 years. Children with extremely severe TS have benefited after several years of treatment with clonidine, and only slight increases in medication have been required. The major side effect of clonidine is sedation; it appears early in the course of treatment, especially if the dose is increased quickly, but abates after several weeks. A few patients have dry mouth, but children less often than adults. Clonidine continues to decrease salivary flow even after years of treatment (Selinger *et al.*, 1984). Rarely, patients complain that things are "too bright," perhaps due to impairment of pupillary constriction. At higher doses, there may be hypotension and dizziness; this is more likely if clonidine is given at high doses quite early or if it is increased to over 0.4 or 0.5 mg/day. At lower doses, blood pressure is not clinically affected, although a fall of several mm Hg in diastolic and systolic pressure can be detected. Slight prolongation of the PR interval on the electrocardiogram has been noted, but has not been considered of significance. No other medical or clinical side effects have emerged.

An EKG and routine blood studies should be obtained before clonidine is administered. No alterations in standard blood chemistry measures or hemogram have been identified. The combined use of haloperidol and clonidine has not yet been examined in controlled studies, and only anecdotal information is available. The combination has been used in two clinical situations: (1) for patients whose symptoms are not fully controlled on haloperidol, or who are having serious side effects when medication is increased, yet who cannot discontinue haloperidol because of the severity of symptoms; and (2) for patients on clonidine who have inadequate control of motor and phonic symptoms. It appears that patients can be managed with smaller doses of haloperidol when clonidine is added; on the other hand, haloperidol may improve tic control for some patients on clonidine. Small doses of both medications are used when the drugs are combined, and no serious side effects have been reported other than those seen with the drugs used individually.

4.4.2c. Pimozide. Pimozide is a potent neuroleptic widely used in Europe for the treatment of psychosis. Several clinical studies have suggested pimozide to be as effective as haloperidol in the treatment of TS and possibly less sedating; controlled comparisons are required (Shapiro and Shapiro, 1982a, 1984; Ross and Moldofsky, 1977; Shapiro et al., 1983; Moldofsky and Brown, 1982). Pimozide is a diphenylbutylpiperidine derivative, chemically distinct from haloperidol, clonidine, or the phenothiazines. Its mode of action appears to be preferential blocking of postsynaptic dopamine (D_2) receptors (Seeman and Lee, 1975; Nose and Takemoto, 1975). Pimozide was an effective therapeutic agent in a double-blind, crossover design comparing it with placebo (Shapiro and Shapiro, 1984). Side effects are similar to those encountered with haloperidol, but may be less severe and appear to be tolerable for many patients. Individual patients who have not had a favorable result with haloperidol or clonidine occasionally report dramatic improvement with pimozide. It may be a useful addition to the pharmacological agents for TS. Treatment is initiated at 1 mg/day, and dosage may be gradually increased to a maximum of 6–10 mg/day (0.2 mg/kg) for children and 20 mg/day for adults. Pimozide has a long half-life (55 hr), and once-daily dosage may be feasible. Major side effects are similar to those of haloperidol, and include sedation, pseudoparkinsonism, akathisia, insomnia, and dizziness, as well as depression, nervousness, and other adverse behavioral effects. Anticholinergic agents are useful. TD should be considered a likely long-term risk until proven otherwise (Shapiro and Shapiro, 1984).

Pimozide causes EKG changes in up to 25% of patients, including T-wave inversion, U waves, QT prolongation, and bradycardia. EKG changes are observable within 1 week and at doses as low as 3 mg/day. The manufacturer recommends discontinuation of pimozide with the occurrence of T-wave inversion or U waves, seen in up to 20% of patients; dosage should not be increased if there is prolongation of the QT interval (corrected). Discontinuation of pimozide appears to bring normalization of the EKG within 1 week. Several cardiac deaths have occurred in physically healthy patients receiving pimozide. In addition to usual clinical and laboratory monitoring, patients receiving pimozide should receive an EKG before treatment, monthly during dosage increases, and at 3-month intervals thereafter (Shapiro and Shapiro, 1984).

4.4.2d. Phenothiazines and Other Medications. Haloperidol was thought to have a specific therapeutic effect in TS, but experience suggests that some patients have a comparable response to phenothiazines (Borison et al., 1982). When equivalent doses are used and side effects are similar, haloperidol may be no more useful than phenothiazines. On the other hand, phenothiazines have no greater value than haloperidol. When a patient cannot tolerate haloperidol, a trial with a phenothiazine may be indicated.

Substituted benzylamines (e.g., metapropamide) have been used in Europe with some success, but pseudoparkinsonian side effects and altered kidney function have limited their broad use. Agents that affect cholinergic function are not commonly used in the treatment of TS. Intravenous physostigmine has been used to study cholinergic mechanisms; even those investigators observing a reduction in TS symptoms have been unable to apply agents like physostigmine clinically (Stahl and Berger, 1980, 1981). Lecithin had no benefit in controlled trials or anecdotal reports (Rosenberg and David, 1982). Agents affecting serotonergic function have not been useful, but there are few rigorous studies (Van Woert et al., 1977a,b, 1982). It is likely that medications with increasingly specific modes of action will become available during the next several years for the treatment of TS.

4.4.2e. Choice of Medication. The clinician's choice of initial drug is a difficult decision. The greatest cumulative experience is with haloperidol, so that its therapeutic benefits and side effects are well defined. Clonidine may be preferred as a first drug because of its limited side effects and positive effect on attention; however, when a rapid response is needed, haloperidol is more effective. Clonidine has less immediate and dramatic therapeutic effects, and they are less extensively defined. Until more evidence accumulates, or other drugs become available, individual clinical experience will determine which drug should be given an initial several-month course. If a patient is started on haloperidol, discontinuation may be difficult because of withdrawal symptoms which are not attenuated by clonidine at usual doses. Some clinicians have added low-dose clonidine to low-dose haloperidol with good results, but no controlled studies have been reported. Whether pimozide will become an alternative to haloperidol will depend on the seriousness and frequency of side effects when it is more widely used; the association with cardiac death and the limited study with children suggest caution.

When used alone, antidepressant medications either aggravate or fail to improve TS symptoms. However, if a TS patient develops a serious depression, the use of an antidepressant can be added to ongoing TS treatment (haloperidol, clonidine) with good results. Both haloperidol and clonidine may cause lowered spirits or dysphoria, and assessment of depression may be difficult. A period of no medication might be considered before the addition of an antidepressant, especially if depression appears soon after the use of medication and with no apparent psychosocial precipitant. Minor tranquilizers have no apparent benefit on tic symptomatology; however, individual patients have benefited when they are used to alleviate anxiety or improve sleep.

4.4.3. Academic Intervention and Genetic Counseling

Attentional and learning problems necessitate educational intervention for children with TS. They may require special tutoring, a learning laboratory, a self-contained classroom, or special day or residential school settings, depending on the severity of academic and associated behavioral problems. It may be difficult to convince a school district of the need for special school provisions when a bright TS patient does not have specific learning disabilities but has attentional problems limiting his optimal functioning. TS is an uncommon disorder, and schools need to be informed about the nature of TS and its effects on attention and learning; the physician must be active as a child's advocate.

Parents and older TS patients increasingly inquire about the genetic risk for siblings and offspring. The precise mode of inheritance is still not known, so only general advice is possible. Birth into a family with a first-degree relative (parent or sibling) with TS increases the risk of disorder for the child from one in many hundreds or thousands to one in four or five. The risk is much higher for male offspring. Genetic counseling requires tact and sensitivity about the meaning of the information to a young adult with TS. The children of a mother with TS have an especially high risk, and judicious concern is required when counseling the TS mother who desires a child. At present, there is no method for prenatal diagnosis. It is important to emphasize the uncertainties of genetic counseling, as well as the increasing knowledge about treatment.

4.4.4. TS Patients with Multiple Handicaps

The adolescent or adult with long-standing, severe TS and multiple associated social and academic difficulties presents complex treatment challenges. It is not uncommon for these most severely afflicted individuals to have few personal or social resources and to have intensely ambivalent relations with their exhausted families. Disentangling what is "Tourette's" and what are the manifold consequences of chronicity, disorganization, and various medications may be a major, long-term therapeutic task. Patients may no longer know what is under their control, in any sense of this term, and what is primarily a manifestation of their TS. Reconstructing their experience and trying to understand what they are doing is a goal of the therapeutic work. Medication side effects and withdrawal-emergent effects confuse matters and make it difficult to assess any intervention. Most pathetic are the young adults who exhibit self-mutilation, such as poking their eyes or biting their cheeks or banging their heads, during TS crises; other patients become chronically dependent and unable to function on their own, yet have nobody to whom to turn. For the young adult who has had a serious interference with school achievement, socialization, and personality development, a thorough rehabilitation program is required. The patient may need vocational guidance, a halfway-house program, psychotherapy, family counseling, and advocacy, in addition to judicious use of medication. Even in desperate situations, therapeutic commitment combined with the patient's determination and courage may lead to satisfying therapeutic results. The treatment is facilitated if there is a therapeutic team which can be mutually supportive and can work together to find social and financial resources during the many months when the patient may be dependent and demanding.

Episodes of exacerbation are to be expected. Months of hard-won progress may seem to dissipate in days without a trace. It is natural for the physician to become disappointed and angry during these exacerbations, as symptoms return and a patient seems to crumble. The patient may sense the physician's attitude; when he becomes enraged and utterly discouraged, the treatment relationship may end. Clinicians, like parents, may cajole, bribe, and threaten. The physician may not know how to set "limits" that can be used by the patient to regain a sense of inner control, because he recognizes that such behavioral approaches are sometimes an expression of anger. However, if a therapeutic alliance can be maintained, it is possible to weather the storm and for this shared experience to strengthen the treatment relationship as the patient restabilizes.

5. OVERVIEW

Clinical investigators have achieved substantial progress in the generation of more effective pharmacological treatments for psychiatric disorders in childhood. At the same time, it must be recognized that attaining the rapid rate of development required to match the needs of children hinges on the nurturance of two activities. Valid and reliable assessment procedures must be employed if clinicians are to make accurate judgments concerning the efficacy of new therapies. This requires that the investigator sustain the delicate balance between targeted clinical measures and a comprehensive evaluation that is optimal for the patient, and that he deploy these measures in the face of the multiple clinical influences that create pressure to discard formal measures in the name of urgency and simplicity. In the end, sophisticated neurobiological research is always vulnerable to foundering on associated uninterpretable clinical data. It is clear, for example, that the complex brain mechanisms underlying the regulation of attention, learning, and motor activity will not be clarified in the absence of precise measures of the accompanying clinical phenomena.

On the other side, it is imperative that clinical investigators grappling with the neuropsychiatric disorders of childhood employ the best new methods developed by the ballooning basic neurobiology enterprise. These advances have made it possible to design and utilize ever-improving technologies for the assessment and treatment of these children. Clinical investigators who keep pace with these developments will be able to take advantage of them to unravel the confusing problems facing us and facilitate the optimal development of the children we care for.

Acknowledgments

We are grateful to Ms. M. Easton, Mr. L. Richardson, and Mrs. A. Cooper for preparation of the manuscript. We appreciate the support of research described in this chapter by the Office of Mental Retardation and Developmental Disabilities, State of New York; The Rosenstiel Foundation; The Joseph L. Shulman Foundation; The Gateposts Foundation; MHCRC Grant MH 30929; NICHD Grant HD 03008; CCRC Grant RR 00125.

6. REFERENCES

ABIKOFF, H., and GITTELMAN, R., 1985, Hyperactive children treated with stimulants: Is cognitive training a useful adjunct? *Arch. Gen. Psychiatry* **42**:953–961.

ACKERMAN, P. T., DYKMAN, R. A., HOLCOMB, P. I., and McCRAY, D. S., 1982, Methylphenidate effects on cognitive style and reaction time in four groups of children, *Psychiatry Res.* **7**:199–213.

AGHAJANIAN, G. K., 1978, Feedback regulation of central monoaminergic neurons: evidence from single cell recording studies, in: *Essays in Neurochemistry and Neuropharmacology*, Vol. 3 (M. B. H. Youdim, W. Lovenberg, D. F. Sharman, and J. R. Lagnado, eds.), John Wiley, New York.

AMAN, M. G., 1980, Psychotropic drugs and learning problems—A selective review, *J. Learning Disabil.* **13**:87–97.

AMAN, M. G., 1982, Psychotropic drugs in the treatment of reading disorders, in: *Reading Disorders: Varieties and Treatments* (R. N. Malatesha and P. G. Aaron, eds.), Academic Press, New York.

AMAN, M. G., and WERRY, J. S., 1982, Methylphenidate and diazepam in severe reading retardation, *Child Psychiatry* **21**:31–37.

AMERY, B., MINICHIELLO, M. D., and BROWN, G. L., 1984, Aggression in hyperactive boys: Response to d-amphetamine, *J. Am. Acad. Child Psychiatry* **23**:291–294.

ANGRIST, B., 1983, Psychoses induced by central nervous system stimulants and related drugs, in: *Stimulants: Neurochemical, Behavioral, and Clinical Perspectives* (I. Creese, ed.), Raven Press, New York.

ANGRIST, B., and SUDILOVSKY, A., 1978, Central nervous system stimulants: Historical aspects and clinical effects, in: *Stimulants*, Vol. 11, *Handbook of Psychopharmacology* (L. L. Iversen, S. D. Iversen, and S. H. Snyder, eds.), Plenum Press, New York, pp. 99–165.

ANTELMAN, S. M., and CAGGIULA, A. R., 1977, Norepinephrine-dopamine interactions and behavior: A new hypothesis of stress-related interactions between brain norepinephrine and dopamine is proposed, *Science* **195**:646–653.

BAKER, H., JOH, T. H., and REIS, D. J., 1980, Genetic control of the number of midbrain dopaminergic neurons in inbred strains of mice: Relationship to size and neuronal density of the striatum, *Proc. Natl. Acad. Sci. USA* **77**:4369–4373.

BARKLEY, R. A., and CUNNINGHAM, C. E., 1978, Do stimulant drugs improve the academic performance of hyperkinetic children? *Clin. Pediatr.* **17**:85–92.

BECKER-MATTES, A., MATTES, J., ABIKOFF, H., and BRANDT, L., 1985, State-dependent learning in hyperactive children on methylphenidate, *Am. J. Psychiatry* **142**:455–459.

BERGEN, D., TANNER, C. M., and WILSON, R., 1982, The electroencephalogram in Tourette syndrome, *Ann. Neurol.* **11**:382–385.

BERRY, C. A., SHAYWITZ, S. E., and SHAYWITZ, B. A., 1985, Girls with attention deficit disorder: A silent minority? A report on behavioral and cognitive characteristics, *Pediatrics* **76:**801–809.
BIEL, J. H., and BOPP, B. A., 1978, Amphetamines: Structure–activity relationships, in: *Handbook of Psychopharmacology*, Vol. 11 (L. L. Iversen, S. D. Iversen, and S. H. Snyder, eds.), Plenum Press, New York, pp. 1–38.
BLACKLIDGE, V., and EKBLAD, R., 1971, The effectiveness of methylphenidate hydrochloride (Ritalin) on learning and behavior in public school educable mentally retarded children, *Pediatrics* **47:**923–926.
BLOMBERG, P. A., KOPIN, I. J., GORDON, E. K., MARKEY, S. P., and EBERT, M. H. 1980, Conversion of MHPG to vanillylmandelic acid, *Arch. Gen. Psychiatry* **37:**1095–1098.
BOEHME, R. E., and CIARANELLO, R. D., 1982, Genetic control of dopamine and serotonin receptors in brain regions of inbred mice, *Brain Res.* **266:**51–65.
BOGOMOLNY, A., ERENBERG, G., and ROTHNER, D., 1982, Behavioral effects of haloperidol in young Tourette syndrome patients, in: *Advances in Neurology*, Vol. 35 (A. J. Friedhoff and T. N. Chase, eds.), Raven Press, New York.
BORISON, R. L., ANG, L., CHANG, S., DYSKEN, M., CAMATY, J. E., and DAVID, J. M., 1982, New pharmacological approaches in the treatment of Tourette syndrome, in: *Advances in Neurology*, Vol. 35 (A. J. Friedhoff and T. N. Chase, eds.), Raven Press, New York.
BRADLEY, C., 1937, The behavior of children receiving benzedrine, *Am. J. Psychiatry*, **94:**577–585.
BRADLEY, C., and GREEN, E., 1940, Psychometric performances of children receiving amphetamine (benzedrine) sulfate, *Am. J. Psychiatry*, **97:**388–394.
BROWN, G. L., EBERT, M. H., MIKKELSEN, E. J., BUCHSBAUM, M., and BUNNEY, W. E., JR., 1979, Dopamine agonist piribedil in hyperactive children, presented at annual meeting of American Psychiatric Assoc., Chicago, 1979, *Syllabus and Scientific Proceedings*, pp. 254–255.
BROWN, G. L., EBERT, M. H., HUNT, R. D., and RAPOPORT, J. L., 1981, Urinary 3-methoxy 4-hydroxyphenylglycol and homovanillic acid response to D-AMPH in hyperactive children, *Biol. Psychiatry* **16:**779–787.
BRUUN, R. D., 1982a, Dysphoric phenomena associated with haloperidol treatment of Tourette syndrome, in: *Advances in Neurology*, Vol. 35 (A. J. Friedhoff and T. N. Chase, eds.), Raven Press, New York.
BRUUN, R. D., 1982b, Clonidine treatment of Tourette syndrome, in: *Advances in Neurology*, Vol 35 (A. J. Friedhoff and T. N. Chase, eds.), Raven Press, New York.
BRUUN, R. D., 1984, Gilles de la Tourette's syndrome: An overview of clinical experience, *J. Am. Acad. Child Psychiatry* **23:**126–133.
BUCHSBAUM, M. S., HAIER, R. J., SOSTEK, A. J., WEINGARTNER, H., ZAHN, T. P., SIEVER, L. J., MURPHY, D. L., and BRODY, L., 1985, Attention dysfunction and psychopathology in college men, *Arch. Gen. Psychiatry* **42:**354–360.
BUCK, S. H., and YAMAMURA, H. I., 1982, Neuropeptides in normal and pathological basal ganglia, in: *Advances in Neurology*, Vol. 35 (A. J. Friedhoff and T. N. Chase, eds.), Raven Press, New York.
BUNNEY, B. S., 1984, Antipsychotic drug effects on the electrical activity of dopaminergic neurons, *Trends Neurosci.* **7:**212–215.
BUNNEY, B. S., and AGHAJANIAN, G. K., 1978, d-Amphetamine-induced depression of central dopamine neurons: evidence for mediation by both autoreceptors and striato-nigral feedback pathway, *Naunyn Schmiedelbergs Arch. Pharmacol.* **304:**255–261.
BUNNEY, B. S., and DERIEMER, S., 1982, Effect of clonidine on dopaminergic neuron activity in the substantia nigra: Possible indirect mediation by noradrenergic regulation of the serotonergic raphe system, in: *Advances in Neurology* (A. J. Friedhoff and T. N. Chase, eds.), Raven Press, New York.

BURD, L., KERBESHIAN, J., WIKENHEISER, M. and FISHER, W., 1986, Prevalence of Gilles de la Tourette's syndrome in North Dakota adults, *Am. J. Psychiatry* **143**:787–788.

BUTLER, I. J., KOSLOW, S., SEIFERT, W. et al., 1979, Biogenic amine metabolism in Tourette syndrome, *Ann. Neurol.* **6**:37–39.

CAINE, E. D., LUDLOW, C. L., POLINSKY, R. J., and EBERT, M. H., 1984, Provocative drug testing in Tourette's syndrome: d- and 1-amphetamine and haloperidol, *J. Am. Acad. Child Psychiatry* **23**(2):142–147.

CANTWELL, D. P., 1985, Hyperactive children have grown up: What have we learned about what happens to them? *Arch. Gen. Psychiatry* **42**:1026–1028.

CANTWELL, D. P., and SATTERFIELD, J. H., 1978, The prevalence of academic underachievement in hyperactive children, *J. Pediatr. Psychol.* **3**:168–171.

CAPARULO, B. K., COHEN, D. J., ROTHMAN, S. L., et al., 1981, Computed tomographic brain scanning in children with developmental neuropsychiatric disorders, *J. Am. Acad. Child Psychiatry* **20**:338–357.

CHARLES, L., SCHAIN, R., and ZELNIKER, T., 1981, Optimal dosages of methylphenidate for improving the learning and behavior of hyperactive children, *Dev. Behav. Pediatr.* **2**:78–81.

CHASE, C. H., SCHMITT, R. L., RUSSELL, G., and TALLAL, P., 1984, A new chemotherapeutic investigation: Piracetam effects on dyslexia, *Ann. Dyslexia* **34**:29–48.

CIARANELLO, R. D., BARCHAS, R., KESSLER, S., and BARCHAS, J. D., 1972, Catecholamines: Strain differences in biosynthetic enzyme activity in mice, *Life Sci.* **2**:565–572.

COHEN, D. J., and LECKMAN, J. F., 1984, Tourette's syndrome: Advances in treatment and research. Introduction, *J. Am. Acad. Child Psychiatry* **23**:123–125.

COHEN, D. J., SHAYWITZ, B. A., CAPARULO, B. K., YOUNG, J. G., and BOWERS, M. B., Jr.,1978, Chronic, multiple tics of Gilles de la Tourette's disease: CSF acid monoamine metabolites after probenecid administration, *Arch. Gen. Psychiatry* **35**:245–250.

COHEN, D. J., SHAYWITZ, B. A., YOUNG, J. G., CARBONARI, C. M., NATHANSON, J. A., LIEBERMAN, D., BOWERS, M. B., JR., and MAAS, J. W., 1979a, Central biogenic amine metabolism in children with the syndrome of chronic multiple tics of Gilles de la Tourette: Norepinephrine, serotonin, and dopamine, *J. Am. Acad. Child Psychiatry* **18**:320–341.

COHEN, D. J., YOUNG, J. G., NATHANSON, J. A., and SHAYWITZ, B. A., 1979b, Clonidine in Tourette's syndrome, *Lancet*, **2**:551–553.

COHEN, D. J., DETLOR, J., YOUNG, J. G., and SHAYWITZ, B. A., 1980, Clonidine ameliorates Gilles de la Tourette syndrome, *Arch. Gen. Psychiatry* **37**:1350–1357.

COHEN, D. J., DETLOR, J., SHAYWITZ, B. A., and LECKMAN, J. F., 1982, Interaction of biological and psychological factors in the natural history of Tourette syndrome: A paradigm for childhood neuropsychiatric disorders, in: *Gilles de la Tourette Syndrome, Advances in Neurology*, Vol. 35 (A. J. Friedhoff and T. N. Chase, eds.), Raven Press, New York, pp. 31–40.

COMINGS, D. E., and COMINGS, B. G., 1984, Tourette's syndrome and attention deficit disorder with hyperactivity: Are they genetically related? *J. Am. Acad. Child Psychiatry* **23**(2):138–146.

COMINGS, D. E., and COMINGS, B. G., 1985a, Tourette syndrome: Clinical and psychological aspects of 250 cases, *Am. J. Hum. Genet.* **37**:435–450.

COMINGS, D. E., GURSEY, B. T., AVELINO, E., KOPP, U., and HANIN, I., 1982, Red blood cell choline in Tourette syndrome, in: *Advances in Neurology*, Vol. 35 (A. J. Friedhoff and T. N. Chase, eds.), Raven Press, New York.

COMINGS, D. E., COMINGS, B. G., DEVOR, E. J., and CLONINGER, C. R., 1984, Detection of a major gene for Gilles de la Tourette syndrome, *Am. J. Hum. Genet.* **36**:586–600.

CONE, T. E., and WILSON, L. R., 1981, Quantifying a severe discrepancy: A critical analysis, *Learning Disabil. Q.* **4**:359–371.

CONNERS, C. K., 1972, Psychological effects of stimulant drugs in children with minimal brain dysfunction, *Pediatrics* **49:**702–708.
CONNERS, C. K., 1985, Methodological and assessment issues in pediatric psychopharmacology, in: *Diagnosis and Psychoparmacology of Childhood and Adolescent Disorders* (J. M. Wiener, ed.), John Wiley, New York, pp. 69–110.
CONNERS, C. K., and TAYLOR, E., 1980, Pemoline, methylphenidate, and placebo in children with minimal brain dysfunction, *Arch. Gen. Psychiatry* **37:**922–930.
CONNERS, C. K., ROTHCHILD, G., EISENBERG, L., SCHWARTZ, L. S., and ROBINSON, E., 1969, Dextroamphetamine sulfate in children with learning disorders: effects on perception, learning, achievement, *Arch. Gen. Psychiatry* **21:**182–190.
CONNERS, C. K., TAYLOR, E., MEO, G., KURTZ, M. A., and FOURNIER, M., 1972, Magnesium pemoline and dextroamphetamine: A controlled study in children with minimal brain dysfuntion, *Psychopharmacologia* **26:**321–336.
CONRAD, W. G., DWORKIN, E. S., SHAI, A., and TOBIESSEN, J. E., 1971, Effects of amphetamine therapy and prescriptive tutoring on the behavior and achievement of lower class hyperactive children, *J. Learning Disabil.* **4:**45–53.
CREESE, I., 1983, Classical and atypical antipsychotic drugs: New insights, *Trends Neurosci.* **6:**479–481.
DENCKLA, M. B., 1979, Childhood learning disabilities, in: *Clinical Neuropsychology* (K. M. Heilman and E. Valenstein, eds.), Oxford University Press, New York.
DENCKLA, M. B., BEMPORAD, J. R., and MACKAY, M. C., 1976, Tics following methylphenidate administration: A report of 20 cases, *JAMA* **235:**1349–1351.
DIMOND, S. J., and BROUWERS, E. Y. M., 1976, Increase in the power of human memory in normal man through the use of drugs, *Psychopharmacology* **49:**307–309.
DOUGLAS, V. I., 1983, Attentional and cognitive problems, in: *Developmental Neuropsychiatry* (M. Rutter, ed.), The Guilford Press, New York, pp. 280–329.
DYKMAN, R. A., ACKERMAN, P. T., and MCCRAY, D. S., 1980, Effects of methylphenidate on selective and sustained attention in hyperactive, reading disabled and presumably attention disordered boys, *J. Nerv. Ment. Dis.* **168:**745–752.
EASTGATE, S. M., WRIGHT, J. J., and WERRY, J. S., 1978, Behavioral effects of methylphenidate in 6-hydroxydopamine-treated rats, *Psychopharmacology* **58:**157–159.
EDELBROCK, C., COSTELLO, A. J., and KESSLER, M. D., 1984, Empirical corroboration of attention deficit disorder, *J. Am. Acad. Child Psychiatry* **23:**285–290.
ELDRIDGE, R., SWEET, R., LAKE, C. R., ZIEGLER, M., and SHAPIRO, A. K., 1977, Gilles de la Tourette's syndrome: Clinical, genetic, psychologic, and biochemical aspects in 21 selected families, *Neurology* **27:**115–124.
ELKINS, R., RAPOPORT, J., ZAHN, T., BUCHSBAUM, M., WEINGARTNER, H., KOPIN, I., LANGER, D., and JOHNSON, C., 1981, Acute effects of caffeine in normal prepubertal boys, *Am. J. Psychiatry* **138:**178–183.
ERINOFF, L., MACPHAIL, R. C., HELLER, A., and SEIDEN, L. S., 1979, Age-dependent effects of 6-hydroxydopamine on locomotor activity in the rat, *Brain Res.* **164:**195–205.
FAWCETT, J., MAAS, J. W., and DEKIRMENJIAN, H., 1972, Depression and MHPG excretion. Response to dextroamphetamine and tricyclic antidepressants, *Arch. Gen. Psychiatry* **26:**246–251.
FEINBERG, M., and CARROLL, B. J., 1979, Effects of dopamine agonists and antagonists in Tourette's disease, *Arch. Gen. Psychiatry* **36:**979–985.
FERGUSON, H. B., and RAPOPORT, J. L., 1983, Nosological issues and biological validation, in: *Developmental Neuropsychiatry* (M. Rutter, ed.), The Guilford Press, New York, pp. 369–384.
FINK, J. S., and REIS, D. J., 1981, Genetic variations in midbrain dopamine cell number: Parallel with differences in responses to dopaminergic agonists and in naturalistic behaviors mediated by central dopaminergic system, *Brain Res.* **222**(2):335–349.

FINK, J. S., and SMITH, G. P., 1979, Decreased locomotor and investigatory exploration after denervation of catecholamine terminal fields in the forebrain of rats, *J. Comp. Physiol. Psychol.* **93**:34.

FINK, J. S., and SMITH, G. P., 1980a, Mesolimbicocortical dopamine terminal fields are necessary for normal locomotor and investigatory exploration in rats, *Brain Res.* **199**:359–384.

FINK, J. S., and SMITH, G. P., 1980b, Relationships between selective denervation of dopamine terminal fields in the anterior forebrain and behavioral responses to amphetamine and apomorphine, *Brain Res.* **201**:107–127.

FINK, J. S., and SMITH, G. P., 1980c, Mesolimbic and mesocortical dopaminergic neurons are necessary for normal exploratory behavior in rats, *Neurosci. Lett.* **17**:61–65.

FINK, J. S., SWERDLOFF, A., JOH, T. H., and REIS, D. J., 1979, Genetic differences in ^{3}H-spiroperidol binding in caudate nucleus and cataleptic response to neuroleptic drugs in inbred mouse strains with different numbers of midbrain dopamine neurons, *Neurosci. Abstr.* **5**:647.

FINNERTY, R. J., SALTYS, J. J., and COLE, J. O., 1971, The use of *d*-amphetamine with hyperkinetic children, *Psychopharmacologia* **21**:302–308.

FOG, R., PAKKENBERG, REGEUR, L., and PAKKENBERG, B., 1982, "Tardive" Tourette syndrome in relation to long-term neuroleptic treatment of multiple tics, in: *Advances in Neurology,* Vol. 35 (A. J. Friedhoff and T. N. Chase, eds.), Raven Press, New York.

GADOW, K. D., 1981, Prevalence of drug treatment for hyperactivity and other childhood behavior disorders, in: *Psychological Aspects of Drug Treatment for Hyperactivity* (K. D. Gadow and J. Loney, eds.), Westview Press, Boulder, CO, pp. 13–76.

GADOW, K. D., 1983, Effects of stimulant drugs on academic performance in hyperactive and learning disabled children, *J. Learning Disabil.* **16**:190–299.

GAN, J., and CANTWELL, D. P., 1982, Dosage effects of methylphenidate on paired associate learning: Positive/negative placebo responders, *J. Am. Acad. Child Psychiatry* **21**:237–242.

GARFINKEL, B., WENDER, P., SLOMAN, L., O'NEIL, J., and GOLOMBEK, H., 1983, Tricyclic antidepressant and methylphenidate treatment of attention deficit disorder in children, *J. Am. Acad. Child Psychiatry* **22**:343–348.

GITTELMAN, R., 1980, Indications for the use of stimulant treatment in learning disorders, *J. Am. Acad. Child Psychiatry* **19**:623–636.

GITTELMAN, R., and FEINGOLD, I., 1983, Children with reading disorders. I. Efficiency of reading remediation, *J. Child Psychol. Psychiatry* **24**:167–191.

GITTELMAN-KLEIN, R., and KLEIN, D. F., 1976, Methylphenidate effects in learning disabilities, *Arch. Gen. Psychiatry* **33**:655–664.

GITTELMAN, R., KLEIN, D. F., and FEINGOLD, I., 1983, Children with reading disorders. II. Effects of methylphenidate in combination with reading remediation, *J. Child Psychol. Psychiatry* **24**:193–212.

GITTELMAN, R., MANNUZZA, S., SHENKER, R., and BONAGURA, N., 1985, Hyperactive boys almost grown up. I. Psychiatric status, *Arch. Gen. Psychiatry* **42**:937–947.

GLOWINSKI, J., TASSIN, J. P., and THIERRY, A. M., 1984, The mesocortico-prefrontal dopaminergic neurons, *Trends Neurosci.* **7**:415–418.

GOETZ, C. G., and KLAWANS, H. L., 1983, Stimulant-induced chorea: Clinical studies and animal models, in: *Stimulants: Neurochemical, Behavioral and Clinical Perspectives* (I. Creese, ed.), Raven Press, New York.

GOLDEN, G. S., 1974, Gilles de la Tourette's syndrome following methylphenidate administration, *Dev. Med. Child Neurol.* **16**:76–78.

GOLDENRING, J. R., WOOL, R. S., SHAYWITZ, B. A., BATTER, D. K., COHEN, D. J., YOUNG, J. G., and TEICHER, M. H., 1980, Effects of continuous gastric infusion of food dyes on developing rat pups, *Life Sci.* **27**:1897–1904.

GOLDMAN-RAKIC, P. S., 1984, The frontal lobes: Uncharted provinces of the brain, *Trends Neurosci.* **7**:425–429.

GOYETTE, C. H., CONNERS, C. K., and ULRICH, R. F., 1978, Normative data on revised Conners parent and teacher rating scales, *J. Abnorm. Child Psychol.* **6**:221–236.

GROVES, P. M., 1983, A theory of the functional organization of the neostriatum and the neostriatal control of voluntary movement, *Brain Res. Rev.* **5**:109–132.

GROVES, P. M., and TEPPER, J. M., 1983, Neuronal mechanisms of action of amphetamine, in: *Stimulants: Neurochemical, Behavioral, and Clinical Perspectives* (I. Creese, ed.), Raven Press, New York.

HALPERIN, J. M., GITTELMAN, R. KLEIN, D. F., and RUDEL, R. G., 1984, Reading disabled hyperactive children: A distinct subgroup of attention deficit disorder with hyperactivity? *J. Abnorm. Child Psychol.* **12**:1–14.

HANIN, I., MERIKANGAS, J. R., MERIKANGAS, K. R., et al., 1979, Red-cell choline and Gilles de la Tourette syndrome, *N. Engl. J. Med.* **301**:661–662.

HECHTMAN, L., WEISS, G., and PERLMAN, T., 1984, Young adult outcome of hyperactive children who received long-term stimulant treatment, *J. Am. Acad. Child Psychiatry* **23**:261–269.

HEFFNER, T. G., and SEIDEN, L. S., 1983, Impaired acquisition of an operant response in young rats depleted of brain dopamine in neonatal life, *Psychopharmacology* **79**:115–119.

HELFGOTT, E., RUDEL, R. G., and KRIEGER, J., 1984, Effect of piracetam on the single word and prose reading of dyslexic children, *Psychopharmacol. Bull.* **20**:688–690.

HOFFMAN, S., ENGLEHARDT, D., MARGOLIS, R., POLIZO, P., WAIZER, J., and ROSENFELD, R., 1974, Response to methylphenidate in low socioeconomic hyperactive children, *Arch. Gen. Psychiatry* **30**:354–359.

HOY, E., WEISS, G., MINDE, K., and COHEN, N., 1978, The hyperactive child at adolescence: Emotional, social, and cognitive functioning, *J. Abnorm. Child Psychol.* **6**:311–324.

HUESSY, H., and GENDRON, R., 1970, Prevalence of the so-called hyperkinetic syndrome in public school children of Vermont, *Acta Paediatr.* **37**:243–248.

HUESSY, H. R., METOYER, M., and TOWNSEND, M., 1974, Eight–ten year follow-up of 84 children treated for behavioral disorder in rural Vermont, *Acta Paedopsychiatr.* **40**(6):230–235.

HUNT, R. D., MINDERAA, R. B., and COHEN, D. J., 1985, Clonidine benefits children with attention deficit disorder and hyperactivity: Report of a double-blind placebo-crossover trial, *J. Am. Acad. Child Psychiatry* **24**:617–629.

IRWIN, M., BELENDIUK, K., McCLOSKEY, K., and FREEDMAN, D. X., 1981, Tryptophan metabolism in children with attention deficit disorder, *Am. J. Psychiatry* **138**:1082–1085.

IVERSEN, S. D., 1977, Brain dopamine systems and behavior, in: *Handbook of Psychopharmacology*, Vol. 8, *Drugs, Neurotransmitters, and Behavior* (L. L. Iversen, S. D. Iversen, and S. H. Snyder, eds.), Plenum Press, New York, pp. 333–384.

IVERSEN, S. D., and KOOB, G. F., 1977, Behavioral implications of dopaminergic neurons in the mesolimbic system, in: *Advances in Biochemical Psychopharmacology*, Vol. 16 (E. Costa and G. L. Gessa, eds.), Raven Press, New York, pp. 209–214.

JACOBS, B. L., TRULSON, M. E., HEYM, J., and STEINFELS, G. F., 1982, On the role of CNS serotonin in the motor abnormalities of Tourette Syndrome: Behavioral and single-unit studies, in: *Advances in Neurology* (A. J. Friedhoff and T. N. Chase, eds.), Raven Press, New York.

JASTAK, J. F. and JASTAK, S. R., 1978, *The Wide Range Achievement Test,* Jastak Associates, Wilmington, DE.

KAVALE, K., 1982, The efficiency of stimulant drug treatment for hyperactivity: A meta-analysis, *J. Learning Disabil.* **15**:280–289.

KEHNE, J. H., GALLAGER, D. W., and DAVIS, M., 1985, Spinalization unmasks clonidine's α_1-adrenergic mediated excitation of the flexor reflex in rats, *J. Neurosci.* **5**:1583–1590.
KELLY, P. H., 1977, Drug-induced motor behavior, in: *Handbook of Psychopharmacology*, Vol. 8, *Drugs, Neurotransmitters, and Behavior* (L. L. Iversen, S. D. Iversen, and S. H. Snyder, eds.), Plenum Press, New York, pp. 295–331.
KEOGH, B. K., 1971, Hyperactivity and learning disorders: Review and speculation, *Exceptional Children* **38**:101–110.
KHAN, A. U., and DEKIRMENJIAN, H., 1981, Urinary excretion of catecholamine metabolites in hyperkinetic child syndrome, *Am. J. Psychiatry* **138**(1):108–110.
KIDD, K. K., PRUSOFF, B. A., and COHEN, D. J., 1980, Familial pattern of Gilles de la Tourette syndrome, *Arch. Gen. Psychiatry* **37**:1336–1339.
KLAWANS, H. L., GOETZ, C. G., and PERLIK, S., 1980, Tardive dyskinesia: Review and update, *Am. J. Psychiatry* **137**:900–908.
KLAWANS, H. L., NAUSIEDA, P. A., GOETZ, C. G., TANNER, C. M., and WEINER, W. J., 1982, Tourette-like symptoms following chronic neuroleptic therapy, in: *Advances in Neurology*, Vol. 35 (A. J. Friedhoff and T. N. Chase, eds.), Raven Press, New York.
KNIGHTS, R. M., and HINTON, G. G., 1969, The effects of methylphenidate (Ritalin) on the motor skills and behavior of children with learning problems, *J. Nerv. Ment. Dis.* **148**:643–653.
KNOTT, P. J., and HUTSON, P. H., 1982, Stress-induced stereotypy in the rat: Neuropharmacological similarities to Tourette syndrome, in: *Advances in Neurology*, Vol. 35 (A. J. Friedhoff and T. N. Chase, eds.), Raven Press, New York.
KOOB, G. F., DEL FIACCO, M., and IVERSEN, S. D., 1977, Dissociable properties of dopamine neurons in the nigrostriatal and mesolimbic dopamine systems, in: *Advances in Biochemical Psychopharmacology*, Vol. 16 (E. Costa and G. L. Gessa, eds.), Raven Press, New York, pp. 589–595.
KOSLOW, S. H., and CROSS, C. K., 1982, Cerebrospinal fluid monoamine metabolites in Tourette syndrome and their neuroendrocrine implications, in: *Advances in Neurology*, Vol. 35 (A. J. Friedhoff and T. N. Chase, eds.), Raven Press, New York.
KRAGER, J., SAFER, D., and EARHARDT, J., 1979, Medication used to treat hyperactive children: Follow-up survey results, *J. School Health* **49**:317–321.
KUCZENSKI, R., 1983, Biochemical actions of amphetamine and other stimulants, in: *Stimulants: Neurochemical, Behavioral, and Clinical Perspectives* (I. Creese, ed.), Raven Press, New York.
LAHEY, B. B., SCHAUGHENCY, E. A., STRAUSS, C. C., and FRAME, C. L., 1984, Are attention deficit disorders with and without hyperactivity similar or dissimilar disorders? *J. Am. Acad. Child Psychiatry* **23**:302–309.
LAMBERT, N. M., and SANDOVAL, J., 1980, The prevalence of learning disabilities in a sample of children considered hyperactive, *J. Abnorm. Child Psychol.* **8**:33–50.
LAMBERT, N. M., SANDOVAL, J., and SASSONE, D., 1978, Prevalence of hyperactivity in elementary school children as a function of social system definers, *Am. J. Orthopsychiatry* **48**:446–463.
LANGER, D. H., RAPOPORT, J. L., BROWN, G. L., EBERT, M. H., and BUNNEY, W. E., JR., 1982, Behavioral effects of carbidopa-levodopa in hyperactive boys, *J. Am. Acad. Child Psychiatry* **21**(1):8–10.
LANGER, D., RAPOPORT, J., EBERT, M., LAKE, C. R., and NEE, L., 1985, Pilot trial of mianserin hydrochloride for childhood hyperactivity, in: *The Psychobiology of Childhood: Profiles in Current Issues* (B. Shopsin and L. Greenhill, eds.), Spectrum Publications, New York.
LECKMAN, J. F., COHEN, D. J., DETLOR, J., YOUNG, J. G., HARCHERIK, D., and SHAYWITZ, B. A., 1982, Clonidine in the treatment of Tourette syndrome: A review of data, in:

Advances in Neurology, Vol, 35 (A. J. Friedhoff and T. N. Chase, eds.), Raven Press, New York.

LECKMAN, J. F., DETLOR, J., HARCHERIK, D. F., et al., 1983, Acute and chronic treatment in Tourette syndrome: A preliminary report on clinical response and effect on plasma and urinary catecholamine metabolites, growth hormone, and blood pressure, *J. Am. Acad. Child Psychiatry* **22**:433–440.

LECKMAN, J. F., COHEN, D. J., GERTNER, J. M., ORT, S., and HARCHERIK, D. F., 1984, Growth hormone response to clonidine in children ages 4–17: Tourette's syndrome vs. children with short stature, *J. Am. Acad. Child Psychiatry* **23**:174–181.

LEES, A. J., FERNANDO, J. C. R., and CURZON, G., 1979, Serotonergic involvement in behavioral response to amphetamine at high dosage, *Neuropharmacology* **18**:153–158.

LLOYD, K. G., 1978, Neurotransmitter interactions related to central dopamine neurons, in: *Essays in Neurochemistry and Neuropharmacology,* Vol. 3 (M. B. H. Youdim, W. Lovenberg, D. F. Sharman, and J. R. Lagnado, eds.), Wiley, New York, pp. 129–207.

LONEY, J., LANGHORE, J. E., and PATERNITE, C. E., 1978, An empirical basis for subgrouping the hyperkinetic/minimal brain dysfunction syndrome, *J. Abnorm. Psychol.* **87**:431–441.

LONEY, J., KRAMER, J., and MILICH, R., 1981, The hyperactive child grows up: Prediction of symptoms, delinquency, and achievement at follow-up, in: *Psychosocial Aspects of Drug Treatment for Hyperactivity* (K. Gadow and J. Loney, eds.), Westview Press, Boulder, CO.

LOWE, T. L., COHEN, D. J., DETLOR, J., KREMENITZER, M. W., and SHAYWITZ, B. A., 1982, Stimulant medications precipitate Tourette's syndrome, *JAMA* **247**:1729–1731.

LYON, M., and ROBBINS, T. W., 1975, The action of central nervous system stimulant drugs: a general theory concerning amphetamine effects, in: *Current Developments in Psychopharmacology,* Vol. 2, Halsted Press, New York, pp. 80–163.

MAAS, J. W., and LECKMAN, J. F., 1983, Relationships between central nervous system noradrenegic function and plasma and urinary MHPG and other norepinephrine metabolites, in: *MHPG: Basic Mechanisms and Psychopathology* (J. W. Maas, ed.), Academic Press, New York.

MAAS, J. W., HATTOX, S. E., GREENE, N. M., and LANDIS, D. H., 1979, 3-Methoxy-4-hydroxphenethyleneglycol (MHPG) production by human brain *in vivo, Science* **205**:1025–1027.

MATTIS, S., 1978, Dyslexic syndromes: A working hypothesis that works, in: *Dyslexia: An Appraisal of Current Knowledge* (A. L. Benton and D. Pearl, eds.), Oxford University Press, New York.

MATTIS, S., FRENCH, J. H., and RAPIN, I., 1975, Dyslexia in children and young adults: Three independent neuropsychological syndromes, *Dev. Med. Child Neurol.* **17**:150–163.

MAURER, R. G., and STEWART, M. A., 1980, Attention deficit without hyperactivity in a child psychiatry clinic, *J. Clin. Psychiatry* **417**:232–233.

MENDELSON, W., JOHNSON, N., and STEWART, M. A., 1971, Hyperactive children as teenagers: A follow-up study, *J. Nerv. Ment. Dis.* **153**:273–279.

MIKKELSON, E., LAKE, C. R., BROWN, G. L., ZIEGLER, M. G., and EBERT, M. H., 1981, The hyperactive child syndrome: Peripheral sympathetic nervous system function and the effect of d-amphetamine, *Psychiatr. Res.* **4**(2):157–169.

MILLER, F. E., HEFFNER, T. G., KOTAKÉ, C., and SEIDEN, L. S., 1981, Magnitude and duration of hyperactivity following neonatal 6-hydroxydopamine is related to the extent of brain dopamine depleted, *Brain Res.* **229**:123–132.

MINDE, K., WEISS, G., and MENDELSON, N., 1972, A 5 year follow-up study of 91 hyperactive school children, *J. Am. Acad. Child Psychiatry* **11**:595–610.

MOLDOSKY, H., and BROWN, G.M., 1982, Tics and serum prolactin response to pimozide in Tourette syndrome, in: *Advances in Neurology,* Vol. 35 (A. J. Friedhoff and T. N. Chase, eds.), Raven Press, New York.

MOORE, K. E., 1978, Amphetamines: Biochemical and behavioral actions in animals, in: *Handbook of Psychopharmacology*, Vol. II, *Stimulants* (L. L. Iversen, S. D. Iversen, and S. H. Snyder, eds.), Plenum Press, New York, pp. 41–98.

NEIMARCK, E., SLOTNICK, N. and ULRICH, T., 1971, Development of memorization strategies, *Dev. Psychol.* **5**:427–432.

NIELSEN, E. B., EISON, M. S., LYONS, M., and IVERSEN, S. D., 1983, Hallucinating behaviors in primates produced by around-the-clock amphetamine treatment for several days via implanted capsules, in: *Ethopharmacology: Primate Models of Neuropsychiatric Disorders* (K. A. Miczek, ed.), Liss, New York, pp. 79–100.

NOSE, T., and TAKEMOTO, H., 1975, The effect of penfluridol and some psychotropic drugs on monoamine metabolism in central nervous system, *Eur. J. Pharmacol.* **31**:351–359.

PAULS, D. L., COHEN, D. L., HEIMBUCH, R., DETLOR, J., and KIDD, K. K., 1981, Familial pattern and transmission of Gilles de la Tourette syndrome and multiple tics, *Arch. Gen. Psychiatry* **38**:1085–1090.

PEARSON, D. E., TEICHER, M. H., SHAYWITZ, B. A., COHEN, D. J., YOUNG, J. G., and ANDERSON, G. M., 1980, Environmental influences on body weight and behavior in developing rats after neonatal 6-hydroxydopamine, *Science* **209**:715–717.

PELHAM, W. E., 1983, The effects of psychostimulants on academic achievement in hyperactive and learning disabled children, *Int. Acad. Res. Learning Disabil.* **3**:1–48.

PELHAM, W. E., BENDER, M. E., CADDELL, J., BOOTH, S., and MOORER S. H., 1985, Methylphenidate and children with attention deficit disorder: Dose effects on classroom academic and social behavior, *Arch. Gen. Psychiatry* **42**:948–952.

PORRINO, L. J., RAPOPORT, J. L., BEHAR, D., SCEERY, W., ISMOND, D. R., and BUNNEY JR., W. E., 1983a, A naturalistic assessment of the motor activity of hyperactive boys, I. Comparison with normal controls, *Arch Gen Psychiatry* **40**:681–687.

PORRINO, L. J., RAPOPORT, J. L., BEHAR D., IMOND, D. R., and BUNNEY JR., W. E., 1983b, A naturalistic assessment of the motor activity of hyperactive boys, II. Stimulant drug effects, *Arch. Gen. Psyciatry* **40**:688–693.

QUINN, P. O., and RAPOPORT, J. L., 1975, One-year follow-up of hyperactive boys treated with imipramine or methylphenidate, *Am. J. Psychiatry*, **132**:241–245.

RAPOPORT, J. L., QUINN, P. O., BRADBARD, G., RIDDLE, D., and BROOKS, E., 1974, Imipramine and methylphenidate treatments of hyperactive boys, *Arch. Gen. Psychiatry* **30**:789–793.

RAPOPORT, J., BUCHSBAUM, M., ZAHN, T., WEINGARTNER, H., LUDLOW, L., and MIKKELSEN, E., 1978a, Dextroamphetamine: Behavioral and cognitive effects in normal prepubertal boys, *Science* **199**:560–563.

RAPOPORT, J. L., MIKKELSEN, E. J., EBERT, M. H., BROWN, G. L., WEISE, V. K., and KOPIN, I. J., 1978b, Urinary catecholamines and amphetamine excretion in hyperactive and normal boys, *J. Nerv. Ment. Dis.* **166**(10):731–737.

RAPOPORT, J., BUCHSBAUM, M., WEINGARTNER, H., ZAHN, T., LUDLOW, C., BARTKO, J., and MIKKELSEN, E. J. 1980, Dextroamphetamine: Cognitive and behavioral effects in normal and hyperactive boys and normal adult males, *Arch. Gen. Psychiatry* **37**:933–943.

RAPOPORT, J. L., BERG, C. J., ISMOND, D. R., ZAHN, T. P., and NEIMS, A., 1984, Behavioral effects of caffeine in children: Relationship between dietary choice and effects of caffeine challenge, *Arch. Gen. Psychiatry* **41**(11):1073–1079.

RAPOPORT, M. D., MURPHY, H. A., and BAILEY, J. S., 1982, Ritalin vs. response cost in the control of hyperactive children: A within-subject comparison, *J. Appl. Behav. Anal.* **15**:205–216.

RAPOPORT, M. D., DUPAUL, G. J., STONER, G., BIRMINGHAM B. K., and MASSE, G., 1985, Attention deficit disorder with hyperactivity: Differential effects of methylphenidate on impulsivity, *Pediatrics* **76**:938–943.

REIS, D. J., BAKER, H., and FINK, J. S., 1982, Genetic control of the number of dopamine neurons in mouse brain: Its relationship to brain morphology, chemistry, and behavior, in: *Genetic Strategies in Psychobiology and psychiatry* (E. S. Gerhson, S. Matthyse, X. O. Breakfield, and R. Ciarnanello, eds.), Boxwood Press, Pacific Grove, CA.

REIS, D. J., FINK, J. S., and BAKER, H., 1983, Genetic control of the number of dopamine neurons in the brain: Relationship to behavior and responses to psychoactive drugs, in: *Genetics of Neurological and Psychiatric Disorders* (S. S. Kety, L. P. Rowland, R. L. Sidman, and S. W. Matthysse, eds.), Raven Press, New York.

REYNOLDS, C. R., 1981, The fallacy of "two years below grade level for age" as a diagnostic criterion for reading disorders, *J. School Psychol.* **19**:350–358.

RIDDLE, K. D., and RAPOPORT, J. L., 1976, A 2-year follow-up of 72 hyperactive boys, *J. Nerv. Ment. Dis.* **162**:126–134.

RIE, D. R., and RIE, H. E., 1977, Recall, retention and Ritalin, *J. Consult. Clin. Psychol.* **45**:967–972.

RIE, H. E., RIE, E. D., STEWART, S., and AMBUEL, P., 1976, Effects of methylphenidate on underachieving children, *J. Consult. Clin. Psychol.* **44**:250–260.

ROBBINS, T. W., 1984, Cortical noradrenaline, attention, and arousal, *Psychol. Medi.* **14**:13–21.

ROBBINS, T. W., and SAHAKIAN, B. J., 1979, "Paradoxical" effects of psychomotor stimulant drugs in hyperactive children from the standpoint of behavioral pharamcology, *Neuropharmacology* **18**:931–950.

ROSENBERG, G. S., and DAVIS, K. L., 1982, Precursors of acetylcholine: Considerations underlying their use in Tourette syndrome, in: *Advances in Neurology,* Vol. 35 (A. J. Friedhoff and T. N. Chase, eds.), Raven Press, New York.

ROSS, M. S., and MOLDOFSKY, H., 1977, Comparison of pimozide with haloperidol in Gilles de la Tourette syndrome, *Lancet* **1**:103.

ROSS, R. A., JUDD, A. B., PICKEL, V. M., JOH, T. H., and REIS, D. J., 1976, Strain-dependent variations in number of midbrain dopaminergic neurons, *Nature* **264**:654–656.

RUDEL, R. G., and HELFGOTT, E., 1984, Effect of piracetam on verbal memory of dyslexic boys, *J Am. Acad. Child Psychiatry* **23**:695–699.

RUTTER, M., 1983, Behavioral studies: Questions and findings on the concept of a distinctive syndrome, in: *Developmental Neuropsychiatry* (M. Rutter, ed.), The Guilford Press, New York, pp. 259–279.

RUTTER, M., and YULE, W., 1975, The concept of specific reading retardation, *J. Child Psychol. Psychiatry* **16**:181–197.

SANDBERG, S. T., WIESELBERG, M., and SHAFFER, D., 1980, Hyperkinetic and conduct problem children in a primary school population. Some epidemiological considerations, *J. Child Psychol. Psychiatry* **21**:293–311.

SATIN, M. S., WINSBERG, B. G., MONETTI, C. H., SVERD, J., and FOSS, D. A., 1985, A general population screen for attention deficit disorder with hyperactivity, *J. Am. Acad. Child Psychiatry* **24**:756–764.

SATTERFIELD, J. H., CANTWELL, D. P., SAUL, R. E., LESSER, L. I., and PODOSIN, R. L., 1973, Response to stimulant drug treatment in hyperactive children: prediction from EEG and neurological findings, *J. Aut. Child. Schizo.* **3**:36–48.

SATTERFIELD, J., SATTERFIELD, B., and CANTWELL, D., 1981, Three-year multimodality treatment study of hyperactive boys, *J. Pediatrics* **98**:650–655.

SATTERFIELD, J. H., HOPE, C. M., and SCHELL, A. M., 1982, A prospective study of delinquency in 110 adolescent boys with attention deficit disorder and 88 normal adolescent boys, *Am. J. Psychiatry* **139**:119–120.

SEEMAN, P., and LEE, T., 1975, Antipsychotic drugs: direct correlation between clinical potency and presynaptic action on dopamine neurons, *Science* **188**:1217–1219.

SEGAL, D. S., and SCHUKIT, M. A., 1983, Animal models of stimulant-induced psychosis, in: *Stimulants: Neurochemical, Behavioral, and Clinical Perspectives*, Raven Press, New York.

SELEMON, L. D., and GOLDMAN-RAKIC, P. S., 1985, Longitudinal topography and interdigitation of corticostriatal projections in the rhesus monkey, *J. Neurosci.* **5:**776–794.

SELINGER, D., COHEN, D. J., ORT, S., ANDERSON, G. M., CARUSO, K. A., and LECKMAN, J. F., 1984, Parotid salivary response to clonidine in Tourette's syndrome: Indicator of adrenergic responsivity, *J. Am. Acad. Child Psychiatry* **23:**392–398.

SHAFFER, D., and GREENHILL, L., 1979, A critical note on the predictive validity of "the hyperkinetic syndrome," *J. Child Psychol. Psychiatry* **20:**61–72.

SHAFFER, D., O'CONNER, P. A., SHAFER, S. Q., and PRUPIS, S., 1983, Neurological "soft signs": Their origins and significance for behavior, in: *Developmental Neuropsychiatry* (M. Rutter, ed.), The Guilford Press, New York, pp. 144–163.

SHAFFER, D., SCHONFELD, I., O'CONNOR, P. A., STOKMAN, C., TRAUTMAN, P. SHAFER S., and NG, S., 1985, Neurological soft signs: Their relationship to psychiatric disorder and intelligence in childhood and adolescence, *Arch. Gen. Psychiatry* **42:**342–351.

SHAPIRO, A. K., and SHAPIRO, E., 1981, Do stimulants provoke, cause or exacerbate tics or Tourette syndrome? *Compr. Psychiatry* **22(3):**265–273.

SHAPIRO, A. K., and SHAPIRO, E., 1982*b*, Clinical efficacy of haloperidol, pimozide, penfluridol, and clonidine in the treatment of Tourette syndrome, in: *Gilles de la Tourette Syndrome. Advances in Neurology*, Vol. 35 (A. J. Friedhoff and T. N. Chase, eds.), Raven Press, New York, pp. 383–386.

SHAPIRO, A. K., and SHAPIRO, E., 1984, Controlled study of pimozide vs. placebo in Tourette's syndrome, *J. Am. Acad.Child Psychiatry* **23(2):**161–173.

SHAPIRO, A. K., SHAPIRO, E., WAYNE, H. L., and CLARKIN, J., 1973*a*, Organic factors in Gilles de la Tourette's syndrome, *Br. J. Psychiatry* **122:**659–664.

SHAPIRO, A. K., SHAPIRO, E., and WAYNE, H. L. 1973*b*, Treatment of Gilles de la Tourette's syndrome with haloperidol: Review of 34 cases, *Arch. Gen. Psychiatry*, **28:**92–96.

SHAPIRO, A. K., SHAPIRO, E., BRUNN, R. D., and SWEET, R. D., 1978, *Gilles de la Tourette's Syndrome*, Raven Press, New York.

SHAPIRO, A. K., SHAPIRO, E., and EISENKRAFT, G. J., 1983, Treatment of Gilles de la Tourette syndrome with pimozide, *Am. J. Psychiatry* **140:**1183–1186.

SHAPIRO, E., and SHAPIRO, A. K., 1982*a*, Tardive dyskinesia and chronic neuroleptic treatment of Tourette patients, in: *Advances in Neurology*, Vol. 35 (A. J. Friedhoff and T. N. Chase, eds.), Raven Press, New York.

SHAPIRO, T., 1985, Developmental considerations in psychopharmacology: The interaction of drugs and development, in: *Diagnosis and Psychopharmacology of Childhood and Adolescent Disorders* (J. M. Wiener, ed.), Wiley, New York, pp. 51–68.

SHAPIRO, T., and PERRY, R., 1976, Latency revisited: The age of seven plus or minus one, *Psychoanal Study Child.* **31:**79–105.

SHAYWITZ, B. A., and PEARSON, D. E., 1978, Effects of phenobarbital on activity and learning in 6-hydroxydopamine-treated rat pups, *Pharmacol. Biochem. Behav.* **9:**173–179.

SHAYWITZ, B. A., YAGER, R. D., KLOPPER, J. H., and GORDON, J. W., 1976*a*, Paradoxical response to amphetamine in developing rats treated with 6-hydroxypopamine, *Nature* **261:**153–155.

SHAYWITZ, B. A., YAGER, R. D., and KLOPPER, J. H., 1976*b*, Selective brain dopamine depletion in developing rats: An experimental model of minimal brain dysfunction, *Science* **191:**305–308.

SHAYWITZ, B. A., GORDON, J. W., KLOPPER, J. H., and ZELTERMAN, D., 1977*a*, The effect of 6-hydroxydopamine on habituation activity in the developing rat pup, *Pharmacol. Biochem. Behav.* **6:**391–396.

SHAYWITZ, B. A., COHEN, D. J., and BOWERS, M. B., JR., 1977*b*, CSF monoamine metabolites in children with minimal brain dysfunction: Evidence for alteration of brain dopamine, *J. Pediatr.* **90**:67–71.

SHAYWITZ, B. A., KLOPPER, J. H., and GORDON, J. W., 1978, Methylphenidate in 6-hydroxdopamine-treated developing rat pups, *Arch. Neuro.* **35**:463–469.

SHAYWITZ, B. A., TEICHER, M. H., COHEN, D. J., ANDERSON, G. M., YOUNG, J. G., and LEVITT, P., 1984, Dopaminergic, but not noradrenergic mediation of hyperactivity and performance deficits in the developing rat pup, *Psychopharmacology* **82**:73–77.

SHAYWITZ, S. E., HUNT, R. D., JATLOW, P., COHEN, D. J., YOUNG, J. G., PIERCE, R. N., ANDERSON, G. M., and SHAYWITZ, B. A., 1982, Psychopharmacology of attention deficit disorder: Pharmacokinetic, neuroendocrine, and behavioral measures following acute and chronic treatment with methylphenidate, *Pediatrics* **69**:688–694.

SHEKIM, W. O., DEKIRMENJIAN, H., and CHAPEL, J. L., 1977, Urinary catecholamine metabolites in hyperkinetic boys treated with d-amphetamine, *Am. J. Psychiatry* **134**(11):1276–1279.

SHEKIM, W. O., and DEKIRMENJIAN, H., 1978, Catecholamine metabolites in nonhyperactive boys with arithmetic learning disability: A pilot study, *Am. J. Psychiatry* **135**:490–491.

SHEKIM, W. O., DEKIRMENJIAN, J., and CHAPEL, J. L., 1979a, Urinary MHPG excretion in minimal brain dysfunction and its modification by d-amphetamine, *Am. J. Psychiatry* **136**(5):667–671.

SHEKIM, W. O., DEKIRMENJIAN, H., CHAPEL, J. L., JAVAID, J., and DAVIS, J. M., 1979b, Norephinephrine metabolism and clinical response to dextroamphetamine in hyperactive boys, *J. Pediatr.* **95**:389–394.

SHEKIM, W. O., KASHANI, J., BECK, N., CANTWELL, D. P., MARTIN, J., ROSENBERG, J., and COSTELLO, A., 1985, The prevalence of attention deficit disorders in a rural midwestern community sample of nine-year-old children, *J. Am. Acad. Child Psychiatry* **24**:765–770.

SHETTY, T., and CHASE, T. N., 1978, Central monoamines and hyperkinesis of childhood, *Neurology* **26**:1000–1002.

SILVER, L. B., 1981, The relationship between learning disabilities, hyperactivity, distractibility, and behavior problems: A clinical analysis, *J. Am. Acad. Child Psychiatry* **20**:385–397.

SIMEON, J., WATERS, B., RESNICK, M., FIEDOROWICZ, C., TRITES, R., VOLAVKA, J., and SIMEON, S., 1979, Clinical and EEG effects of piracetam on children with learning disorders, in: *International Symposium on Nootropic Drugs*, Sociedade de Medicina e Cirurgia de Rio de Janeiro, pp. 81–88.

SIMEON, J., WATERS, B., and RESNICK, M., 1980, Effects of piracetam in children with learning disorders, *Psychopharmacol. Bull.* **16**:65–66.

SINGER, H. S., TUNE, L. F., BUTLER, I. J., ZACZEK, R., and COYLE, J. T., 1982, Clinical symptomatology, CSF neurotransmitter metabolites, and serum haloperidol levels in Tourette syndrome, in: *Advances in Neurology*, Vol. 35 (A. J. Friedhoff and T. N. Chase, eds.), Raven Press, New York.

SKIRBOLL, L. R., GRACE, A. A., and BUNNEY, B. S., 1979, Dopamine auto- and post-synaptic receptors: Electrophysiological evidence for differential sensitivity to dopamine agonists, *Science* **206**:80–82.

SLOVITER, R. S., DRUST, E. G., and CONNOR, J. D., 1978, Evidence that serotonin mediates some behavioral effects of amphetamine, *J. Pharmacol. Ther.* **206**:348–352.

SOLANTO, M. V., 1986, Behavioral effects of low-dose methylphenidate in childhood attention deficit disorder: Implications for a mechanism of stimulant drug action, *J. Am. Acad. Child Psychiatry* **25**:96–101.

SORENSON, C. A., VAYER, J. S., and GOLDBERG, C. S., 1977, Amphetamine reduction of motor activity in rats after neonatal administration of 6-hydroxydopamine, *Biol. Psychiatry* **12**:133–137.

SPRAGUE, R. L., and SLEATOR, E. K., 1977, Methylphenidate in hyperkinetic children: Differences in dose effects on learning and social behavior, *Science* **198**:1274–1276.

SPRAGUE, R. L., BARNES, K. R., and WERRY, J. S., 1970, Methylphenidate and thioridazine: Learning, reaction time, activity, and class room behavior in disturbed children, *Am. J. Orthopsychiatry* **40**:615–28.

STAHL, S. M., and BERGER, P. A., 1980, Cholinergic treatment in the Tourette syndrome, *N. Engl. J. Med.* **302**:1311.

STAHL, S. M., and BERGER, P. A., 1981, Physostigmine in Tourette syndrome: Evidence for cholinergic underactivity, *Am. J. Psychiatry* **138**:240–242.

STAHL, S. M., and BERGER, P. A., 1982, Cholinergic and dopaminergic mechanisms in Tourette syndrome, in: *Advances in Neurology*, Vol. 35 (A. J. Friedhoff and T. N. Chase, eds.), Raven Press, New York.

STEGNICK, A. J., 1972, The clinical use of piracetam: A new nootropic drug, The treatment of symptoms of senile involution, *Arzneim.-Forsch. Drug Res.* **22**:975–977.

STEPHENS, R., PELHAM, W. E., and SKINNER, R., 1984, The state-dependent and main effects of pemoline and methylphenidate on paired-associate learning and spelling in hyperactive children, *J. Consult. Clin. Psychol.* **52**:104–113.

STEWART, M. A., CUMMINGS, C., SINGER, S., and DEBLOIS, C. S., 1981, The overlap between hyperactive and unsocialized aggressive children, *J. Child. Psychol. Psychiatry* **22**:35–45.

STOOF, J. C., DIJKSTRA, H., and HILLEGERS, J. P. M., 1978, Changes in the behavioral response to a novel environment following lesioning of the central dopaminergic system in rat pups, *Psychopharmacology* **57**:163–170.

SWANSON, J., and KINSBOURNE, M., 1976, Stimulant related state-dependent learning in hyperactive children, *Science* **192**:1354–1356.

SWANSON, J., and KINSBOURNE, M., 1979, The cognitive effects of stimulant drugs on hyperactive (inattentive) children, in: *Attention and The Development of Cognitive Skills* (G. Hale and M. Lewis, eds.), Plenum Press, New York, pp. 249–274.

SWANSON, J. M., KINSBOURNE, M., ROBERTS, W., and ZUCKER, K., 1978, Time-response analysis of the effect of stimulant medication on the learning ability of children referred for hyperactivity, *Pediatrics* **61**:21–29. 1978.

TRULSON, M. E., and JACOBS, B. L., 1979, Long-term amphetamine treatment decreases brain serotonin metabolism: Implications for theories of schizophrenia, *Science* **205**:1295–1297.

VAN ROSSUM, J. M., BROEKKAMP, C. L. E., and PIJNENBURG, A. J. J., 1977, Behavioral correlates of dopaminergic function in the nucleus accumbens, in: *Advances in Biochemical Psychopharmacology*, Vol 16 (E. Costa and G. L. Gessa, eds.), Raven Press, New York, pp. 201–207.

VAN WOERT, M. H., ROSENBAUM, D., HOWIESON, J., and BOWERS, M. B., JR., 1977a, Long-term therapy of myoclonus and other neurologic disorders with L-5-hydroxytryptophan and carbidopa, *N. Engl. J. Med.* **296**:70–75.

VAN WOERT, M. H., YIP, L. C., and BALIS, M. E., 1977b, Purine phosphoribosyltransferase in Gilles de la Tourette syndrome, *N. Engl. J. Med.* **296**:210–212.

VAN WOERT, M. H., ROSENBAUM, D., and ENNA, S. J., 1982, Overview of pharmacological approaches to therapy for Tourette syndrome, in: *Advances in Neurology*, Vol. 35 (A. J. Friedhoff and T. N. Chase, eds.), Raven Press, New York.

VOLKMAR, F. R., LECKMAN, J. F., DETLOR, J., HARCHERIK, D. F., PRICHARD, J. W., SHAYWITZ, B. A., and COHEN, D. J., 1984, EEG abnormalities in Tourette's syndrome, *J. Am. Acad. Child Psychiatry* **23**:352–353.

WEINGARTNER, H., RAPOPORT, J. L., BUCHSBAUM, M. S., BUNNEY, W. E., EBERT, M. H., MIKKELSEN, E. J., and CAINE, E. D., 1980, Cognitive processes in normal and hyperactive children and their response to amphetamine treatment, *J. Abnorm. Psychol.* **89**:25–37.

WEINGARTNER, H., LANGER, D., GRICE, J., and RAPOPORT, J., 1982, Acquisition and retrieval of information in amphetamine treated hyperactive children, *Psychiatry Res.* **6:**21–29.

WEISS, G., 1983, Long-term outcome: Findings, concepts, and practical implications, in: *Developmental Neuropsychiatry* (M. Rutter, ed.), The Guilford Press, New York, pp. 422–436.

WEISS, G., MINDE, K., DOUGLAS, V., WERRY, J., and SYKES, D., 1971, Comparison of the effects of chlorpromazine, dextroamphetamine, and methylphenidate on the behavior and intellectual functions of hyperactive children, *Can Med. Assoc. J.* **104:**20–25.

WEISS, G., KRUGER, E., DANIELSON, U., and ELMAN, M., 1975, Effect of long term treatment of hyperactive children with methylphenidate, *Can. Med. Assoc. J.* **112:**159–165.

WEISS, G., HECHTMAN, L., PERLMAN, T., HOPKINS, J., and WENAR, A., 1979, Hyperactives as young adults. A controlled prospective ten-year follow-up of 75 children, *Arch. Gen. Psychiatry* **36:**675–681.

WEISS, G., HECHTMAN, L., MILROY, T., and PERLMAN, T., 1985, Psychiatric status of hyperactives as adults: A controlled prospective 15-year follow-up of 63 hyperactive children, *J. Am. Acad. Child Psychiatry* **24:**211–220.

WENDER, P. H., EPSTEIN, R. S., KOPIN, I. J., and GORDON, E. K., 1971, Urinary monamine metabolites in children with minimal brain dysfunction, *Am. J. Psychiatry* **127:**1411–1415.

WERRY, J. S., and SPRAGUE, R. L., 1974, Methylphenidate in children, effects of dosage, *Aust. N.Z. J. Psychiatry* **8:**9–19.

WILSHER, C. R., and MILEWSKI, J., 1983, Effects of piracetam on dyslexics verbal conceptualizing ability. *Psychopharmacol. Bull.* **19:**3–4.

WILSHER, C. R., ATKINS, G., and MANFELD, P., 1979, Piracetam as an aid to learning in dyslexia: Preliminary report, *Psychopharmacologia* **65:**107–109.

WILSHER, C. R., ATKINS, G., and MANFELD, P., 1984, Effect of piracetam on dyslexics' reading ability, *J. Learning Disabil.* **18:**19–25.

WOLRICH, M., DRUMMOND, T., SALOMON, M. K., O'BRIEN, M. L., and SIVAGE, C., 1978, Effects of methylphenidate alone and in combination with behavior modification procedures on the behavior and academic performance of hyperactive children, *J. Abnorm. Child Psychol.* **6**(1)**:**149–161.

YOUNG, J. G., 1981, Methylphenidate-induced hallucinations: Case histories and possible mechanisms of action, *J. Dev. Behav. Pediatr.* **2:**35–38.

YOUNG, J. G., 1985, The neurobiology of memory and learning in childhood, in: *Psychiatry* (J. O. Cavenar, Jr., and R. Michels, eds.), Lippincott, Philadelphia.

YOUNG, J. G., COHEN, D. J., HATTOX, S. E., KAVANAGH, M. E., ANDERSON, G. M., SHAYWITZ, B. A., and MAAS, J. W., 1981a, Plasma free MHPG and neuroendocrine responses to challenge doses of clonidine in Tourette's syndrome: Preliminary report, *Life Sci.* **29:**1467–1475.

YOUNG, J. G., COHEN, D. J., KAVANAGH, M. E., LANDIS, H. D., SHAYWITZ, B. A., and MAAS, J. W., 1981b, Cerebrospinal fluid, plasma, and urinary MHPG in children, *Life Sci.* **28:**2837–2845.

YOUNG, J. G., COHEN, D. J., SHAYWITZ, S. E., CAPARULO, B. K., KAVANAGH, M. E., HUNT, R. D., LECKMAN, J. F., ANDERSON, G. M., DETLOR, J., HARCHERIK, D., and SHAYWITZ, B. A., 1982, Assessment of brain function in clinical pediatric research: Behavioral and biological strategies, *Schizophrenia Bull.* **8**(2)**:**205–235.

YOUNG, J. G., COHEN, D. J., ANDERSON, G. M., and SHAYWITZ, B. A., 1984, Neurotransmitter ontogeny as a perspective for studies of child development and pathology, in: *The Psychobiology of Childhood* (L. Greenhill and B. Shopsin, eds.), Spectrum Publications, New York.

YOUNG, J. G., LEVEN, L. I., KNOTT, P. J., LECKMAN, J. F., and COHEN, D. J., 1985, Tourette's syndrome and tic disorders, in: *Diagnosis and Psychopharmacology of Childhood and Adolescent Disorders* (J. M. Wiener, ed.), Wiley, New York.

Yu-Cun, S., and Wang, Y-F., 1984, Urinary 3-methoxy-4-hydroxyphenylglycol sulfate excretion in seventy-three schoolchildren with minimal brain dysfunction syndrome, *Biol. Psychiatry* **19**:861–870.

Zametkin, A., Brown, G., Karoum, G., Rapoport, J., Chuang, L., Langer, D., and Wyatt, R., 1984a, Urinary phenylethylamine response to *d*-amphetamine in boys with attention deficit disorder, *Am. J. Psychiatry* **141**:1055–1058.

Zametkin, A. J., Karoum, F., Rapoport, J. L., Brown, G. L., and Wyatt, R. J., 1984b, Phenylethylamine excretion in attention deficit disorder, *J. Am. Acad. Child Psychiatry* **23**:310–314.

Zametkin, A. J. Karoum, F., Linnoila, M., Rapoport, J. L., Brown, G. L., Chuang, L-W., and Wyatt, R. J., 1985a, Stimulants, urinary catecholamines, and indoleamines in hyperactivity: A comparison of methylphenidate and dextroamphetamine, *Arch. Gen. Psychiatry* **42**:251–255.

Zametkin, A., Rapoport, J. L., Murphy, D. L., Linnoila, M., and Ismond, D., 1985b, Treatment of hyperactive children with monoamine oxidase inhibitors. I. Clinical efficacy, *Arch. Gen Psychiatry* **42**:962–966.

Zametkin, A., Rapoport, J. L., Murphy, D. L., Linnoila, M., Karoum, F., Potter, W. Z. and Ismond D. 1985c, Treatment of hyperactive children with monoamine oxidase inhibitors. II. Plasma and urinary monoamine findings after treatment, *Arch. Gen. Psychiatry* **42**(1b):969–973.

# 3

STRUCTURE, PROCESS, AND MECHANISM: CASE STUDIES IN THE PSYCHOPHARMACOLOGY OF FEEDING

John E. Blundell

1. INTRODUCTION

In the area of physiological psychology, the study of mechanisms controlling food intake has always occupied a central position. Indeed, one of the first elaborate accounts of a central theory of drive used feeding as the primary example of a motivated behavior (Morgan, 1943). With the change in emphasis in theorizing from a neuroanatomical mode of the 1950s to a largely neurochemical mode of the 1970s, an increasing penetration of physiological psychology by pharmacological techniques and ideas has occurred. In turn, this has led to a large number of studies on the effect of drugs on food intake. A casual inspection of the literature indicates that over the years hundreds of chemical agents have been shown to adjust food consumption in experimental animals. The most frequent form of adjustment is a suppression of intake. This seductive array of data suggests that the "behavioral pharmacology of feeding" is a research area in a healthy state of development. However, this prolifera-

---

John E. Blundell • BioPsychology Laboratories, Psychology Department, University of Leeds, Leeds LS2 9JT, United Kingdom.

tion of numbers may be misleading for, as in other areas of psychopharmacology, it is relatively easy to obtain statistically significant effects by drug administration, and consequently, it is easy to demonstrate some relationship between a drug and food consumption. It is worth noting that not all such events elucidate the action of a drug or the operation of systems controlling feeding. How is it possible to make sense of the numbers? Indeed, the problematic issue in this field is to provide appropriate interpretations for the ever-increasing number of grams of food eaten or left unconsumed by animals after drug treatment (Blundell, 1981a). The argument presented in this chapter will be that it is possible to develop a cohesive theoretical framework to improve understanding of the pharmacological manipulations of feeding. This argument is based on two major themes:

First, explanatory power can be enhanced by a close examination of the structure of behavior (e.g., Fentress, 1976; Blundell, 1981b). Often, experiments involving sophisticated pharmacological or neurochemical manipulations fail to achieve full potential, since only coarse shifts in behavior have been measured. Of course, a detailed description of structure alone will not readily advance thinking, but a knowledge of *structure* is important when it is used to illuminate *process* and *mechanism* (to be defined later). In other words, structure provides insight into the way in which behavior is organized and how its expression is controlled.

Second, the argument promotes a movement away from the notion of simple cause–effect relationships underlying the control of feeding and the design of experiments involving pharmacological agents (e.g., Blundell, 1982a). This strategy is in keeping with the encouragement Waddington (1977) gave scientists: to abandon the study of rigid causes and effects and instead to interpret the world in terms of interacting processes. Evidence will be provided later to demonstrate that the study of feeding represents a classic example of chains of interactions, which only arbitrarily can be segmented into cause–response units. The undertaking to consider behavior as complex interactions does not render the investigation of feeding less precise, but it does have implications for the design and interpretation of experiments.

It is intended that these two themes taken together will allow a clearer conceptualization of the design of future research. This exercise need not entail the construction of an exclusive psychopharmacological theory, for it seems appropriate, given our current level of knowledge, to incorporate psychopharmacological data within a broader framework of biobehavioral processes. Accordingly, this chapter will seek to develop an expanded theoretical network and to show how pharmacological manipulations penetrate the fabric of interrelationships surrounding feeding activities. The ultimate goal must be to use the psychopharmacological method to disclose the mode of action of mechanisms responsible for the control of feeding behavior.

2. CONTROL OF FEEDING: A FIRST LOOK

In the last 25 years, theory in feeding research has been directed by two major influences. The first of these was the development of experimentation within the tradition of the physiology of regulation. This emphasized the principle of homeostasis and on the maintenance of body weight as a convenient index of regulation. Food intake, measured according to calories or weight of feed consumed, was conceived in quantitative terms as one of the agents *controlled* in the interests of body weight *regulation*. Consequently, the activity of feeding was relegated to a secondary and lowly position as the instrument supplying calories to the body. Many experiments were designed to examine the relationship between caloric intake and body weight (following a variety of treatments) on the belief that this would shed light on the physiological mechanisms responsible for regulation. Although this forceful line of research has produced advances in knowledge of the physiology of regulation, the emphasis on the function of food intake has had the effect of restraining research on the truly behavioral aspects of feeding. The argument to be presented here is that a behavioral analysis of feeding activity can illuminate processes and mechanisms involved in control and regulation. More recently, interest has shifted to assign a more prominent position to energy utilization in the regulation of body weight (e.g., Keesey, 1980; Rothwell and Stock, 1979).

The second major influence has come from central theories of motivation, among which the most widely elaborated was the dual-center approach of Stellar (1954). This theoretical arrangement was broader in scope and more detailed than has often been recognized, and many of the complex operating features have been passed over by researchers in favor of a much simpler, but experimentally more convenient picture. For example, Stellar's notion of a center was a functional entity that did not carry with it the idea of a small, concentrated, fixed physical locus in the brain. In addition, Stellar emphasized the role of a central motivational mechanism as an integrator of inputs through interoceptive (physiological) and exteroceptive (environmental) channels. Although Stellar drew attention to the position of the brain within a larger system, the most dramatic pieces of experimental evidence had the effect of encouraging researchers on motivation to go directly to the brain. Only one aspect of Stellar's theory was enthusiastically taken up, and this directed almost two decades of research to an examination of the consequences of stimulating and inactivating specific zones within the hypothalamus.

Taken together, these two influences meant that the study of the control of food intake, often regarded as equivalent to the study of the motivation for eating, was tied, on the one hand, to investigations of body weight regulation and, on the other, to the properties of centers in the brain. It was from within this climate that early studies on the pharmacology of feeding emerged. For example, one family of investigations was concerned with the way in which drugs and chemicals affected specific hypothalamic loci while another cluster dealt with longer-term effects on body weight. These themes, along with their associated experimental designs, may be regarded as a paradigm; in turn, this paradigm determined research strategies. In simplified form, it meant that motivation of feeding was the study of hunger, expressed through specific brain centers in the interests of regulating body weight. Recently, two authors have suggested the desirability of shifting the paradigm to allow alternative research strategies to invade the field. First, Smith (1982) proposed that motivational theory should take up the phenomenon of satiety rather than hunger as its central theme. Such a proposition focuses attention upon the cessation of eating rather than its inception and upon the consequences of consumption rather than its antecedents. This suggestion has obvious implications for the design and interpretation of experiments. Second, Blundell (1981*b*, 1982*b*) proposed that feeding theory could advance by readjusting attention toward qualitative (as opposed to quantitative) aspects of feeding, in particular, toward the study of food preferences and nutrient selection. This proposal would also have implications for experimental design especially by the introduction of the variable of elective food choice into feeding experiments. Interestingly, both these proposals advocate a prominent place for behavioral structure in the development of knowledge about mechanisms. Two comments should be added to qualify the above propositions. First, the strategies referred to had already been used by many researchers before the particular themes were characterized in the above fashion. Second, the idea that either of these propositions constitutes a true paradigm shift may be debatable, but they certainly contribute to a clear shift of emphasis within feeding research. This shift is critical for the design and interpretation of pharmacological experiments, but before dealing with this issue, it will be useful to construct a foundation of evidence about the effects of drugs and chemicals on feeding.

3. DRUGS AND FOOD INTAKE

The study of this topic falls within the subdiscipline of behavioral pharmacology, an area that embraces research in both applied and pure science and incorporates three major purposes (e.g., Thompson and Schuster, 1968). First, behavioral pharmacology of feeding has grown along with the increasing interest of pharmaceutical companies in the development of antiobesity drugs. This enterprise has needed testing procedures to determine which of the thousands of new pharmaceutical compounds display clinically desirable behavioral activity. Since drugs are developed primarily for social and economic motives, and not for the convenience of theoretical biology, preliminary testing of drugs is dominated by pragmatic considerations, and there are obvious practical reasons why any potential compound can receive only limited attention. Accordingly, the "screening problem" has promoted the development of quick and simple procedures for the rapid classification of many compounds and for the evaluation of their potential usefulness in clinical practice. A second purpose of behavioral pharmacology involves the use of detailed behavioral procedures to act as a behavioral assay for investigating the mechanisms of drug action. When subjected to refined analysis, many categories of behavior reveal a complex structure, parts of which are extremely sensitive to manipulation without necessarily being accompanied by crude shifts in the "total quantity of behavior." This is true of food consumption, and changes in subtle features of the pattern of feeding behavior may be used to shed light upon the mode of action of the drug causing the change. A third and major purpose of behavioral pharmacology is the use of drugs as tools to explore the relationship between physiological happenings and behavioral events. In this way, drugs can be used as pharmacological scalpels to dissect the components of natural systems governing food consumption and to reveal the properties of this system. Under certain circumstances, drugs can show how biological systems function. To achieve this purpose, behavioral pharmacology of feeding must be concerned as much with overeating (hyperphagia) as with undereating (hypophagia).

From the outset, it is clear that the system that controls food consumption involves a complex network in which metabolic, neural, and hormonal signals are integrated into a coherent pattern. It follows that adjustments in food intake may occur following pharmacological manipulations at many points in the system (e.g., Blundell, 1980; Blundell and Rogers, 1978; Sullivan and Comai, 1978; Sullivan and Gruen, 1985). Consequently, the interpretation of the effect of a drug on food intake is often not obvious. For example, eating may be altered by drugs that directly modify sensory receptors or that indirectly influence the perception of gustatory and olfactory stimuli. In addition, drugs acting on digestive activities or modifying the physicochemical characteristics of the stomach may alter the processing of ingested nutrients and affect the act of eating itself. Alternatively, pharmacological agents may interfere with nutrient absorption chemically or prevent the formation of an end product of digestion or, by some physicochemical effect, affect absorption in the intestine. It is known from the results of bypass surgery of the intestine in animals (Sclafani *et al.,* 1978) and humans (Mills and Stunkard, 1976) that intervention at this level produces dramatic changes in food consumption and in taste perception. Moreover, certain compounds known to modify lipid synthesis may exert additional effects on food intake (e.g., Sullivan *et al.*, 1974) by adjusting the internal metabolic signals through which the brain is believed to receive information about the state of storage tissue. Food intake could also be modified as a result of the action of a drug on energy expenditure, either directly through thermogenesis or indirectly through a change in behavioral activity.

Within the brain, drugs may influence the tendency to feed by affecting a variety of processes. For example, the peripheral signals of the state of the body may be changed so that a certain distortion occurs when metabolic information is translated into neural activity. Additionally, the neural circuits that integrate different sources of information may be affected, and of course, drugs may alter the neural coding of the motivational output for eating. Although not frequently mentioned, pharmacological manipulation could affect in an unknown way the neural mechanisms that mediate in the learned relationships between food stimuli and feeding responses.

Consequently, a variety of general routes by which the administration of drugs to experimental animals could alter the pattern of food intake exist. Initially, therefore, the observation that a pharmacological manipulation changes food consumption tells us very little about the possible mechanism involved.

3.1. Suppression of Food Intake

Many agents have been reported to reduce food intake when injected, usually peripherally, into experimental animals. These agents include neurotransmitters, hormones, amino acids and other precursors of transmitters, peptides and other neuromodulators, metabolites of digestion, certain chemical fractions of blood and urine, synthetic compounds (such as anorexic drugs), receptors blockers, reuptake blockers, and direct receptor agonists. This variety should not be surprising, since the overall feeding system is extensive and such compounds could interfere with the functioning of the system at many points. Table 1 provides some examples of compounds that can reduce food consumption. Since these agents were peripherally injected, the precise site of action is difficult to determine in the absence of further critical experiments. Moreover, although in certain cases the mechanism of action appears obvious, it should be considered that, in most studies, food consumption was measured over a brief interval of time in food-deprived animals. Consequently, injected compounds may appear to be anorexic by impeding the

TABLE 1
Various Agents That Reduce Food Intake

Substance	Comments	Reference
Satiated blood portions	Blood from free-feeding rats. 26 ml injected in 2 ml portions reduced intake of sweetened milk (30-min test) of rats fed 30 min every day for 24 days	Davis et al., 1967
Satietin	Peptide extracted from human plasma injected i.v. or intraventric. reduces food intake of rats deprived for 96 hr	Knoll, 1979
Anorexic urine	Peptide (pyroGlu-His-Gly-OH) extracted from urine of anorexia nervosa patients. Injected to female free-feeding mice. 50% decrease in daily food intake. Effect persists for year	Trygstad et al., 1978
Glucose and glycerol	40% glucose by gastric intubation decreases intake at 2, 7, and 24 hr. 40% glyercol decreases intake over 24 hr	Glick, 1980
(−) Hydroxycitrate	Female rats, daily 3-hr feeding. 0.33 nm/kg hydrosycitrate orally twice daily. Decreased intake accounts for reduction in body weight and body lipids	Sullivan et al., 1974
Threochlorocitrate	Slows gastric emptying. Oral administration reduces food intake in rats and dogs	Sullivan et al., 1981
Atropine	Rats deprived 17 hr. Sham feeding with gastric fistula (liquid diet). Atropin methyl nitrate (2–250 mg/kg) dose-related decrease in intake	Lorenz et al., 1978
Epinephrine/norepinephrine	Rats, high-carbohydrate diet for 1 hr/day. Epinephrine—0.1, 0.15, and 0.2 mg/kg. Norepinephrine—0.1, 0.15 mg/kg. 5 min before. 0.15 dose reduces intake by 71% and 34%, respectively	Russek et al., 1967
Amphetamine(A)/mazindol(M)	Rats, 6 hr feeding per day, 2 hr test. Drugs given immediately before. A—1.25 mg/kg; M—7.5 mg/kg—effects blocked by ventral noradrenergic bundle lesions	Garattini and Samanin, 1976

(continued)

TABLE 1 (*Continued*)

Substance	Comments	Reference
Mazindol, lisuride, piribedil, nomifensine, and apomorphine	Rats, 4 hr/day feeding. Drugs injected i.p. at various times before start of 1 hr test. All drugs reduce intake—effect blocked by pimozide	Carruba *et al.*, 1980
Serotonin (5-HT)	Zucker rat and lean rats, VMH-lesioned rats. 14 g food/day between 9 and 2. 5-HT—12.5 mg/100 g—5 min prior to 2 hr test. Decreased eating in all groups	Bray and York, 1972
Tryptophan	50 mg/kg tryptophan i.p. Rats—eatometer—Noyes pellets. Free-feeding rats—decrease in meal size and 24-hr intake. 16-hr deprivation decrease in size of first large meal and increase in postmeal interval	Latham and Blundell, 1979
5-Hydroxytryptophan (5-HTP)	Rats deprived 18 hr 5-HTP—30/60/90 mg/kg i.p.—dose-related decrease. Free feeding with eatometer 30 mg/kg decreases meal size and 24-hr intake	Blundell and Latham, 1980
Fenfluramine, quipazine, ORG 6582, m-CPP (5-HT agonists and uptake blockers)	Rats 4-hr feeding per day. Injections immediately before 1-hr test. All agents reduce intake	Samanin *et al.*, 1980; Garattini, 1978
Estrogens	Ovariectomized female rats—unrestricted access to food. Estradiol benzoate—2.0 g and estrone benzoate—20.0 g reduce daily intake	Wade, 1975
Cholecystokinin	Rats—5.5-hr deprivation. CCK—2.5–40 Ivy Dog U/kg (15 min before test) decreases intake in first 30 min	Gibbs *et al.*, 1973
Bombesin	Rats—15-hr deprivation, liquid food sham feeding. Synthetic bombesin 2–256 mg/kg decreases intake in first 15 min of 60-min test	Martin and Gibbs, 1980
Enterogastrone	Mice—17-hr deprivation, liquid diet. Hormone given 10–15 min after onset of feeding (0.1–1.0 mg) decreases intake for 30–60 min	Schally *et al.*, 1967

(*continued*)

TABLE 1 (*Continued*)

Substance	Comments	Reference
Somatostatin (SS)	Rats deprived early in light part of cycle. 4/5 hr later given i.p. 1 mg SS. Decreases intake in 30-min test	Lotter *et al.*, 1981
Thyrotropin-releasing hormone (TRH)	Rats, TRH (10–20 mg/kg i.p.) 20-hr deprivation, 1-hr test, 30-min data given. Injection immediately before test reduces intake	Vogel *et al.*, 1979
Calcitonin	Rats—25–50 U/kg decrease 24-hr food intake. Rats given 30-min period of eating/day—maximum inhibition when 12.5 U/kg given 4.5–8.3 hr before	Freed *et al.*, 1979
Prostaglandins	$F_2\alpha$—1 mg/kg i.p. to rats fed for 2 hr/day. Suppressed intake for 30 min. Also effective in satiated and partially satiated rats	Doggett and Jawaharlal, 1977a
Prostaglandin precursors	Rats deprived 22 hr. Arachidonic, linolenic, and linoleic acids decrease intake for 30–60 min. Effect blocked by indomethacin and paracetamol	Dogget and Jawaharlal, 1977b
Cocaine and coca extracts	Rats 1 hr feeding/day on ground chow. Cocaine 3.45–27.6 mg/kg i.p. or p.o. reduces intake, as does chloroform extraction layer of coca	Bedford *et al.*, 1980
	Rats 5-hr feeding period. Cocaine—10/15/15 mg/kg i.p. Dose-dependent decrease in first hours—no effect no total intake	Balopode *et al.*, 1979
Muscimol and EOS	Rats—condensed milk for 30 min each day. 0.5/1.0/2.0 mg/kg muscimol—dose-related decrease	Cooper *et al.*, 1980
THIP (GABA agonist)	Fasted rats, i.v. THIP gives dose-dependent decrease	Blavet *et al.*, 1982
Naloxone	Rats 48-hr deprivation, 2-hr measurement. Food intake reduced by naloxone 1.0–10.0 mg/kg. No effect in mouse (24 hr deprivation)	Holtzman, 1974
Tetrahydrocannabinol (THC)	Male rats, 6-hr feeding/day. THC (2.5 and %.0 mg/kg) markedly	Sofia and Barry, 1974

(*continued*)

TABLE 1 (*Continued*)

Substance	Comments	Reference
β-Phenylethylamine	decreases food intake in first 2 hr with carryover to next 4 hr Rats—(50 or 100 mg/kg) gives 20% reduction in 24-hr food intake	Dourish, 1982
Cathinone	(−) Isomer reduces milk intake in 15-min test	Foltin *et al.*, 1982
Cathine (phenylpropanolamine)	Dose of 4 mg/kg decreases carrot consumption (5-hr tests) in deprived rats	Zelger and Carlini, 1980
Isoproterenol	Anorexia produced by systemic injections and blocked by perifornical propranolol	Leibowitz, 1970
Salbutamol	Rats, 4-hr feeding schedule. Drug 2.5, 5.0, 10.0, 20.0 mg/kg—15 min before test. All doses reduce intake in 1-hr test	Borsini *et al.*, 1982
Benzodiazepine inverse agonists (eg., CGS 8216)	Nondeprived rats fed high-palatability food. Dose-dependent reduction in 30-min test	Cooper and Estall, 1985

animal's behavior rather than by acting physiologically upon a natural regulatory system.

3.2. Enhancement of Food Intake

Hundreds of chemical agents can reduce food intake, whereas a much smaller number can increase intake. There are probably two major reasons for this—one methodological and one theoretical. First, failure to eat is a passive response, which may merely indicate a sort of abstinence by default. That is, any interference with the natural expression of behavior may lead to a decline in intake (particularly in short tests). Second, it is reasonable to suppose that a number of routes may mediate the inhibition of eating. It follows that the involvement of any one of these routes by means of a pharmacological agent centrally or peripherally applied should inhibit eating. In other words, stimulation of one particular system will be a *sufficient* but not a *necessary* condition for inhibition. However, if one inhibitory system is blocked pharmacologically or neurochemically, other systems continue to function and to express inhibition. Consequently, it may be difficult to observe an augmentation of food intake through a process of disinhibition. Alternatively, if a pharmacological agent acts on a facilitatory system to induce eating, this will be countered by functioning inhibitory processes, and only a brief potentiation may be observed.

Despite these limitations, a number of notable instances illustrate that pharmacological agents can produce increases in eating and gains in body weight. Some of these phenomena are both sizable and robust, and they include the effects of clinically important groups of compounds such as antipsychotic drugs, antidepressant drugs, and minor tranquilizers (Table 2). All three of the most common categories of minor tranquilizers, barbiturates (Watson and Cox 1976), meprobamate (Soubrie et al., 1975), and the benzodiazepines (Poschel, 1971) increase food intake markedly in animals tested in a wide variety of situations (Cappell et al., 1972; Randall et al., 1960). Probably the most dramatic of these effects involves the widely used benzodiazepines diazepam (Valium) and chlordiazepoxide (Librium). These drugs have been found to stimulate eating in mice (Soubrie et al., 1975), rats (Wise and Dawson, 1974), cats (Mereu et al., 1976), and horses (Brown et al., 1976) with an intensity sometimes bordering on voraciousness. It is possible that benzodiazepines may induce eating indirectly by altering emotional circumstances related to feeding (Soper and Wise, 1971; Tye et al., 1976), although it has been suggested that this class of compounds has a specific action on central mechanisms influencing hunger or satiety (Margules and Stein, 1967). Indeed, it has been suggested that benzodiazepines can be considered "hunger-mimetic" agents (Cooper, 1980), although, as noted previously, there appear to be notable differences between various benzodiazepine compounds (File, 1980).

Although not widely recognized, benzodiazepine-induced eating also occurs in humans (Goodman and Gilman, 1970), and both chlordiazepoxide and diazepam have been reported to bring about increases in appetite and weight gain apparently unrelated to improvements in mental state (Edwards, 1977). In addition, obesity in psychiatric hospital populations maintained on major tranquilizers is well known and considered to be a serious complication of drug therapy (Amdisen, 1964; Holden and Holden, 1970). Instances of severe weight gain are known to occur with the use of phenothiazines and butyrophenones linked to an increase in appetite (Robinson et al., 1975). It has also been reported that patients who gain weight on phenothiazine medication display a markedly increased rate of eating (Blundell et al., 1980). These observations are consistent with the results of animal studies showing changes in food intake following treatment with chlorpromazine (Reynolds and Carlisle, 1961; Stolerman, 1970). In addition, weight gain can occur with lithium (Vendsborg et al., 1976) and amitryptiline therapy (Paykel et al., 1973), an effect that

TABLE 2
Various Agents That Increase Food Intake

Substance	Comments	Reference
Hyperphagic urine	Peptide fraction extracted from urine of anorexia nervosa patients. During posttreatment period, mice overate and became obese	Trygstad et al., 1978
Chloralose	Male rats, powdered diet. α-Chloralose 2.5–50 mg/kg i.p. Increased intake at 15 and 25. Latency decreased during dark phase	Booth and Nicholls, 1974
Meprobamate (M)	Rats—22-hr deprivation/2-hr feeding—isolated. M—100 mg/kg oral administration. 17% increase in intake. Barbiturate and chlordiazepoxide also effective	Bainbridge, 1968
Barbiturates	Male rats, fully satiated, 1-hr intake. Increased intake with sodium pentobarbital (9.5 mg/kg and phenobarbital (40 mg/kg)	Watson and Cox, 1976
Benzodiazepines	Male rats, mice—liquid food. Diazepam, chlordiazepoxide, oxazepam, nitrazepam, lorazepam all increase intake, and decrease latency (except nitrazepam). Also barbiturates, meprobamate	Soubrie et al., 1975
Neuroleptics Chlorpromazine (CPZ)	Rats—free-feeding. CPZ 4 mg/kg s.c. or intragastric increases food intake on first day. So-called first day hyperphagia	Robinson et al., 1975
Promazine	0.5 mg/kg (250 mg) i.v. to adult horse. Eating within 30 min and increase in 1-hr intake	Brown et al., 1976
Clozapine	Male rats, free-feeding—pellet food. Intragastric clozapine (10–20 mg/kg) increases intake in 2-hr test immediately after injection	Antelman et al., 1977
5-HT antagonists Cyproheptadine	Rats, overnight deprivation, 6-hr feeding—continuous recording. 12.5 mg/kg increases size and duration of first meal	Baxter et al., 1970
Methysergide	Rats, 16-hr deprivation then feed for 1 hr. Methysergide 2.0 mg/kg s.c. increases intake in following hours	Blundell and Leshem, 1974
WA 335-BS	Cats 2.5-hr test. 2.5 mg/kg p.o. increases intake	Kahling et al., 1975
Opiate agonists	Free-feeding rats. Ethylketocyclazocine (kappa	Sanger and McCarthy, 1981

(continued)

TABLE 2 (*Continued*)

Substance	Comments	Reference
	receptor) 0.1/10.0 mg/kg and the enkephaline analog RX 783030 (mu receptor). Increase eating at 1, 2, 4 hr	
Clonidine	Rats, ad lib food—measures at 6, 24 hr 300 g/kg for more than 3 days increase eating at 6 hr period	Atkinson et al., 1978
	Rats—choice of diets. Tests in dark period—50 min, 60 min, 75 min. Clonidine 25, 50, 100 g/kg i.p. increases food intake (and protein)	Mauron et al., 1980
	Stumptail macaques. 0.1 mg/kg intramuscularly for 7 days increases daily food intake	Schlemmer et al., 1979
Yohimbine	Rats, diet choice. Mild (1-hr) deprivation before dark period. Yohimbine (10 mg/kg) massive increase in intake during 50-min test	Mauron et al., 1980
Insulin	Rats, protamine zinc insulin, 2 s.c. injections/day. 10 U/day doubles intake on chow and high-fat diet	Panksepp et al., 1975
2-Deoxy-*d*-glucose	Rabbit, free-feeding, intravenous administration. Decreased latency to first meal and threefold increase in food intake in first hour	Gonzalez and Novin, 1974
5-*Thio*-glucose	Rats, nondeprived, 6-hr test period Intracardiac infusion. 5-TG increased intake at third of dose of 2-DG	Slusser and Ritter, 1980
Androgens	Gonadectomized male rats, free-feeding, s.c. injections of testosterone, dihydrotestosterone, androstenidione daily for 10 days increase food intake and body weight	Rowland et al., 1980
Formamidines	Rats. Formamidine (Amitraz) and chlordimeform, normally pesticides, increase intake during day when potential to feed is slow	Pfister et al., 1978
Caffeine	Male mice, daytime feeding, 2-hr test. Increased intake with 10, 20, 40 mg/kg	Dobrzanski and Doggett, 1976
Tifluodom (opioid-benzodiazepine)	Free-feeding rats, tested during light period. 0.5, 1.0, and 2.0 mg/kg increase intake over 0–4 hr. Effect blocked by naloxone	Jackson and Sewell, 1984

(*continued*)

TABLE 2 (*Continued*)

Substance	Comments	Reference
8-*OH*-DPAT (putative 5-HT, agonist)	Nondeprived rats. Very low doses (15–60 g/kg) increase food intake. Higher doses elicit feeding plus locomotion and stereotypy	Dourish *et al.*, 1985

seems to be associated with a preference for carbohydrates (Morgan, 1977; see Blundell, 1980, for a review).

A further class of compounds believed to increase food intake and weight gain are serotonergic antagonists. For example, the serotonin (and histamine) antagonist cyproheptadine (Miller, 1963) has been said to increase appetite in asthmatic children (Bergen, 1964), in underweight adults (Noble, 1969), and in a patient with anorexia nervosa (Benady, 1970) and has been reported to increase both weight and height (Idelsohn, 1967). Although it has been suggested that cyproheptadine influences food intake only under special experimental conditions, definite increases in food consumption (Baxter *et al.*, 1970) and in body weight (Ghosh and Parvathy, 1973) have been demonstrated in rats. Taken together, these experiments illustrate that pharmacological manipulations not only suppress food intake but also lead to its enhancement.

4. INTERPRETATION OF PHARMACOLOGICAL ACTION

The traditional way in which a mechanism of action has been investigated in pharmacological studies on feeding involves four steps. The procedure may be outlined for the case of a suppression of intake. (1) The drug inhibits food consumption during a brief feeding test. (2) In other experiments, the drug is shown to exert a specific action on brain chemistry (often the biogenic amines). (3) Direct or indirect intervention in the amine system antagonizes the inhibitory effect of the drug on food intake. (4) This particular amine is involved in anorexia. One of the major experimental strategies in this area of research is to antagonize a drug-induced suppression by means of a direct intervention in the brain (a specific stereotaxic lesion or the injection of a neurotoxin) or an indirect intervention by means of a peripherally administered pharmacological agent. The philosophy usually adopted for understanding these effects exists in a strong and weak form. The *strong* argument is that the neurochemical systems manipulated to antagonize drug-induced anorexia must be implicated in the neural control of food intake. The *weak* argument is that the particular neurochemical adjusted merely mediates the effect of the drug. If the strong argument is accepted, it must overcome the logical objection that, before a neurochemical mechanism can be implicated in feeding control, it must be shown that the drug-induced inhibition of intake makes use of the natural feeding control system. Evidence can be assembled on this issue in a number of ways. For example, the drug effect can be monitored when feeding is provoked by a physiological stimulus such as glucoprivation (induced by injections of 2-deoxy-d-glucose) or insulin-induced hypoglycemia. Another procedure is to examine the structure of behavior to determine the extent to which the drug-induced changes resemble those that occur during natural cycles of hunger and satiety. This latter approach is the one that has been adopted by the author and that will be described in this chapter. The approach rests upon the recognition that feeding behavior represents one element within a biopsychological system for the management of an organism's nutritional requirements (Blundell, 1984a); behavior is therefore not isolated but interacts with other elements in the system (Blundell and Hill, 1986). A structural approach also draws attention to the importance of the expression of behavior in context and time.

5. CONTEXTUAL AND TEMPORAL DIMENSIONS OF BEHAVIOR

The eating behavior of animals can be said to represent an adaptive response arising from demands in various parts of the biopsychological feeding system. This simple notion embraces two important aspects of the experimental study of feeding: a recognition, first, that feeding behavior is different from food intake and, second, that feeding behavior can be defined according to contextual and temporal dimensions. In many studies on the effects of drugs or physiological manipulations on feeding, the dependent variable is derived by simply measuring the weight of food taken from a container over a brief period of time. However, it is apparent that mammalian food intake comprises complex behavior sequences and constitutes a discontinuous process in which periods of eating alternate with periods of noneating. These qualitative features give character to ingestive behavior and draw attention to the distinction between food intake and feeding behavior, which can only be understood through a detailed analysis of the feeding response. Although measurement of the sheer bulk of food consumed may shed light upon certain features of energy balance, it seems likely that a more detailed analysis of the "behavioral flux" (Blundell and McArthur, 1981) will be required to determine how psychological processes exert a moment-to-moment control over feeding activity.

Feeding regarded as behavior (i.e., with a definable structure in addition to mass) can be monitored along two dimensions—the contextual and the temporal. The contextual dimension determines the nature of the elements displayed and includes all aspects of the environment, including the presence of a home area, predators, competitors, stressors, and ambient temperature, together with the physical form of the available food and its composition. This last item is particularly important, since in the study of feeding behavior in the laboratory, animals are usually fed a single, uniform composite-chow diet. However, the contextual qualities of food can be varied in a number of ways, including changes in the macronutrient composition of the diet, the number of choices available, and sensory and hedonic aspects (embracing variety and palatability), together with the location and accessibility of food. Changing these contextual aspects may completely alter the effect of a drug (Blundell *et al.*, 1986; Levine *et al.*, 1985; Moses and Wurtman, 1984; Rowland and Bartness, 1982) or other manipulation (Collier *et al.*, 1977) upon feeding. Clearly, the number of choices available, their form (e.g., liquid, powder, pellet, mash, granule), and their location will determine the type of behavior that an animal must display in order to eat.

In addition to the nature of the actual behavioral elements involved, the structure of behavior is revealed by the distribution of these elements over time (Wiepkema, 1971a,b). This temporal dimension reflects the pattern of feeding and is composed of feeding and nonfeeding elements. Analysis can occur at the macro- or microlevels (Blundell and Latham, 1982). Accordingly, the structure of behavior reflects the operation of important contextual variables influencing food intake and contains the resolving power to indicate the buildup and decay of underlying physiological events. In this way, the structure of behavior can be a useful tool in determining the process invoked during particular experimental manipulations.

6. STRUCTURE, PROCESS, AND MECHANISM

The central theme of this chapter is the proposition that an examination of behavioral structure of feeding can provide insights into the operation of the systems controlling food consumption. What exactly is meant by this? It has been noted previously that in laboratory studies on experimental animals, scores of chemical compounds have been reported to alter food intake following their peripheral injection. The most frequent alteration is reduction of intake, although a smaller number of chemical compounds increase intake. In addition, it is usually implied that the change in food intake is engendered by action on some underlying process such as hunger or satiation. However, the interpretation of chemically induced alterations in food intake is not obvious. The most attractive explanation is that the chemical agents act upon some aspect of the natural process by which animals match their food intake to nutritional requirements. For reductions in food intake, however, the change may be the result of some nonspecific, nonphysiological impediment to the act of eating. For example, animals (and humans) may be prevented from eating by an inability to articulate the motor movements of eating, by the displacement of eating by the intrusion of normal or pathological acts, or by a diversion of attention to other aspects of the environment (Blundell, 1979a; Smith and Gibbs, 1979). The crucial question is whether chemically induced suppression of feeding reflects the operation of the natural process of satiation. In order to identify an action upon a natural physiological process, more evidence is required than a mere change in the total amount of food consumed. One technique is to analyze changes in the structure of behavior. The organization of units of behavior into a sequence is not arbitrary, but reflects a relationship between internal dispositions and environmental constraints. The organization of behavior can, therefore, be considered adaptive. However under circumstances that reflect disease or adverse environmental conditions, the structure of behavior would be expected to change and could be considered pathological or haphazard. Therefore, an examination of the structure of behavior can be used to identify adaptive responses of "natural" processes and distorted responses brought about by "pathological" physiological or environmental conditions.

In a number of areas of behavior, the *structure* of a behavioral sequence can be used to indicate the occurrence of certain underlying *processes*. In turn, these processes (that guide the articulation of behavior) are activated by specific *mechanisms*. Of course, a number of mechanisms may occur conjointly to govern the smooth running of a process. For example, in sexual behavior of rats, the copulatory sequence of mounts, intromissions, and ejaculation of the male constitutes an adaptive sequence (Adler, 1969; Bermant, 1961), which reflects the operation of processes linking physiological dispositions and environmental variables. Various parameters derived from the structure of the copulatory sequence can be altered by hormonal manipulation or procedures that affect the brain. Adjustments to the structure reflect changes in the processes of sexual motivation or consummatory capacity, and mechanisms involved in these processes can be inferred from the experimental manipulations (Beach, 1976, 1979). When feeding behavior is considered, the

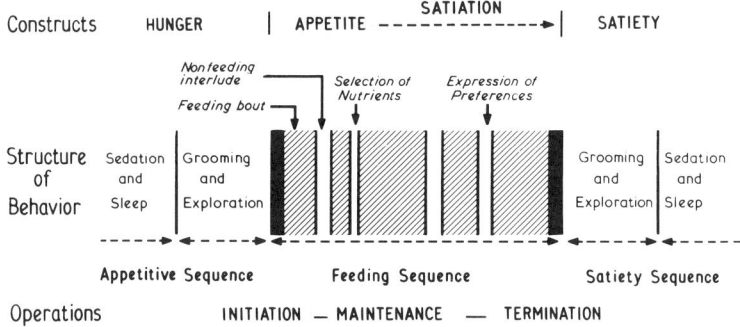

FIG. 1. Representation of the structure of behavior relevant for the analysis of feeding.

organizational structure of the behavioral sequence of feeding, grooming, and resting that concludes an episode of eating indicates the development of the process of satiation, and the agency (e.g., hormonal, neurochemical) that provoked the behavioral change indicates the mechanism (Antin *et al.*, 1975; Blundell and McArthur, 1981; Smith and Gibbs, 1976). Accordingly, the structure of behavior can be used to determine whether the effect of a drug (or other physiological manipulation) on food intake is mediated by a natural process or a pathological condition. It follows from this that drugs can be used as tools to investigate the operation of mechanisms that control the articulation of natural processes. Figure 1 is a representation of the structure of behavior sequence and illustrates the potential for using changes in behavior structure as a dependent variable. On the understanding that the structure of behavior is not arbitrary or capricious but is related in a meaningful way to processes (labeled as constructs in Fig. 1), alterations in behavior sequences can be used to deduce the mode of action of pharmacological manipulations. It should be emphasized that a behavioral approach to the analysis of drug action is not an alternative to biochemical investigations; ideally, the two approaches should be used in conjunction to allow the disclosure of synchrony between the neurochemical and behavioral flux.

7. METHODOLOGICAL DEVELOPMENTS

In recent years, a number of experimental devices have been introduced as alternatives to food deprivation for the instigation of eating or overeating. These procedures include tail pinch-induced eating, muscimol injections into the dorsal raphe nuclei, and a sucrose supplement to the diet (see Sclafani, 1985, for a review). However, the developments that will be briefly described here are those that monitor the fine structure of feeding behavior, under meaningful contextual conditions, in detail. They have all been useful in disclosing the operation of processes such as hunger and satiation, or specific food selection. Moreover, these procedures, in conjunction with judicious pharmacological manipulation, can be used to shed light on the specific neurochemical mechanisms that articulate the processes. Among the most important methodological features are the following:

7.1. Free-Feeding Animals

This involves the use of animals fed *ad libitum* in drug studies as an alternative to the commonly used severe food deprivation and cyclical feeding regimens. The rationale behind the avoidance of severe food deprivation schedules has been set out elsewhere (Moran, 1975; Blundell and Latham, 1979a).

7.2. Microanalysis of the Structure of Feeding Behavior

Feeding is an episodic activity in which the episodes of eating (bouts), nonfeeding episodes, and the relationship between these variables, can be measured. The procedure appears to have been first used for drug studies in animals by Blundell and Latham (1977). In this use of the technique, the behavior of rats during a 1-hr period was exhaustively recorded in six categories: eating, drinking, grooming, locomotor activity, and resting. From these records, together with the weight of food, it was possible to derive the following parameters: total food intake (g), duration of time spent eating (min), number of eating bouts (n), size of bouts (g), duration of bouts (min), and the local rate of eating (g/min). The purpose of this fine analysis was to reveal certain subtle differences between the effects of drugs not revealed by a simple measure of the amount of food consumed and the action of drugs on processes underlying eating. Using this procedure, clear differences have been observed between agents acting on serotonergic systems (fenfluramine, ORG 6582, Lilly 110140, tryptophan, and 5-hydroxytryptophan), neuroleptics (pimozide, α-flupenthixol), and catecholaminergic compounds (e.g., amphetamine and mazindol) Blundell and Latham, 1978, 1979b, 1980). This type of analysis has prompted the suggestion that serotonin systems are involved in the mechanism of satiation. The technique has also been used in a very short feeding test to examine the actions of chlordiazepoxide (Cooper, 1980) and spiperone (Cooper et al., 1979) and to investigate the involvement of β-receptors in amphetamine anorexia (Willner and Towell, 1982a) and the action of amphetamine following chronic antidepressant treatment (Willner and Towell, 1982b). In later sections, the use of microanalysis to investigate the action of opioid blockers and to identify specific and nonspecific anorexic actions will be described.

7.3. Macroanalysis of Feeding Patterns

The continuous monitoring of long-term eating patterns in *free-feeding* rats never forcibly subjected to periods of deprivation identifies the meal as the unit of feeding. From the basic variable can be computed the parameters of meal size, meal duration, meal frequency, intermeal interval, and various other measures that describe the pattern of feeding behavior (for a review, see Blundell and Latham, 1982). The procedure has been used to study the action of amphetamine (Borbely and Waser, 1966) and to compare the effects of amphetamine and fenfluramine (Blundell and Leshem, 1975; Blundell et al., 1976). Interestingly, the action of fenfluramine was characterized by a reduction in meal size, which suggested that the drug was acting to promote the process of satiation and therefore cause an early termination of eating. This effect has been confirmed many times (Blundell and Latham, 1978; Burton et al., 1981; Davies, 1976; Davies et al., 1983; Grinker et al., 1980).

This type of analysis over long periods of time permits alterations in behavioral parameters to be matched against the time course of drug concentration in blood (Blundell et al., 1975). In addition, distinctive profiles produced by different drugs can be revealed. As noted previously, amphetamine and fenfluramine can be readily separated. In addition, the dopamine receptor blockers give rise to quite different profiles characterized by a slow rate of eating and a large increase in meal size (Blundell and Latham, 1978). The profiles of tryptophan (Latham and Blundell, 1979) and 5-hydroxytryptophan (Blundell and Latham, 1979c) can be distinguished, whereas the opioid antagonists naloxone (McLaughlin and Baile, 1984) and naltrexone (Kirkham, 1985) produce a profile different from that of serotoninergic agonists and dopamine antagonists.

Accordingly, macroanalysis of meal patterns provides a useful strategy in the pharmacology of feeding in the following ways: the sensitivity of the technique (1) permits distinctions to be made between different compounds with similar effects on total food consumed, (2) sheds light on the mode of action of drugs assessed under normal physiological conditions, and (3) provides information on the way in which drugs influence different aspects of feeding through the processes of hunger, appetite, satiation, and satiety.

7.4. Variety and Palatability of Food

The use of foods characterized by their variety and palatability has encouraged interest in a form of experimental obesity (Sclafani and Springer, 1976; Sclafani, 1978) that appears to have features in common with the development of obesity in humans. The use of a highly palatable cafeteria diet in pharmacological research permits distinctions to be made between drugs acting on hunger and appetite and assessment of the action of drugs on the hedonic value of food. In addition, the manipulation of the contextual dimension in this way has made it clear that not all of the so-called anorexic drugs suppress intake equally when different types of food are offered. For example, it has been demonstrated that the opiate receptor blocker naloxone exerts a greater suppressing effect on the consumption of snack food than laboratory chow (Apfelbaum and Mandenoff, 1981). The effect also occurs with naltrexone (Mandenoff et al., 1982) and signifies a more potent effect when the diet induces hyperphagia. Interestingly, amphetamine is a less potent anorexic agent with a varied diet than with chow, but the action of the opiate blockers is matched by dl-fenfluramine (Bowden et al., 1983), which also suppresses the level of weight gain (Kirby et al., 1978). It is clear that the use of varied and palatable foods in conjunction with pharmacological manipulation has opened up a new area of feeding research and has provided an original method of investigating processes and mechanisms.

7.5. Motivation Measured by Instrumental Performance

In assessing drug action, it is useful to monitor not only the act of eating itself but also the willingness to obtain food. This willingness is normally referred to as the hunger drive, and it may be measured by training rats to make an instrumental response to obtain food. There is an extensive literature on the use of lever pressing in operant chambers under the control of complex reinforcement schedules as a means of measuring various motivational parameters. One other type of easily monitored response is running along a straight-arm maze from a start chamber to a goal box. This device permits the measurement of a number of parameters, including latency to emerge (from the start chamber), speed of running (along the alley), latency to eat (in the goal box), amount of food consumed (on each trial), and cumulative food intake (over a series of trials). This procedure allows simultaneous monitoring of temporal changes in appetitive motivation and in the development of satiation (consummatory response). In earlier experiments, it had been demonstrated that amphetamine and fenfluramine produce quite distinctive effects on runway performance (Thurlby and Samanin, 1981; Thurlby et al., 1983).

This technique will be referred to later to illustrate further the dependence of drug action upon contextual factors.

7.6. Nutritional Aspects of Eating

In the literature on control of food intake, an overwhelming number of studies have involved the purely quantitative aspects of ingestion (weight of food consumed or its energy value); a much smaller number of experiments have been concerned with qualitative aspects of ingestion such as food selection. In pharmacological studies of feeding, nutritional aspects of the food were not taken into consideration until the late 1970s. It is, however, quite clear that the actual composition of food, i.e., its nutritional content, is an important determinant of intake and that drugs are likely to exert different effects upon diets varying in nutritional composition. One important consequence of considering nutritional aspects of eating is the recognition of the phenomenon of dietary self-selection. When offered a choice of diets varying in macronutrient composition, experimental animals will voluntarily self-select intakes of protein, fat, and carbohydrate (for reviews, see Lat, 1967; Overmann, 1976; Blundell, 1983). Experimentation using pharmacological agents to modify dietary self-selection really began with the report that *dl*-fenfluramine and fluoxetine—two drugs that influence serotonin metabolism—gave rise to a protein-sparing effect if given rats that were offered a choice between high- and low-protein diets (Wurtman and Wurtman, 1977). However, experimentation in this field is hindered by a variety of methodological problems (Blundell, 1983), and the effect of pharmacological treatment can be modulated by a number of factors, including food deprivation (Blundell and McArthur, 1979), age (McArthur and Blundell, 1983), and the nature of the diet (McArthur and Blundell, 1986).

A number of pharmacological agents, peptides, hormones, and neurotransmitters have been shown to adjust the intake of protein, carbohydrate, or fat (see Blundell, 1983, for review). When used in conjunction with a continuous monitoring system for monitoring behavioral structure (Blundell and McArthur, 1981), the dietary self-selection procedure can provide crucial information about the manner in which pharmacological treatments adjust food consumption.

Of course, the most important reason why the nutritional aspect of foods must be seriously considered is because the composition of food can influence brain neurotransmitters, which are frequently the substrate through which drugs are believed to exert their effects. For example, food can influence serotonin synthesis in two ways: by supplying the neurotransmitter amino acid precursor (tryptophan) in quantities sufficient to increase (or decrease) the plasma pool size or by changing plasma concentrations of the large neutral amino acids (valine, leucine, isoleucine, tyrosine, phenylalanine), which compete with tryptophan for the same carrier-mediated transport system into the brain. It is for this reason that food high in carbohydrates, consumed by fasted rats, increase brain tryptophan levels and accelerate serotonin synthesis (Fernstrom and Faller, 1978; Glaeser et al., 1983). Consequently, it may be clearly expected that the action of drugs influencing food intake will be modulated by the nature of the diet offered. Indeed, it has even been reported that drugs that facilitate serotonin transmission have a potent anorexic effect with a high-carbohydrate food, but the anorexia is abolished when a low-carbohydrate diet is available (Moses and Wurtman, 1984).

8. CASE STUDIES IN THE PHARMACOLOGICAL ANALYSIS OF FEEDING

The examples given in this section have been chosen to illustrate the value of using a structuralist approach to investigate the causes of the effects of drugs upon food intake and to explore the nature of the processes and mechanisms underlying eating by using drugs as tools. Obviously, the two issues are interrelated. As noted earlier, measurement of the temporal dimension of feeding assumes increased power when experimental manipulations are made simultaneously in the contextual dimension.

8.1. Serotonin Manipulations and the Structure of Feeding Behavior

It has been recognized for a number of years that pharmacological treatments that alter the metabolism and disposition of serotonin can change food consumption. This was noted in certain early experiments (e.g., Soulairac, 1963), and subsequent advances in the development of serotoninergic drugs made possible studies that revealed an apparent covariation between serotonin activity and food intake: Treatments that produced an increase in serotoninergic synaptic activity depressed food intake, whereas drugs that reduced serotoninergic function tended to facilitate intake. This field of research has been specifically reviewed on several occasions (Blundell, 1977, 1979b, 1984b) and has formed part of larger reviews on the pharmacology of feeding (Blundell, 1982a; Coscina, 1977; Hoebel, 1977; Leibowitz, 1980) and on the mechanisms of anorexic drug action (Garattini, 1978). It has been suggested that serotonin may act reciprocally with dopamine (Blundell and Latham, 1978; McDermott et al., 1977), and a number of models have suggested an interaction between serotonin and other neuromodulators and neurotransmitters (Blundell, 1980; Hoebel and Leibowitz, 1981; Morley, 1980; Morley and Levine, 1983).

However, although it is quite clear that pharmacological and neurological manipulations of serotoninergic systems change food intake in experimental animals, the interpretation of these changes is not obvious. For example, many treatments do not distinguish between a central or peripheral site of action, the particular role of serotonin in modifying consumption is not specified, nor is it known whether the effect of the experimental treatment represents a true physiological adjustment of the processes that match eating behavior to nutritional requirements or whether the change in food intake is simply the result of some nonspecific perturbation. In order to define a role (or roles) for serotonin in the control of feeding, it is necessary to go beyond the covariation of serotonin activity and the amount of food consumed and investigate the processes that articulate eating behavior. It will be argued here that one important experimental strategy involves analysis of the structure of feeding behavior.

8.1.1. Microstructural Analysis

The basis of this approach has been described earlier (Section 7.2), and in this section, certain experimental findings will be used to illustrate how the microstructure of behavior differentiates between different drug treatments and shows how drugs may operate to reduce the amount of food consumed. For example, the effects of equianorectic doses of the serotoninergic drug *dl*-fenfluramine have been compared with those of three other anorectic drugs—*d*-amphetamine, mazindol, and diethylpropion—whose actions are mediated largely via catecholaminergic mechanisms. Although these compounds similarly suppress food intake, they differed on a number of microstructural parameters (Blundell and Latham, 1978). On the one hand, it was revealed that *d*-amphetamine markedly increased the latency to the initiation of eating and actually caused rats to increase the rate of consumption. On the other hand, *dl*-fenfluramine noticeably slowed the rate of eating. It has since been demonstrated that this slow rate of eating is reliably displayed by neuroleptics such as pimozide and α-flupenthixol, by serotonin reuptake blockers such as ORG 6582 (Sugrue et al., 1976) and Lilly (110140) (Fuller and Wong, 1977), and by compounds such as 5-hydroxytryptophan (5-HTP) (Blundell and Latham, 1979*b,c*). However, it is clear that the slow rate of eating need not invariably *cause* the reduction in food intake. For example, pimozide does not necessarily produce anorexia—when the rate of eating is slowed, the animals compensate by increasing the time spent eating, so no deficit in food intake occurs. However, with a serotonergic drug such as fenfluramine, rats do not compensate for the slow eating rate by increasing eating time. Consumption is curtailed independently of the rate of eating (Blundell and Latham, 1980).

Consequently, analysis of the microstructure of feeding has revealed that serotonergic manipulations are characterized by a normal latency to initiate consumption, a slow rate of eating, and an early termination of intake. The specificity of these effects is demonstrated by their antagonism by methergoline (Blundell and Latham, 1980). This distinctive pattern of effects suggests an action that hastens the termination of eating rather than an action that blocks its initiation. This may be interpreted as a facilitation of the process of satiation.

8.1.2. Meal Pattern Analysis

This procedure appears to have been first used in drug studies about 17 years ago (Borbely and Waser, 1966) when the active drug (amphetamine) was delivered via the rat's drinking water. Since that time, the serotoninergic drug *dl*-fenfluramine has been the most frequently used pharmacological tool. The initial study that compared the effects of amphetamine and fenfluramine demonstrated that these drugs displayed quite different profiles when meals were monitored continuously over 24-hr periods in nondeprived rats (Blundell and Leshem, 1975; Blundell *et al.*, 1976). Interestingly, the effect of fenfluramine was characterized by a reduction in meal size, which suggested that the drug was acting to promote the process of satiation and therefore cause an early termination of eating. This effect has now been confirmed many times in a number of separate studies (Blundell and Latham, 1978; Davies, 1976; Grinker *et al.*, 1980; Burton *et al.*, 1981; Davies *et al.*, 1983). In keeping with the initial observation of Blundell and Leshem (1975), it has recently been confirmed that the "effects of fenfluramine are specific to meal size with a negligible effect upon meal initiation" (Davies *et al.*, 1983). However, it is useful in a case like this to display the actual data—automatically collected and recorded—to verify the qualitative description and to explain the nature of the structural analysis. For this reason, a computer printout record has been included (Fig. 2) to allow the reader to inspect the detailed nature of the structural changes brought about by *dl*-fenfluramine. These data describe the feeding pattern of a rat over a 2-day period. In this example, the first day (bouts 1–12) is the control day and the second day (bouts 13–23) is the experimental day on which the rat received an intraperitoneal injection of *dl*-fenfluramine (5.0 mg/kg). The printout provides information about all parameters of the meal profile. Reading from left to right (Fig. 2), we begin with the bout number (i.e., meal num-

SLOT:1 ANIMAL:4 EATING DATA FILE:FENFB 5

BOUT NO		START TIME	END TIME	INTERVAL PRE	INTERVAL POST	DURN SECS	NO.	WT. GM	W/I-RATIO PRE	W/I-RATIO POST	AVE. G/M	MDN G/M	MDN IPI	SIQ RNG
1	N	5	6	5	81	71	10	40	0	4	33	47	51	7
2	N	87	95	81	233	278	47	188	23	8	40	42	56	11
3	N	328	336	233	107	312	51	204	8	19	39	42	56	10
4	N	443	455	107	252	399	66	264	24	10	39	42	57	8
5	N	707	721	252	152	509	65	260	10	17	36	40	60	10
6	N	873	885	152	258	421	67	268	17	10	38	40	60	10
7	N	1143	1149	258	32	213	38	152	5	47	42	46	52	8
8	N	1181	1191	32	392	316	46	184	57	4	34	36	65	9
9	D	1583	1593	392	295	347	57	228	5	7	39	43	55	8
10	D	1888	1897	295	176	329	57	228	7	12	41	42	57	8
11	D	2073	2085	176	207	413	59	236	13	11	34	38	63	14
12	D	2292	2310	207	194	606	72	288	13	14	28	34	69	17
13	N	104	120	194	101	563	28	112	5	11	11	20	115	71
14	N	221	230	101	108	327	12	48	4	4	8	12	191	157
15	N	338	341	108	387	142	12	48	4	1	20	23	102	20
16	N	728	737	387	233	336	17	68	1	2	12	34	70	9
17	N	970	978	233	243	320	24	96	4	3	18	35	67	24
18	D	1221	1232	243	52	431	52	208	8	40	28	32	73	13
19	D	1284	1291	52	42	260	27	108	20	25	24	25	96	15
20	D	1333	1339	42	527	206	29	116	27	2	33	32	74	10
21	D	1866	1876	527	245	326	41	164	3	6	30	32	75	9
22	D	2121	2127	245	109	222	36	144	5	13	38	38	62	8
23	D	2236	2244	109	77	296	37	148	13	19	30	34	69	6

BOUT NO	QUARTER-BOUT MDN'S 1	2	3	4	QUARTER-BOUT IBI'S NO. & SECS DURN. 1 (NO.)	1 (SECS)	2 (NO.)	2 (SECS)	3 (NO.)	3 (SECS)	4 (NO.)	4 (SECS)
1	0	0	0	0	0	0	1	5	0	0	2	20
2	49	53	56	57	0	0	0	0	2	21	0	0
3	59	49	63	55	1	11	0	0	1	10	0	0
4	52	56	56	60	2	23	0	0	1	6	1	9
5	59	57	70	64	3	104	0	0	2	32	0	0
6	58	59	61	60	2	91	1	6	0	0	2	20
7	58	60	48	49	1	12	0	0	0	0	1	7
8	65	66	61	65	1	7	0	0	1	3	1	9
9	52	51	56	63	1	9	1	6	1	18	1	11
10	55	54	65	57	1	18	0	0	0	0	1	7
11	59	74	51	69	1	6	2	14	2	22	3	26
12	68	68	65	69	2	23	2	14	2	17	3	76
13	104	115	288	118	2	71	0	0	4	186	3	58
14	0	0	0	0	2	156	1	29	1	48	1	35
15	0	0	0	0	1	57	1	16	0	0	0	0
16	0	0	0	0	2	45	1	12	0	0	1	184
17	81	59	52	67	1	184	0	0	1	6	2	148
18	84	69	86	70	1	101	1	8	1	30	0	0
19	86	96	97	98	1	28	0	0	0	0	0	0
20	70	74	66	53	1	10	0	0	0	0	0	0
21	77	66	75	81	1	12	1	9	0	0	0	0
22	62	67	73	60	1	14	0	0	0	0	0	0
23	69	68	69	58	3	47.	0	0	0	0	0	0

DAY NO.	NIGHT-TIME BOUTS NO	WT.	AV. WT.	AV. RTE	DAY-TIME BOUTS NO.	WT.	AV. WT.	AV. RTE	OVER WHOLE DAY NO.	WT.	AV. WT	AV. RTE	NT:DY RATIOS NO.	WT.	TTL RDGS	UNIT SIZE	WT/GAP-RATIO PRE-	POST
1	8	1560	195	41	4	980	245	39	12	2540	211	41	20	15	635	40	15	13
2	5	372	74	24	6	688	148	32	11	1260	114	28	8	4	315	40	8	11

MEAL-SIZE DISTRIBUTION – TOTALS & % BY WT.

0-19		20-39		40-59		60-79		80-99		100-119		120-139		140+	
1	2	1	6	6	50	4	43	0	0	0	0	0	0	0	0
3	13	6	57	2	30	0	0	0	0	0	0	0	0	0	0

ERRORS= 2

FIG. 2. Example of a computer printout of data from 2 days of continuous monitoring of feeding. This eating data file displays the exact start and finish of every meal, the duration and size of each meal, rates of eating during the meals, pre- and postmeal ratios, and summaries of each day's data. Here, the animal received a control injection on the first day and *dl*-fenfluramine (5.0 mg/kg) on the second. The drug clearly reduced meal size and the rate of eating.

ber). The second column indicates whether the meal was taken at night (N) or during the day (D). The next two columns give the actual start and end times of meals in decimal hours. The fifth and sixth columns give the pre- and postmeal interval in decimal hours. The seventh column gives meal duration, and columns eight and nine, the number of pellets and weight in grams consumed during a meal; the next two columns give pre- and postmeal ratios.

The remaining 16 columns of the eating data file (Fig. 2) examine intrameal events and are based on an analysis of the interpellet intervals. The major parameter derived from these data is the intrameal eating rate. This is computed from the weight of one food pellet divided by the median interpellet interval, which is computed from all interpellet intervals occurring within a meal. Quarter-bout medians are also computed, as there is evidence that feeding rates may be high at the start of meals and lower at the end (Wiepkema, 1971a; Le Magnen, 1971). Indeed, the rate of eating, calculated from the median interpellet interval, is slower over the second half of the meal than the first. This is probably one indicator of the development of satiation.

It is therefore interesting that one major effect of *dl*-fenfluramine is to slow the eating rate, a phenomenon also displayed by other agents that increase serotonin metabolism (Blundell and Latham, 1978) with the exception of tryptophan, which, although it reduced meal size, appeared to have no effect on feeding rate (Latham and Blundell, 1979). It should also be noted that drugs blocking dopamine receptors (e.g., pimozide and α-flupenthixol) also reduce eating rate, but unlike serotonergic agents, they lead to an increase in meal size (Blundell and Latham, 1978). This indicates that the slow rate of eating brought about by 5-HT agents does not necessarily reduce food intake.

The effect of *dl*-fenfluramine on eating rate can be more easily demonstrated by reference to plots of log survivor functions of interpellet intervals (Fig. 3). This measure is calculated to reveal the "break-point" in the distribution of interpellet intervals, thereby providing an objective criterion for the choice of intermeal interval. Changes in the slope of the log survivor function indicate a change in the probability of an event occurring (see Cox and Lewis, 1966). The slope also provides an indicator of the rate of events, and it is clear in Fig. 3 that *dl*-fenfluramine flattens the slope of the log survivor curve and, therefore, slows the rate of eating (during the night period). Consequently, in free-feeding rats *dl*-fenfluramine displays two major effects: a reduction in meal (or bout) size and a reduction in the intrameal rate of eating (Blundell and Latham, 1978; Burton et al., 1981).

Here mention should also be made of the effects of serotonin, which, when injected peripherally, will reduce food intake (Soulairac, 1963; Bray and York, 1972; Pollock and Rowland, 1981; Fletcher and Burton, 1984).

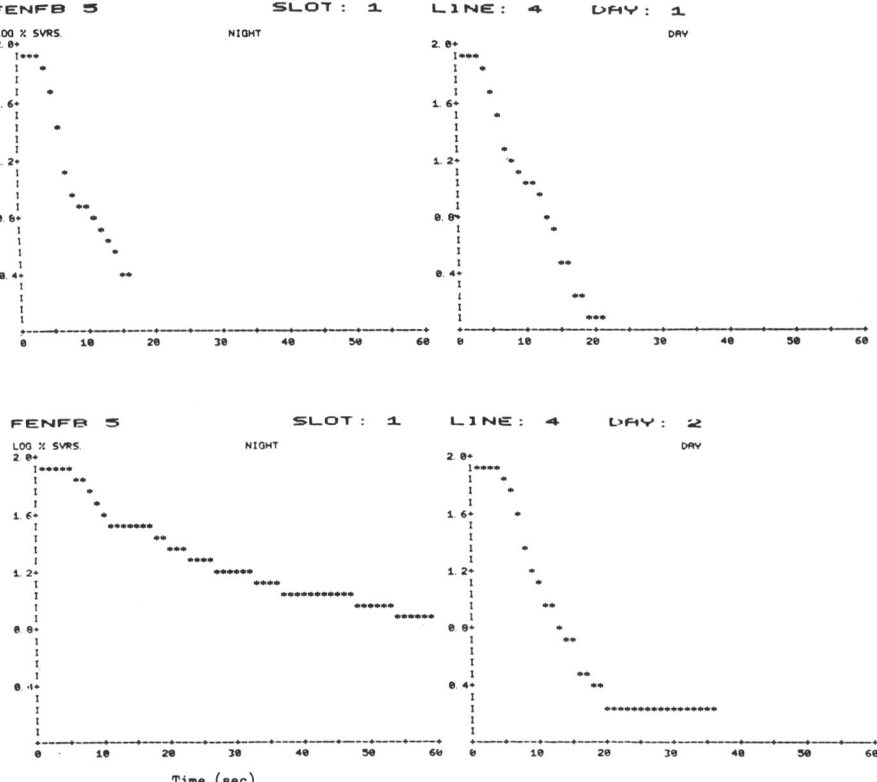

FIG. 3. Example of computer printouts of log survivor plots of interpellet intervals after saline treatment (top) and dl-fenfluramine (bottom). The drug (injected at the beginning of the dark phase) notably increased the size of the interpellet intervals (reduced the rate of eating) during the night period.

Using automated control apparatus, similar to that described earlier, Fletcher (1985) has shown that peripheral injections of 5-HT reduce bout duration and bout size, an effect similar to that previously demonstrated with fenfluramine. However, 5-HT did not reduce the eating rate, an effect similar to that demonstrated for tryptophan (Latham and Blundell, 1979). How should these findings be interpreted?

Since peripheral injections of 5-HT are unlikely to lead to any direct effect of 5-HT on brain receptors, the reduction in meal size appears to be mediated peripherally. This is consistent with the observation that the effect of 5-HT on food intake is blocked by xylamidine, a 5-HT receptor blocker that does not cross the blood–brain barrier (Fletcher, 1985). However, the nature of the peripheral mechanism involved is not yet clear, but it does not appear to involve the rate of gastric emptying. This is demonstrated by the finding that methysergide blocks the anorectic action of 5-HT but has no effect on the slowing of gastric emptying (Fletcher 1985). In addition, a peripheral mechanism does not appear able to account for the effects of *dl*-fenfluramine, since the anorectic action is not blocked by xylamidine (Fletcher, 1985).

Moreover, there is now substantial evidence on the effects of serotonergic modulation following direct central administration of serotonin. Using an eatometer procedure similar to that described earlier, it has been reported that low doses of serotonin infused into the paraventricular nucleus exert effects on feeding profiles quite similar to those displayed following peripheral administration, i.e., no effect on the latency to begin eating, a clear reduction in meal size, and a significant reduction in the rate of eating (Grinker *et al.*, 1982; Shor-Posner *et al.*, 1986).

Taken together, these findings suggest that both central and peripheral activation of 5-HT stores can produce changes in the structure of eating behavior, the most prominent adjustment being a reduction in meal (or bout) size. The change in eating rate appears to be centrally mediated. The specificity of these effects is evidence against a general behavioral suppressing action of 5-HT facilitation and suggests a more subtle intervention in the feeding process.

8.1.3. Dietary Self-Selection

Serotonergic manipulations can also alter the structure of feeding behavior when the choice of diets is adjusted (i.e., when rats are offered more than one type of food). Although this experimental model has been used for many years (e.g., Richter, 1943), until recently the phenomenon had been ignored in pharmacological investigations of feeding in which animals are generally maintained on a single composite diet containing a balanced mixture of essential nutrients. However, interest in pharmacological aspects of voluntary self-selection has been promoted by theoretical developments concerning the role of neurotransmitter systems in the regulation of protein and carbohydrate intake (see Anderson, 1979; Wurtman *et al.*, 1981; Li and Anderson, 1984; Ashley, 1985; Blundell, 1983). Brain serotonin is postulated to play a major role in determining macronutrient (dietary) selection by means of a mechanism that links nutrient composition of the diet to amino acid profiles in plasma, which, in turn, helps to determine tryptophan uptake into the brain and thereby modulates 5-HT synthesis (see Wurtman *et al.*, 1981, for details). Consequently, experimental manipulations of central 5-HT would be expected to alter an animal's selection of dietary macronutrients. Considerable methodological difficulties militate against unambiguous outcomes of experiments in this area (see Blundell, 1983, for review), and there is not universal accord among researchers (Blundell, 1984a). However, in general, the administration of pharmacological agents that facilitate synaptic 5-HT activity tends to promote a "protein-sparing" (Hirsch *et al.*, 1982) or a "carbohydrate-suppressive" (Moses and Wurtman, 1984) effect. However, the composition and number of diets appear critical, since other researchers have reported a decrease in fat intake following serotonergic manipulation (Orthen-Gambill and Kanarek, 1982) by *dl*-fenfluramine. When diets are varied in voluntary choice experiments, it is clear that a number of variables are implicated. They include the concentrations of macronutrients in the diets; the odor, taste, and texture of the diets; the acceptability of the diet to the rat; the familiarity and novelty of the diets; and the number of choices available. All these factors, acting individually or collectively, may influence a rat's choice of a particular food. Considering the complexity of these variables in the contextual dimension, it is surprising that even limited agreement has been obtained about the action of 5-HT manipulations. Taken together, the results suggest that central 5-HT tends to facilitate protein selection or depress preference for carbohydrate (Leibowitz and Shor-Posner, 1986).

8.1.4. Diet Selection and Feeding Profiles: Appetitive and Satiety Sequences

It is clear that the measurement of the end result of a rat's choices from two diets or more is not an alternative to monitoring of temporal changes. The techniques of nutrient selection and meal pattern analysis can be combined. In addition, the use of videotaped records of behavior allows a microstructural analysis of feeding and nonfeeding episodes. These procedures have been combined within a single experimental system (Fig. 4). Comparing the action of *d*-amphetamine and *dl*-fenfluramine has revealed certain interesting features of pharmacological manipulation on behavioral structure (Blundell and McArthur, 1981). On the one hand, amphetamine produced a severely fragmented sequence of behavior in which the structure of the meal was only loosely defined. On the other hand, *dl*-fenfluramine gave rise to a clear meal structure within which the rats spent more time eating the high-protein diet than the high-carbohydrate diet. The drug did not markedly disturb the structure of the appetitive or meal phases of the feeding cycle. However, the detailed monitoring of the structure of behavior disclosed one important aspect of the effects of serotonergic manipulation through arousal. Although *dl*-fenfluramine did notably increase the amount of time each rat spent resting, the rest periods did not intrude upon the meal phase of the cycle but appeared in their appropriate place in the sequence of behaviors forming the satiety phase. In other words, *dl*-fenfluramine extended the periods of rest that normally intervene between meals (Danguir *et al.*, 1979), but the tendency to rest did not interfere with the rat's ability to eat. This

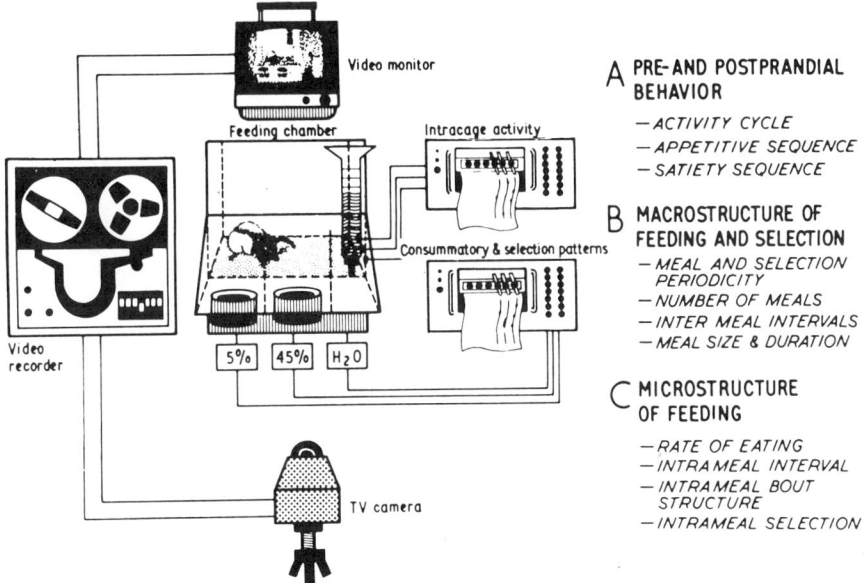

FIG. 4. Plan of the technique for the computer-logged continuous monitoring of diet selection, meal patterns, and appetitive and satiety sequences of behavior.

means that the anorectic action was not brought about by drowsiness. This observation is quite crucial to an understanding of the action of serotonergic drugs and illustrates two methodological issues: first, the importance of measuring different behaviors (e.g., eating and resting) simultaneously rather than in independent experiments and, second, the value of monitoring temporal changes in the structure of behavior.

8.1.5. Dietary-Induced Obesity

This topic is included here to illustrate how knowledge of the structure of behavior can help interpret studies on drugs and dietary-induced hyperphagia.

In recent studies (Hill et al., 1983; Blundell et al., 1986), we have examined the effect of the d-isomer of fenfluramine on food intake and weight gain during the dynamic and plateau phases of dietary-induced obesity. In two separate experiments, d-fenfluramine was given continuously to rats for 76 days during the dynamic phase of obesity (Experiment 1) or for 36 days, once a plateau phase of obesity had been reached (Experiment 2). The drug was given in the drinking water at a concentration of 0.057 mg/ml, and the rats received the normal diet of chow plus a cafeteria diet of bread, chocolate, biscuits, and beef fat. A control group

TABLE 3
d-Fenfluramine and Cafeteria-Induced Weight Gain[a]

	Experiment 1		Experiment 2
	36 days	76 days	36 days
Cafeteria	0.28(0.04)	0.16(0.03)	0.75(0.05)[b]
Chow	0.25(0.03)	0.14(0.02)	0.18(0.06)

[a] Effect of *d*-fenfluramine on weight loss during dynamic (Experiment 1) and plateau (Experiment 2) phases of dietary-induced obesity. The figures in the body of the table are the mean (SE) body weight losses for the treated animals compared with placebo-treated controls. The values indicate the body weight (g) lost per day per mg/kg of drug.
[b] $t = 6.772, p < 0.01$.

received tap water without drug, and separate groups of animals were maintained on laboratory chow for comparison. Consequently, the experimental design conformed to a 2×2 format with drug conditions (*d*-fenfluramine and water) and two diet conditions (cafeteria and normal chow).

The major outcome of the study is shown in Table 3. Since individual animals consumed differing quantities of water and therefore received differing amounts of the drug, measures of food intake and body weight were standardized to allow meaningful comparisons to be made among treatments.

The results disclosed an interesting pattern of effects. *d*-Fenfluramine significantly reduced food intake in both cafeteria-fed rats and the chow-fed control group, and this was accompanied by a marked loss of body weight. However, the potency of the drug (i.e., its capacity to reduce body weight compared with a placebo) was much greater in the plateau phase of obesity (Experiment 2) than in any of the other groups. In other words, although *d*-fenfluramine will reduce body weight over considerable periods of time in cafeteria- or chow-fed animals, it appears to be most effective in animals that have already been made obese. What is the explanation for this enhanced effectiveness? One possibility is that the action is mediated via adjustments in behavioral structure. It has been demonstrated repeatedly that one of the major actions accounting for the anorexic effect of serotonergic manipulations is a reduction in meal size. Moreover, it has been demonstrated that the development of dietary-induced obesity is associated with gradual changes in meal patterns (Rogers and Blundell, 1984). In particular, the plateau phase of obesity is characterized by a feeding pattern composed of a small number of large meals. Consequently, any pharmacological agent suppressing meal size may be expected to exert a potent effect in animals eating large, infrequent meals.

8.1.6. Summary of Findings

The studies discussed in this section have indicated how an analysis of behavioral structure can enhance understanding of the action of serotonergic manipulations upon food intake. In a number of studies using tryptophan (Latham and Blundell, 1979), 5-HTP (Blundell and Latham, 1979a; Fletcher, 1985), 5-HT (Fletcher, 1985), 5-HT uptake blockers (Blundell and Latham, 1978), fenfluramine (see above), and cyproheptadine (Baxter et al., 1970), it has been shown that a major effect of serotonin is to adjust meal size. Some manipulations also exert an effect upon intrameal eating rate and upon satiety ratios (ratio of meal size to postmeal interval—e.g., Latham and Blundell 1979). The behavioral sequences preceding and following a meal are preserved after fenfluramine administration, with a potentiation and elongation of the intermeal sleep period (Blundell and McArthur, 1981). Taken together, these and other findings suggest that 5-HT manipulations do not contaminate or distort the normal sequence of feeding activities. The results are consistent with an action upon the development of the process of satiation and a prolongation of the state of satiety.

8.2. Behavioral Analysis of the Effects of Opioid Antagonists on Feeding

It is more than 10 years since Holtzman (1974) demonstrated that the opioid antagonist naloxone decreased food intake in rats. Since that time, more than 40 papers have described the effects of either naloxone or naltrexone on food intake, and these compounds have come to be regarded as anorexic agents. Indeed, naloxone reduces intake when feeding is induced by starvation, noradrenaline injections into the paraventricular nucleus, muscimol injections into the dorsal raphe, and administration of 2-deoxy glucose and by stress (see Morley and Levine, 1985), in addition to suppressing spontaneous food intake in free-feeding rats. However, there are certain peculiarities about the anorexic profile of naloxone. For example, dose–response studies have demonstrated a quite mild anorexic action and a shallow dose–response curve for naloxone and other opioid antagonists (Sanger, 1981), and doses of naloxone as high as 80 mg/kg fail to suppress intake totally (unpublished data). This action of opioid antagonists is in sharp contrast to that of other well-known pharmacological anorexic agents, which generally show steep dose–response curves and frequently complete block eating. Naloxone does appear to reduce food intake, but what are the processes responsible for this effort and does it constitute a natural or an unnatural inhibition of eating? In order to investigate these issues, the action of naloxone was subjected to a series of behavioral analyses.

8.2.1. Naloxone and the Microstructure of Behavior

In this study, rats were tested under mild (6-hr) food deprivation and received three doses of naloxone (1.0, 2.5, and 5.0 mg/kg) and saline in a counterbalanced order. After the presentation of food, each animal's behavior was monitored for 30 min. The behavior was logged by means of a hand-held keyboard connected in parallel to a Nova 840 minicomputer and a Campden event recorder. Behavior was exhaustively recorded in the following categories: eating, drinking, grooming, sniffing, walking, rearing, and resting/inactive. The number of episodes and the duration of each individual episode were recorded.

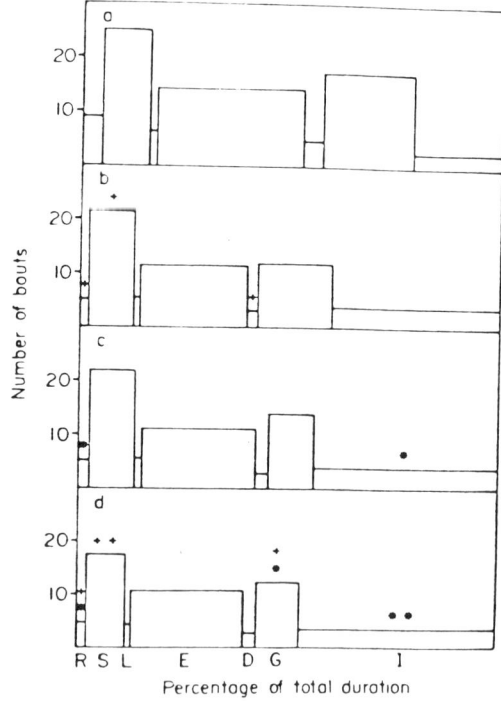

FIG. 5. Behavioral profiles for 6-hr-deprived rats over 30 min following i.p. injections of saline (a) or 1.0 (b), 2.5 (c), or 5.0 (d) mg/kg of naloxone. The mean number of bouts and mean duration, as a percentage of the total duration of the test, are given for each recorded behavior. The behavior categories for each dose are rearing (R), sniffing (S), locomotion (L), eating (E), drinking (D), grooming (G), and resting/inactivity (I). $*p < .05$, $**p < .01$ (percent total duration) and $^+p < .05$, $^{++}p < .01$ (number of bouts), difference from control using paired t test (two-tailed), $n = 8$.

The behavioral profiles produced by the four treatments are shown in Fig. 5. and a difference between the saline- and naloxone-treated animals is apparent. However, differences between the various doses of naloxone are less obvious, a finding that mirrors the weak dose–response effect on food intake. Considering the number of bouts of each behavior after naloxone treatment, there is a reduction in all categories with the exception of resting/inactivity, which, in contrast, is increased at all doses. Similar adjustments occur with regard to the total duration of each behavior, active behaviors (sniffing, rearing, grooming, eating, and drinking) being reduced below control values while the duration of resting is increased in a dose-related manner. The increase in resting associated with the decline in active behaviors could suggest that naloxone may simply be inhibiting food intake through an overall sedative action. However, further inspection of the parameters of the microstructure of eating shows clearly that this is not the case.

As shown in Table 4, measures of latency to the first contact with food and to the initiation of eating were reduced in a manner related to the dose of naloxone. This means that following naloxone treatment rats approach food more quickly and begin eating sooner. Moreover, a comparison of the latency to the end of the *final* eating bout and latency to the onset of the *first* bout of resting indicates that naloxone treatment

TABLE 4
Effects of Naloxone on Eating and Resting over 30 Min after 6-Hr Food Deprivation[a]

		Dose (mg/kg^{-1}, i.p.)		
	Saline	1.0	2.5	5.0
Total intake (g)	2.95	1.95	1.90*	1.80**
	(0.44)	(0.49)	(0.44)	(0.33)
Eating rate (g min^{-1})	0.32	0.23	0.23	0.22*
	(0.04)	(0.04)	(0.04)	(0.02)
Duration of eating (min)	9.59	9.12	8.00	6.82
	(2.00)	(2.34)	(1.76)	(0.97)
Duration of resting (min)	6.57	9.27	12.45	15.56
	(1.38)	(3.28)	(2.38)	(1.90)
Latency to onset of eating (min)	3.28	1.03	2.21	0.91
	(1.88)	(0.37)	(0.98)	(0.21)
Latency to end of final eating bout (min)	19.25	18.32	12.57	11.51*
	(1.68)	(3.52)	(2.68)	(1.33)
Latency to onset of first resting bout (min)	23.85	20.63	17.13	14.90*
	(2.15)	(3.24)	(2.25)	(1.55)

[a]Values for total intake and eating rate are means (SEM) for eight rats. All other values are means (SEM) for six rats. *$p < .005$, **$p < .01$ difference from control using t test for repeated measures (two-tailed).

gave rise to the increase in resting only *after* the rats had finished eating. Taken together, these findings suggest that a simple sedative explanation does not account for the suppression of eating by naloxone. It is clear that sedation did not impede the onset of eating, nor did it subsequently interfere with the expression of feeding. Bouts of eating were not delayed by the animal falling asleep or resting.

However, these findings are somewhat puzzling. Naloxone both increases the speed of initiation of eating and hastens the termination of eating (within the 30-min test period). On the one hand, the early cessation of eating followed by a long period of resting is consistent with an action of naloxone to promote satiation, since resting and sleeping after feeding is a natural behavioral response. On the other hand, the rapid reaction to food at the beginning of the test period suggests an action to enhance hunger. The shortening of the latency to initiate eating after naloxone was subsequently confirmed by examining the effect of the drug in a novel environment—an experimental manipulation intended to extend the eating latency. Under these circumstances, naloxone reduced time to first contact with food and reduced the latency for the initiation of feeding bouts of varying duration (see Kirkham and Blundell, 1984).

On the basis of the behavioral adjustments noted in this observational study, naloxone appears to exert a dual action on feeding. The drug hastens the initiation of eating but also brings about an early termination. This dual action helps to explain certain puzzling effects of naloxone. For example, the shallow dose–response function could arise from naloxone-intensifying processes controlling the initiation *and* termination of eating, thereby creating a mild net increase in food intake. It has also been reported that low doses of naloxone produce reliable (but statistically nonsignificant) increases in intake (Levine, 1983), while under certain experimental circumstances, naloxone may give rise to overeating (Shimomura *et al.*, 1982). Furthermore, the inhibition by naloxone of eating in humans with no effect on reported hunger (Trenchard and Silverstone, 1983) suggests an ambivalent or unusual action of the drug on the feeding process. The dual action of naloxone can be interpreted as an action on both hunger and satiation. Since overall food intake is generally reduced after naloxone treatment, it follows that the effect on satiation is usually the stronger, although certain experimental circumstances may favor the disclosure of the hunger effect. This behavioral profile demonstrates that naloxone is quite different in its mode of action from more traditional anorexic drugs such as amphetamine or fenfluramine. Indeed, considered as an anorexic agent, naloxone seems to be in a class of its own.

8.2.2. Motivation Assessed in the Runway

In order to further investigate the processes involved in naloxone's action, measures were made of the effects of the drug on instrumental performance in the runway. The technique has been described earlier (Section 7.5), and in this study, the effects of naloxone and naltrexone were compared with equianorectic doses of d-fenfluramine and amphetamine. The rats were trained in the runway and given food to maintain them at 85% of normal body weight. On test days, the rats were given 15 trials in the runway and allowed to eat for 2 min in the goal box at the end of each trial. This method was devised in order to monitor the development of satiation under control conditions and following drug administration. The technique proved capable not only of distinguishing between drugged and nondrugged rats but also of distinguishing between the actions of individual drugs. For naloxone and naltrexone, levels of runway performance (latency to emerge, running speed, latency to eat) were initially quite similar to those for saline-treated animals. Initially,

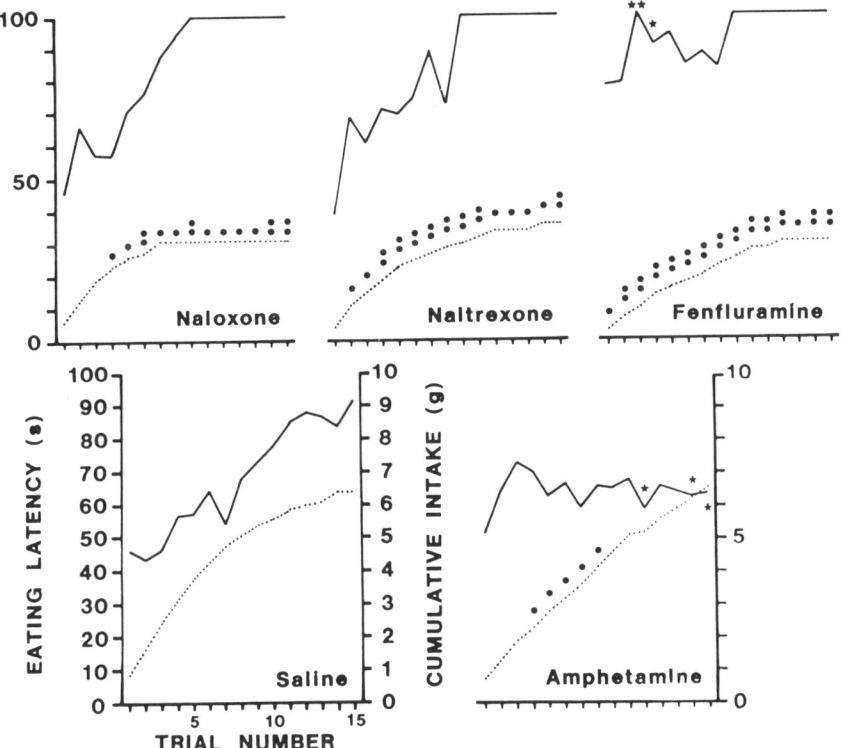

FIG. 6. Overall latency to eat (—) and cumulative food intake (· · · ·) over 15 runway trials after saline, naloxone (5.0 mg/kg), naltrexone (2.5), d-fenfluramine (1.5), and d-amphetamine (1.0). *$p < .05$, **$p < .01$ (latency); ·$p < .05$, :$p < .01$ (intake)—significantly different from saline (Newman–Keuls test for multiple comparisons following ANOVA). Overall latency—time from raising the door of the starting chamber to the initiation of eating in the goal box. Note that the anorexic action of d-amphetamine is completely eliminated.

food intake per trial was also normal. In the control condition, a typical satiation curve was demonstrated, with mean intake per trial declining over time. This effect is clearly shown in Fig. 6, which also indicates that a measure of motivational performance (overall latency to eat) changes in similar fashion. Thus, the development of satiation is reflected in both runway performance and food consumed. Both naloxone and naltrexone facilitate the development of satiation as reflected in lengthening of the latency to eat and a decline in the amount of food consumed. It is important that neither of these opioid blockers reduced the motivation to eat before feeding had been initiated. There was no evidence of any motivational deficit that might have reduced the tendency to initiate the primary instrumental or consummatory response. Consequently, the action of these opioid antagonists appears to depend upon food consumption; the drugs seem to augment the feedback resulting from ingestion, and this intensifies the process of satiation (Kirkham and Blundell, 1986).

8.2.3. Macroanalysis of Feeding Patterns

It follows from the outcome of the previous two studies that naloxone and naltrexone should exert certain specific effects upon meal patterns in accordance with their augmentation of satiation. Accordingly, the effects of these drugs were analyzed in free-feeding rats maintained in automated feeding chambers (see Section 7.3). The findings for naloxone are illustrated in Table 5 and indicate that the effect of the drug is limited to the first two meals consumed after drug administration. The dominant effect of naloxone is to reduce the sizes of the first two meals, and this is quite consistent with the postulated action upon the process of satiation. In addition, the elongation of the first postmeal interval leads to a marked change in the size of the satiety ratio. In other words, the effect of naloxone is to reduce meal size (satiation) and to strengthen the period of

TABLE 5
Naloxone-Induced Alterations to Meal Parameters of Free-Feeding Rats during Dark Phase (Meals 1–3)[a]

Meal number	Treatment	Meal duration (min)	Meal size (g)	Eating rate (g/min)	Postmeal interval (hr)	Satiety ratio
1	Saline	6.12 ± 0.87	1.62 ± 0.08	0.34 ± 0.03	0.90 ± 0.12	1.92 ± 0.26
	Naloxone	2.39 ± 0.68**	0.54 ± 0.08***	0.30 ± 0.03	1.30 ± 0.39	0.60 ± 0.27*
2	Saline	7.69 ± 2.71	1.71 ± 0.20	0.33 ± 0.04	0.74 ± 0.14	2.62 ± 0.52
	Naloxone	5.28 ± 1.66	0.68 ± 0.06**	0.25 ± 0.03	0.96 ± 0.18	1.18 ± 0.38
3	Saline	7.40 ± 3.74	1.35 ± 0.37	0.33 ± 0.02	2.45 ± 0.91	1.07 ± 0.20
	Naloxone	6.74 ± 1.94	0.84 ± 0.15	0.32 ± 0.04	0.71 ± 0.16	1.43 ± 0.43

[a] All values are the mean (± SEM) of six rats.
*$p < .05$, **$p < .01$, ***$p < .001$: significantly different from control values using t test for repeated measures (two-tailed).

inhibition over further eating (satiety). The time course of this effect is in keeping with the known duration of action of naloxone.

The effects of naltrexone were similar, but not identical, to those of naloxone. Action was limited to the first two meals of the feeding profile, but although naltrexone reduced meal size, this was not statistically significant; the drug did, however, significantly prolong the postmeal intervals of the first two meals.

These findings confirm and extend previous analyses of the action of these opioid antagonists. The analysis of the structure of behavior and its modulation with time has revealed new information about naloxone and naltrexone not available with the simple measurement of food consumption. Moreover, changes in the structure of behavior have been used to determine the action upon particular processes. Taken together, the three different procedures provide good evidence for the involvement of an opioidergic mechanism in the process of satiation. The difference between the action of these opioid antagonists and serotonin agonists appears to be that the former augment the development of satiation, whereas the latter have the capacity to initiate as well as to amplify the process. In turn, this difference suggests that these two sets of agents act at different points in the satiety cascade.

8.3. Behavioral Calibration of Natural and Abnormal Anorexia

One of the most intriguing problems in the analysis of drug-induced anorexia is how to evaluate the "natural" or "pathological" action of a drug on food intake. This involves differentiating between the inhibition of food consumption arising from a specific intervention in a physiological system controlling nutritional requirements and that resulting from nonspecific changes leading to the suppression or contamination of behavior. It was noted earlier that temporal changes in the structure of behavior can be used as a behavioral assay of the development of satiation. Consequently, by inhibiting food intake by agents believed to exert nonspecific or unphysiological actions and simultaneously monitoring behavior changes, it becomes possible to diagnose pseudosatiation. This technique has been referred to as behavioral calibration (Blundell *et al.*, 1985).

A study was designed to calibrate the behavioral structure characterizing anorexia and to define behavior representative of normal or abnormal conditions. Treatments were chosen that, by general agreement, may be regarded as inducing normal or contaminated processes. A comparison was made between the effects on behavioral structure of a reduction in food intake brought about by prefeeding (normal ingestion by mouth) and two agencies believed to depress consumption by mechanisms not involved in the development of satiation. Note that the term satiation is reserved for the cessation of food consumption arising as a result of food ingestion. The two agencies chosen were injections of lithium chloride, which is commonly believed to induce intestinal discomfort and nausea, and the adulteration of food with bitter-tasting quinine hydrochloride, which produces an aversive response. During the experiment, animals were placed on a cyclic regimen of 20 hr of food deprivation followed by 28 hr of access to food. During the first hour of feeding, the animals were placed in a glass observation tank, during which time each rat's behavior was continuously observed and recorded by a trained observer. The animal's activities were classified into seven mutually exclusive categories—eating, drinking, sniffing (while otherwise inactive), walking, grooming, rearing, and resting—and the observer recorded the onset, duration, and termination of these behavioral events by pressing buttons on a hand-held control panel. The coded keys were connected on-line to a Data General NOVA 840 minicomputer and a Campden event recorder. The data collected in this way were processed to provide the microparameters of eating behavior. In addition to these specific feeding parameters, which have previously been shown to be sensitive indicators of a variety of experimental manipulations, computation was also made of the amount of time taken up by feeding and the various nonfeeding activities. The duration of the behaviors recorded was plotted over time to reveal the sequential changes in behavior as eating progressed and eventually ceased during the 1-hr test period. Plotting the data in this way was designed to disclose the emergence of a pattern of behavior characterizing the development of satiation.

A within-subjects design was employed, and each animal was tested under each of the four conditions. A counterbalanced order of presentation (Latin square) was used to minimize order effects. The treatment comprised a control condition and three experimental conditions each titrated to produce equianorectic effects, i.e., an intake approximately 50% of the control value for the 1-hr test. The first experimental treatment was a prefeed (PF) of the test food, amounting to 70% of the control 1-hr intake, and given 1 hr before the start of the feeding test. The amount of the prefeed varied between 4.4 and 5.0 g for individual animals. The second treatment was an intraperitoneal injection of lithium chloride (LC) at a dose (60 mg/kg) selected on the basis of a dose–response study carried out before the start of the experiment proper. The third treatment involved adulteration of the test food with quinine (Q) at a concentration of 0.04%, a value again derived from earlier dose–response studies. It was expected that each experimental treatment would produce an equivalent suppression of intake during the 1-hr test period. The effects of the treatments upon food intake and feeding parameters during the 1-hr test session are shown in Table 6. The experimental conditions brought about significant changes in food consumption ($F[3,18]$

TABLE 6
Food Intake and Feeding Parameters Recorded during a 1-Hr Feeding Test in 20-Hr Deprived Rats[a]

	Food intake (g)**	Duration of eating (min)**	Number of eating bouts*	Latency to eat (min)**	Local eating rate (g/min)**
Control	6.60	16.07	21.57	0.43	0.430
	(0.26)	(1.44)	(2.58)	(0.22)	(0.03)
Prefeed	3.27	6.57	16.14	4.68	0.566
	(0.52)	(1.16)	(2.87)	(1.63)	(0.09)
Lithium	3.89	13.55	13.71	0.99	0.296
	(0.40)	(1.76)	(2.92)	(0.23)	(0.02)
Quinine	4.13	12.88	26.29	0.83	0.380
	(0.45)	(1.75)	(5.55)	(0.29)	(0.09)

[a]Each value is the mean (+SE) of seven subjects. *$p < .05$, **$p < .01$ ANOVA.

$= 26.8; p < .01$), and amounts consumed after each treatment were significantly less than the control value. It can be seen that the experimental treatments each reduced food consumption by approximately 50%. Table 6 also indicates that the treatments produced marked changes in the various parameters of feeding behavior with significant differences noted on each variable (smallest $F = 4.07, p < .05$). *Post hoc* comparisons with the Newman–Keuls test revealed that PF was significantly different from all other conditions on duration of eating and latency; Q increased and LC decreased the number of eating bouts; and both Q and LC reduced the local rate of eating. The effects of the treatments upon feeding and the other recorded categories of behavior are shown in Tables 7 and 8. Table 7 illustrates the percentage of time allocated to each behavior during the 1-hr test, and it can be seen that the treatment brought about marked changes in most categories. Significant treatment effects are as noted with smallest $F = 3.04, p < 0.05$. Table 8 shows changes in the number of

TABLE 7
Percentage of Time Spent on the Seven Monitored Behaviors during the 1-Hr Test Period

	Rearing**	Walking	Sniffing*	Grooming*	Resting	Eating**	Drinking**
Control	10.59	1.26	17.18	23.04	17.92	26.78	3.24
Prefeed	17.81	2.25	25.99	23.44	17.21	10.94	2.36
Lithium	4.91	1.46	24.75	14.87	28.53	22.59	2.89
Quinine	12.58	1.42	25.40	14.99	21.86	21.47	2.29

*$p < .05$, **$p < .01$ ANOVA.

TABLE 8
Mean (+SE) Number of Separate Bouts of Observed Behaviors during the 1-Hr Test Period

	Rearing**	Walking*	Sniffing**	Grooming*	Resting	Eating*	Drinking	Total**
Control	55.71	28.57	98.14	40.71	52.29	21.57	7.29	304.29
	(10.30)	(7.61)	(12.94)	(8.65)	(5.26)	(2.58)	(1.64)	(34.64)
Prefeed	101.29	50.57	156.29	46.00	52.14	16.14	4.43	426.86
	(15.75)	(9.73)	(18.83)	(9.97)	(7.02)	(2.87)	(0.92)	(50.03)
Lithium	39.14	24.57	92.86	23.71	46.57	13.71	6.57	247.14
	(11.66)	(5.23)	(15.33)	(3.00)	(5.76)	(2.92)	(2.81)	(35.70)
Quinine	81.43	33.86	133.14	36.14	47.71	26.29	5.71	364.29
	(11.60)	(5.70)	(16.45)	(7.84)	(8.60)	(5.55)	(1.89)	(46.32)

*$p < .05$, **$p < .01$ ANOVA.

bouts of each activity, and again it can be seen that the treatment gave rise to changes in most behaviors. From these data, it is possible to characterize the way in which each experimental treatment brought about a reduction in food consumption. The PF anorexia was associated with increased latency and a short duration of quite rapid feeding. The reduction of feeding was accompanied by changes in behavioral categories of rearing and sniffing—the increased number of bouts signifying an active behavior pattern. The LC anorexia was brought about by a reduced number of bouts of eating and a markedly reduced local rate of eating. This reduced eating was associated with a marked decrease in grooming and an increase in resting. The Q anorexia was typified by a large number of brief bouts of feeding involving a slow eating rate. The eating profile was again accompanied by a decrease in grooming and an increase in resting.

These data indicate that the experimental treatments produced widespread changes in the duration and number of episodes of eating and other behaviors. However, the method of behavioral analysis also revealed temporal changes in behavior. In Fig. 7, the temporal profiles of the three major categories of behavior—eating, grooming, and resting—implicated in the development of satiation are plotted. Differences between the two pathological treatments and the two normal conditions are immediately apparent and reflect the changes in grooming and resting shown in Table 7. The results of this study have been described at some length because of the methodological importance attached to the possibility of distinguishing between satiation and pseudosatiation.

The study has shown that the three anorexic treatment conditions (PF, Q, and LC) not only reduced the amount of food consumed in the 1-hr test but also produced clear alterations in the structure of feeding behavior. Moreover, although the treatments produced approximately equivalent reductions in the amount of food eaten, they gave rise to dis-

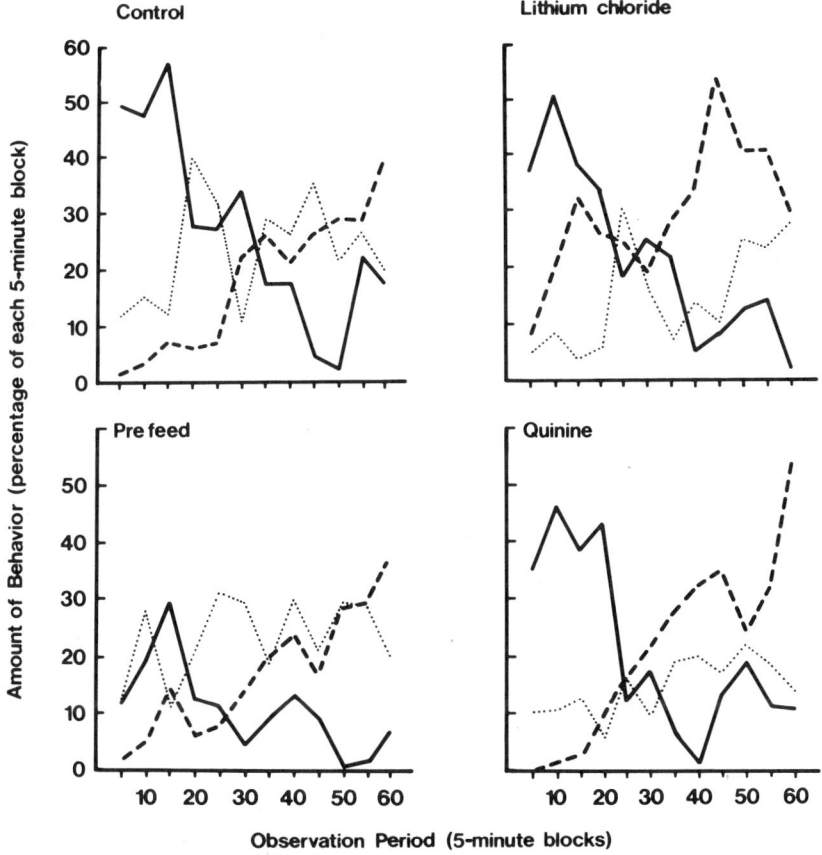

FIG. 7. Temporal profiles of the three behaviors—eating (—), grooming (· · · ·), and resting (- - -)—chiefly implicated in the development of satiation. Data are plotted as percentages of times occupied by each behavior in each 5-min block over the course of the 1 hr test.

tinctive adjustments to the measured parameters of the act of eating. Consequently, agents that produce anorexia via different mechanisms (defined here as normal or pathological) can be readily identified by their effects upon the structure of behavior. The data disclosed clearly apparent differences between the behavioral effects of the PF treatment and the effects engineered by LC and Q. However, as would be expected, certain differences were observed between LC and Q treatments. The reduced number of bouts of eating brought about by LC and the large number of very brief bouts seen with Q are quite understandable in the light of the presumed mechanisms of action of these treatments.

In addition to changes in the structure of actual eating events, the three treatments gave rise to significant alterations in nonfeeding activities. This indicates that anorexia not only affects food intake and feeding behavior but also involves associated aspects of the behavioral repertoire. Moreover, there was again a clear difference between the effects of PF (a so-called normal treatment) and LC and Q (considered pathological treatments). Taken together, these sets of data indicate that analysis of the structure of behavior (feeding and nonfeeding) is sensitive to the action of various anorexic treatments. More important, changes in behavioral structure provide a means of diagnosing whether a suppression of food intake is brought about through activation of a normal physiological process or whether it arises from physiological disturbance (LC) or contamination (Q).

Although definite differences have been demonstrated in the type and frequency of occurrence of behavioral events between various anorexic treatments, a further clear and meaningful difference was disclosed by the temporal profiles (Fig. 7). These profiles also cast light upon the relationship between the experimental treatments and the natural development of satiation. In the behavioral sequence of satiety described by Smith, Gibbs, and co-workers, cessation of eating is associated with an increase in grooming followed by resting. This pattern has also been shown in the transition from a feeding phase to a satiety phase recorded in conjunction with meal taking in nondeprived animals (Blundell and McArthur, 1981). This sequence is again well illustrated by the C and PF conditions in Fig. 7. In both cases, the onset and rise of the profile of resting is preceded by a period in which grooming is the dominant behavior. However, this sequence is disturbed following the Q and LC treatments. In keeping with the increased occurrence of resting and the decreased frequency of grooming (Table 7) brought about by LC and Q, the profiles in Fig. 7 show that as feeding begins to decline there is a sharp rise in resting to the exclusion of grooming. In the case of LC, there is a marked peak of resting before grooming appears, and in the Q condition, resting increases sharply and grooming never reaches an appreciable level. Neither in LC or Q does grooming act as a transition behavior between eating and resting. It may justifiably be argued that the behavioral profiles for the C and PF conditions reflect the operation of the natural process of satiation, i.e., the cessation of food intake arising from the consequences of ingestion. In contrast, the profiles for LC and Q represent a diagnosis of the symptoms of anorexia not dependent upon a normal process of satiation. Taken together, the parameters of feeding behavior, the frequencies of associated behaviors, and the qualitative pattern of the temporal profiles indicate that an analysis of the structure of behavior can distinguish between anorexia due to the operation of satiation and anorexia engendered by a physiological or environmental impediment.

Of course, it should be kept in mind that there cannot be a total separation between the consequences of normal and pathological anorexic treatments. First, rats in the LC and Q conditions did consume a certain amount of food, and therefore, weak postingestive effects on behavior would be expected. Second, even normal satiation (following a substantial period of food deprivation) may involve a mild degree of intestinal discomfort, and third, it is widely accepted that satiety involves a decline in the hedonic value of food. When these common elements of the normal and pathological treatments are allowed for, the differences observed in the frequency of behaviors and in the temporal sequence are striking.

What are the implications of these results for the pharmacological manipulation of eating and, in particular, for drug-induced anorexia? Behavioral calibration permits the identification of anorexia brought about by adverse circumstances (physiological or environmental). Consequently, by monitoring the effects of drugs on the structure of behavior, it should be possible to determine whether a drug stops eating by facilitating a normal process of satiation or by creating abnormal physiological (metabolic or sensory) conditions. Inspection of the results of studies already carried out suggests that the massive increase in locomotor activity and the decrease in grooming induced by amphetamine are not compatible with the normal operation of satiation. This feature, together with other unusual aspects of the action of peripherally administered amphetamine on food intake, suggests that amphetamine should no longer be considered a reference compound for drug-induced anorexia. The studies on *dl*-fenfluramine and other compounds acting upon serotoninergic systems have revealed a behavioral profile quite different from that of amphetamine. The constellation of behavioral changes induced by racemic fenfluramine appears a little ambiguous, incorporating changes typical of normal satiation and abnormal anorexia. The drug reduced the rate of eating, slightly increased resting, but did not change grooming. Examination of the temporal profile of behavioral adjustments, however, indicated that the increase in resting occurred at the end of the satiety sequence and did not interfere with the development of satiation. The changes in behavioral structure induced by racemic fenfluramine do not place it in the same category as LC or Q. Similar reasoning can be used to classify the anorexia induced by opioid antagonists (Section 8.2). Here again, the onset of resting did not occur until eating had terminated, indicating a preservation of the natural sequence of behaviors occurring during satiation. It is apparent from the results of this study and other experiments on the effects of drugs on behavioral structure that there are a number of behavioral profiles that can represent abnormal anorexia as opposed to the natural anorexia brought about by premature onset of satiety or intensification of the process of satiation. For example, the profiles of LC and Q (present experiment) are quite different from behavioral changes brought about by amphetamine (Blundell and Latham, 1980) and by bombesin (Gibbs *et al.,* 1981; Kulkovsky *et al.,* 1982), but all of these are readily distinguishable from C and PF (present experiment) and earlier related studies of fenfluramine (Blundell and Latham, 1978), naloxone (Kirkham and Blundell, 1984), and cholecystokinin (Antin *et al.,* 1975). In addition, it also seems likely that the behavioral profiles of anorexia-inducing drugs will not necessarily always fit neatly into normal or pathological categories. This will arise from the tendency of drugs to exert multiple effects—in part facilitating a natural process involved in the control of food intake and in part creating abnormal physiological circumstances. Moreover, although the results of behavioral analysis can provide a sensitive indicator of a drug's action, the characterization of a drug's effect on feeding should also include other aspects of its relationship to eating, such as a preference for particular macronutrients (see Section 7.6), an effect on dietary-induced hyperphagia (Section 7.4), and the influence on meal parameters of free-feeding animals (Section 7.3). The results of the present study, however, show that changes in behavioral structure can be calibrated to define normal and abnormal anorexic patterns. The structure reflects the operation of underlying processes, which, in turn, can be linked to specific mechanisms.

9. CONTROL OF FEEDING: A SECOND LOOK

It is now more than 30 years since the postulation of the dual-center (or multifactorial) theory of motivation (Stellar, 1954). During this period, there has been a massive increase in knowledge in the field of neuroscience and a corresponding advance in the database relating to the control of food intake. What role have drugs played in this advancement?

9.1. Impact of Pharmacological Studies

One of the main features of pharmacological agents is their capacity to be used as tools to manipulate particular neurochemical systems selectively. In terms of experimental procedures, drugs are very convenient devices in that they can provoke large changes in consumption (at least in the short term—see Section 3), and this has given rise to a massive amount of data. However, the ease of manipulating food consumption by drug administration carries with it a number of methodological implications. First, drugs as tools are not always specific—they may have effects on more than one neurotransmitter system (which may depend on the dose) and they may exert effects at multiple sites in the brain. Second, when administered parenterally, drugs may act both within the brain and in the periphery. Third, when experiments are designed in a simple stimulus (drug)–response (food intake) fashion, the outcome will rarely cast light upon the processes that mediate in the matching of an organism's feeding activity to its nutritional requirements. Often experimenters conclude their reports with the observation that the results may indicate some role for transmitter X (influenced by the drug) in the overall control of intake. Such a conclusion, even couched in such vague and tentative language, is often unwarranted, since frequently no attempt has been made to assess the proper meaning of the change in consumption observed. Is the change consistent with energy metabolism, with the physiological handling of particular nutrients, or with the functions and integration of different behaviors?

Even the classic pharmacological strategy of agonist–antagonist effect, or stimulation–blockade, does not overcome these objections. Certainly, this strategy does increase confidence in the identity of the systems involved, but it does not disclose the function of the system nor does it reveal whether the change in food consumption is a meaningful behavioral shift or an artifactual behavioral upheaval. The use of specialized classic pharmacological procedures for *in vitro* tissue preparations in experiments on the whole freely behaving organism is appropriate, but additional methodological provisions are required. It has been argued in this chapter that drug studies on feeding should be embraced within a clear conceptual framework embodying a manifest methodology. The thesis proposed here is represented by the framework of a biopsychological system and a methodology that emphasizes the meaningfulness of behavioral structure—expressed in accordance with particular contextual and temporal conditions.

9.2. A Paradox: The Orexic and Anorexic Effects of Amphetamine

Many of the difficulties inherent in the interpretation of drug effects on food consumption can be illustrated by an inspection of the consequences of amphetamine administration. For more than 40 years, amphetamine has been regarded as the standard anorectic drug. It is, of course, true that amphetamine can reduce food intake, but in other domains of research, locomotor activity and stereotypy have been considered major behavioral targets (e.g., Costa and Garattini, 1970). Moreover, in recent years, it has been shown that amphetamine does not invariably have a consistent effect on food consumption. For example, in deprived rats, amphetamine actually increases the rate of eating (an enhancing effect) while diminishing total food intake (a suppressant effect) (Blundell and Latham, 1978, 1980). In addition, amphetamine has been shown to increase food consumption paradoxically. This has been observed when very low doses of the drug are given mice (Dobrzanski and Doggett, 1976) or rats (Blundell and Latham, 1978) that have not been subjected to food deprivation. The phenomenon has also been shown to occur in cats (Wolgin *et al.,* 1976) and rats (Stricker and Zigmond, 1976) in which sedating lateral hypothalamic lesions have been produced, and it has occasionally been reported in food-deprived animals (Holtzman, 1974).

It is also apparent that the modulation of the action of amphetamine does not depend invariably upon some internal physiological readjustment. Although amphetamine anorexia can be attenuated by 6-hydroxydopamine lesions of the ventral noradrenergic bundle (Ahlskog, 1974) or by the administration of neuroleptic drugs (e.g., Burridge and Blundell, 1979), this effect can also be completely antagonized by measuring food consumption in a runway (see Fig. 5, Section 8.2). Add to these pieces of evidence the fact that amphetamine has a marked effect on nutrient selection in food choice experiments (Blundell and McArthur, 1979), and the action of amphetamine appears strongly as a context-dependent phenomenon. This picture of the effects of amphetamine can be represented by the model shown in Fig. 8. The action of amphetamine varies according to the circumstance—changes in internal state, alterations in environ-

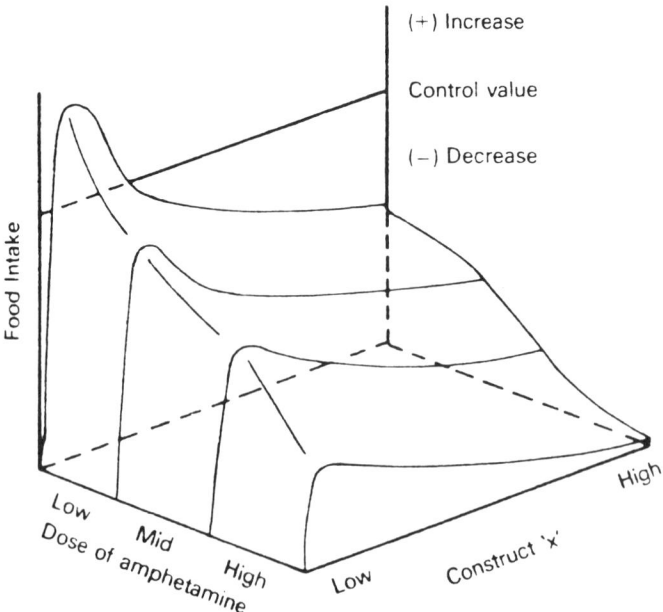

FIG. 8. Conceptualization of the range of quantitative effects of amphetamine.

mental demands—and the prevailing conditions can either attenuate or reverse the widely known typical anorexic effect. The conceptualization devised to account for these varied effects of amphetamine is founded on the assumption that the drug's effects can only be properly interpreted by considering its action within a system; changing the values of elements within the system modulates the final outcome. Such a conceptualization is only possible because of the large amount of data available on amphetamine—the most frequently used drug in feeding experiments. As other drugs are used under different experimental circumstances, their effects may best be interpreted through a system approach. Already, the reported modulation of the anorexic action of fenfluramine by the nutrient composition of the diet (Moses and Wurtman, 1984) suggests that fenfluramine anorexia is also context dependent. The current scientific way of thinking about drug–feeding relationships promotes the idea of drugs with particular profiles, exerting selective effects on food consumption. Experiments are, therefore, designed to capitalize on these effects and to confirm them. However, if the prevailing view were changed to embrace context-dependent effects and system modulation of a drug's action, the experiments would be designed differently and the behavioral pharmacology of feeding would be radically reshaped.

9.3. Models of Feeding Control

In recent years, the widespread use of pharmacological procedures (including central and peripheral administration) has led to the identification of certain agents having particularly potent effects on food consumption and to the definition of certain very sensitive central sites of action. The most reliable and powerful effects appear to be mediated via hypothalamic sites—particularly the paraventricular nucleus and the perifornical area (see Liebowitz, 1980, for a review). These zones appear to contain α_2-adrenoceptive sites and β-adrenoceptive sites, respectively. This arrangement has been confirmed by the judicious use of central microinjection procedures in conjunction with peripheral drug administration. The identity of these sites has been derived from the use of the agonist–antagonist pharmacological methods. Further studies with serotonergic compounds have disclosed a clear 5-HT modulation of the α-adrenoceptors in the paraventricular nucleus. In turn, these data, together with data from lesion studies, suggest a central model for the interplay of various aminergic systems that influence food consumption (Hoebel and Leibowitz, 1981). A similar conceptualization based on a temporal rather than spatial interaction has also been put forward to account for the effects produced by drugs with differing neurochemical actions (e.g., Blundell, 1981a, 1982b). Are these models an advance on the dual-center concept proposed 30 years ago? Progress has been made in two ways. First, the newer models are more detailed and more specific about the nature of the brain elements involved and the moment-to-moment control of eating. Second, the recent conceptualizations admit a greater complexity in the crucial mechanisms. This is reflected in the notion of an interaction between active elements, the final outcome being dependent upon the state of a number of neuromodulatory components.

In addition to the conceptualizations mentioned earlier, major contributions have been made to central models through the work of Morley and of Hoebel. Morley has been responsible for giving credibility to the role of peptides in the central control of eating. A large series of experiments have demonstrated that many peptides can actively influence food ingestion when applied directly to the brain. Two groups of peptides increase feeding after central injection: the opioid peptide family (β-endorphin, dynorphin, and α-neoendorphin) and the pancreatic polypeptide family (human pancreatic polypeptide, neuropeptide Y, and peptide YY). More than a dozen peptides bring about a decrease in eating after central injection (e.g., Morley et al., 1985; Morley and Levine, 1985). From the outset, Morley attempted to embrace the large number of active peptides within one central integrative model, and this gave rise to a series of conceptualizations of ever-increasing complexity (e.g., Morley, 1980; Morley and Levine, 1983). One major feature of these models was the attempt to relate the peptides to the amine neurotransmitters. Hoebel has also made specific suggestions regarding the interrelationships between peptide and amine systems in the brain (Hoebel, 1984). The principle underlying the construction of such models is the notion of a cascade, with food ingestion initiating a sequence of neurochemical events. For experimental purposes, the cascade can be interrupted at various points to adjust consumption.

These models clearly recognize, and attempt to embrace, a complex set of interactions within the brain. Since the elements in these models can usually be manipulated by peripherally injected compounds (directly or indirectly), the active sites and systems are directly relevant to pharmacological approaches to feeding.

There is one further distinction between the recent models and the dual-center hypothesis. The notion of two critical nuclei in the hypothalamus, where experimental manipulation could produce such dramatic changes, had the effect of concentrating attention on the relationship between these two zones and behavior to the relative exclusion of other aspects of the system. Consequently, many experiments were carried out with little regard for the physiological processes that accompany food ingestion. In contrast, recently developed models—operating from a wider experimental base—have incorporated a link between central amine/peptide systems, peripheral metabolic events, and selective behavioral adjustment. For example, the activity of α- and β-adrenoceptive elements in the hypothalamus has been linked to the metabolism of carbohydrates and protein (Leibowitz and Shor-Posner, 1986) and the activity in the pituitary–adrenal axis—particularly the release of corticosterone (Leibowitz, 1986a). In turn, the up-and-down regulation of α-adrenergic receptor activity in the hypothalamus has been related to the structural patterning of feeding behavior—both eating episode cycles during night and day and the direction of behavior embodied in food choices (Leibowitz, 1986b). It is the anchoring of brain events—at one end in metabolism and at the other end in behavioral structure—which gives a central model its credibility.

Consequently, the models of feeding currently being generated reflect the theme of this chapter. Researchers who use pharmacological manipulations should recognize the existence of a system that embraces both metabolism and behavior. In this domain, drugs can continue to be valuable tools to elucidate the relationships between structure, processes, and mechanisms.

ACKNOWLEDGMENTS

I am grateful to Micah Leshem, Colin Latham, Peter Rogers, Bob McArthur, Tim Kirkham, and Andy Hill for scientific collaboration on the empirical studies and on the development of ideas described in this chapter. I thank Betty Fowbert for help with the preparation of the text.

10. REFERENCES

ADLER, N. T., 1968, Effects of the male's copulatory behavior on successful pregnancy of the female rat, *J. Comp. Physiol. Psychol.* **69:**613–622.

AHLSKOG, J. E., 1974, Food intake and amphetamine anorexia after selective forebrain norepinephrine loss, *Brain Res.* **82:**211–240.

AMDISEN, A., 1964, Drug-produced obesity. Experiences with chlorpromazine, perphenazine and clopenthixol, *Dan. Med. Bull.* **11:**182–189.

ANDERSON, G. H., 1979, Control of protein and energy intake: role of plasma amino acids and brain neurotransmitters, *Can. J. Physiol. Pharmacol.* **57:**1043–1057.

ANTELMAN, S. M., BLACK, C. A., and ROWLAND, N. E., 1977, Clozapine induces hyperphagia in undeprived rats, *Life Sci.* **21:**1747–1750.

ANTIN, J., GIBBS, J., HOLT, J., YOUNG, R. C., and SMITH, G. P., 1975, Cholecystokinin elicits the complete behavioural sequence of satiety in rats, *J. Comp. Physiol. Psychol.* **89:**784–790.

APFELBAUM, M., and MANDENOFF, A., 1981, Naltrexone suppresses hyperphagia induced in the rat by a highly palatable diet, *Pharmacol. Biochem. Behav.* **15:**89–91.

ASHLEY, D. V. M., 1985, Factors affecting the selection of protein and carbohydrate from a dietary choice, *Nutr. Res.* **5:**555–571.

ATKINSON, J., KIRCHERTZ, E. J., and PETERS-HAEFELI, L., 1978, Effect of peripheral clonidine on ingestive behaviour, *Physiol. Behav.* **21:**73–77.

BAINBRIDGE, J. G., 1968, The effect of psychotropic drugs on food reinforced behaviour and on food consumption, *Psychopharmacologia* (Berlin) **12**:204–213.

BALOPOLE, D. E., HANSULT, C. D., and DORPH, D., 1979, Effect of cocaine on food intake in rats, *Psychopharmacology* **64**:121–122.

BAXTER, M. G., MILLER, A. A., and SOROKO, F. E., 1970, The effect of cyproheptadine on food consumption in the fasted rat, *Br. J. Pharmacol.* **39**:229–230P.

BEACH, F. A., 1976, Sexual attractivity, proceptivity and receptivity in female mammals, *Horm. Behav.* **7**:105–138.

BEACH, F. A., 1979, Animal models for human sexuality, in: *Sex, Hormones and Behaviour,* Ciba Foundation Symposium 62 (new series), Excerpta Medica, Amsterdam, pp. 113–132.

BEDFORD, J. A., LOVELL, D. K., TURNER, C. E., ELSOHLY, M. A., and WILSON, M. C., 1980, The anorexic and actometric effects of cocaine and two coca extracts, *Pharmacol. Biochem. Behav.* **13**:403–408.

BENADY, D. R., 1970, Cyproheptadine hydrochloride (Periactin) and anorexia nervosa: A case report, *Br. J. Psychiatry* **117**:681–682.

BERGEN S. S., 1964, Appetite stimulating properties of cyproheptadine, *Am. J. Dis. Child.* **108**:270–274.

BERMANT, G., 1961, Response latencies of female rats during sexual intercourse, *Science* **133**:1771–1773.

BLAVET, N., DE FEUDIS, F. V., and CLOSTRE, F., 1982, THIP inhibits feeding behaviour in fasted rats, *Psychopharmacology* **76**:75–78.

BLUNDELL, J. E., 1977, Is there a role for serotonin (5-hydroxytryptamine) in feeding? *Int. J. Obesity* **1**:15–42.

BLUNDELL, J., 1979a, Hunger, appetite and satiety—Constructs in search of identities, in: *Nutrition and Lifestyles* (M. Turner, ed.), Applied Science Pub., London, pp. 21–42.

BLUNDELL, J. E., 1979b, Serotonin and feeding, in: *Serotonin in Health and Disease,* Vol. 5 (W. B. Essman, ed.), Spectrum, New York, pp. 403–450.

BLUNDELL, J. E., 1980, Pharmacological adjustment of the mechanisms underlying feeding and obesity, in: *Obesity* (A. J. Stunkard, ed.), Saunders, Philadelphia, pp. 182–207.

BLUNDELL, J. E., 1981a, Biogrammar of feeding: Pharmacological manipulations and their interpretations, in: *Progress in Theory in Psychopharmacology* (S. J. Cooper, ed.), Academic Press, London, pp. 233–276.

BLUNDELL, J. E., 1981b, Deep and surface structures: A qualitative approach to feeding, in: *The Body Weight Regulatory System: Normal and Disturbed Mechanisms* (L. A. Cioffi, W. P. T. James, T. Van-Itallie, eds.), Raven Press, New York, pp. 73–82.

BLUNDELL, J. E., 1982a, Neuroregulators and feeding: Implication for the pharmacological manipulating of hunger and appetite, *Rev. Pure Appl. Pharmacol. Sci.* **3**(4):381–462.

BLUNDELL, J. E., 1982b, Factors regulating food intake: From causes to interactions, *Aliment. Nutr. Metab.* **3**:7–19.

BLUNDELL, J. E., 1983, Processes and problems underlying the control of food selection and nutrient intake, in: *Nutrition and the Brain,* Vol. 6 (R. J. Wurtman and J. J. Wurtman, eds.), Raven Press, New York, pp. 164–221.

BLUNDELL, J. E., 1984a, Systems and interactions: An approach to the pharmacology of eating and hunger, in: *Eating and Its Disorders* (A. J. Stunkard and E. Stellar, eds.), Raven Press, New York, pp. 39–65.

BLUNDELL, J. E., 1984b, Serotonin and appetite, *Neuropharmacology* **32**:1537–1552.

BLUNDELL, J. E., and HILL, A. J., 1986, Biopsychological interactions underlying the study and treatment of obesity, in: *The Psychosomatic Approach: Contemporary Practice of Whole Person Care* (M. J. Christie and P. G. Mellett, eds.), Wiley, New York, pp. 115–138.

BLUNDELL, J. E., and LATHAM, C. J., 1977, Pharmacological modification of eating behaviour. Proceedings of 6th Int. Congress on Physiology of Food and Fluid Intake, Paris, 1977.

BLUNDELL, J. E., and LATHAM, C. J., 1978, Pharmacological manipulation of feeding behaviour: Possible influences of serotonin and dopamine on food intake, in: *Central Mechanisms of Anorectic Drugs* (S. Garattini and R. Samanin, eds.), Raven Press, New York, pp. 83–109.

BLUNDELL, J. E., and LATHAM, C. J., 1979a, Pharmacology of food and water intake, in: *Chemical Influences on Behaviour* (S. Cooper and K. Brown, eds.), Academic Press, London, pp. 201–254.

BLUNDELL, J. E., and LATHAM, C. J., 1979b, Serotonergic influences on food intake: Effect of 5-hydroxytryptophan on parameters of feeding behaviour in deprived and free-feeding rats, *Pharmacol. Biochem. Behav.* **11**:431–437.

BLUNDELL, J. E., and LATHAM, C. J., 1979c, Sensitivity of the behavioural assay for measuring the action of drugs on feeding: Effects of tryptophan and 5-hydroxy-tryptophan, *Br. J. Pharmacol.* **66**:482P.

BLUNDELL, J. E., and LATHAM, C. J., 1980, Characterisation of adjustments to the structure of feeding behaviour following pharmacological treatment: Effects of amphetamine and fenfluramine and the antagonism produced by pimozide and methergoline, *Pharmacol. Biochem. Behav.* **12**:717–722.

BLUNDELL, J. E., and LATHAM, C. J., 1982, Behavioural pharmacology of feeding, in: *Drugs and Appetite* (T. Silverstone, ed.), Academic Press, London, pp. 41–80.

BLUNDELL, J. E., and LESHEM, M. B., 1974, The effect of serotonin manipulation in rats with lateral hypothalamic lesions. Proceedings, Fifth International Conference on Physiology of Food and Fluid Intake, Jerusalem, 1974.

BLUNDELL, J. E., and LESHEM, M. B., 1975, Analysis of the mode of action of anorexic drugs, in: *Recent Advances in Obesity Research I* (A. Howard, ed.), Newman, London, pp. 368–371.

BLUNDELL, J. E., and MCARTHUR, R. A., 1979, Investigation of food consumption using a dietary self-selection procedure: Effects of pharmacological manipulations and feeding schedules, *Br. J. Pharmacol.* **67**:436P–438P.

BLUNDELL, J. E., and MCARTHUR, R. A., 1981, Behavioural flux and feeding: Continuous monitoring of food intake and food selection and the video-recording of appetitive and satiety sequences for the analysis of drug action, in: *Anorectic Agents, Mechanisms of Action and of Tolerance* (S. Garattini, ed.), Raven Press, New York.

BLUNDELL, J. E., and ROGERS, P. J., 1978, Pharmacological approaches to the understanding of obesity, *Psychiatr. Clin. North Am.* **1**:629–650.

BLUNDELL, J. E., CAMPBELL, D. B., LESHEM, M. B., and TOZER, R., 1975, Comparison of the time course of the anorexic effects of amphetamine and fenfluramine with drug levels in blood, *J. Pharm. Pharmacol.* **27**:187–192.

BLUNDELL, J. E., LATHAM, C. J., and LESHEM, M. B., 1976, Differences between the anorexic actions of amphetamine and fenfluramine—Possible effects on hunger and satiety, *J. Pharm. Pharmacol.* **28**:471–477.

BLUNDELL, J. E., TOMBROS, E., ROGERS, P. J., and LATHAM, C. J., 1980, Ecological analysis of feeding: Implications for the pharmacological manipulation of food intake in animals and man, *Prog. Neuropsychopharmacol.* **4**:319–326.

BLUNDELL, J. E., ROGERS, P. J., and HILL, A. J., 1985, Behavioural structure and mechanisms of anorexia: Calibration of natural and abnormal inhibition of eating, *Brain Res. Bull.* **15**:371–376.

BLUNDELL, J. E., HILL, A. J., and KIRKHAM, T. C., 1986, Dextrofenfluramine and eating behaviour in animals: action on food selection, motivation and body weight, in: *Human*

Body Weight (S. Bender and L. J. Brookes, ed.), Churchill-Livingstone, London, pp. 233–239.

BOOTH, D. A., and NICHOLLS, J., 1974, Behavioural specificity of chloralose-induced feeding in the rat, *Psychopharmacologia* (Berlin) **39**:145–150.

BORBELY, A., and WASER, P. G., 1966, Das fressverhalten der Ratte. Haufigkeit und Gewicht der Mahlzeiten unter dem Einfluss von Amphetamin, *Psychopharmacologia* **9**:373–381.

BORSINI, F., BENDOTTI, C., THURLBY, P., and SAMANIN, R., 1982, Evidence that systemically administered salbutamol reduces food intake in rats by acting on central beta-adrenergic sites, *Life Sci.* **30**:905–911.

BOWDEN, C., WHITE, K., and TUTWILER, G., 1983, Inhibition of energy intake of cafeteria fed rats by mechanistically different anorectic agents. Proceeding of IV Int. Cong. on Obesity, New York, Oct. 5–8, 1983, p. 35A.

BRAY, G. A., and YORK, D. A., 1972, Studies on food intake in genetically obese rats, *Am. J. Physiol.* **223**:176–179.

BROWN, R. F., HOUPT, K. A., and SCHRYVER, H. F., 1976, Stimulation of food intake in horses by diazepam and promazine, *Pharmacol. Biochem. Behav.* **5**:495–497.

BURRIDGE, S. L., and BLUNDELL, J. E., 1979, Amphetamine anorexia: Antagonism by typical but not atypical neuroleptics, *Neuropharmacology* **18**:453–457.

BURTON, M. J., COOPER, S. J., and POPPLEWELL, D. A., 1981, The effect of fenfluramine on the microstructure of feeding and drinking in the rat. *Br. J. Pharmacol.* **72**:621–633.

CAPPELL, H., LEBLANC, A. E., and ENDRENYI, L., 1972, Effects of chlordiazepoxide and ethanol on the extinction of a conditioned taste aversion, *Physiol. Behav.* **9**:167–169.

CARRUBA, M. O., RICCIARDI, S., MULLER, E. E., and MANTEGAZZA, P., 1980, Anorectic effect of Lisuride and other ergot derivatives in the rat, *Eur. J. Pharmacol.* **64**:133–141.

COLLIER, G., HIRSCH, E., and KANAREK, R., 1977, The operant revisited, in: *Handbook of Operant Behaviour* (W. K. Honig and J. E. R. Staddon, eds.), Prentice-Hall, Englewood Cliffs, NJ.

COOPER, B. R., HOWARD, J. L., WHITE, H. L., SOROKO, F., INGOLD, K., and MAXWELL, R. F., 1980, Anorexic effect of ethalolamine-*o*-sulfate and muscimol in the rat: Evidence that GABA inhibits ingestive behaviour, *Life Sci.* **26**:1997–2002.

COOPER, S. J., 1980, Benzodiazepines as appetite-enhancing compounds, *Appetite* **1**:7–19.

COOPER, S. J., and ESTALL, L. B., 1985, Behavioural pharmacology of food, water and salt intake in relation to drug actions at benzodiazepine receptors, *Neurosci. Biobehav. Rev.* **9**:5–19.

COOPER, S. J., SWEENEY, K. F., and TOATES, F. M., 1979, Effects of Spiperone on feeding performance in a food preference test, *Psychopharmacology* **63**:301–305.

COSCINA, D. V., 1977, Brain amines in hypothalamic obesity, in: *Anorexia Nervosa* (R. A. Vigersky, ed.), Raven Press, New York, pp. 97–107.

COSTA, E., and GARATTINI, S., 1970, *Amphetamines and Related Compounds*, Raven Press, New York.

COX, D. R., and LEWIS, P. A. W., 1966, *The Statistical Analysis of Series of Events*, Methuen, London.

DANGUIR, J., NICOLAIDIS, S., and GERARD, H. 1979, Relations between feeding and sleep patterns, *J. Comp. Physiol. Psychol.* **93**:820–830.

DAVIES, R. F., 1976, Some neurochemical and physiological factors controlling free feeding patterns in the rat, Ph.D. thesis, McGill University, Montreal.

DAVIES, R. F., ROSSI, J., PANKSEPP, J., BEAN, N. J., and ZOLOVICK, A. J., 1983, Fenfluramine anorexia: A peripheral locus of action, *Physiol. Behav.* **30**:723–730.

DAVIS, J. D., GALLAUGHER, R. L., and LADOVE, R., 1967, Food intake controlled by a blood factor, *Science.* **156**:1247–1248.

DOBRZANSKI, S., and DOGGETT, N. S., 1976, The effects of (+)-amphetamine and fenfluramine on feeding in starved and satiated mice, *Psychopharmacology* **48**:283–286.

DOGGET, N. S., and JAWAHARLAL, K., 1977a, Some observations on the anorectic activity of prostaglandin F_2, *Br. J. Pharm.* **60**:409–415.
DOGGETT, N. S., and JAWAHARLAL, K., 1977b, Anorectic activity of prostaglandin precursors, *Br. J. Pharm.* **60**:417–423.
DOURISH, C. T., 1982, Phenylethylanmine-induce anorexia in the albino rat, in: *The Neural Basis of Feeding and Reward* (B. G. Hoebel and D. Novin, eds.), Haer Institute, Brunswick, pp. 543–549.
DOURISH, C. T., HUTSON, P. H., and CURZON, G., 1985, Low doses of the putative serotonin agonist 8-hydroxy-2 (Di-*n*-propylamino) Tetralin (8-OH-DPAT) elicit feeding in the rat, *Psychopharmacology* **86**:197–204.
EDWARDS, J. G., 1977, Unwanted effects of psychotropic drugs IV. Drugs for anxiety, *Practitioner* **219**:117–21.
FENTRESS, J. C., 1976, Dynamic boundaries of patterned behaviour: Interaction and self-organization, in: *Growing Points in Ethology* (P. G. Bateson and R. A. Hinde, eds.), Cambridge University Press, London, pp. 135–169.
FERNSTROM, J. D., and FALLER, D. V., 1978, Neutral amino acids in the brain: Changes in response to food ingestion, *J. Neurochem.* **30**:1531–1538.
FILE, S. E., 1980, Effects of benzodiazepines and naloxone on food intake and food preference in the rat, *Appetite* **1**:215–224.
FLETCHER, P. J., 1985, Serotonin in the control of feeding behaviour, Ph.D. thesis, University of Sussex.
FLETCHER, P. J., and BURTON, M. J., 1984, Effects of manipulations of peripheral serotonin on feeding and drinking in the rat, *Pharmacol. Biochem. Behav.* **20**:835–840.
FOLTIN, R. W., WOOLVERTON, W. L., and SCHUSTER, C. R., 1982, Effects of psychomotor stimulants, alone or in pairs, on milk drinking in the rat after intraperitoneal and intragastric administration, *J. Pharm. Exp. Ther.* **226**:411–418.
FREED, W. J., PERLOW, M. J., and WYATT, R. J., 1979, Calcitonin: Inhibitory effect on eating, *Science* **206**:850–852.
FULLER, R. W., and WONG, D. T., 1977, Inhibition of serotonin reuptake, *Fed. Proc.* **36**:2154–2158.
GARATTINI, S., 1978, Importance of serotonin for explaining the action of some anorectic agents in: *Recent Advances in Obesity Research: 11* (G. A. Bray, ed.), Newman, London, pp. 433–441.
GARATTINI, S., and SAMANIN, R., 1976, Anorectic drugs and neuro-transmitters, in: *Food Intake and Appetite* (T. Silverstone, ed.), Dahlem Konferenzem, Berlin, pp. 82–208.
GHOSH, M. N., and PARVATHY, S., 1973, The effect of cyproheptadine on water and food intake and on body weight in fasted adult and weanling rats, *Br. J. Pharmacol.* **48**:328–329P.
GIBBS, J., YOUNG, R. C., and SMITH, G. P., 1973, Cholecystokinin elicits satiety in rats with open gastric fistulas, *Nature* **245**:323–325.
GIBBS, J., KULKOVSKY, P. J., and SMITH, G. P., 1981, Effects of peripheral and central bombesin on feeding behaviour of rats, *Peptides* **2**:179–183.
GLAESER, B. S., MATHER, T. J., and WURTMAN, R. J., 1983, Changes in brain levels of acidic, basic and neutral amino acids after consumption of single meals containing various proportions of protein, *J. Neurochem.* **41**:1016–1021.
GLICK, Z., 1980, Food intake of rats administered with glycerol, *Physiol. Behav.* **25**:621–626.
GONZALEZ, M. F., and NOVIN, D., 1974, Feeding induced by intracranial and intravenously administered 2-deoxy-D-glucose, *Physiol. Psychol.* **2**:326–330.
GOODMAN, L. S., and GILMAN, A., 1970, *The Pharmacological Basis of Therapeutics*, 4th ed., Macmillan, New York.

GRINKER, J. A., DREWNOSKI, A., ENNS, M., and KISSILEFF, H., 1980, Effects of d-amphetamine and fenfluramine on feeding patterns and activity of obese and lean Zucker rats, *Pharmacol. Biochem. Behav.* **12**:265–275.

GRINKER, J. A., MARINESCU, C., and LEIBOWITZ, S. F., 1982, Effects of central injections of neurotransmitters and drugs on freely-feeding rats, *Soc. Neurosci. Abstr.* **8**:604.

HILL, A., ROGERS, P., and BLUNDELL, J., 1983, Effect of an anorexic drug (d-fenfluramine) on body weight and food intake during the dynamic and plateau phases of dietary-inducted obesity in rats: more potent drug action in obese animals. Proceedings of IV Int. Congress on Obesity, New York, October 5–8, 1983, p. 11A.

HIRSCH, J. A., GOLDBERG, S., and WURTMAN, R. J., 1982, Effect of (+) or (−) - enantiomers of fenfluramine or norfenfluramine on nutrient selection by rats, *J. Pharm. Pharmacol.* **34**:18–21.

HOEBEL, B. G., 1977, Pharmacologic control of feeding, *Annu. Rev. Pharmacol. Toxicol.* **17**:605–621.

HOEBEL, B. G., 1984, Neurotransmitters in the control of feeding and its rewards: Monoamines, opiates and brain-gut peptides, in: *Eating and Its Disorders* (A. J. Stunkard and E. Stellar, eds.), Raven Press, New York, pp. 15–38.

HOEBEL, B. G., and LEIBOWITZ, S. F., 1981, Brain monoamines in the modulation of self-stimulation, feeding, and body weight, in: *Brain, Behaviour and Bodily Disease* (H. A. Weiner, M. A. Hofer, and A. J. Stunkard, eds.), Raven Press, New York, pp. 103–142.

HOLDEN, J. M. C., and HOLDEN, V., 1970, Weight changes with schizophrenic psychosis and psychotropic drugs therapy, *Psychosomatics* **1**:551–561.

HOLTZMAN, S. G., 1974, Behavioural effects of separate and combined administration of naloxone and d-amphetamine, *J. Pharmacol. Exp. Ther.* **189**:51–60.

IDELSHON, F., 1967, Experience with cyproheptadine hydrochloride as a nonhormonal anabolic. Its effect on the body weight of pediatric patients, *Oriental Med.* **185**:824–826.

JACKSON, H. C., and SEWELL, R. D. E., 1984, The role of opioid receptor sub-types in tifluodom-induced feeding, *J. Pharm. Pharmacol.* **29**:683–686.

KAHLING, VON J., ZIEGLER, H., and BACHAUSE, H., 1975, Zentrale Wirkungen von WA335-BS, einer substanz mit peripherer Antiserotonin und Antihistamin-wirkung, *Arzneim.-Forsch* **25**:1737–1744.

KEESEY, R. E., 1980, A set-point analysis of the regulation of body weight, in: *Obesity*, (A. J. Stunkard, ed.), Saunders, Philadelphia, pp. 144–165.

KIRBY, M. J., PLEECE, S. A., and REDFERN, P. H., 1978, The effect of fenfluramine on obesity in rats—a new method for the screening of potential anti-obesity agents, *Br. J. Pharmacol.* **64**:442P.

KIRKHAM, T. C., 1985, Investigation of opioid mechanisms in the control of feeding behaviour, Ph.D. thesis, University of Leeds.

KIRKHAM, T. C., and BLUNDELL, J. E., 1984, Dual action of naloxone on feeding revealed by behavioural analysis: Separate effects on initiation and termination of eating, *Appetite* **5**:45–52.

KIRKHAM, T. C., and BLUNDELL, J. E., 1986, Effect of naloxone and naltrexone on the development of satiation measured in the runway: Comparisons with d-amphetamine and d-fenfluramine, *Pharmacol. Biochem. Behav.* **25**:123–128.

KNOLL, J., 1979, Satietin: A highly potent anorexigenic substance in human serum, *Physiol. Behav.* **23**:497–502.

KULKOVSKY, P. J., GIBBS, J., and SMITH, G. P., 1982, Behavioural effects of bonbesin administration in rats, *Physiol. Behav.* **28**:505–512.

LAT, J., 1967, Self-selection of dietary components, in: *Handbook of Physiology*, Vol. 1, *Alimentary Canal* (F. Code, ed.), American Physiology Society, Washington, DC.

LATHAM, C. J., and BLUNDELL, J. E., 1979, Evidence for the effect of tryptophan on the pattern of food consumption in free feeding and food deprived rats, *Life Sci.* **24**:1971–1978.

LEIBOWITZ, S. F., 1970, Reciprocal hunger-regulating circuits involving alpha- and beta-adrenergic receptors located, respectively, in the ventromedial and lateral hypothalamus, *Proc. Natl. Adac. Sci. USA* **67**:1063–1070.

LEIBOWITZ, S. F., 1980, Neurochemical systems of the hypothalamus—Control of feeding and drinking behaviour and water-electrolyte excretion, in: *Handbook of the Hypothalamus*, Volume 3, Dekker, New York, pp. 299–437.

LEIBOWITZ, F. F., 1986a, Brain monoamines and peptides: Role in the control of eating behaviour, *Fed. Proc.* **45**:1396–1403.

LEIBOWITZ, S. F., 1986b, Hypothalamic serotonin in the control of eating behavior, *Adv. Biosci.* **60**:343–352.

LEIBOWITZ, S. F., and SHOR-POSNER, G., 1986, Monoamine meal patterns in the rat, in: *Psychopharmacology of Eating Disorders: Theoretical and Clinical Advances* (M. O. Carruba and J. E. Blundell, eds.), Raven Press, New York.

LE MAGNEN, J., 1971, Advances in studies on the physiological control and regulation of food intake, in: *Progress in Physiological Psychology* (E. Stellar and J. M. Sprague, eds.), Academic Press, London, pp. 203–261.

LEVINE, A., 1983, Species diversity in opioid feeding systems. Proceedings of the 4th International Congress on Obesity, New York, October 4–8.

LEVINE, A. S., MORLEY, J. E., KNEIP, J., GRACE, M., and BROWN, D. M., 1985, Environment modulates naloxone's suppressive effect on feeding in diabetic and non-diabetic rats, *Physiol. Behav.* **34**:391–393.

LI, E. T. S., and ANDERSON, G. H., 1984, 5-hydroxytryptamine: A modulator of food composition but not quantity? *Life Sci.* **34**:2453–2460.

LORENZ, D., MARDI, P., and SMITH, G. P., 1978, Atropine methyl nitrate inhibits sham feeding in the rat, *Pharmacol. Biochem Behav.* **8**:405–407.

LOTTER, E. C., KRINSKY, R., MCKAY, J. M., TRENEER, C. M., PORTE, D., and WOOD, S. C., 1981, Somatostatin decreases food intake of rats and baboons, *J. Comp. Physiol.* **95**:278–287.

MANDENOFF, A., FUMERON, F., APFELBAUM, M., and MARGULES, D. L., 1982, Endogenous opiates and energy balance, *Science* **215**:1536–1538.

MARGULES, D. L., and STEIN, L., 1967, Neuroleptics v. tranquillizers: Evidence from animals of mode and site of action, in: *Neuropsychopharmacology* (H. Bril, J. O. Cole, P. Deniker, H. Hippius, and P. B. Bradley, eds.), Excerpta Medica, Amsterdam, pp. 108–120.

MARTIN, C. F., and GIBBS, J., 1980, Bombesin elicits satiety in sham feeding rats, *Peptides* **1**:131–134.

MAURON, C., WURTMAN, J. J., and WURTMAN, R. J., 1980, Clonidine increases food and protein consumption in rats, *Life Sci.* **27**:781–791.

MCARTHUR, R. A., and BLUNDELL, J. E., 1983, Protein and carbohydrate self-selection: Modification of the effects of fenfluramine and amphetamine by age and feeding regimen, *Appetite* **4**:113–124.

MCARTHUR, R. A., and BLUNDELL, J. E., 1986, Dietary self-selection and intake of protein and energy is altered by the texture of the diets, *Physiol. Behav.* **38**:315–319.

MCDERMOTT, L. J., ALHEID, G. F., HALARIS, A. E., and GROSSMAN, S. P., 1977, A correlational analysis of the effects of surgical transections of three components of the MFB on ingestive behaviour and hypothalamic, striatal, and telencephalic amine concentrations, *Pharmacol. Biochem.* **6**:203–214.

MCLAUGHLIN, C. L., and BAILE, C. A., 1984, Feeding behaviour responses of Zucker rats to naloxone, *Physiol. Behav.* **32**:755–761.

MEREU, G. P., FRATTA, W., GESSA, P., and GESSA, G. L., 1976, Voraciousness induced in rats by benzodiazepines, *Psychopharmacology* **47**:101–103.

MILLER, J. A., 1963, Serotonin antagonist cyproheptadine, *Ann. Allergy* **21**:588–592.

MILLS, M. J., and STUNKARD, A. J., 1976, Behavioural changes following surgery for obesity, *Am. J. Psychiatry* **133**:527–531.

MORAN, G., 1975, Severe food deprivation: Some thoughts regarding its exclusive use, *Psychol. Bull.* **82**:543–557.

MORGAN, C. T., 1943, *Physiological Psychology*, McGraw-Hill, New York.

MORGAN, R., 1977, Three weeks in isolation with two schizophrenic patients, *Br. J. Psychiatry* **131**:504–513.

MORLEY, J. E., 1980, The neuroendocrine control of appetite: The role of the endogenous opiates, cholecystokinin, TRH, gamma-amino-butyric-acid and the diazepam receptor, *Life Sci.* **27**:355–368.

MORLEY, J. E., and LEVINE, A. S., 1983, The central control of appetite, *Lancet* **i**:398–401.

MORLEY, J. E., and LEVINE, A. S., 1985, The pharmacology of eating behaviour, *Ann. Rev. Pharmacol. Toxicol.* **25**:127–146.

MORLEY, J. E., LEVINE, A. S., GOSNELL, B. A., and KRAHN, D. D., 1985, Peptides as central regulators of feeding, *Brain Res. Bull.* **14**:511–519.

MOSES, P. L., and WURTMAN, R. J., 1984, The ability of certain anorexic drugs to suppress food consumption depends on the nutrient composition of the test diet, *Life Sci.* **35**:1297–1300.

NOBLE, R. E., 1969, Effect of cyproheptadine on appetite and weight gain in adults, *JAMA* **209**:2054–2055.

ORTHEN-GAMBILL, N., and KANAREK, R. B., 1982, Differential effects of amphetamine and fenfluramine on dietary self-selection in rats, *Pharmacol. Biochem. Behav.* **16**:303–309.

OVERMANN, S. R., 1976, Dietary self-selection by animals, *Psychol. Bull.* **83**:218–235.

PANKSEPP, J., POLLACK, A., KROST, K., MEEKER, R., and RITTER, M., 1975, Feeding in response to repeated protamine zinc insulin injections, *Physiol. Behav.* **14**:487–493.

PAYKEL, E. S., MUELLER, P. S., and DE LA VERGNE, P. M., 1973, Amitriptyline, weight gain and carbohydrate craving: A side effect, *Br. J. Psychiatry* **123**:501–507.

PFISTER, W. R., ILLINGWORTH, R. M., and YIM, G. K. W., 1978, Increased feeding in rats treated with chlordimeform and related formadines: A new class of appetite stimulants, *Psychopharmacology* **60**:47–51.

POLLOCK, J. D., and ROWLAND, N., 1981, Peripherally administered serotonin decreased food intake in rats, *Pharmacol. Biochem. Behav.* **15**:179–183.

POSCHEL, B. P. H., 1971, A simple and specific screen for benzodiazepine-like drugs, *Psychopharmacologia* **19**:193–198.

RANDALL, L. O., SCHALLEK, W., HEISE, G. A. KEITH, E. F., and BAGDON, R. E., 1960, The psychoactive properties of methaminodiazepoxide, *J. Pharm. Exp. Ther.* **129**:163–171.

REYNOLDS, R. W., and CARLISLE, H. J., 1961, The effect of chlorpromazine on food intake in the albino rat, *J. Comp. Physiol. Psychol.* **54**:354–356.

RICHTER, C. P., 1943, Total self-regulatory functions in animals and human beings, *Harvey Lecture Series* **38**:63–103.

ROBINSON, R. G., MCHUGH, P. R., and FOLSTEIN, M. F., 1975, Measurement of appetite disturbances in psychiatric disorder, *J. Psychiatr. Res.* **12**:59–68.

ROGERS, P. J., and BLUNDELL, J. E., 1984, Meal patterns and food selection during the development of obesity in rats fed on cafeteria diet, *Neurosci. Biobehav. Rev.* **8**:441–453.

ROTHWELL, N. J., and STOCK, M. J., 1979, A role for brown adipose tissue in diet-induced thermogenesis, *Nature* **281**:31–35.

ROWLAND, D. L., PERRINGS, T. S., and THOMMES, J. A., 1980, Comparison of androgenic effects on food intake and body weight in adults rats, *Physiol. Behav.* **24**:205–209.

ROWLAND, N., and BARTNESS, T. J., 1982, Naloxone suppresses insulin-induced food intake in novel and familiar environments, but does not affect hypoglycaemia, *Pharmacol. Biochem. Behav.* **16**:1001–1003.

RUSSEK, M., MOGENSON, G. J., and STEVENSON, J. A. F., 1967, Calorigenic, hyperglycemic and anorexigenic effects of adrenaline and noradrenaline, *Physiol. Behav.* **2**:429–433.

SAMANIN, R., CACCIA, S., BENDOTTI, C., BORSINI, F., BORRONI, E., INVERNIZZI, R., PATACINI, R., and MENNINI, T., 1980, Further studies on the mechanism of serotonin-dependent anorexia in rats, *Psychopharmacology* **68**:99–104.

SANGER, D., 1981, Endorphinergic mechanisms in the control of food and water intake, *Appetite* **2**:193–208.
SANGER, D. J., and MCCARTHY, P. S., 1981, Increased food and water intake produced in rats by opiate receptor agonists, *Psychopharmacology* **74**:217–220.
SCHALLY, A. V., REDDING, T. W., LUCIEN, H. W., and MEYER, J., 1967, Enterogastrone inhibits eating by fasted mice, *Science* **157**:210–211.
SCHLEMMER, R. F., CASPER, R. C., NARASIMHACHARI, N., and DAVIS, J. M., 1979, Clonidine induced hyperphagia and weight gain in monkeys, *Psychopharmacology* **61**:233–234.
SCLAFANI, A., 1978, Dietary obesity, in: *Recent Advances in Obesity Research II* (G. Bray, ed.), Newman, London, pp. 123–132.
SCLAFANI, A., 1985, Animal models of obesity, in: *Dietary Treatment and Prevention of Obesity* (R. T. Frankle, J. Dwyer, L. Morangue, and A. Owen, eds.), Libby, London, pp. 105–123.
SCLAFANI, A., and SPRINGER, D., 1976, Dietary obesity in adult rats: Similarities to hypothalamic and human obesity syndromes, *Physiol. Behav.* **17**:461–471.
SCLAFANI, A., KOOPMANS, H. S., VASSELLI, J. R., and REICHMAN, M., 1978, Effects of intestinal bypass surgery on appetite, food intake, and body weight in obese and lean rats, *Am. J. Physiol.* **234**:E389-E398.
SHIMOMURA, Y., OKU, J., GLICK, Z., and BRAY, G. A., 1982, Opiate receptors, food intake and obesity, *Physiol. Behav.* **28**:441–445.
SHOR-POSNER, G., GRINKER, J. A., MARINESCU, C., BROWN, O., and LEIBOWITZ, S. F., 1986, Hypothalamic serotonin in the control of meal patterns and macro-nutrient selection, *Appetite* **7** (in press).
SLUSSER, P. G., and RITTER, R. C., 1980, Increased feeding and hyperglycaemia elicited by intracerebroventricular 5-thioglucose, *Brain Res.* **202**:474–478.
SMITH, G. P., 1982, Satiety and the problem of motivation in: *The Physiological Mechanisms of Motivation* (D. W. Pfaff, ed.), Springer-Verlag, New York.
SMITH, G. P., and GIBBS, J., 1976, Cholecystokinin and satiety: Theoretic and therapeutic implications, in: *Hunger: Basic Mechanisms and Clinical Implications* (D. Novin, W. Wyrwicka, and G. Bray, eds.), Raven Press, New York, pp. 349–355.
SMITH, G. P., and GIBBS, J., 1979, Postprandial satiety, *Prog. Psychobiol. Physiol. Psychol.* **8**:179–242.
SOFIA, R. D., and BARRY, H., 1974, Acute and chronic effects of Δ 9-tetrahydrocannabinol on food intake by rats, *Psychopharmacologia* **39**:213–222.
SOPER, W. Y., and WISE, R. A., 1971, Hypothalamically induced eating: Eating from noneaters with diazepam, *T.I.T.J. Life Sci.* **1**:79–84.
SOUBRIE, P., KULKARNI, S., SIMON, P., and BOISSIER, J. R., 1975, Effects des anxiolytiques sur la prise de nouriture de rats et de souris places en situation novelle ou familiere, *Psychopharmacologia* **45**:203–210.
SOULAIRAC, A., 1963, Neurological factors in the control of the appetite, in: *International Review of Neurobiology* (C. C. Pfeiffer and J. R. Smythies, eds.), Academic Press, New York, pp. 303–346.
STELLAR, E., 1954, The physiology of motivation, *Psychol. Rev.* **61**:5-23
STOLERMAN, I. P., 1970, Eating, drinking and spontaneous activity in rats after the administration of chlorpromazine, *Neuropharmacology* **9**:405–411.
STRICKER, E. M., and ZIGMOND, M. J., 1976, Recovery of function after damage to central catecholamine-containing neurons: A neurochemical model for the lateral hypothalamic syndrome in: *Progress in Physiological Psychology*, Vol. 6 (J. M. Sprague and A. N. Epstein, eds.), Academic Press, New York, pp. 121–188.
SUGRUE, M. F., GOODLET, I., and MIREYLEES, S. E., 1976, On the selective inhibition of serotonin uptake in vivo by ORG 6582, *Eur. J. Pharmacol.* **40**:121–130.
SULLIVAN, A. C., and COMAI, K., 1978, Pharmacological treatment of obesity. *Int. J. Obesity* **2**:167–189.

SULLIVAN, A. C., and GRUEN, R. K., 1985, Mechanisms of appetite modulation by drugs, *Fed. Proc.* **44**:139–144.
SULLIVAN, A. C., TRISCARI, J., HAMILTON, J. G., and MILLER, O. N., 1974, Effect of (−) hydroxycitrate upon the accumulation of lipid in the rat: II. Appetite, *Lipids* **9**:129–134.
SULLIVAN, A. C., GUTHRIE, R. W., and TRISCARI, J., 1981, Chlorocitric acid, a novel anorectic agent with a peripheral mode of action, in: *Anorectic Agents, Mechanisms of Action and of Tolerance* (S. Garattini, ed.), Raven Press, New York, pp. 143–158.
THOMPSON, T., and SCHUSTER, C. R., 1968, *Behavioural Pharmacology*, Prentice-Hall, Englewood Cliffs, NJ.
THURLBY, P. C., GRIMM, V. E., and SAMANIN, R., 1983, Feeding and satiation observed in the runway: The effects of *d*-amphetamine and *d*-fenfluramine compared, *Pharmacol. Biochem. Behav.* **18**:841–846.
THURLBY, P. L., and SAMANIN, R., 1981, Effects of anorectic drugs and prior feeding on food-rewarded runway behaviour, *Pharmacol. Biochem. Behav.* **14**:799–804.
TRENCHARD, E., and SILVERSTONE, J. T., 1983, Naloxone reduces the food intake of human volunteers, *Appetite: J. Intake Res.* **4**:43–50.
TRYGSTAD, O., FOSS, I., EDMINSON, P. H., JOHANSEN, J. H., and REICHELT, K. L., 1978, Humoral control of appetite: A urinary anorexigenic peptide. Chromatographic patterns of urinary peptides in anorexia nervosa, *Acta Endocrinol.* **89**:196–208
TYE, N. C., NICHOLAS, D. J., and MORGAN, M. J., 1976, Chlordiazepoxide and preference for free food in the rat, *Pharmacol. Biochem. Behav.* **3**:1149–1151.
VENDSBORG, P. B., BECH, P., and RAFAELSON, O. J., 1976, Lithium treatment and weight gain, *Acta Psychiatr. Scand.* **53**:139–147.
VOGEL, R. A., COOPER, B. R., BARLOW, T. S., PRANGE, A. J., MUELLER, R. A., and BREESE, G. R., 1979, Effects of thyrotropin-releasing hormone on locomotor activity, operant performance and ingestive behaviour, *J. Pharmacol. Exp. Ther.* **208**:161–168.
WADDINGTON, C. H., 1977, *Tools for Thought*, Paladin, St. Albans.
WADE, G., 1975, Some effects of ovarian hormones on food intake and body weight in female rats, *J. Comp. Physiol. Psychol.* **88**:183–193.
WATSON, P. J., and COX, J. S., 1976, An analysis of barbiturate-induced eating and drinking in the rat, *Physiol. Psychol.* **4**:325–332.
WIEPKEMA, P. R., 1971a, Positive feedbacks at work during feeding, *Behaviour* **39**:266–273.
WIEPKEMA, P. R., 1971b, Behavioural factors in the regulation of food intake, *Proc. Nutr. Soc.* **30**:142–149.
WILLNER, P., and TOWELL, A. D., 1982a, Microstructural analysis of the involvement of beta-receptors in amphetamine anorexia, *Pharmacol. Biochem. Behav.* **17**:252–262.
WILLNER, P., and TOWELL, A. D., 1982b, The effects of chronic tricyclic antidepressant treatment on anorexia mediated by presynaptic dopamine receptors, *Soc. Neurosci. Abstr.* **8**:358.
WISE, R. A., and DAWSON, V., 1974, Diazepam-induced eating and lever pressing for food in sated rats, *J. Comp. Physiol. Psychol.* **86**:930–941.
WOLGIN, D. L., CYTAWA, J., and TEITELBAUM, P., 1976, The role of activation in the regulation of food intake, in: *Hunger: Basic Mechanisms and Clinical Implications* (D. Novin, W. Wyrwicka, and G. Bray, eds.), Raven Press, New York, pp. 179–191.
WURTMAN, J. J., and WURTMAN, R. J., 1977, Fenfluramine and fluoxetine spare protein consumption while suppressing caloric intake by rats, *Science* **198**:1178–1180.
WURTMAN, R. J., HEFTL, F., and MELAMED, E., 1981, Precursor control of neurotransmitter synthesis, *Pharmacol. Rev.* **32**:315–335.
ZELGER, J. C., and CARLINI, E. A., 1980, Anorexigenic effects of 2 amines obtained from 'Catha edulis' Forsk (Khat) in rats, *Pharmacol. Biochem. Behav.* **12**:701–706.

4

THE PSYCHOPHARMACOLOGY OF AGGRESSION

Klaus A. Miczek

1. RECENT HISTORY OF PSYCHOPHARMACOLOGICAL AGGRESSION RESEARCH

Understanding the biological and environmental determinants of aggressive behavior is the goal of many scientists, ranging from anthropologists to zoologists. Psychopharmacological issues and methods have contributed to and benefited from this area of research relatively recently. Before some major findings and areas of active psychopharmacological aggression research are summarized, it will be useful to refer briefly to the theoretical and methodological roots of the current work.

1.1. Psychiatric Research Questions

Clinical concerns with highly aggressive individuals are most often the starting point for inquiries into neurobiological mechanisms that may mediate aggressive behavior patterns. The clinical practitioner looks toward experimental aggression research with the hope of learning about more rational treatment options (Cloninger, 1983; Eichelman, 1977; Lion, 1975; Sheard, 1983, 1984; Tupin, 1985). In the clinical setting,

---

Klaus A. Miczek • Department of Psychology, Tufts University, Medford, Massachusetts, 02155.

aggression is approached as a psycho- or sociopathology that requires treatment.

Initially, it is important to learn whether the clinically encountered aggressive behavior pattern is a pathology in itself or a symptom of a more pervasive disorder. Several important neurological diseases such as epilepsy are associated with so-called uncontrollable aggressive acts (e.g., Monroe, 1978). A host of affective disorders, e.g., psychosis, depression, and phobic anxiety, include often violent, aggressive outbursts. A further, up to now unresolved question has to explore whether pathological aggressive acts are based on neural mechanisms that are distinct from those mediating nonpathological forms of aggression (Sheard, 1983). Are pathological aggressive acts on a continuum with nonpathological aggressive behavior or, alternatively, do they constitute separate phenomena mediated by distinct, presumably abnormal neural processes?

Closely aligned with psychiatric concerns are the objectives of work in the pharmaceutical industry. Generally, no therapeutic agents have

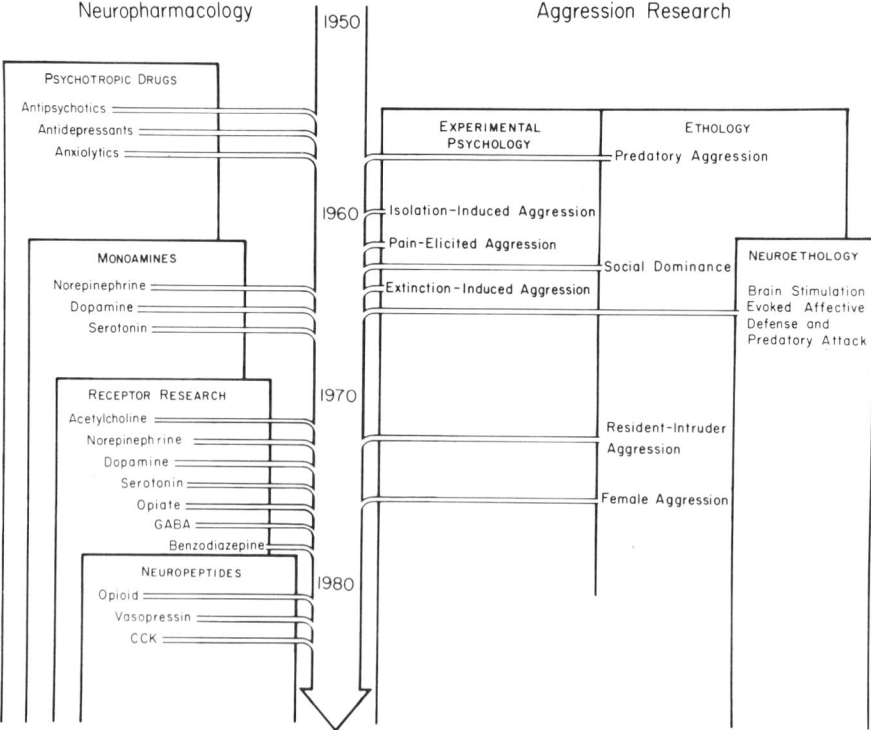

FIG. 1. Major developments during the past three decades that influenced psychopharmacological research on aggression. The historical roots for neuropharmacology, experimental psychology, and ethology can be traced back considerably further.

been developed that may be used specifically in the treatment of pathological aggressive behavior or in controlling symptoms of aggression and hostility that are part of complex affective disorders. Exceptions to this general pattern are several so-called antiaggressive drugs that have been promoted in recent years, such as Sch 12679 (Itil and Mukhopadhay, 1978), YG 19-256 (Owen, 1980), and fluprazine (Olivier *et al.*, 1984; Bradford *et al.*, 1984).

During the 1960s and 1970s preclinical experimental preparations were developed for the purpose of modeling features of human aggressive behavior (Fig. 1). Almost every major class of drugs has been investigated in different *models* of aggressive behavior, mainly in isolated mice and in rats that were exposed to pain, but also in fish, pigeons, cats, and primates (e.g., Sheard, 1977; Eichelman, 1978). In the absence of sufficient knowledge about common causative factors and common functions of aggression in a given animal species and in humans, the internal and predictive validity of most laboratory models of aggression remains a matter of contention (e.g., Miczek and Winslow, 1987*a*).

Unusual aggressive behavior in the course of addiction to certain drugs and during withdrawal represents yet another serious clinical and societal problem (Crowley, 1983; Tinklenberg and Stillman, 1970). The goal of rationally managing aggressive behavior in the context of drug abuse has prompted the development of experimental preparations that allow the systematic study of aggression during drug dependence and withdrawal. In addition to providing significant insights into the mechanisms of drug dependence, these experimental preparations also help delineate mechanisms mediating aggressive and defensive behavior.

1.2. Origins of Behavioral Methodology

Major conceptual and methodological roots for behavioral aggression research can be traced to experimental psychology (e.g., Dollard *et al.*, 1939; Buss, 1961; Bandura, 1973; Kelly, 1974) and ethology (e.g., Tinbergen, 1968; Marler, 1976; Eibl-Eibesfeldt, 1961; Fig. 1).

Exposure to aversive living conditions such as deprivation of social contact or, alternatively, crowding, restricted access to limited resources such as food, presentation of aversive stimuli such as electric shock pulses, and omission or intermittency of scheduled reinforcement are among the most frequent experimental manipulations for engendering aggressive behavior that have been the focus of psychologically oriented work. These *environmental* manipulations are usually performed in placid and domesticated laboratory animals, which rarely, if ever, exhibit aggressive behavior. To evoke or to induce some act of aggression by exposing an otherwise nonaggressive individual to aversive environmental events has led to the view that aggressive behavior represents an *anti*social activity.

The ethological study of aggressive behavior, originating with field observations, recognized that every species that can fight will fight, under appropriate conditions (Scott, 1958). Attack toward a territorial intruder or toward an unfamiliar group member, defense of the young, and attack and threat in the context of group formation and maintenance or in competition for mates, preferred foods, or niches include some of the most often studied aggression-provoking situations from an ethological perspective. The elaborate behavioral repertoire for aggressive behavior, organized in predictable sequences of pursuit, threat, attack, defense, flight, and submission, prompted the broader term *agonistic behavior* in order to capture the many behavioral elements in conflict situations (Scott, 1966). The ethological analysis examines not only the phylogenetic and ontogenetic origin, but also the *adaptive* significance of aggressive behavior.

A further development within the ethological framework are neuroethological methods. Originating with the pioneering studies by Hess (1928), direct electrical or chemical stimulation of neural foci may evoke integrated sequences of attack and defensive behavior as well as predatory attack in several animal species; moreover, electrical neuronal activity accompanying aggressive or defensive behavior may be recorded. The brain stimulation-evoked aggressive behavior parallels, in many respects, the behavior engendered under field conditions.

Considering the differences in psychiatric, experimental–psychological, and ethological research objectives and approaches, it is not surprising that the term "aggression" assumes multiple meanings and loses much of its communicative value, if no operational definition is provided.

1.3. Emerging Neuroscientific Objectives

Since the type of aggressive behavior may be pathological, antisocial, or, alternatively, adaptive in nature, the study of neural mechanisms of aggression and drug action thereon presents a highly varied picture. As in other areas of behavioral pharmacology (e.g., Kelleher and Morse, 1968), traditionally two strategies have been pursued. Type I studies use drugs as tools for characterizing the neural mechanisms that underlie a specific aggressive behavior. This type of research assumes that the research tool, i.e., the mechanism of drug action, is well understood. Type II research uses selected aggressive acts as a means to screen for a specific class of drugs or even to serve as markers for a specific neurotransmitter. The underlying assumption for this type of research is that the selected behavior and its neural basis are adequately described. Type II studies are problematic, since it is generally appreciated that the mechanisms for even the simplest aggressive act are complex and incompletely understood. Nowadays, mostly pragmatic research, such as screening for antidepressant drugs by blocking the mouse-killing response of rats (see below), use the type II strategy.

In their enthusiasm, psychopharmacological aggression researchers attempted to link modifications in a *single* neurotransmitter to changes in aggressive behavior. At varying times, each of the known brain biogenic amines was suspected to represent the "code" for aggression; for example, the "aggressive monoamines" (Eichelman *et al.*, 1973), hypothalamic acetylcholine (e.g., Smith *et al.*, 1970), or alternatively, serotonin (e.g., Valzelli and Garattini, 1968) were suggested as being critically significant in the control of aggressive behavior. Around 1970, the single neurotransmitter control code was expanded initially to a "neurochemical dualism" and eventually to a multitransmitter control of aggressive behavior (e.g., Reis, 1974; Avis, 1974; Pradhan, 1975; Daruna, 1978). Just as a nerve cell membrane may be either excited or inhibited, and a neurotransmitter may be either excitatory or inhibitory at the *cellular* level, aggressive behavior was said to be under excitatory and inhibitory control by functionally opposite neurotransmitters. Being guided by autonomic nervous system pharmacology, the first candidates for *behavioral* excitation and inhibition were norepinephrine and acetylcholine, which were later supplanted by dopamine and serotonin. The concept of exciting and inhibiting aggressive behavior by opponent neurotransmitters, although attractively simple, is presently yielding to a more realistic view.

The discovery of peptides, steroids, and amines, as well as their neurochemically differentiated receptors in anatomically circumscribed brain structures, provided an opportunity for matching the behavioral complexities of aggressive interactions.

2. FRAMEWORK FOR BEHAVIORAL ANALYSIS OF AGGRESSION

Most behavioral preparations for psychopharmacological aggression research are derived originally from at least three conceptual and methodological frameworks: experimental–psychological, neurological, and ethological approaches to aggression. A review of the essential features of the representative experimental protocols will help in understanding the behavioral phenomena produced with each procedure.

2.1. Experimental–Psychological Approach

To engender aggressive behavior under controlled laboratory conditions, pervasive as well as discrete environmental manipulations have been used; these range from prolonged isolated housing to the delivery of painful electric shock pulses. After exposure to a specific reinforcement history, omission of reinforcement often leads to aggressive behavior. Alternatively, providing the opportunity to engage in aggressive behavior may serve as a reinforcing event, i.e., maintaining behavior that leads to aggressive behavior.

2.1.1. Isolation-Induced Aggression

The most often used behavioral method in preclinical psychopharmacological research on aggressive behavior is to isolate mice and, subsequently, examine their interactions with a stimulus animal (e.g., Malick, 1979). When confronted with another mouse, the isolated adult male mouse chases, threatens, and attacks the opponent or, alternatively, engages in defensive and flight reactions (e.g., Ginsburg and Allee, 1942; Scott and Fredericson, 1951; Brain and Nowell, 1970; Krsiak, 1975b). Several important variables determine the proportion of animals showing aggressive behavior, the intensity and frequency of aggressive behavior, as well as the stability and pattern of the behavior; among the most important variables are the duration of the isolation period (Valzelli, 1969; Banerjee, 1971a; Thurmond, 1975; Cairns *et al.*, 1985), the developmental stage at which isolated housing occurs (Cairns and Nakelski, 1971; Goldsmith *et al.*, 1976), the strain of mice (Brain, 1975; DaVanzo *et al.*, 1966), the number of mice tested (Welch and Welch, 1969; Valzelli, 1969; Hadfield, 1982), the experience of the isolated mouse with fighting behavior (Scott, 1966; DaVanzo *et al.*, 1966), the social experience, sex, age, and hormonal and neural condition of the stimulus animal (Parmigiani and Brain, 1983; Denenberg *et al.*, 1973; Brain and Poole, 1976; Brain *et al.*, 1981b), the duration of the encounter (Janssen *et al.*, 1960; Thurmond, 1975), and the size of the test environment, as well as the familiarity of the animals with the cage (e.g., Malick, 1979).

Not all mice become aggressive after being housed in isolation: A varying proportion of isolated mice exhibits defensive and flight responses instead of attack and threat behavior when confronting a nonaggressive stimulus animal (e.g., Krsiak, 1975b). Since the behavioral sequelae of isolated housing may include opposite modes of agonistic behavior, attack or flight, it is often difficult to interpret neurochemical and endocrinological data in isolated mice. In order to link, for example, a profile of brain catecholamine or serotonin activity, as well as pituitary, adrenal, and gonadal hormone secretions, in isolated mice to aggressive behavior, it is necessary to study only those animals that actually show this behavior (e.g., Anton *et al.*, 1968; Maengwyn-Davies *et al.*, 1973; Tizabi *et al.*, 1979; Valzelli, 1973b).

The behavioral measurements of isolation-induced aggression began with coarse single indices (e.g., Malick, 1979) and have become considerably more detailed and informative, including, most recently, sequential analysis of the behavior pattern (e.g., Brain *et al.*, 1984; Poshivalov and Khodko, 1984; Jones and Brain, 1985). Rating scales that engender a score of "aggressiveness" (e.g., Valzelli *et al.*, 1967), the proportion of animals exhibiting aggressive behavior (e.g., Cairns and Scholz, 1973; Tizabi *et al.*, 1980a,b; Thurmond, 1975), the duration or frequency of aggressive episodes during a fixed-time test (e.g., Maengwyn-Davies *et al.*, 1973; Karczmar *et al.*, 1978; Hadfield *et al.*, 1982), or the time for the first attack to occur represent examples of the all-or-none type of measurement. More recent research has provided detailed ethological recordings of the many characteristic acts, postures, and movements that constitute aggressive behavior (e.g., Brain and Nowell, 1970; Krsiak, 1975b, 1979; Miczek and O'Donnell, 1978; Olivier and van Dalen, 1982; Poshivalov, 1982). This latter approach permits a direct, concurrent assessment of drug effects on aggressive and nonaggressive behavioral elements, informing on the specificity of drug action (Miczek and Krsiak, 1979).

The value of studying aggressive behavior by isolated mice for psychopharmacology derives from the predictive and internal validity of this experimental preparation. That isolation-induced aggression may model a psychopathology (e.g., Valzelli, 1973b; Garattini and Valzelli, 1981) has been questioned; many behavioral, pharmacological, and endocrinological features of isolated mice appear to be similar to those of resident mice who exclude other adult males from their established territories (Brain, 1975; Crawley *et al.*, 1975; Miczek and O'Donnell, 1978). Formidable projects have explored whether drug effects on isolation-induced aggression in mice selectively identify antipsychotics or neuroleptics (e.g., Janssen *et al.*, 1960) or anxiolytics (e.g., Ross and Ogren, 1976; Garattini and Valzelli, 1981) or antidepressants (e.g., Delini-Stula and Vassout, 1981; Malick, 1979). However, drugs of all therapeutic classes decrease isolation-induced aggression and differ only in their degree of behavioral specificity.

2.1.2. Pain-Induced Aggression

Much research, especially during the 1960s and 1970s, used a protocol of delivering electric shock pulses to a pair of rats or mice through the grid floor of a test cage and measuring drug effects on the resulting aggressive–defensive reactions (e.g., Sheard, 1981). In further variations of this protocol, restrained monkeys, rats, or mice are presented with electric shock to their tail, which usually evokes biting responses directed toward an inanimate object placed in front of the animal.

Pain-induced aggression or shock-induced fighting, first described in rats (O'Kelly and Steckle, 1939), is produced by brief duration electric shock pulses of moderate intensity (2 mA) and scrambled polarity, presented every other second via the bars of a grid floor of a small experimental chamber that accommodates a pair of rats (e.g., Ulrich and Azrin,

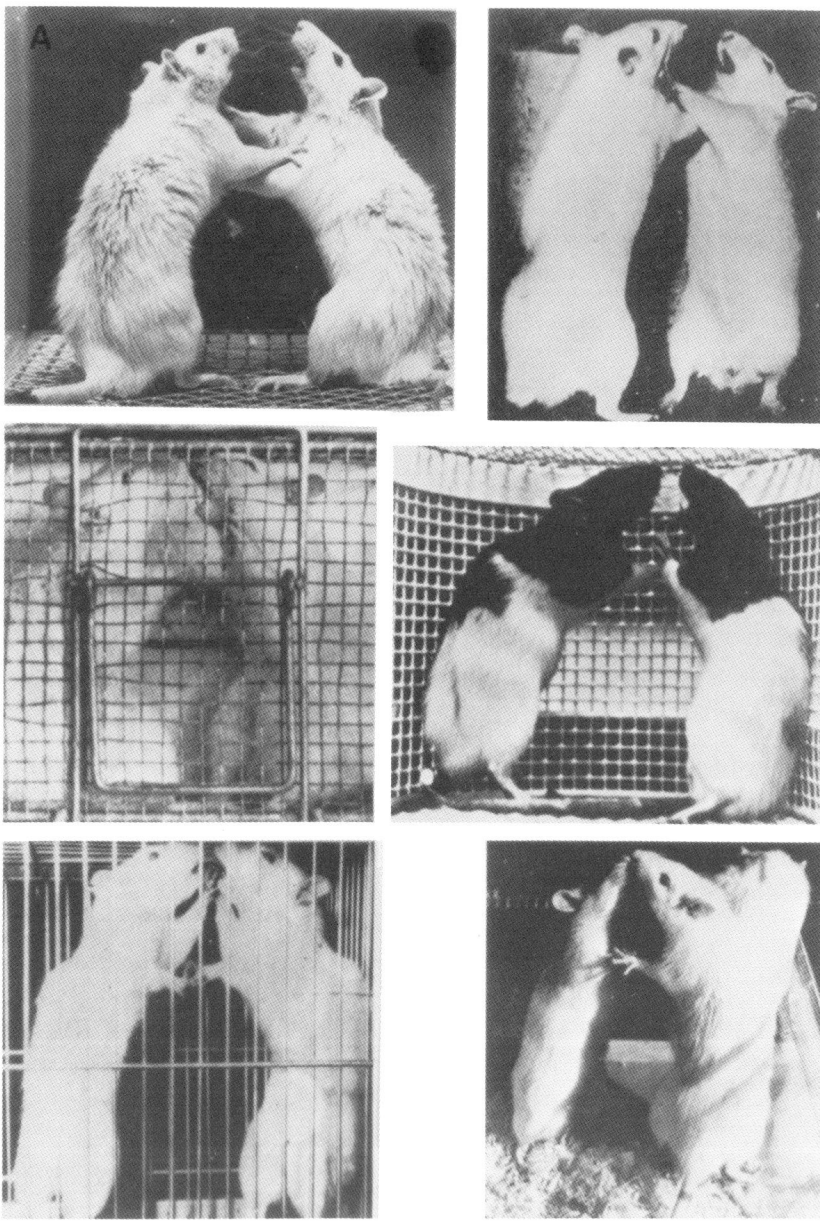

FIG. 2. Mutual upright postures, referred to in varying terminology, during different kinds of experimental manipulations: (A) (Top left) A dominant and a subordinate rat during an extinction-induced aggression test (from Miczek, 1974). (Top right) Two male rats while being exposed to pulses of electric shock through the grid floor, in "stereotyped fighting posture" (Ulrich and Azrin, 1962). (Center left) Two male rats after being injected intravenously with 1 mg/kg apomorphine, in fighting position (Senault, 1970). (Center right) Two male rats, 30 min after being injected subcutaneously with 20 mg/kg apomorphine, in an "aggressive attitude" (McKenzie, 1971). (Bottom left) Two rats, after being deprived of rapid-eye-movement sleep for 4 days and then injected with 10 mg/kg of delta-9-tetra-

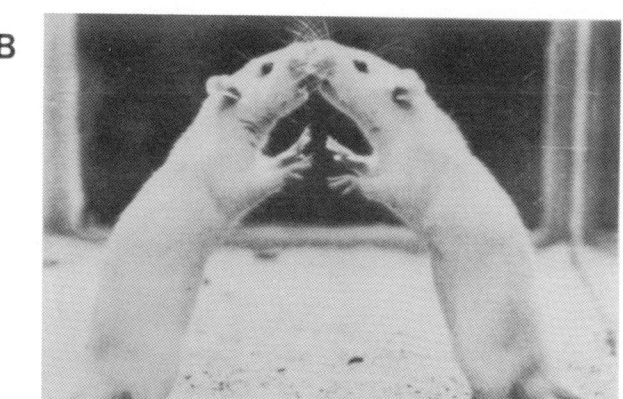
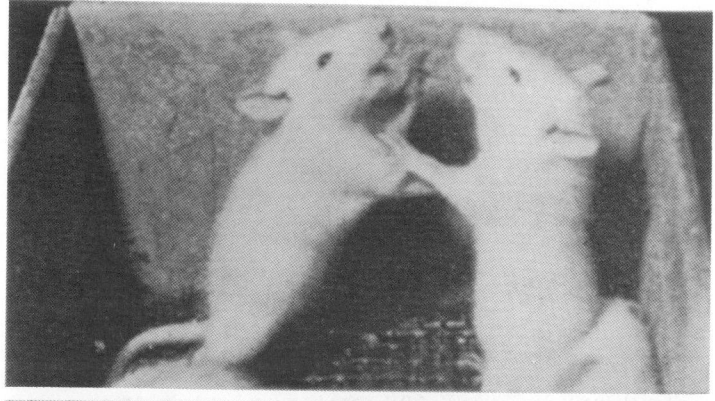
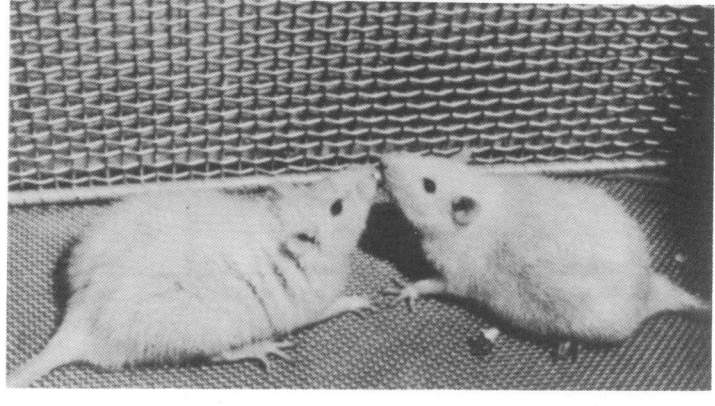

hydrocannabinol, showing "mutual upright posture" (Carlini, 1977). (Bottom right) Two male rats, about 30 min after intraperitoneal injection of 8 mg/kg para-chloroamphetamine, showing "bizarre social behavior" (Korf and Kuiper, 1971). (B) (Top) Two rats, injected with the peripheral decarboxylase inhibitor Ro-4602 and L-dopa (316 μmol/kg), showing "peculiar" and "bizarre" social behavior (Lammers and van Rossum, 1968). (Center) Two male weanling Wistar rats, after being injected subcutaneously with 2.5 mg/kg apomorphine, showing "fighting" (Schneider, 1968). (Bottom) Two rats, after subcutaneous injection of a monoamine oxidase inhibitor followed by 25 mg/kg L-dopa, showing "mutual aggressiveness or rage" (Randrup and Munkvad, 1969b).

1962; Ulrich et al., 1965). Further relevant variables that determine the so-called shock-induced fighting behavior are the rats' age, sex, hormonal status, previous experience with other rats and with aversive stimulation, and intact vibrissae (Ulrich, 1966; Conner and Levine, 1969; Powell et al., 1971; Maier et al., 1972; Thor et al., 1974).

The topography of the rats' behavior elicited by electric shock pulses has often inspired such anthropomorphic terms as "boxing posture," "sparring," and "exchanging blows," but actually includes an upright posture with both opponents facing each other, heads angled upward, mouth open, forepaws moving up and down, and audible vocalizations (Fig. 2). These behavioral elements are characteristic of a rat *defending* against an attacking opponent or a predator (Blanchard et al., 1978; Blanchard and Blanchard, 1984). However, pairs of mice and rats appear to differ in their response to painful electroshock; in addition to assuming the defensive upright posture in reaction to foot shock (Kimbrel, 1969), mice also engage in offensive biting attacks (Tedeschi et al., 1959; Legrand and Fielder, 1973; Brain et al., 1981a; Heller, 1984). It is also possible to record automatically the mice's bites toward each other or toward an inanimate sensor in reaction to electroshock to their tails (Puglisi-Allegra and Renzi, 1977; Wagner et al., 1983). An early method for presenting painful electric shocks and automatically measuring the evoked bites toward a rubber hose was developed for restrained squirrel monkeys (Hutchinson et al., 1966).

The usefulness of evoking aggressive or defensive responses by painful stimuli for psychopharmacological aggression research has been problematic. The procedure permits systematic variations of the parameters of the aversive stimulus and adequate quantification of a selected aspect of aggressive or defensive behavior. Under circumscribed conditions, painful aversive stimuli may evoke reactions that are subsumed under the general label *aggression* (Scott and Fredericson, 1951; Berkowitz, 1983). The nature of the behavior, its functional significance, and how it relates to the remainder of the behavioral repertoire of agonistic behavior, however, are often unclear (e.g., Hutchinson, 1983; Blanchard and Blanchard, 1984). Any drug effect on pain-induced aggression may be the result of a complex interaction between changes in pain perception, reactions to the stress of restraint and exposure to electric shock pulses, and also, processes specific to defense and aggression (Sheard, 1981).

2.1.3. "Frustration"-Induced Aggression and Aggression as Adjunct to Schedule-Controlled Behavior

In spite of its high face validity, aggressive behavior that results from failing to obtain reinforcement is less frequently investigated in psychopharmacological studies than isolation- or pain-induced aggression (e.g.,

Kelly, 1974; Miczek and Winslow, 1987a); the most systematic current experimental work is actually conducted with human subjects (e.g., Cherek, 1981; Cherek *et al.*, 1983, 1984).

Psychological theorists propose "frustration" as the hypothetical construct that results from the discontinuation or omission of scheduled reinforcement and that engenders aggressive behavior (e.g., Dollard *et al.*, 1939). Operationally, once a behavioral response has been reinforced constantly, complete omission of reinforcement (i.e., *extinction*) may result in aggressive behavior if an appropriate target is available (e.g., Azrin *et al.*, 1966; Thompson and Bloom, 1966; Miczek, 1974; Dantzer *et al.*, 1980). More subtle manipulations of the response–reinforcement relationship by schedules of reinforcement that specify *intermittent* reinforcement contingencies also generate aggressive behavior and provide information on concurrent nonaggressive behavior (e.g., Looney and Cohen, 1982; Cherek *et al.*, 1973; Hutchinson *et al.*, 1968; Knutson, 1970; Webbe *et al.*, 1974). One of the hallmarks of research on extinction- or schedule-induced aggressive responses is the accurate, objective, and often automated behavioral measurement technique. A criterion response such as the pigeon's peck or a monkey's bite is automatically recorded (e.g., Looney and Cohen, 1982).

When aggressive responses occur during the performance of behavior that is under the control of a specific schedule of reinforcement, then the aggressive behavior is called *adjunctive* (Falk, 1977). Adjunctive behavior is usually excessive, i.e., it occurs at a homeostatic cost and varies in nature according to the available opportunities. At present, it is unclear how general or specific the behavioral activation is that results from intermittent reinforcement schedules. Drug effects on aggressive behavior that occurs as an adjunct to schedule-controlled behavior may be similar to those on other types of adjunctive behavior and not specific to aggression.

2.2. Neurological Approach

In order to approach aggressive behavior as a function of specific neural processes, direct experimental manipulations of these processes are necessary to evoke, under controlled laboratory conditions, behavior that is characteristic for a given animal species. Hess (1928, 1948) showed that attack and defense can be elicited in otherwise placid cats by delivering microampere pulses to discrete subcortical sites. The discovery of brain tumors in individuals with uncontrollable outbursts of violent behavior was an important impetus for the use of experimental lesions of neural structures in animals to reproduce comparable behavioral phenomena. A complex, rarely studied, and poorly understood relationship appears to exist between certain epileptic disorders and aggressive behavior (e.g., Mirsky and Harman, 1974).

2.2.1. Brain Stimulation-Evoked Aggression

A sophisticated research methodology permits psychopharmacological studies of several species-specific patterns of aggressive and defensive behavior as they are evoked by intracranial electrical stimulation (e.g., Delgado, 1963; Flynn *et al.*, 1979; Kruk *et al.*, 1979; Bandler, 1982*a,b*; Siegel and Edinger, 1983). Most research has been performed in cats and involved electrical stimulation of either the medial or lateral hypothalamus, the first resulting in affective defense and the latter in a quiet biting attack.

The behavioral and autonomic phenomena elicited by stimulation of sites in the medial hypothalamus and connected subcortical structures of cats were originally labeled *affektive Abwehr* by Hess (1948), but subsequently they were varyingly referred to as *affective aggression, emotional behavior, defensive attack,* or *rage;* the stimulated cat hisses and spits, shows piloerection in the back region and tail, dilates the pupils, retracts the ears, bares teeth and claws, and arches the back, and if provoked, strikes defensively (Hess and Brügger, 1943). In psychopharmacological studies, one of these behavioral elements is usually selected as criterion behavior, most often hissing vocalizations, and drug effects are assessed in terms of how the current threshold for evoking hissing is altered (e.g., Fukuda and Tsumagari, 1983; Funderburk *et al.*, 1970; Baxter, 1968*a,b*; MacDonnell *et al.*, 1971).

The cat's quiet biting attack or predatory attack as evoked by lateral hypothalamic stimulation is less often used in psychopharmacological research, presumably because the relative lack of autonomic nervous system activity may suggest less affective components of the behavior (Wasman and Flynn, 1962; Berntson *et al.*, 1976). Changes in the amount of current necessary to evoke the biting reflex, as well as in latency for the behavior to occur, are the primary indices of drug action (e.g., Dubinsky *et al.*, 1973; Katz, 1980; MacDonnell and Fessock, 1972; Marini *et al.*, 1979*b*).

A less frequently used methodological variation of the electrical brain stimulation method has been extended to rats as subjects. Although predatory attack and killing can be elicited by electrically stimulating hypothalamic sites in rats (e.g., Vergnes and Karli, 1969, 1970; Woodworth, 1971; Panksepp, 1971*a*), only sparse pharmacological data have been obtained with this difficult preparation (e.g., Panksepp, 1971*b*). More recently, attack leaps and bites were reliably evoked by electrical hypothalamic stimulation of rats from the Dutch WE-zob strain directed toward a stimulus rat (Koolhaas, 1978; Kruk et al., 1979), and initial systematic drug effects were studied (Kruk et al., 1984; Olivier et al., 1984). However, the behavior evoked by brain stimulation in rats is determined by various environmental and experiential variables and may reflect considerable anatomical plasticity (e.g., Valenstein et al., 1970).

2.2.2. Brain Lesion-Induced Aggression

Spurred by histopathological findings of brain tumors in violent patients (e.g., Mark and Ervin, 1970), the lesion, or ablation method, has been applied to experimental aggression research. Experimental destruction of more or less discrete brain areas in rats, as well as in other animals, may elicit behavioral phenomena that have been viewed as forms of aggression. Particularly, lesions of the lateral septal forebrain area, the medial hypothalamus, the olfactory bulbs, or the dorsal and median raphe nuclei in laboratory rats lead to dramatic behavioral changes, sometimes referred to as *rage, emotional behavior, hyperreactivity, hyperdefensiveness* (e.g., Brady and Nauta, 1953; Miczek and Grossman, 1972; Cain, 1974; Albert and Walsh, 1982, 1984). The behavioral elements induced by brain lesions have been characterized to be of a defensive nature (e.g., Albert and Walsh, 1982). These behavioral changes are typically assessed by rating the animal's reactivity to a set of sensory stimuli and assigning a score on a scale. Pharmacological manipulations of lesion-induced aggressive–defensive reactions attempt to screen a variety of agents from different therapeutic classes, although with limited selectivity (e.g., Sofia, 1969b; Malick, 1970b; Ueki et al., 1972b). In spite of its apparent face validity, the lesion method for inducing aggressive behavior is problematic for psychopharmacological studies because of the coarse quantification of the behavior and because the tissue damage changes the blood–brain barrier and uptake mechanisms.

2.2.3. Toxin- and Drug-Induced Aggression

The impetus for studying drug-induced aggression often comes from societal and medical concerns with violent behavior in the context of drug abuse and exposure to environmental toxins. The behavioral starting point for studies on aggressive behavior induced by some pharmacological or toxicological treatment is usually a domesticated laboratory animal without history of aggressive behavior. A remarkably wide range of substances and treatment regimens have been associated with the appearance of a variety of aggressive and defensive behaviors; it will be useful to consider first, catecholaminergic agonists and neurotoxins; later, hallucinogens and cholinomimetics; and eventually, serotonin depletors and synthesis inhibitors.

The early observations by Chance (1946a) on "defensive encounters" in groups of laboratory mice injected with large doses of amphetamine (i.e., more than 10 mg/kg, s.c.) have been confirmed (e.g., Rolinski, 1973) and extended also to rats (e.g., Lammers and van Rossum, 1968; Randrup and Munkvad, 1969a,b). Behaviorally, rats or mice treated with near-toxic doses of amphetamine assume upright postures facing each other, vocalize, and move their forelimbs up and down; these phenomena are illustrated in Fig. 2 and have been called *bizarre social behavior, rage,* or *aggressiveness*. Similar responses can be induced by very high doses of L-dopa, apomorphine and clonidine, and methylxanthines, as well as MAO inhibitors and reuptake blockers, particularly after catecholamine synthesis has been blocked (e.g., Senault, 1968, 1970; McKenzie, 1971; Dlabac, 1973; Gianutsos and Lal, 1976a; Fog, 1969; Scheel-Krüger and Randrup, 1968; Morpurgo, 1968; Maj *et al.*, 1979, 1980; Ozawa *et al.*, 1975; Sakata and Fuchimoto, 1973a,b; Yen *et al.*, 1970). Pharmacological treatment with apparently opposite neurochemical effects, namely, administration of the neurotoxin 6-hydroxydopamine (6-OHDA), also increases irritability and, under certain circumstances, induces the peculiar defensive behavior illustrated in Fig. 2 (Nakamura and Thoenen, 1972; Thoa *et al.*, 1972a,b,c; Coscina *et al.*, 1973). However, since high amphetamine doses may result in the endogenous formation of 6-OHDA (Seiden and Vosmer, 1984), a new interpretation is required for the mechanisms of so-called stimulant-induced aggression. Also, brain serotonin appears to interact with apomorphine- and clonidine-induced aggression; not only do serotonergic drugs modulate apomorphine- and clonidine-induced acts and postures (Rolinski and Herbut, 1979; Hahn *et al.*, 1982), but *p*-chloroamphetamine, a 5-HT depletor, may also induce "bizarre" aggressive behavior by itself (Korf and Kuiper, 1971; Gianutsos and Lal, 1975).

The spectrum of pharmacological treatments that may induce elements of aggressive and defensive reactions in laboratory animals also includes hallucinogens (see pp. 254, 259). For example, lysergic acid diethylamide phencyclidine, mescaline, and cannabinoids, usually at very high doses and in conjunction with exposure to severe stress, such as electric foot shock, food deprivation, deprivation of rapid-eye-movement sleep, or after catecholamine depletion, may induce in a certain percentage of laboratory rats unusual acts and postures that resemble defensive reactions as shown in Fig. 2 (e.g., Schneider, 1968; Carlini and Masur, 1969; Carlini, 1977; Musty and Consroe, 1982; Sbordone and Carder, 1974; Musty *et al.*, 1976; Fujiwara *et al.*, 1984; Votava, 1969).

Withdrawal from chronic exposure to opiates is a further pharmacological treatment that may induce elements of aggressive and defensive behavior in laboratory animals (e.g., Lal, 1975b; Gianutsos and Lal, 1976a). Similar to the previously mentioned forms of drug-induced aggression, morphine withdrawal aggression can be enhanced by various manipulations that lead to more dopamine release, block reuptake, and activate dopamine receptors (Gianutsos and Lal, 1978). Behaviorally, morphine-withdrawal aggression in rats is similar to stimulant- and hallucinogen-induced forms of behavior (see Fig. 2).

The stressful nature of near-toxic doses of acutely or chronically administered catecholaminergic agonists, hallucinogens, or cytotoxic agents or of withdrawal from opiates, often in combination with environmental stressors, appears to necessitate a major role of the catecholamines in the peripheral and central nervous system in these unusual behavioral reactions. The catecholaminergic component in responses to stress may also be critical in the aggressive and defensive behavior induced by such environmental toxins as bronopol or trimethyltin (e.g., Neiminen and Mottonen, 1975; Dyer et al., 1982). The behavioral outcome of pharmacological insults, such as by the neurotoxin 6-OHDA or withdrawal from morphine, appears to depend on the previous history of social and aggressive behavior; monkeys that are dominant in their free-ranging troops become socially incapacitated after 6-OHDA treatment (Redmond et al., 1973); profound depletion of catecholamines by 6-OHDA left the behavior of isolated aggressive mice largely unaltered, but increased aggressive behavior in previously nonaggressive animals (Pöschlova et al., 1976); mice without experience of fighting show a large increase in attack behavior during withdrawal from morphine, but those with a history of aggressive behavior fail to alter their behavior during morphine withdrawal (Kantak and Miczek, in press).

The validity of drug-induced aggression appears problematic because of the unusual behavioral phenomenology, lack of generality beyond domesticated laboratory animals, and the inappropriate context. Mescaline-, amphetamine-, and morphine-withdrawal–induced aggressive responses in rats, particularly during exposure to electric foot shock, have been proposed to represent incidences of "pathological" aggression (Sbordone et al., 1981). The acts and postures resulting from drug treatments are behavioral fragments, isolated from the context of aggressive interactions, without a clear indication of functional significance, prompting such terms as *bizarre* and *ambiguous*.

2.2.4. Drug-Induced Killing

Only a small proportion of laboratory rats kill mice, even after starvation (Karli, 1956). It is not clear whether *predatory behavior* would be a more adequate term for the omnivorous rat's killing response toward mice; when mouse killing, or muricide, is induced by drug treatment, irritability and defensive reactions may be significant in the initiation of this response (Karli, 1981).

Early interest in acetylcholine and aggressive behavior (e.g., Allikmets, 1974) was supported by demonstrations that cholinomimetic drugs (e.g., carbachol) or acetylcholinesterase inhibitors (e.g., physostigmine) could induce killing behavior in a certain proportion of rats or cats, often after some delay (Smith *et al.*, 1970; Bandler, 1970; Berntson and Leibowitz, 1973; Vogel and Leaf, 1972; Miczek, 1976*b*). Intrahypothalamic injections of carbachol in cats may, however, also result in heightened defensive or "rage" reaction (Romaniuk, 1974; Romaniuk *et al.*, 1973, 1974).

After blockade of serotonin synthesis at the tryptophan hydroxylase step, cytotoxic destruction of serotonin-containing neurons, or consumption of trytophan-low diet, a sizable number of nonkiller rats start to kill mice (e.g., Sheard, 1969; Vergnes *et al.*, 1977; Vergnes, 1980; Vergnes and Kempf, 1982; Gibbons *et al.*, 1978, 1979; Applegate, 1980). A limiting condition for the initiation of killing behavior by depletion or destruction of serotonin neurons appears to be how familiar the animals are with their potential prey before drug treatment (e.g., Marks *et al.*, 1977; Vergnes and Kempf, 1981). Moreover, the degree of serotonin depletion and its time course are poorly related to the initiation of killing, if at all (e.g., Miczek *et al.*, 1975). Curiously, carnivores such as grasshopper mice or cats show either an impaired predatory killing response or no effect after tryptophan hydroxylase inhibition (Dubinsky *et al.*, 1973; McCarty *et al.*, 1976).

Drug-induced killing has been of interest not only as a phenomenon for delineating brain–behavior relationships (Karli, 1981), but also for pragmatic reasons. It appears that many antidepressant drugs, but also psychomotor stimulants and anticholinergics, block mouse-killing behavior in laboratory rats (e.g., Horovitz *et al.*, 1966; Howard *et al.*, 1981).

2.2.5. Aggression Associated with Seizure Activity

In spite of the frequently asserted association between convulsive phenomena and acts of violence and aggression (e.g., Monroe, 1978; Mark and Ervin, 1970), there is little agreement in the clinical literature on a direct relationship between temporal lobe disease and violence (e.g., Mirsky and Harman, 1974; Kligman and Goldberg, 1975; Eichelman, 1983). Only a few experimental preparations may be relevant to this important issue. Increased epileptic excitability or "kindling" may be produced by high-frequency electrical stimulation of amygdaloid or hippocampal sites, which culminate eventually in motor convulsions. Such kindling stimulation of the amygdala or hippocampus in rats causes them to resist capture and overreact to touch (Pinel *et al.*, 1977) and kill mice with shorter latencies (McIntyre, 1978). However, in cats, kindling stimulation of the amygdala suppressed the killing response and shifted the animals to defensive reactions (Adamec and Stark-Adamec, 1983). The effects of kindling stimulation of amygdaloid sites may also be assessed from the threshold for the current that is necessary to evoke either a predatory attack or an affective defense by hypothalamic stimulation (Siegel, 1984). The direction in which threshold current is modulated appears to depend on the location of the seizure focus and on which type of behavior is elicited.

Unfortunately, the complex association between seizure activity and aggressive behavior has not been a topic of preclinical experimental research in psychopharmacology. The clinical success with anticonvulsant drugs in treating violent individuals is promising but needs to be substantiated (Monroe, 1975; Eichelman, 1983).

2.3. Ethological Approach

Although ethological work had its origin in field research, many critical features of this approach have been reproduced under controlled laboratory conditions. During the past decade, much preclinical research on the psychopharmacology of aggression has been influenced by ethological concepts and methods (e.g., Miczek *et al.*, 1984*b*). Following the lead of Chance and his students (Chance and Silverman, 1964; Chance, 1968; Mackintosh *et al.*, 1977), the focus on biologically valid behavior and situational context and on detailed quantitative records and analysis of species-specific behavior patterns has become the methodological hallmark of the more recent "ethopharmacological" aggression research (e.g., Miczek and Krsiak, 1979; Miczek and Winslow, 1987*a;* Poshivalov and Khodko, 1984).

2.3.1. Status-Related Aggression

Success or failure in aggressive interactions in species that form groups leads to social stratifications that are often referred to as hierarchy or dominance order. A group member's social status or rank in an established group is determined by several factors, such as age, genealogical position, sex, physical prowess, and success in situations of conflict (e.g., Hinde, 1983). Aggression within an established group occupies actually only a small segment of an individual's entire behavioral "budget." For example in groups of squirrel monkeys, less than 5% of the behavioral repertoire is accounted for by agonistic behavior (Fig. 3; Winslow and Miczek, 1985). The elements of agonistic behavior shown in conflict situations within established groups have been identified and catalogued for

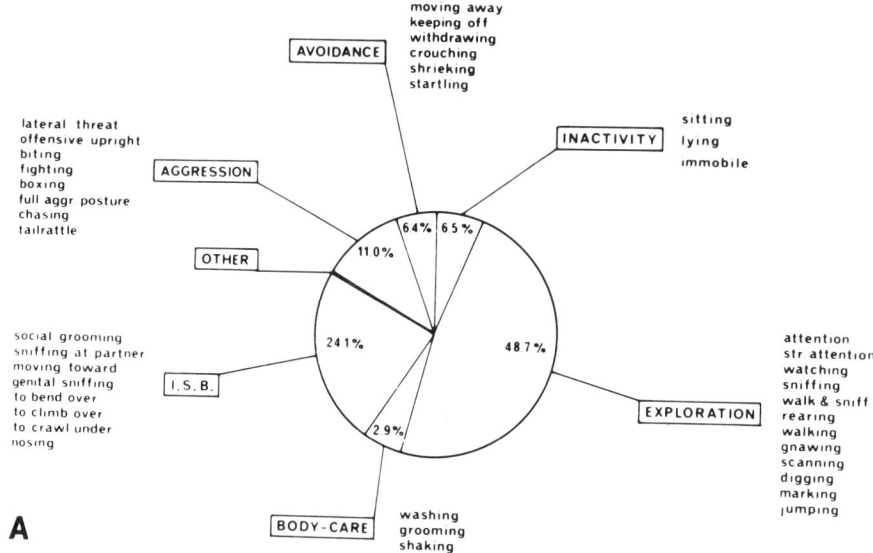

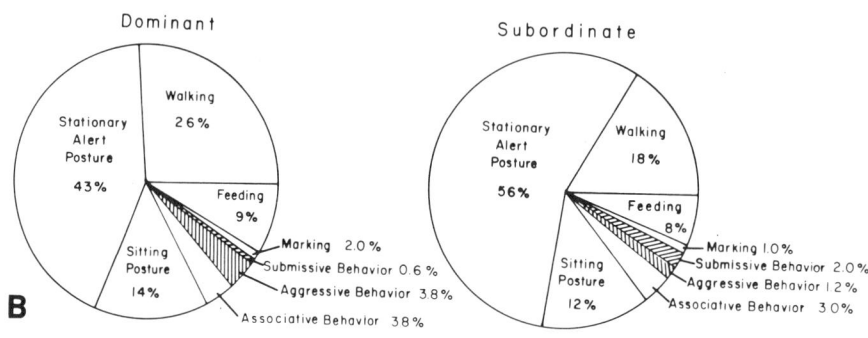

FIG. 3. (A) Activity budget for rats. Mean percentage of time spent on seven behavioral categories in a 15-min confrontation of male resident Wezob rats ($n = 8$) with a male Wistar intruder. The behavioral elements belonging to each category are shown (from Olivier et al., 1984). (B) Activity budgets for dominant and subordinate squirrel monkeys living in established groups: the proportion of time spent walking, sitting, in stationary alert posture, feeding, marking, aggressive, associative, and submissive behaviors. (From Winslow and Miczek, 1985.)

most species that are commonly subjects in preclinical psychopharmacological research, such as rats (Barnett, 1975; Grant and Mackintosh, 1963), cats (Leyhausen, 1960), rhesus monkeys (Sade, 1967; Altmann, 1962), and squirrel monkeys (Hopf et al., 1974). During the past decade, microprocessor-based data collection technology has led to important methodological advances. The reliability and speed of encoding and analyzing formidable amounts of observational data have been greatly improved, and novel ways of detecting drug action on sequences and patterns of behavior are now possible (e.g., Miczek and Krsiak, 1979; Smith and Byrd, 1983; Hendrie and Bennett, 1983; DePaulis, 1983; Poshivalov *et al.*, 1979; Jones and Brain, 1985).

The significance of aggressive behavior as it occurs in an unambiguously defined social context for psychopharmacological studies appears to be profound; in addition to the long-known endocrine differences between high- and low-ranking group members (e.g., Sassenrath, 1971; Rose *et al.*, 1971; Sapolsky, 1982; Steklis *et al.*, 1985), the recent demonstrations of differential activity in synthetic and metabolic enzymes for catecholamines and serotonin between dominant and subordinate animals are especially consequential for drug action (e.g., Raab and Oswald, 1980; Raleigh *et al.*, 1984, 1985; Kraemer, 1985).

2.3.2. Resident–Intruder Aggression

In species that feature complex social organizations as well as in those where adult members largely live solitary excluding others from their territory, an unfamiliar intruder provokes intense and frequent aggression (e.g., Wilson, 1975). Even under controlled laboratory conditions using domesticated animals, such as mice, rats, hamsters, or cats, the confrontation with an unfamiliar adult animal leads to attack, threat, and pursuit by the resident toward the intruder (e.g., Crawley *et al.*, 1975; Blanchard *et al.*, 1975; Miczek, 1978, 1979b; Hoffmeister and Wuttke, 1969; Payne and Swanson, 1970). The major advantages of studying aggressive behavior between residents and intruders are the validity of the behavior and the context that generates the behavior; the reliability with which aggressive behavior occurs in this context, even in laboratory animals; the elaborate behavioral repertoire encompassing all salient elements of attack and threat, as well as defense, submission, and flight; and the absence of such potentially confounding variables as isolated housing, restraint, food deprivation, exposure to electric shock pulses, extensive conditioning history, or adaptation to a novel test environment.

In the early days of experimental preclinical research, resident–intruder aggression was used to screen for psychoactive drugs but in an unusual species, fish (Abramson and Evans, 1954; Walaszek and Abood, 1956), and with impressionistic accounts of the behavioral changes. During the past decade, prototypes of virtually all major classes of drugs have been studied with regard to their effects on resident–intruder aggression (e.g., Olivier and van Dalen, 1982; Poshivalov, 1982; Miczek and Winslow, 1987a). From a behavioral viewpoint, several features of these recent studies are notable; the comprehensive analysis of the behavioral repertoire has made it possible to identify those elements, whether agonistic or nonagonistic, that are the primary targets of drug action and thereby has made it possible to assess the behavioral specificity and "cost" of the drug effect; the selective pharmacological manipulation of either opponent provides information on drug effects that differentiate between the resident's attack and threat behavior and the intruder's defense, submission and flight; monitoring the behavior of both the pharmacologically manipulated animal and the opponent reveals subtle behavioral changes that occur in a drug-free animal interacting with a drugged animal.

2.3.3. Maternal Aggression

What is known about the psychopharmacology of aggression has, until recently, been limited to the male of the species. This serious deficiency in clinical as well as preclinical work is not the least the result of the persistent belief that aggression is a male-specific phenomenon. That females of various species are aggressive, often equal to, and sometimes in excess of, males, has now been documented, although the literature is still very sparse (Floody, 1983; Svare and Mann, 1983). Defense and dispersal of the young are the most apparent functions of female aggression during lactation; however, a very important function of female aggression derives from interactions among female rivals and leads to the suppression of reproductive success by the submissive animal (Floody, 1983).

The most common procedure for studying aggression by females focuses on the lactation period and examines the female's interactions with an intruder animal. Especially in the latter portion of pregnancy and the early portion of lactation, a high incidence of aggressive behavior is exhibited by female mice, rats, and hamsters toward either a male or female intruder (Erskine *et al.*, 1978; Gandelman, 1972; Ogawa and Makino, 1984; Siegel *et al.*, 1983; Wise, 1974; Hood, 1984). Maternal aggression in mice appears to depend on the suckling stimulation from the pups (Svare and Gandelman, 1976). However, ovariectomized female rats and hamsters without any reproductive experience attack a female intruder (DeBold and Miczek, 1981, 1984; Vandenbergh, 1971). Behaviorally, maternal aggression is intense and frequent; it includes the same acts and postures that are displayed by males; female rats and mice direct their bites frequently toward the opponent's snout, which may suggest a defensive nature of this behavior (DeBold and Miczek, 1981).

The few pharmacological studies on maternal aggression that exist up to now have selected the level of aggressive behavior that is shown during a given portion of the lactation period as the baseline for drug manipulations (e.g., Olivier *et al.*, 1985; Brain and Al-Maliki, 1979; Mann *et al.*, 1980; Wise and Pryor, 1977; Ieni and Thurmond, 1985). The systematic fluctuation of aggressive behavior during the course of the lactation period points to a complex dependence on hormonal mechanisms and presents unusual methodological challenges for pharmacological work.

When drugs alter maternal aggression, their primary site of action may be on those hormonal mechanisms rather than directly on the central nervous system (CNS). Nonetheless, female aggression constitutes a significant although much neglected phenomenon, the neurochemical mechanisms of which need to be explored (Miczek and DeBold, 1983).

2.3.4. Predatory Aggression

From an ethological viewpoint, it may be a contradiction to combine predatory and aggressive behavior, both subserving separate functions and involving different behavioral, physiological, and neural processes (e.g., O'Boyle, 1974; Rossi, 1975; Polsky, 1975). Yet, several observations have emerged that differentiate attacking and killing of a prey from feeding (e.g., Yoshimura and Miczek, 1983). Sometimes, the term *interspecies aggression* has been applied to predatory attack and antipredator defense, to differentiate it from the more commonly studied forms of *intraspecies aggression* (e.g., Huntingford, 1976). After considering earlier electrical brain stimulation-evoked "quiet biting attack" and drug-induced killing (see above), it may be appropriate to note that the predatory attack and kill, as it is characteristic for certain animal species, is often the focus of experimental psychopharmacological work.

The rat's attack on a mouse and its eventual mouse-killing response represent the form of predatory aggression that is most frequently studied in laboratory research (e.g., Karli, 1956; O'Boyle, 1974; van Hemel, 1975; Rossi, 1975; Kreiskott, 1969). This research tradition is unusual, since only a few laboratory rats kill mice (e.g., Walsh, 1982), the killing behavior cannot be induced in all rats even after severe food deprivation (e.g., Karli, 1956; Paul *et al.*, 1971), and even wild rats, being omnivorous and capable of killing small mammals, birds, and fish, engage infrequently in mouse killing (Barnett, 1975). Moreover, when the killing response is initially displayed by a laboratory rat, it is not in the form of a "quiet" stalking attack, but includes signs of strong sympathetic activity that suggest nonpredatory components of the behavior (Karli, 1981).

Psychopharmacological interests in mouse-killing behavior follow two lines, either to induce the killing response in nonkiller rats by a given pharmacological treatment (see above) or to block this behavior pharmacologically (Barr *et al.*, 1976). The blockade of mouse-killing behavior has been proposed as a preclinical screen for drugs with antidepressant properties (e.g., Horovitz *et al.*, 1965) and continues to be used (e.g., Howard *et al.*, 1981; Shibata *et al.*, 1984), although psychomotor stimulant and anticholinergic drugs are detected as "false positives" (e.g., Barnes *et al.*, 1967).

Predatory behavior in carnivorous species such as cats, ferrets *(Putorius furio)*, and grasshopper mice (*Onychomys leucogaster* and *torridus*) has been investigated to a considerably lesser extent than mouse killing by rats in psychopharmacological research. Interestingly, antidepressant, anxiolytic, antipsychotic, anticholinergic, and psychomotor stimulant drugs as well as serotonin-depleting agents, alter predatory behavior in these species not at all, or often in opposite direction to the killing behavior by rats (e.g., Cole and Wolf, 1970; Leaf *et al.,* 1978; Schmidt and Apfelbach, 1977; Schmidt, 1979, 1980; McCarty *et al.,* 1976). These findings suggest important pharmacological and possibly neurobiological differences between mouse killing in rats and predatory behavior by carnivores.

3. PRECLINICAL AND CLINICAL AGGRESSION RESEARCH

The purpose of discussing preclinical and clinical research findings concurrently is mainly heuristic. In spite of some notable exceptions, it has been difficult to establish behavioral, neuroanatomical, and neuropharmacological homologies or even just analogies between human and nonhuman aggressive behavior. The following discussion will address first a group of pharmacological agents that are known for their antiaggressive properties and that are the major therapeutic drugs for the treatment of pathological aggression. A further group of drugs is known mainly for its abuse potential and is often linked to enhanced aggressive and violent behavior. As will become obvious, the differentiation between these two groups of drugs is quite artificial. For example, benzodiazepines and barbiturates are discussed in the group of drugs with antiaggressive properties, whereas alcohol is grouped with the drugs of abuse; all three classes of drugs, however, share many similarities in behavioral profile and possibly even common mechanisms of action.

3.1. Antiaggressive Drug Treatments

The most significant issue in evaluating the antiaggressive effects of a given drug concerns their behavioral specificity (e.g., Miczek and Krsiak, 1979). Any drug, given at appropriate parameters, may decrease aggressive behavior; however, drugs differ greatly in how specifically and selectively they affect aggressive versus nonaggressive behavior. Stated in economic terms, at which behavioral costs are the antiaggressive effects obtained? Traditionally, the preclinical research strategies compare the dose range at which aggressive behavior is decreased with the doses that decrease nonaggressive behavior; the analysis is rarely pursued further to determine whether the decrease in nonaggressive motor activity is the result of sedation, neuromuscular impairment, or other forms of incapacitation. Only recently, quantitative ethological analyses have been performed to identify the varied sources for antiaggressive drug effects (e.g., Poshivalov and Khodko, 1984; Olivier *et al.*, 1984; Miczek and Winslow, 1987*a*). Moreover, impairment of nonaggressive motor activities should be considered only as a preliminary step in the assessment of behavioral specificity of antiaggressive drug effects. It is quite likely that so-called antiaggressive effects may occur in the same dose range that affects maternal, sexual, play, or other associative behavior patterns. These more extensive behavioral comparisons have rarely been made.

3.1.1. Antipsychotic Drugs

Phenothiazines and butyrophenones, as the classic or typical antipsychotic or neuroleptic drugs, are the most frequently used agents in the treatment of pathologically aggressive individuals, particularly in emergency situations. This usage pattern is surprising in light of the poor specificity of their antiaggressive effects, as is already evident from the preclinical studies. With the advent of so-called atypical antipsychotic agents with fewer and potentially less disruptive side effects, the antiaggressive effects of the antipsychotic drugs continue to be of interest (e.g., Itil and Seaman, 1978; Tupin, 1985).

3.1.1a. Preclinical Data. Antiaggressive effects of phenothiazines and butyrophenones have been found consistently since the discovery of these drugs in many preclinical tests. This "calming" (*ergo* tranquilizing) and sedating effect was particularly apparent in feral animals (e.g., Das *et al.*, 1954; Walaszek and Abood, 1956; Lister *et al.*, 1971) and may have led to the widespread use of these drugs in veterinary medicine (e.g., Niemegeers *et al.*, 1974).

The initial critical question concerns the specificity of the antiaggressive effects of the antipsychotic drugs (e.g., Miczek and Krsiak, 1979; Malick, 1979; Valzelli, 1979; Miczek and Winslow, 1987*a*). As an illustrative example, Table 1 summarizes the effects of chlorpromazine, the prototypic phenothiazine, on aggressive behavior by isolated mice; defensive reactions by squirrel monkeys or pairs of rats or mice during exposure to painful electric shocks; affective–defensive reactions by cats due to electrical brain stimulation; irritability and defensive behavior in rats after electrolytic or toxic insult to brain tissue; and killing behavior by rats. For comparison, in the second column of Table 1, the doses of chlorpromazine are given at which decreases in motor activity are seen. All the more detailed studies address the issue of behavioral specificity by comparing the effects on aggressive responses with those on nonaggressive motor activity. However, opposite conclusions on the behavioral specificity of the effects of antipsychotic drugs on aggressive behavior are reached

TABLE 1
Doses of Chlorpromazine for Decreasing Aggression and Nonaggressive Motor Activity[a]

Aggression	Nonaggressive motor activity	Reference
Isolation-induced aggression		
In mice		
ED50[b] 10 p.o.	ED50 10 p.o.	Yen *et al.*, 1959
ED50 0.99 s.c.	ED50 1.43 s.c.	Janssen *et al.*, 1960
ED50 11.3 p.o.	N/S	Cook and Weidley, 1960
ED50 12.5 p.o.	N/S	Gray *et al.*, 1961
0.5, 1.2 i.p.	4, 8 i.p.	Scriabine and Blake, 1962
ED50 9.6 p.o.	ED50 25.5 p.o.	Cole and Wolf, 1966
ED50 1.54 i.p.	ED50 5 i.p.	DaVanzo *et al.*, 1966
2.5 i.p.	10 i.p.	Valzelli *et al.*, 1967
ED50 2 p.o.	N/S	Boissier *et al.*, 1968
ED50 2.35 p.o.	ED50 14.3 p.o.	Hoffmeister and Wuttke, 1969
2 i.p.	4 i.p.	Le Douarec and Broussy, 1969
ED50 1.6 i.p.	ED50 0.7 i.p.	Sofia, 1969*b*
ED50 2 i.p.	ED50 0.7 i.p.	Dubinsky *et al.*, 1973
ED50 1.7 i.p.	>1.7 i.p.	Malick, 1979
2, 5 s.c.	2.5 i.p.	Delini-Stula and Vassout, 1979
1, 2.5, 5 s.c.	N/S	Benton, 1984
Pain-induced aggression		
In mice		
ED50 6.8 p.o.	ED50 4.7 p.o.	Tedeschi *et al.*, 1959
ED50 4.2 p.o.	N/S	Chen *et al.*, 1963
5 i.p.	5 i.p.	Kostowski, 1966
ED50 1.77 p.o.	ED50 14.3 p.o.	Hoffmeister and Wuttke, 1969
ED50 3.4 i.p.	ED50 0.7 i.p.	Sofia, 1969*b*
ED50 10.8 p.o.	ED50 4.7 p.o.	Tedeschi *et al.*, 1969
ED50 1.1	N/S	Barkov, 1973
In rats		
5 i.p.	>5 i.p.	Brunaud and Siou, 1959
ED50 3.5	N/S	Barkov, 1973
1–10 s.c.	N/S	Powell *et al.*, 1973
In hamsters		
ED70 16 p.o.	N/S	Kreiskott, 1963
In squirrel monkeys		
0.5–2 s.c.	>2 s.c.	Emley and Hutchinson, 1983*b*
Brain stimulation-induced affective defense in cats		
>3 i.v.	N/S	Kido *et al.*, 1967
>5 i.p.	5 i.p.	Baxter, 1968*b*
>5 i.p.	2.5, 5 i.p.	Funderburk *et al.*, 1970
>8 i.p.	8 i.p.	Dubinsky and Goldberg, 1971
ED50 5 i.p.	N/S	Fukuda and Tsumagari, 1983
Brain lesion-induced irritability		
In mice		
>2 i.p.	N/S	Kletzkin, 1969

(continued)

TABLE 1
(Continued)

Aggression	Nonaggressive motor activity	Reference
In rats		
ED50 6.8 i.p.	ED50 3.1 i.p.	Horovitz et al., 1963
ED50 12.1 i.p.	N/S	Malick et al., 1969
ED50 11.3 i.p.	ED50 1.9 i.p.	Goldberg, 1970
5, 10 i.p.	5, 10 i.p.	Ueki et al., 1972b
Drug-induced aggression		
In mice		
dl-Dopa		
ED50 2.4 i.p.	N/S	Yen et al., 1970
In rats		
Apomorphine		
16 i.p.	N/S	Senault, 1970
6-OHDA		
ED50 5.09 i.p.	ED50 1.46 i.p.	Nakamura and Thoenen, 1972
Isocarboxazid/Imipramine		
5 i.p.	N/S	Zetler and Hauer, 1975
Mouse killing		
In rats		
25 i.p.	2–15 i.p.	Karli, 1958, 1959a,b
ED50 5.5 i.p.	ED50 3.7 i.p.	Horovitz et al., 1966
>50	10–50	Loiselle and Capparell, 1967
ED50 9 i.p.	ED50 1.7 i.p.	Sofia, 1969a
ED50 5.6 i.p.	ED50 1.9 i.p.	Goldberg, 1970
5	N/S	Valzelli and Bernasconi, 1971
5, 10 i.p.	5, 10 i.p.	Ueki et al., 1972b
5–20 i.p.	N/S	Delini-Stula and Vassout, 1979
10 s.c.	N/S	Shibata et al., 1984
In cats		
>8 i.p.	N/S	Leaf et al., 1978

[a] All doses are expressed in mg/kg; N/S = data not specified.
[b] ED50 = Effective dose that decreased behavior either in 50% of the subjects or by 50% from the control level.

because the measurements of motor activity vary widely in sensitivity and because the experimental manipulations, types of aggressive behavior, species, and sophistication of assessing aggressive behavior differ markedly. For example, the median effective doses of chlorpromazine for decreasing isolation-induced aggression in mice differ up to 10-fold between experiments (e.g., Janssen et al., 1960, versus Cole and Wolf, 1966); even larger differences are seen in the corresponding doses that decrease nonaggressive motor activity. In general, those tests that require *active* behavioral initiative detect suppressive effects of chlorpromazine at considerably lower doses than those that measure *reactive* behavior.

A limited degree of behavioral specificity in the antiaggressive effects of chlorpromazine appears to exist in some isolated aggressive mice and pain-exposed mice, rats, and monkeys (Table 1); under most conditions, however, this drug decreases aggressive and defensive behavior only at doses equal to or in excess of those that sedate or impair motor activity. This lack in specificity of chlorpromazine effects is particularly apparent with regard to aggressive–defensive reactions that are evoked by electrical stimulation of discrete brain structures, irritable and defensive reactions that are induced by electrolytic or toxic insults to brain tissue, or killing behavior by rats or cats (Table 1).

The development of antipsychotic drugs with fewer detrimental side effects than those characteristic of chlorpromazine has met with partial success; many other phenothiazines, butyrophenones, and so-called atypical neuroleptics decrease aggressive and defensive responses only at doses that are closely similar to or even larger than those that suppress nonaggressive motor activity. Haloperidol, pimozide, spiramide, and several phenothiazine derivatives decrease most often nonspecifically (1) isolation-induced aggressive behavior; (2) aggressive–defensive responses in reaction to electric foot shock or as a result of morphine withdrawal, 6-hydroxydopamine infusions, or noradrenergic stimulant drugs; (3) self-directed biting due to pemoline or amphetamine injections; (4) rage reactions due to brain lesions; and (5) mouse killing (Hasselager *et al.*, 1972; Hegstrand and Eichelman, 1983; Hodge and Butcher, 1975; Malick, 1979; Mueller *et al.*, 1982; Mueller and Nyhan, 1982; Nakamura and Thoenen, 1972; Niemegeers *et al.*, 1974; Reis and Fuxe, 1964; Rolinski and Kozak, 1979; Rolinski, 1973; Vergnes and Karli, 1963; Barnett *et al.*, 1974). However, chronic administration of haloperidol renders rats "supersensitive" to the aggression-provoking effects of low doses of the dopamine receptor agonist apomorphine (Gianutsos *et al.*, 1974*a*).

Ethological analyses began to provide new insights into the nature of the behavioral changes as the result of treatment with antipsychotic drugs (e.g., Chance and Silverman, 1964; Silverman, 1965*a,b*; Krsiak and Steinberg, 1969). By studying animals in ethologically valid situations of social conflict and by measuring various salient elements of aggressive, defensive, flight, and also nonagonistic behavior, the behavioral effects of antipsychotic drugs can be delineated more adequately, and more specific questions about the mediating neurobiological mechanisms may be posed. It has become apparent that antipsychotic drugs pervasively suppress many aggressive, social, sexual, maternal, and play behaviors by the individual who initiates these activities (e.g., Zwirner *et al.*, 1975; Beatty *et al.*, 1984; Sieber *et al.*, 1982; Olivier and van Dalen, 1982; Olivier *et al.*, 1984; Poshivalov, 1974; Miczek and Yoshimura, 1982; Yoshimura and Ogawa, 1984). A prominent effect of antipsychotic drugs at moderate doses appears to be an increase in the latency to approach, to threaten, and to attack the opponent or the prey and to shift the behavioral activities from rapid short-duration acts to prolonged postures (e.g., Silverman, 1965a,b, 1966a; Schmidt and Apfelbach, 1977). An intruder or a prey may be less provoking to an animal treated with antipsychotic drugs. Once the episode of fighting or prey capture has been initiated, the composition or sequence of behavioral events remains largely unaltered by antipsychotic drugs up to higher, incapacitating dose levels (Miczek et al., 1982, unpublished observations; Gay and Clark, 1976). The execution of certain aggressive and predatory responses may actually be facilitated by some antipsychotic drugs (e.g., Knight et al., 1963; Schmidt, 1979, 1983).

Defensive responses and escapes in reaction to attack, to painful environmental stimuli, or to direct neural stimulation are unaltered up to large doses of antipsychotic drugs. Earlier studies with phenothiazines already indicated that defensive reactions to electric shock are insignificantly altered by nonincapacitating drug doses (e.g., Table 1). It is even possible to facilitate escape behavior in rats by chlorpromazine (Chance and Silverman, 1964; Silverman, 1965a,b) and to induce the display of submissive postures in Mongolian gerbils by haloperidol (Thiessen and Upchurch, 1981; Upchurch and Schallert, 1982).

When an individual interacts with an opponent who has been treated with a phenothiazine or a butyrophenone, significant changes in the aggressive and social behavior of the drug-free animal occur; chlorpromazine- or haloperidol-treated mice and monkeys provoke fewer attacks from a dominant drug-free opponent (Cairns and Scholz, 1973; Miczek and Yoshimura, 1982; Miczek, unpublished observations); continuous treatment of a dominant mouse with droperidol not only suppresses the treated animal's attack behavior, but also allows the emergence of more frequent attacks by a rival within the group (Poshivalov, 1980). These indirect changes in aggressive behavior that are brought about by the drug treatment of the opponent have marked clinical and societal implications; however, their source remains to be elucidated.

An exception to the general insensitivity of defensive and escape responses to the effects of antipsychotic drugs are the observations in animals that exhibit these types of responses without being aversively stimulated; Krsiak (1975b) has coined the term *timid* to refer to mice that actively engage in a pattern of behavior that is normally seen only in reaction to attacks by an opponent. Chlorpromazine specifically reduces the active display of defensive and escape responses in these timid mice.

In sum, antipsychotic drugs decrease aggressive behavior that is actively initiated at markedly lower doses than defensive and escape behavior in reaction to socially or environmentally aversive stimuli. This pattern of effects parallels the long-known differential effects on conditioned avoidance and escape behavior (e.g., Courvoisier et al., 1953; Cook and Weidley, 1957). With the discovery of different subtypes of dopamine receptors, as well as agonist and antagonist drugs for these subtypes, it will be important to learn about the respective role of these receptor subtypes in various aggressive behavior patterns (e.g., Schmidt, 1983).

3.1.1b. Clinical Data. The most frequently used drugs for treating or more adequately controlling violent aggressive behavior include the phenothiazines, butyrophenones, and thioxanthines; individuals of both sexes, from childhood to advanced age and diagnosed as psychotics, depressives, hyperactives, schizophrenics, mentally retarded, nonpsychotic character-disordered delinquents, amphetamine abusers, and alcoholics, as well as those suffering from organic brain syndrome, have been given these drugs to decrease their assaultive, hostile, and violent behavior (e.g., Itil and Wadud, 1975; Itil, 1981; Leventhal and Brodie, 1981; Pöldinger, 1981; Sheard, 1983; Tupin, 1985). Many studies, mostly in the 1960s and 1970s, established that virtually all phenothiazines, whether of the amino–alkyl (e.g., chlorpromazine), piperidyl–alkyl (e.g., thioridazine, pericyazine), or piperazine–alkyl groups (e.g., perphenazine, trifluoperazine), thioxanthines (e.g., flupenthixol, thiothixene, clopenthixol), butyrophenones (e.g., haloperidol, droperidol, pimozide), or indole derivatives (e.g., molindone), effectively decrease aggressive behavior. Most case reports, open clinical trials, and, more recently, double-blind, placebo-controlled studies focused on psychotics, particularly on schizophrenics, and on patients with organic brain syndromes (Shaw *et al.*, 1963; Ojeda, 1970; Faretra *et al.*, 1970; Rada and Donlon, 1972; Itil and Wadud, 1975; Yesavage, 1982). Additional reports described effectiveness of chlorpromazine, haloperidol, and thioridazine to decrease aggressive behavior in mentally retarded children and adults (Alexandris and Lundell, 1968; Connolly, 1968; Ucer and Kreger, 1969; Llorente, 1969; Le Vann, 1971; Hacke, 1980), children with conduct disorder (Alderton and Hoddinott, 1964; Vialatte, 1966; Cunningham *et al.*, 1968; Schweikert, 1971; Campbell *et al.*, 1982), nonpsychotic patients (Cohen *et al.*, 1968), hostile depressive patients (Overall *et al.*, 1964), and opiate addicts and alcoholics during withdrawal (e.g., Itil and Seaman, 1978), as well as individuals with amphetamine psychosis (Sheard, 1983).

Several negative reports indicate that thioridazine was ineffective in the treatment of hyperactive children (Sprague *et al.*, 1970; Saletu *et al.*, 1975) and actually intensified the violent behavior of mental retardates (Elie *et al.*, 1980); haloperidol and chlorpromazine failed to reduce aggressive behavior of female manic–depressives (Kelly *et al.*, 1976). Sheard (1983) also advised against the use of phenothiazines and butyrophenones in patients with epileptic or intermittent explosive disorders.

In spite of their widespread use, antipsychotic drugs cannot be considered specific antiaggressive drugs, nor do they act specifically on possible neural mechanisms mediating aggressive behavior (Lion, 1975; Leventhal and Brodie, 1981; Pöldinger 1981). The clinical discussion revolves around pragmatic issues, weighing the "costs" and "benefits" of each type of antipsychotic medication. As an initial treatment, especially in an emergency situation when sedative and extrapyramidal side effects are of less concern, intramuscular haloperidol or promazine have been recommended (e.g., Sheard, 1983; Pöldinger, 1981; Tupin, 1985). To reduce the serious complications of long-term maintenance with antipsychotics, such as extrapyramidal symptoms and tardive dyskinesia, preparations such as depo-flupenthixol are given (e.g., Leventhal and Brodie, 1981). Several newer antipsychotic drugs, such as molindone, clozapine, clothiapine, milenperone, melperone, and Sch 12,679, have been used for their antiaggressive effects and possibly less severe sedative effects (DeCuyper *et al.*, 1985a,b; Elie *et al.*, 1980; Hacke, 1980; Pöldinger, 1981; Itil, 1981). Occasionally it has been claimed that certain antipsychotic drugs are more effective in reducing aggressive and hostile behavior such as chlorpromazine in psychotics (e.g., Freyhan 1959) or pericyazine in schizophrenics and nonpsychotic patients (Itil and Seaman, 1978); however, since no controlled comparisons with properly matched samples among various antipsychotic drugs have been made, it is difficult to attribute higher antiaggressive effectiveness to any of the antipsychotic drugs (e.g., Pöldinger, 1981; Leventhal and Brodie, 1981).

Practical issues of control in emergency situations and risks with side effects during long-term maintenance have deflected the questions on the neurobiological mechanisms that may mediate the antiaggressive effects of antipsychotic drugs.

3.1.2. β-Adrenoceptor Blockers

As with the first-generation antipsychotic drugs, beta blockers have begun to be considered systematically in preclinical aggression research only *after* important clinical observations were reported.

3.1.2a. Preclinical Data. Beta blockers have been long neglected in preclinical aggression research. The previous exclusive focus on the antagonism of β-adrenergic receptors in the autonomic nervous system, especially in the cardiovascular system, appears to have obscured any possible site and mechanism of action in the central nervous system. What is known about beta blockers from traditional laboratory tests of animal aggression holds considerable promise. Table 2 summarizes the differential effects of propranolol, a prototypic beta blocking agent, on aggressive behavior in isolated mice, defensive behavior in reaction to electric foot shock in pairs of rats, and mouse-killing behavior by rats. For comparison, the known propranolol effects on nonaggressive motor activity are listed in the second column of Table 2. It is apparent that aggressive and defensive responses are decreased by propranolol at doses that are at least two to four times lower than those necessary to decrease nonaggressive motor

TABLE 2
Doses of Propranolol for Decreasing Aggression and Nonaggressive Motor Activity[a]

Aggression	Nonaggressive motor activity	Reference
Isolation-induced aggression		
In mice		
20 i.p.	N/S	Valzelli et al., 1967
25 i.p.	50 i.p.	Delini-Stula and Vassout, 1979
3.0 s.c.	>5 s.c.	Weinstock and Weiss, 1980
40 i.p.	N/S	Garattini and Valzelli, 1981
Pain-induced aggression		
In mice		
ED50 31.5 s.c.	ED50 21.9 s.c.	Murmann et al., 1966
In rats		
10, 20 i.p.	40 i.p.	Vassout and Delini-Stula, 1977
10, 20 i.p.	N/S	Delini-Stula and Vassout, 1979
10, 20 i.p.	N/S	Sheard, 1979a
5, 10 i.p. bid	N/S	Hegstrand and Eichelman, 1983
Septal lesion-induced aggression		
In rats		
30, 100 s.c.	N/S	Bainbridge and Greenwood, 1971
Drug-induced aggression		
In mice		
Clonidine		
10 i.p.	N/S	Maj et al., 1980
Mouse killing		
In rats		
10, 20 i.p.	40 i.p.	Vassout and Delini-Stula, 1977
10, 20 i.p.	N/S	Delini-Stula and Vassout, 1979
20 s.c.	N/S	Shibata et al., 1983

[a] All doses are expressed in mg/kg; N/S = data not specified.

activity. Moreover, little distinction is made among the types of aggression that are preferentially decreased by propranolol or other centrally active beta blockers (e.g., Vassout and Delini-Stula, 1977).

Beta blockers that do not penetrate into the CNS, such as atenolol or metropolol, fail to alter aggressive behavior in mice (Weinstock and Weiss, 1980; Yoshimura and Ogawa, 1985), suggesting a central site for the antiaggressive effects of beta blockers (e.g., Hara et al., 1983, 1984). Chronic treatment with propranolol or pindolol actually increases pain-induced defensive reactions to electric foot shock, which is paralleled by an increase in B_{max} for β-adrenergic receptors in the cerebral cortex (Hegstrand and Eichelman, 1983). However, it has been questioned whether the antiaggressive effects of beta blockers are actually the result of a blockade of β-adrenergic receptors rather than a blockade of serotonergic receptors (Weinstock and Weiss, 1980).

More extensive ethological studies of propranolol confirm its effective antiaggressive action (e.g., Miczek and DeBold, 1983; Yoshimura and Ogawa, 1985) and also extend the suppressive effects of beta blockers to play fighting (Beatty *et al.,* 1984) and social behavior (Poshivalov, 1981). However, elements of attack and threat behavior appear to be the primary targets of propranolol action; defensive and flight responses of an intruder mouse as well as various types of nonaggressive motor activities are largely unaltered (Miczek and DeBold, 1983). Concurrent monitoring of autonomic activity should reveal at what physiological cost the antiaggressive effects are obtained.

3.1.2b. Clinical Data. A small clinical literature documents antiaggressive effects of propranolol treatment in patients in whom antipsychotic, anxiolytic, antidepressant, or antiepileptic drugs failed to control outbursts of "rage" and belligerent behavior. Starting with Elliott's report (1977), several case studies indicated a marked decline in aggressive behavior, particularly in patients with organic brain disease (Schreier, 1979; Petrie and Ban, 1981; Yudofsky *et al.,* 1981, 1984; Ratey *et al.,* 1983). Two accounts, one a prospective, the other a retrospective study, provide more systematically collected data; seven of eight patients decreased from six to eight daily incidences of assaultive behavior to less than one per day by the fourth week of treatment with up to 520 mg propranolol/day (Greendyke *et al.,* 1984); examination of medical records of 30 children and adolescents with organic brain dysfunctions and uncontrolled rage outbursts revealed a moderate to marked improvement in 24 patients after an individually titrated propranolol treatment (Williams *et al.,* 1982). It is noteworthy that all these patients had been unsuccessfully treated with various other therapeutic drugs.

The limiting conditions for the usefulness of propranolol as an antiaggressive drug derive from this drug's actions on autonomic functions, particularly on the cardiovascular system. Among the most serious side effects of β-adrenergic blockers are low blood pressure, headaches, dizziness, fatigue, insomnia, and depression (e.g., Sheard, 1984).

3.1.3. Barbiturates and Benzodiazepines

Pharmacological classifications identify barbiturates as prototypes of sedative–hypnotic drugs and benzodiazepines as prototypes of anxiolytic drugs. Yet, both types of drugs, as well as alcohol *(vide infra),* share an extensive behavioral profile that includes their effects on aggressive behavior.

3.1.3a. Preclinical Data. In the initial phase of evaluation, the "taming" action of benzodiazepines was already evident when veterinary or laboratory research personnel interacted with feral, laboratory-housed animals such as baboons, rhesus, cynomologous and squirrel monkeys, cats, or minks (Heise and Boff, 1961; Scheckel and Boff, 1966; Coutinho *et al.,* 1971; Bauen and Possanza, 1970; Delgado, 1973; Lister *et al.,* 1971;

Randall *et al.,* 1960; Langfeldt and Ursin, 1971). Similar taming effects of these drugs on animals in zoos pointed to their potential use in veterinary medicine (Heuschele, 1961).

In a second phase of evaluating the antiaggressive effects of the benzodiazepines and barbiturates, the following questions were addressed: How specifically do these drugs decrease aggressive behavior in comparison to nonaggressive motor activity? Which test conditions yield the clearest evidence for specific antiaggressive effects of these drugs? A representative sample of studies, summarized in Tables 3 and 4, shows that barbiturates and benzodiazepines exert antiaggressive effects in various

TABLE 3
Doses of Chlordiazepoxide for Decreasing Aggression and Nonaggressive Motor Activity[a]

Aggression	Nonaggressive motor activity	Reference
Isolation-induced aggression		
In mice		
5, 10 i.p.	20 i.p.	Scriabine and Blake, 1962
ED50 52 p.o.	ED50 415 p.o.	Cole and Wolf, 1966
ED50 >17 i.p.	ED50 17 i.p.	DaVanzo et al., 1966
7.5, 10 i.p.	30 i.p.	Valzelli et al., 1967
ED50 93.2 p.o.	ED50 33.0 p.o.	Hoffmeister and Wuttke, 1969
10, 20 i.p.	40 i.p.	Le Douarec and Broussy, 1969
ED50 23.5 i.p.	ED50 9.2 i.p.	Sofia, 1969b
ED50 15 p.o.	ED50 82 p.o.	Robichaud et al., 1970
54 i.p.	10, 27 i.p.	Weischer and Opitz, 1972
5, 7.5, 15 i.p.	15 i.p.	Valzelli, 1973a
ED50 23.8 i.p.	ED50 32.5 i.p.	Barnett et al., 1974
Pain-induced aggression		
In mice		
1 i.p.	1 i.p.	Kostowski, 1966
ED50 9.99	N/S	Hoffmeister and Wuttke, 1969
ED50 4.2 i.p.	ED50 9.2 i.p.	Sofia, 1969b
ED50 4.7 p.o.	ED50 240 p.o.	Christmas and Maxwell, 1970
ED50 17 p.o.	ED50 82 p.o.	Robichaud et al., 1970
10 p.o.	20 p.o.	Irwin et al., 1971
6.4 i.p.	26.5 i.p.	Goldberg et al., 1973
2–16 i.p.	N/S	Jarvis et al., 1985
In rats		
ED50 35 p.o.	N/S	Christmas and Maxwell, 1970
10, 20 i.p.	40 i.p.	Manning and Elsmore, 1972
In hamsters		
ED70 3.5 p.o.	N/S	Kreiskott, 1963

(continued)

TABLE 3
(Continued)

Aggression	Nonaggressive motor activity	Reference
In squirrel monkeys		
2, 4, 8 s.c.	16, 32 s.c.	Emley and Hutchinson, 1983b
Extinction-induced aggression		
In pigeons		
5 i.m.	>5 i.m.	Moore et al., 1976
Brain stimulation-induced affective defense		
In rats		
10 i.p.	>10 i.p.	Panksepp, 1971a
In cats		
>20 i.p.	N/S	Baxter, 1964b
20 p.o.	N/S	Kido et al., 1967
10 i.p.	N/S	Funderburk et al., 1970
10, 15 i.p.	N/S	Malick, 1970a
Brain lesion-induced irritability		
In rats		
ED50 9.6 i.p.	ED50 5.3 i.p.	Horovitz et al., 1963
ED50 23.8 i.p.	N/S	Malick et al., 1969
ED50 23 i.p.	ED50 7.3 i.p.	Goldberg, 1970
ED50 20 p.o.	N/S	Christmas and Maxwell, 1970
ED50 16 i.p.	>10 i.p.	Goldberg et al., 1973
10, 20 i.p.	20 i.p.	Loizzo and Massotti, 1973
ED 14.1 i.p.	8.2 i.p.	Barnett et al., 1974
Drug-induced aggression		
In mice		
dl-DOPA		
ED50 13 i.p.	N/S	Yen et al., 1970
In rats		
l-Dopa		
>10.6 i.p.	10.6 i.p.	Lammers and van Rossum, 1968
Apomorphine		
32, 64 i.p.	N/S	Senault, 1970
6-OHDA, icv		
ED50 14.8 i.p.	ED50 28.9 i.p.	Nakamura and Thoenen, 1972
Mouse killing		
In rats		
ED50 30 i.p.	20–30 i.p.	Karli, 1961
50–100	>100	Loiselle and Capparell, 1967
ED50 30 i.p.	ED50 5.3 i.p.	Horovitz et al., 1966
ED50 20.5 i.p.	ED50 7.3 i.p.	Goldberg, 1970
ED50 18.7 i.p.	ED50 17.2 i.p.	Barnett et al., 1974
>15 i.p.		Valzelli, 1973a
25, 50, 75 i.p.	N/S	Quenzer and Feldman, 1975
In cats		
>16 i.p.	N/S	Leaf et al., 1978

[a]All doses are expressed in mg/kg; N/S = data not specified.

TABLE 4
Doses of Barbiturates for Decreasing Aggression and Nonaggressive Motor Activity[a]

Aggression	Nonaggressive motor activity	Reference
Isolation-induced aggression		
In mice		
Pentobarbital		
ED50 > 19 i.p.	ED50 19	DaVanzo et al., 1966
ED50 45 p.o.	ED50 41 p.o.	Cole and Wolf, 1966
5 i.p.	N/S	Valzelli et al., 1967
10, 40 i.p.	>10 i.p.	Le Douarec and Broussy, 1969
Phenobarbital		
>50 p.o.	N/S	Yen et al., 1959
ED50 90 p.o.	N/S	Cook and Weidley, 1960
ED50 > 22 i.p.	ED50 22 i.p.	DaVanzo et al., 1966
5 i.p.	N/S	Valzelli et al., 1967
Pain-induced aggression		
In mice		
Phenobarbital		
10 i.p.	10 i.p.	Kostowski, 1966
ED50 37 p.o.	ED50 17.4 p.o.	Tedeschi et al., 1959
Pentobarbital		
30 p.o.	30 p.o.	Irwin et al., 1971
In hamsters		
Phenobarbital		
ED70 10 p.o.	N/S	Kreiskott, 1963
In rats		
Phenobarbital		
80 i.p.	40 i.p.	Crowley, 1972
In squirrel monkeys		
Phenobarbital		
0.5–40 s.c.	0.5–40 s.c.	Emley and Hutchinson, 1983*b*
Brain stimulation-induced affective defense		
In cats		
Phenobarbital		
30 i.v.	N/S	Kido et al., 1967
10–40 i.p.	20, 40 i.p.	Baxter, 1968*b*
40 i.p.	N/S	Malick, 1970*a*
Pentobarbital		
10 i.p.	10 i.p.	Funderburk et al., 1970
Brain lesion-induced irritability		
In rats		
Pentobarbital		
ED50 8.9 i.p.	ED50 9.0 i.p.	Horovitz et al., 1963
ED50 63.5 i.p.	N/S	Malick et al., 1969
20 i.p.	>20 i.p.	Ueki et al., 1972*b*
Drug-induced aggression		
In mice		
dl-Dopa, hexobarbital		
ED50 30–45 i.p.	N/S	Yen et al., 1970

(*continued*)

TABLE 4
(*Continued*)

Aggression	Nonaggressive motor activity	Reference
In rats		
6-OHDA icv,	Pentobarbital	
ED50 8.84 i.p.	ED50 8.72 i.p.	Nakamura and Thoenen, 1972
Isocarboxazid/Imipramine,	Pentobarbital	
10 i.p.	N/S	Zetler and Hauer, 1975
Mouse killing		
In rats		
Pentobarbital		
ED50 10 i.p.	ED50 7.3 i.p.	Horovitz *et al.*, 1966
>20 i.p.	10 i.p.	Ueki *et al.*, 1972a
In rats		
Pentobarbital		
>16 i.p.	N/S	Leaf *et al.*, 1978

*a*All doses are expressed in mg/kg; N/S = data not specified.

laboratory tests of aggression, such as in isolated mice attacking a stimulus animal, in pairs of rats or mice being exposed to electric foot shock, in rats and cats undergoing electrical stimulation of the hypothalamus, and in rats or mice that have been made irritable by CA neurotoxins or high doses of catecholaminergic agonists.

The antiaggressive effects of barbiturates appear to be detected only at doses that also decrease nonaggressive motor activity, whereas a dose separation for antiaggressive effects from those that decrease motor activity is evident for benzodiazepines. Disregarding several important exceptions, antiaggressive effects of chlordiazepoxide may generally be seen at doses that are two to four times lower than those that decrease motor activity. Defensive reactions, such as reactions to electric foot shock, are particularly sensitive to benzodiazepines.

Mouse killing by laboratory rats appears to be less sensitive to the blocking actions of benzodiazepines at nonsedative doses than all other aggressive behaviors. Furthermore, a certain proportion of so-called nonkiller rats are induced to kill mice when treated with benzodiazepines (e.g., Leaf *et al.*, 1975). When killing is suppressed by electrical stimulation of the locus ceruleus, chlordiazepoxide attenuates the suppressive effects of this stimulation and reestablishes the mouse-killing behavior (Kozak *et al.*, 1984). In grasshopper mice (*Onychomys leucogaster*), neither pentobarbital nor chlordiazepoxide significantly decreased predatory attack behavior (Gay and Clark, 1976); chlordiazepoxide actually prolonged the time spent in attacking the prey (Cole and Wolf, 1970). Similarly, benzodiazepines facilitated the predatory attack responses of ferrets (e.g., Apfelbach, 1976, 1978) and induced play behavior in cats interacting with prey (Langfeldt, 1974).

In a comparison of dose ranges for the motor activity-decreasing and antiaggressive effects of barbiturates and benzodiazepines, the relative doses for both effects appeared to be more meaningful than the absolute dosages. As has been pointed out (e.g., Malick, 1978a; Miczek and Krsiak, 1979), the exact dose range depends on many important pharmacological, situational, and measurement parameters, such as the route of administration, drug vehicle, injection–test interval, test duration, specific strain, housing conditions and behavioral history of the test subjects, and the test locale, as well as the reliability and sensitivity of the behavioral measurement. In particular, absolute drug dose levels for decreasing nonaggressive motor activity varied considerably depending on the nature of the test (e.g., photocell versus rotarod) and whether this type of behavior was measured in the same or different animals being examined for antiaggressive effects.

Chronic treatment with various benzodiazepines in groups of mice may increase mortality apparently resulting from injurious fighting (e.g., Fox and Snyder, 1969; Fox et al., 1970; Guaitani et al., 1971). The initial effects of chronic treatment with benzodiazepines included antiaggressive as well as sedative effects; with continued exposure to chlordiazepoxide or diazepam, the sedative effects waned, but the antiaggressive effects persisted (Malick, 1978a; Quenzer et al., 1974). Eventually, even tolerance to the antiaggressive effects of diazepam developed and, most important, aggressive behavior occurred at heightened levels during withdrawal from chronic diazepam treatment (Grant et al., 1985; Miczek, unpublished observations).

In a third phase of research on barbiturates, benzodiazepines, and aggression, more comprehensive pharmacological and behavioral analyses were performed, often with paradoxical results. Extensive dose–effect determinations revealed a bidirectional pattern of changes in aggressive behavior after administration of barbiturates or benzodiazepines; low doses of barbital, pentobarbital, chlordiazepoxide, medazepam, and diazepam often actually *increased* the frequency of attacks by isolated mice, resident male rats, lactating rats, or mice confronting an intruder (Fig. 4; Silverman, 1966b; Miczek, 1974; Poshivalov, 1978; Krsiak, 1975b; Miczek and O'Donnell, 1980; Olivier et al., 1985, 1986), whereas higher doses decreased this behavior. These, as well as several so-called paradoxical clinical observations with benzodiazepines, raised the question of whether benzodiazepines should be viewed as reliable antiaggressive drugs (DiMascio, 1973). Of course, a dose-dependent bidirectional pattern of effects suggests a complex mechanism of action, potentially involving different sites and receptor subtypes.

One of the first contributions of an ethological analysis was the dif-

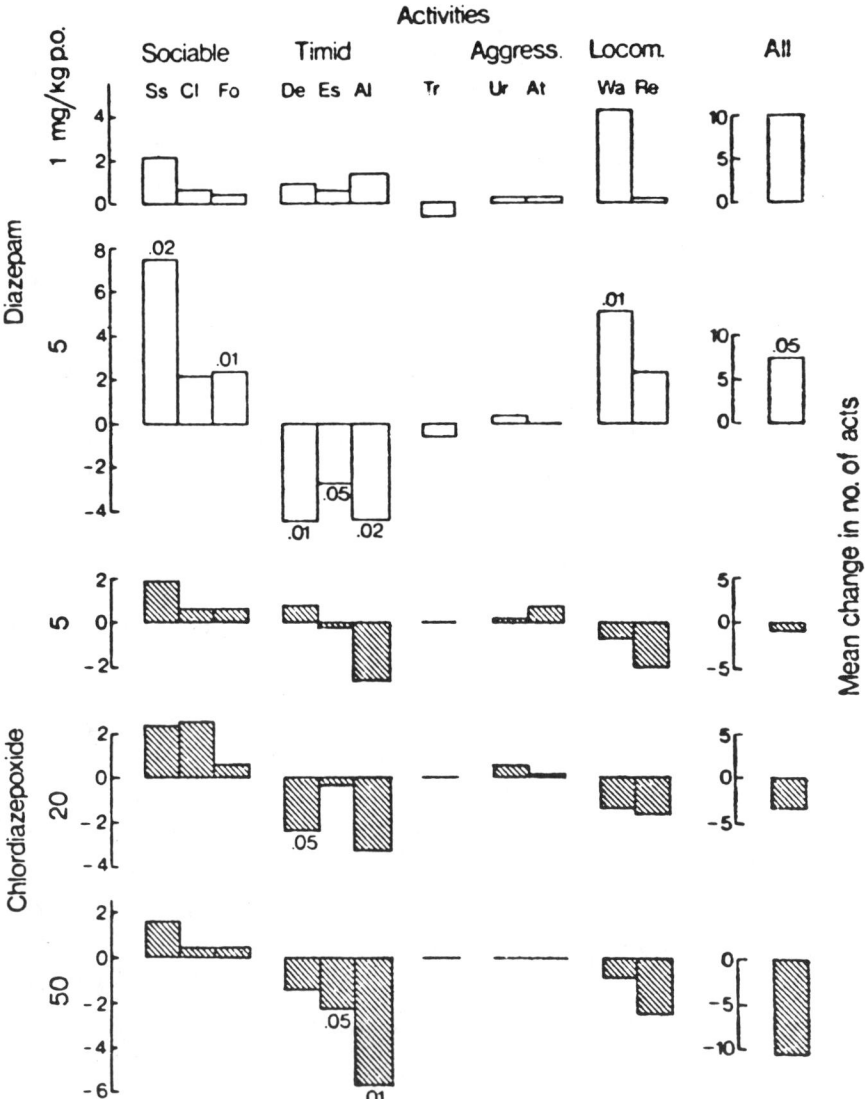

FIG. 4. Behavior of singly housed timid mice given diazepam or chlordiazepoxide in paired interactions with nonaggressive group-housed mice. Ordinate, the number of acts during 4 min expressed as the mean difference from activity in the control interaction. Effects of each dose represent mean results from 8–15 timid mice. (From Krsiak, 1975b.)

ferentiation between the effect of benzodiazepines and barbiturates on attack as compared to the effect on defense and flight (e.g., Chance and Silverman, 1964; Chance, 1968; Krsiak and Steinberg, 1969; Krsiak, 1975b, 1979; Miczek, 1974). Several elements of defensive and flight reactions, usually shown by an animal under attack or, alternatively, after a period of isolated housing, are particularly sensitive to the actions of benzodiazepines and barbiturates (e.g., Langfeldt and Ursin, 1971; Poole, 1973; Crowley et al., 1974; File, 1982, 1984; File and Tucker, 1983; Yoshimura and Ogawa, 1984). Comparisons with the effects of drugs from all major classes led Krsiak to propose that the reduction in defensive and escape reactions may serve as a screen for drugs with anxiolytic properties (Fig. 5; Krsiak, 1974a, 1975a,b; Krsiak et al., 1981, 1984). The flight-reducing effects of benzodiazepines and other anxiolytic drugs persist even after repeated administration (Sulcova et al., 1976), and these effects may be blocked by GABA or benzodiazepine receptor antagonists (Sulcova et al., 1979; Sulcova and Krsiak, 1984). A particularly potent blocking effect of defensive and escape reactions has been seen with the newer benzodiazepine alprazolam (Sulcova, 1985).

The study of benzodiazepine effects in animals with explicit social experiences suggests that success and failure in previous aggressive interactions determine the nature of drug-induced behavioral change. Dominant rats or monkeys may increase their aggressive behavior toward an opponent when given low doses of chlordiazepoxide or diazepam, but subordinate animals do not (e.g., Apfelbach and Delgado, 1974; Miczek, 1974). The study of drug action in socially living animals also reveals that the behavior of the drug-free individuals changes as a function of the opponent's drug state. Subtle changes in social signals may result from treatment with diazepam or chlordiazepoxide that provokes more aggressive behavior from a drug-free opponent (e.g., Dixon, 1982; Miczek, 1974; Delgado et al., 1976).

Changes in brain serotonin (e.g., Valzelli, 1978) or androgen levels (Essman, 1978) were some of the earlier proposed mechanisms for the antiaggressive effects of benzodiazepines. Recently, interest in the effects of benzodiazepines on aggressive behavior has greatly increased, chiefly as the result of the discovery of benzodiazepine receptors (e.g., Braestrup and Squires, 1977). The benzodiazepine receptor site(s) are part of a complex that includes GABA, barbiturate, and picrotoxin receptors and controls chloride ion channels (e.g., Haefely, 1984). Antagonism of the benzodiazepine receptors by Ro 15-1788 antagonizes the effects of diazepam on aggressive behavior, but by itself, Ro15-1788 has only weak, nonsystematic effects on aggressive behavior on isolated mice or resident rats confronting an intruder (Rodgers and Waters, 1984, 1985; Sulcova and Krsiak, 1984; Skolnick et al., 1985; File and Pellow, 1986; Miczek, unpublished data). Ethyl-β-carboline-3-carboxylate, a so-called inverse agonist at the benzodiazepine receptor site, not only decreases aggressive behavior but also antagonizes the effects of diazepam on defensive and flight reactions (Sulcova and Krsiak, 1985; Beck and Cooper, 1986). Social interactions of an associative and affiliative nature as well as exploratory behavior are significantly modulated by Ro15-1788 and other receptor

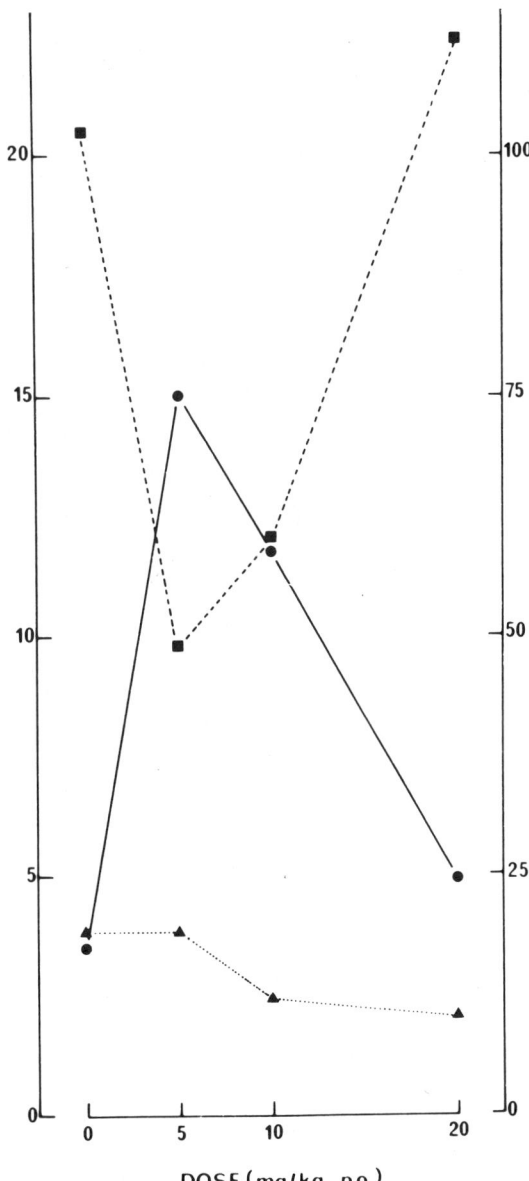

FIG. 5. Effect of chlordiazepoxide (0, 5, 10, and 20 mg/kg, orally) on the number of attacks (●), the number of wounds (▲), and the latency(s) to the first attack (■). Twelve females received each dose in a randomized order 60 min before testing. (From Olivier et al., 1985.)

antagonists as well as inverse agonists (Rodgers et al., 1983; File and Pellow, 1985; File, 1985; Crawley, 1985; Sulcova and Krsiak, 1985).

One of the next critical questions will be to determine whether there are physicochemical features of the benzodiazepine–GABA receptor complex that correspond to features in the profile of physiological and behavioral effects of benzodiazepines and barbiturates. It may be possible to develop substances that separate the pro- and antiaggressive effects as well as the anticonvulsant and muscle-relaxant effects of benzodiazepines and barbiturates.

3.1.3b. Clinical Studies. Antianxiety drugs in the clinical treatment of pathologically violent individuals have been successfully used in various patient and prisoner populations (e.g., Bond and Lader, 1979; Itil and Seaman, 1978; Lion, 1975; Leventhal and Brodie, 1981; Sheard, 1984). A series of uncontrolled, open trials and clinical ratings suggested the effectiveness of chlordiazepoxide, diazepam, and, particularly, oxazepam in reducing aggressive and hostile behavior in chronic psychotic patients (Boyle and Tobin, 1961), chronically ill, depressive, and "anergic schizophrenic" patients (Feldman, 1962), epileptics (Goddard and Lokare, 1970), chronic alcoholics (Gottschalk and Cohn, 1978), anxious outpatients (Rickels and Downing, 1974), and prisoners (Kalina, 1964; Brown, 1978). Several double-blind, placebo-controlled studies established that chlordiazepoxide decreased "overt outward hostility" in asocial and delinquent adolescents (Gleser *et al.*; 1965), impulsive aggressive behavior in schizophrenic patients with a history of physical attack (Monroe and Dale, 1967), and "neurotic hyperaggressiveness" in outpatients (Podobnikar, 1971). In comparison to chlordiazepoxide, oxazepam was more effective in reducing ratings of hostility in outpatients with temper outbursts and assaultive behavior (Lion, 1979). It appears that various patients in different settings benefit from the antiaggressive effects of the benzodiazepines when treatment conditions are adequately managed.

Certain individuals, however, engage in *heightened* aggressive behavior when given benzodiazepines or when abusing barbiturates (e.g., Gossop and Roy, 1976; Tinklenberg *et al.*, 1974, 1976; Tinklenberg and Woodrow, 1974; Paul, 1975). Controversy surrounds the actual frequency and the seriousness of the so-called paradoxical rage reactions associated with benzodiazepines (e.g., Bond and Lader, 1979; Sheard, 1984). Shortly after chlordiazepoxide and diazepam were introduced into clinical practice, several cases that showed increased hostility during treatment with these drugs were reported (e.g., Tobin and Lewis, 1960; Ingram and Timbury, 1960; Murray, 1962; Daly and Kane, 1965). In the late 1960s, a series of studies to investigate the determinants of the hostility and violent behavior associated with one of these drugs were undertaken; these and subsequent studies have led to diametrically opposed conclusions as to the value of benzodiazepines in the treatment of aggressive and hostile behavior (e.g., DiMascio, 1973; Lion, 1975; Itil and Seaman, 1978; Bond and Lader, 1979; Leventhal and Brodie, 1981; Hall and Zisook, 1981).

Case reports on increased aggressive behavior in individuals treated with different kinds of benzodiazepines persist (e.g., Guldenpfennig, 1973; Lion, 1975; Lion *et al.*, 1975a; Greenblatt *et al.*, 1975). Systematic studies, employing self-rating scales or experimenters' ratings, conducted double-blind and placebo-controlled, show statistically reliable increases in aggressive behavior or affective hostility under the benzodiazepine treatment conditions for the research samples as a whole and not limited to certain individuals (e.g., McDonald, 1967; Gardos *et al.*, 1968; Salzman *et al.*, 1969, 1974; DiMascio *et al.*, 1969; Kochansky *et al.*, 1975; Wilkinson, 1985). It appears that the rage and increased hostility in reaction to benzodiazepines may not be paradoxical but rather part of the spectrum of effects produced by these drugs (DiMascio *et al.*, 1969).

The major determinants for the appearance of increased aggressive behavior after benzodiazepines are (1) type of benzodiazepine, oxazepam, for example, being less associated with rage reactions (Kochansky *et al.*, 1975; Salzman *et al.*, 1975); (2) the drug dose (e.g, Azcarate, 1975); (3) the patient's expectations of the drug response; (4) the patient's history of impulse control and hostility; and (5) the nature of the social and environmental setting. These conclusions largely parallel the more recent preclinical data. The physiological processes modulated by behavioral history, anticipatory responses, and social and environmental factors, which make the individual more or less sensitive to the aggression-heightening or aggression-decreasing effects of these drugs, must be studied.

3.1.4. Antidepressant Drugs

The treatment of depressive disorders relies on chemically diverse drugs. The tricyclic antidepressants and the monoamine oxidase inhibitors (MAOI) were the first drugs used and continue to be the major drugs used therapeutically. Lithium, the prototypic drug in the treatment of bipolar depressions, will be discussed in Section 3.1.5. The study of antidepressant drugs and aggressive behavior has been conducted with markedly divergent objectives, ranging from pragmatic, cost-effective, preclinical screens in pharmaceutical laboratories through explorations of the biochemical mechanisms of aggressive behavior to psychodynamic thought that model depressive disorders as forms of self-directed aggression—"aggression turned inward."

3.1.4a. Preclinical Data. In the initial phase of preclinical research with antidepressant drugs, virtually all research protocols relied on *acute* administration of tricyclics of MAOIs. As an example of this research, Table 5 summarizes the antiaggressive effects of acute administration of imipramine, the prototype of the tricyclics, on aggressive behavior. Doses of imipramine that impair motor activity are also included in order to allow an estimate of the behavioral specificity of the antiaggressive effects. Imipramine decreases aggressive behavior by isolated mice, defensive reactions to electric shock by pairs of mice or rats, defensive responses evoked by electrical brain stimulation in cats, and aggressive responses resulting from electrolytic brain lesions or toxic doses only in a behavior-

TABLE 5
Doses of Imipramine for Decreasing Aggression and Nonaggressive Motor Activity[a]

Aggression	Nonaggressive motor activity	Reference
Isolation-induced aggression		
In mice		
ED50 127 p.o.	N/S	Cook and Weidley, 1960
ED50 31.2 i.p.	ED50 44 i.p.	DaVanzo et al., 1966
>20 i.p.	N/S	Valzelli et al., 1967
32 p.o.	N/S	Boissier et al., 1968
20 i.p.	10, 20 i.p.	Le Douarec and Broussy, 1969
ED50 21.7 i.p.	ED50 22.1 i.p.	Sofia, 1969b
ED50 7.1 i.p.		Malick, 1979
ED50 37.4 p.o.		Malick, 1979
25 i.p.	>25 i.p.	Delini-Stula and Vassout, 1979, 1981
Pain-induced aggression		
In mice		
>50 i.p.	N/S	Lapin, 1967
ED50 22 i.p.	ED50 22.1 i.p.	Sofia, 1969b
>20 p.o.	>20 p.o.	Tedeschi et al., 1969
100 p.o.	100 p.o.	Irwin et al., 1971
In rats		
20 i.p.	>20 i.p.	Crowley, 1972
20 i.p.	N/S	Anand et al., 1977
>10 i.p.	N/S	Delini-Stula and Vassout, 1979
Brain stimulation-induced affective defense		
In cats		
8–10 i.p.	N/S	Penaloza-Rójas et al., 1961
>3–12 i.p.	3–12 i.p.	Baxter, 1968b
10 i.p.	N/S	Malick, 1970a
5 i.p.	5 i.p.	Funderburk et al., 1970
Brain lesion-induced irritability		
In rats		
ED50 52.7 i.p.	ED50 23 i.p.	Sofia, 1969b
ED50 52.7 i.p.	N/S	Malick et al., 1969
ED50 52 i.p.	ED50 23 i.p.	Goldberg, 1970
>20 i.p.	10 i.p.	Ueki et al., 1972b
Drug-induced aggression		
In mice		
dl-Dopa		
ED50 11.5 i.p.	N/S	Yen et al., 1970
Clonidine		
10 i.p.	N/S	Maj et al., 1980
In rats		
Apomorphine		
64 i.p.	N/S	Senault, 1970
In cats		
Intraamygdaloid acetylcholine		
5 i.m.	N/S	Allikmets et al., 1969

(*continued*)

TABLE 5
(Continued)

Aggression	Nonaggressive motor activity	Reference
Mouse killing		
In rats		
ED50 8 i.p.	ED50 24 i.p.	Horovitz et al., 1965, 1966
15–40 i.p.	N/S	Didiergeorges et al., 1968
10 i.p.	N/S	Kulkarni, 1968
ED50 8.1 i.p.	ED50 23 i.p.	Sofia, 1969a,b
ED50 4 i.p.	N/S	Barnett et al., 1969
ED50 13.4 i.p.	ED50 23 i.p.	Goldberg, 1970
ED50 13.4 i.p.	N/S	Salama and Goldberg, 1970
10, 20 i.p.	10 i.p.	Ueki et al., 1972b
ED50 8.9 i.p.	ED50 22.5 i.p.	Dubinsky et al., 1973
20 i.p.	N/S	Rolinski, 1975
ED50 5.2 i.p.	N/S	Malick, 1976
10 i.p.	N/S	Valzelli and Bernasconi, 1971, 1976
ED50 11 i.p.	N/S	Yamamoto and Ueki, 1978
10, 25 i.p.	N/S	Delini-Stula and Vassout, 1979

^{a}All doses are expressed in mg/kg; N/S = data not specified.

ally nonspecific manner; the doses of imipramine necessary to decrease aggressive and defensive responses overlap or even exceed those that decrease nonaggressive behavior. This general pattern extends to many other tricyclic antidepressants (e.g., desipramine, chlorimipramine, amitryptyline, iproniazid) and to MAOIs (e.g., pargyline, phenelzine, isocarboxazid, etryptamine, tranylcypromine) (e.g., Welch and Welch, 1968, 1969; Sofia, 1969b; DaVanzo et al., 1966; Valzelli et al., 1967), although occasionally some degree of selectivity in the antiaggressive effects of antidepressants is seen (e.g., Malick, 1979).

An important exception to this rather disappointing set of early observations was the consistent finding that imipramine and other tricyclic antidepressants, as well as MAOIs, block the mouse-killing behavior of rats (Table 5). The blockade of mouse killing ("antimuricidal" effect) is seen at a quarter to a half of the dose required to impair motor activity.

The mechanism for the blockade of mouse killing by antidepressant drugs has become the focus of more recent investigations. Horovitz et al. (1966) originally suggested that the "antimuricidal" effect of antidepressants may be mediated by the action of these drugs on processes in the amygdala. When injected directly into the medial amygdala, imipramine and other tricyclics block mouse killing in so-called natural "killer" rats or in rats induced to kill by olfactory bulbectomy (Leaf et al., 1969; Watanabe et al., 1979; Shibata et al., 1983, 1984); sites in the posterior lateral hypothalamus are also effective targets for the blockade of mouse killing by imipramine (Hara et al., 1983). When mouse killing is induced by a thiamine-deficient diet or by blockade of tryptophan hydroxylase with *para*-chlorophenylalanine (PCPA), tricyclic antidepressants effectively block the killing response (Onodera et al., 1981; Kostowski et al., 1983). However, it appears that other treatments that compromise brain serotonin, such as a tryptophan-free diet, PCPA, *para*-chloramphetamine, or intraraphe injections of 5,7-dihydroxytryptamine, decrease the tricyclics' blockade of the killing response (Marks et al., 1978; Eisenstein et al., 1982; Dubinsky et al., 1973). The blockade of mouse killing by antidepressants with varying anticholinergic activity is not potentiated by antimuscarinic scopolamine (Strickland and DaVanzo, 1986). Imipramine and other tricyclics also attenuated the attack of cats on rats when evoked by electrical stimulation of the lateral hypothalamus (Dubinsky and Goldberg, 1971; Dubinsky et al., 1973a); this latter finding contrasts with the relative lack of effect of antidepressants to alter brain-stimulation-evoked defensive hiss responses in cats (Table 5); in rhesus monkeys, however, intramesencephalic injections of imipramine suppressed brain-stimulation-evoked affective reactions (Allikmets et al., 1968).

Predatory killing by such carnivorous species as cats and ferrets is not affected even by very large doses of imipramine, chlorimipramine, amitriptyline, tranylcypromine, maprotiline, and fluoxetine (Leaf et al., 1978; Schmidt, 1980; Schmidt and Meierl, 1980). These findings are remarkable, since reuptake blockade at neither serotonergic nor noradrenergic presynaptic sites appears to be the critical event for suppression of predatory behavior in carnivores. Apparently, the neurochemical mechanisms mediating predatory killing in laboratory rats and in carnivores differ profoundly.

Increased aggression after antidepressant administration has been observed mostly in drug interaction studies on placid laboratory mice or rats. Behaviorally, these so-called aggressive phenomena are difficult to evaluate, since they comprise elements of behavior, such as indiscriminate biting or upright postures or audible vocalizations (see Fig. 2), that are displayed in an inappropriate context and often associated with additional drug-induced phenomena, such as seizures or motor stereotypes. Imipramine in combination with amphetamine, pargyline, or isocarboxazid (Lapin, 1962; Fog, 1969; Zetler and Hauer, 1975), or alternatively, various MAOIs in combination with L-dopa, amphetamine, or diethyldithiocarbamate (Zetler and Otten, 1969; Randrup and Munkvad, 1969b; Scheel-Krüger and Randrup, 1968; Fog et al., 1970) may produce indiscrimate biting and audible vocalizations in mice or rats. When imipramine or other antidepressants are given for 10–14 days to grouped nonaggressive mice, a subsequent injection of apomorphine (5 mg/kg) or clonidine (20 mg/kg) increased "aggressiveness" (Maj et al., 1979, 1980, 1982). Moreover, in young chicks, imipramine, but not other antidepressants, may induce "aggressive pecking" (Schrold, 1970; Hine et al., 1975b). The nature of the pecking or biting responses induced by antidepressants contrasts with the integrated behavioral sequences characteristic of aggressive interactions. The pharmacological as well as behavioral significance of these drug-induced phenomena has not been elucidated (e.g., Welch and Welch, 1969; Krsiak, 1974b; Miczek and Barry, 1976).

The focus of recent experiments on *chronic* administration of antidepressant drugs has led to a shift away from the acutely induced reuptake blockade at noradrenergic presynaptic terminals as the primary mechanism for their clinically relevant effects. With regard to several aggressive and defensive behaviors, the effects of chronic treatment with antidepressants are often opposite to the effects of acute treatment. After 10 days of imipramine treatment, the current threshold for evoking foot-shock-induced defensive upright reactions was significantly lowered in pairs of rats (Allikmets and Lapin, 1967). The heightened defense has also been demonstrated after repeated administration of various additional tricyclics and MAOIs, as well as such so-called atypical antidepressants as iprindol, mianserine, or maprotiline (Eichelman and Barchas, 1975; Eichelman, 1979; Mogilnicka and Przewlocka, 1981; Mogilnicka et al., 1983; Prasad and Sheard, 1983a,b), although the increased pain-induced defense is not always seen after chronic imipramine (Crowley and Rutledge, 1974). Heightened attack and submission responses are also seen with repeated administration of desmethylimipramine, clomipramine, maprotiline, and amitriptyline in isolated mice and rats (Delini-Stula and Vassout, 1981; Willner et al., 1981) and sometimes even after acute doses of amitryptiline (Kampov-Polevoi, 1978). Whether the intensified aggressive, defensive, and submissive responses in chronically treated animals are mediated by antidepressant-induced changes in noradrenergic or serotonergic receptor sensitivity or uptake processes remains to be explored.

Detailed ethological investigations of the effects of antidepressants on attack and threat, as well as on defense and flight behavior in mice, rats, and hamsters, mainly confirm antiaggressive effects only at high acute doses (Krsiak, 1975b, 1979; Olivier and van Dalen, 1982; Payne et al., 1985), although opposite effects are also reported (e.g., Sieber et al., 1982). Pargyline appears to decrease territorial aggression in the convict cichlid even more effectively than scopolamine (Avis and Peeke, 1979b). So far, there has been no thorough investigation of chronic treatment with antidepressants on aggressive, defensive, and social behavior. This state of affairs is surprising, since animals that are repeatedly attacked and threatened by an opponent exhibit many behavioral and physiological features that are also characteristic of patients with depressive disorders.

3.1.4b. Clinical Data. Most antidepressants are either ineffective in decreasing aggressive behavior or inconsistent in their effects in humans (e.g., Itil and Seaman, 1978). Unipolar depressive disorders are rarely associated with aggressive, violent outbursts. In those depressive patients who are agitated, imipramine and amitriptyline may reduce the hostile, aggressive behavior, but not as effectively as antipsychotics (see p. 210). As a matter of fact, not unlike the so-called paradoxical responses to benzodiazepines (see pp. 222–223), several cases of increased aggressive and hostile behavior have been reported (e.g., Rampling, 1978; Pallmeyer and Petti, 1979).

In addition to the therapeutic application of psychomotor stimulant drugs in hyperactive children (see pp. 274–275), imipramine and amitriptyline have been shown to have led to improved teachers' and parents' ratings for aggressive behavior and conduct problems in these patients (e.g., Winsberg *et al.*, 1972; Waizer *et al.*, 1974; Yepes *et al.*, 1977; Puig-Antich, 1982). However, imipramine may primarily reduce the hyperactivity but not always conduct problems (e.g., Rapoport *et al.*, 1974). In view of the potential side effects of chronic treatment with psychomotor stimulants, antidepressants may be a useful alternative in pediatric psychopharmacology.

Self-directed or autoaggression often occurs in depressive patients. Suicidal tendencies are frequently seen in unpredictably hostile and impulsive depressives (e.g., Montgomery and Montgomery, 1982), and it is this aspect that may be particularly relevant to the treatment of aggressive behavior with antidepressants. It has been claimed that dysfunctions in brain 5-HT, as recorded in subgroups of depressive patients, are related to the mechanisms mediating aggression (e.g., Van Praag, 1982). Low levels of 5-HIAA in the CSF of depressed patients were found to be statistically associated with an increased number of suicide attempts (Asberg *et al.*, 1976). However, homovanillic acid and 3-methoxy-4-hydroxyphenylglycol levels are also very low in patients with a history of suicide attempts. Moreover, the low pretreatment levels of 5-HIAA or MHPG failed to predict the clinical success with either a 5-HT uptake blocker, zimelidine, or a norepinephrine uptake blocker, maprotiline (Montgomery and Montgomery, 1982). Whether the statistical correlation between violent suicide attempts and low 5-HIAA levels in the CSF is predictive of psychopharmacological treatment success with depressives, particularly those with suicidal or hostile tendencies, remains to be explored.

3.1.5. Lithium

Studies on preclinical and clinical effects of lithium at the behavioral and physiological level have been slow in coming. In spite of the lack of commercial incentive, and of the difficulties in identifying sites and mechanisms of action for lithium, its effectiveness in the treatment of mania and depression, and of aggression, has been demonstrated repeatedly.

3.1.5a. Preclinical Data. Concurrent with the first clinical case reports, antiaggressive effects of lithium were evaluated under controlled experimental conditions in laboratory animals (e.g., Weischer, 1969; Sheard, 1970a,b). Table 6 summarizes the dose levels and treatment conditions under which lithium decreases aggressive behavior in isolated mice, defensive reactions to electric footshock in pairs of rats, and irritable and aggressive responses resulting from brain lesions or toxic drug treatment. Lithium is apparently quite toxic at higher doses; more recent studies have monitored the levels of lithium in blood and in brain (e.g., Marini et al., 1979a). Defensive reactions are effectively decreased by nontoxic doses of lithium (e.g., Sheard, 1970a,b; Marini et al., 1979a; Prasad and Sheard, 1982), although enhanced shock- or clonidine-induced

TABLE 6
Doses of Lithium for Decreasing Aggression and Nonaggressive Motor Activity[a]

Aggression	Nonaggressive motor activity	Reference
Isolation-induced aggression		
In mice		
30/1 in H_2O, 2–8 w	N/S	Weischer, 1969
25, p.o, b.i.d.	N/S	Weischer, 1969
0.9% in H_2O, 14 d	N/S	Brain, 1972
40–300 mg/kg i.p.	>300 mg/kg i.p.	Malick, 1978b
0.2, 0.4, i.p., 1–6 d	N/S	Brain and Al-Maliki, 1979
Pain-induced aggression		
In mice		
>0.2, i.p., 4 d	N/S	Brain et al., 1981a
In rats		
5, i.p., 5 d	>5, i.p.	Sheard, 1970b
1–3, i.p.	N/S	Mukherjee and Pradhan, 1976a
0.63 in brain, 28 d in diet	N/S	Marini et al., 1979a
1.5 b.i.d., i.p., 15 d	N/S	Eichelman et al., 1973
5/kg, i.p., 5 d	N/S	McGlone et al., 1980
20/1 in H_2O	N/S	Prasad and Sheard, 1982
Brain lesion-induced irritability		
In rats		
1–3, i.p.	N/S	Mukherjee and Pradhan, 1976b
Drug-induced aggression		
In rats		
PCPA		
5, i.p., 5 d	N/S	Sheard, 1970b
Apomorphine		
2, i.p.	N/S	Allikmets et al., 1979
Mouse killing		
In rats		
>1, 2, i.p., 10 d	2/kg, i.p.	Rush and Mendels, 1975
>3, i.p.	N/S	Mukherjee and Pradhan, 1976b

[a]All doses are expressed in meq/kg; N/S = data not specified.

defensive biting may sometimes be seen at low lithium doses (Bisbee and Cahoon, 1973; Ozawa *et al.*, 1975). Although mouse killing is effectively blocked by tricyclics and MAOIs, lithium fails to alter this behavior in rats and locust killing in mice (Brain and Al-Maliki, 1979). Maternal aggression in mice was not affected by lithium (0.2 meq/day for 4 days; Brain and Al-Maliki, 1979), whereas lithium effectively decreased attack behavior by residential rats or mice toward intruders (Sheard, 1973; Brain and Al-Maliki, 1979).

One of the most intriguing applications of lithium to modifying animal behavior is suppression of predatory behavior in the presence of distinctive taste stimuli *after* the consumption of preylike food. For example, coyotes stop attacking a particular prey after they have eaten only a single meal of lithium-laced meat from that type of prey (Gustavson *et al.*, 1974). This lithium-induced *conditioned taste aversion* has been demonstrated in many animal species, ranging from birds to wolves and including the mouse-killing response of the laboratory rat (Krames *et al.*, 1973; O'Boyle *et al.*, 1973); conditioned taste aversion of predatory behavior, however, cannot be demonstrated in all species (e.g., Langley, 1981). The nausea-inducing properties of lithium have important practical implications. The aversiveness of lithium has already been exploited in the control of predatory attack by certain feral animals on farm animals. However, in situations in which the direct effects of lithium are of interest, the association with stimuli surrounding the drug administration may produce unwarranted "side effects." Lithium alters not only behavior subsequent to drug administration, but also behavior that precedes it. Predatory attack and food intake may be only two examples of lithium-induced conditioned taste aversion, and the range of behaviors to which aversions could be developed may extend beyond these two types. The mechanism by which lithium induces aversions may involve chemoreceptors in the area postrema (McGlone *et al.*, 1980).

A critical question concerns the mechanism by which lithium produces its antiaggressive effects. Brain (1972) proposed that lithium's suppressive effects on androgen production, rather than pituitary–adrenal stimulation, are responsible for the decrease in attack behavior by isolated mice. More recently, brain serotonin systems have been examined as potentially mediating the behavioral and clinical effects of lithium (e.g., Müller-Oerlinghausen, 1985). However, the data on serotonin turnover and reuptake inhibition, particularly during chronic lithium treatment, do not parallel the aggression-decreasing effects in time course (Marini *et al.*, 1979a; Prasad and Sheard, 1982). To what extent the behavioral effects of lithium are mediated by its action on monoamines remains an open question (e.g., Smith, 1985).

3.1.5b. Clinical Data. Cade (1949) renewed the interest in lithium as a beneficial treatment to "control . . . restless impulses and ungovernable tempers," as preferable to prefrontal leukotomy! The therapeutic potential of lithium as an antiaggressive drug has been investigated in individuals with many different psychopathologies and also in violent criminals without psychiatric diagnosis (e.g., Cherek and Steinberg, 1986; Sheard, 1975, 1978, 1984). A series of case studies, as well as a few clinical trials, suggest that a wide range of aggressive individuals, in whom treatment with antipsychotic, antidepressant, sedative–hypnotic, or anxiolytic drugs was ineffective, may benefit from lithium therapy. These individuals range from deaf, mentally retarded and epileptic to psychotic patients and those with antisocial personalities or sociopaths, as well as children and adolescents, who are often hyperactive, severely disturbed, or retarded. The common feature of these cases appears to be that they all include behavioral phenomena that have been labeled "aggressive," "violent," or "hostile" (e.g., Gershon, 1968; Annell, 1969; Dostal and Zvoltsky, 1970; Campbell *et al.*, 1972, 1982; Rifkin *et al.*, 1972; Morrison *et al.*, 1973; Shader *et al.*, 1974; Kerr, 1976; Panter, 1977; Lion *et al.*, 1975*b*; van Putten and Sanders, 1975; Goetzl *et al.*, 1977; Altshuler *et al.*, 1977; Cutler and Heiser, 1978; Dale, 1980). Although suggestive, these reports include individuals with multiple pathologies, maintained concurrently on medication other than lithium; only a few double-blind studies have been reported (Worrall *et al.*, 1975; Sheard *et al.*, 1976; Tyrer *et al.*, 1984; Vetro *et al.*, 1985).

The most systematic evidence for lithium's antiaggressive effects has been gathered in a series of studies with prisoners (Sheard, 1971, 1975; Tupin *et al.*, 1973; Sheard *et al.*, 1976; Sheard and Marini, 1978). The advantage of using hyperaggressive prisoners as subjects is the unambiguous nature of their behavior and the clear dissociation of heightened aggressive behavior from behavioral and affective disorders (Marini and Sheard, 1977). Lithium capsules three times a day significantly reduced violent incidents in 12 volunteer subjects as assessed by the prison staff, who was blind to the treatment conditions, as well as by lower self-ratings of angry affect and tension during the lithium phase of the study (Sheard, 1971). These antiaggressive effects of lithium in aggressive prisoners were confirmed in further open, single-blind studies comparing low and high lithium dose levels and in treatments extending for up to 1.5 years (Tupin *et al.*, 1973; Sheard, 1975). In a major double-blind study in 66 highly aggressive prisoners, using lithium in sustained-release form once a day, progressively fewer reports of major aggressive episodes occurred over the 3-month trial in comparison to the placebo treatment (Sheard *et al.*, 1976); several cases demonstrated a very impressive behavioral change (Sheard and Marini, 1978).

It is clear that only a certain proportion of aggressive individuals respond to lithium treatment; however, the determinants of a satisfactory clinical response to lithium's antiaggressive effects remain unclear. Lithium's antiaggressive effects do not appear to be linked to the drug's toxic effects, increased reaction time, hypothyroidism, decreased serum testosterone, or placebo effects, and most important, there is no obvious connection to an underlying affective disorder (e.g., Marini and Sheard, 1977; Jefferson, 1982). There is a definite need for a double-blind study to assess the antiaggressive effects of lithium at nontoxic levels in clearly diagnosed individuals with unambiguously defined aggressive responses. Without such an assessment, the use of lithium in children and adolescents or epileptics, for example, remains controversial (e.g., Sheard, 1984; Jefferson, 1982).

3.1.6. Anticonvulsants

In the absence of reliable, behaviorally unambiguous experimental preparations for the study of seizure activity and animal aggression, few preclinical data are available on the effects of anticonvulsant drugs on aggressive behavior. Of course, drugs with anticonvulsant properties, such as barbiturates and benzodiazepines, or possibly, lithium, have been used therapeutically to treat epileptic patients (see Sections 3.1.3 and 3.1.5), but it is not clear whether the blockade of seizure activity was the basis for the antiaggressive effect. More than 25 years ago, anticonvulsant and antiaggressive effects were compared directly in mice for several centrally acting drugs (Tedeschi et al., 1959). When electroshock seizures and aggressive–defensive reactions to electric foot shock were used as experimental preparations, the drugs with the most potent anticonvulsant activity, phenobarbital and diphenylhydantoin, required two to five times as high a dose to decrease pain-induced aggression. The anticonvulsant and antiaggressive effects of several classes of drugs were apparently related neither in terms of overlapping dose range nor in potency ranking for both effects.

The effects of agonists and antagonists of γ-aminobutyric acid (GABA) on different kinds of aggressive behavior may be related to those on convulsive activity (e.g., Mandel et al., 1981). However, this possible relationship has never actually been tested. The mechanism of action for diphenylhydantoin's anticonvulsant effects remains to be elucidated, and its effects on different kinds of aggressive behavior need to be explored. Conversely, the potent effects of GABA agonists and antagonists on attack behavior of isolated mice, on pain-induced aggression in mice and rats, and on mouse killing in rats have not been investigated in conjunction with the effects on convulsive activity; they may rather be related to the mechanism of anxiolytic drugs (e.g., DaVanzo and Sydow, 1979; Puglisi-Allegra and Mandel, 1980; Poshivalov, 1981; Sulcova et al., 1978, 1979, 1981; Sulcova and Krsiak, 1980; Delini-Stula and Vassout, 1978; DePaulis and Vergnes, 1983, 1984, 1985; Rodgers and DePaulis, 1982; Potegal et al., 1983).

The rationale for using anticonvulsants clinically to decrease aggressive behavior derives from the possibility that excessive neuronal discharges (ictal responses) and the display of episodic violent behavior (dyscontrol syndrome) have a common mechanism, presumably in the temporal lobe (e.g., Monroe, 1978; Eichelman, 1983). At present, clinical data suggest that treatment with diphenylhydantoin, primidone, and carbamazepine effectively reduced aggressive behavior in most cases (Itil *et al.*, 1967; Bach-Y-Rita *et al.*, 1971; Maletzky, 1973; Blumer *et al.*, 1974; Maletzky and Klotter, 1974; Yaryura-Tobias and Neziroglu, 1975; Monroe, 1975; Monroe *et al.*, 1978; Tunks and Dermer, 1977). In uncontrolled clinical trials with epileptics, the benzazepine derivative Sch-12,679 was found to control severe aggression and outbursts (Itil and Wadud, 1975). Preliminary results from a double-blind study in "persistent dangerous antisocial offenders" suggested an antiaggressive effect of diphenylhydantoin in two individuals over a 6-month period (Covi and Uhlenhuth, 1969). However, double-blind placebo-controlled studies in delinquent youngsters showed that diphenylhydantoin either had no effect or actually increased their aggressive behavior (Lefkowitz, 1969; Conners *et al.*, 1971), leading to the conclusion that antiepileptic drugs are ineffective in decreasing aggressive behavior in children (e.g., Kligman and Goldberg, 1975; Campbell *et al.*, 1982). There is a clear need for data from controlled, double-blind studies to determine whether anticonvulsant drugs decrease episodic violent behavior that is part of a dyscontrol syndrome and other types of aggressive behavior in individuals without evidence of seizurelike activity.

3.1.7. Antiandrogens

Antiandrogenic agents represent a class of substances that differ profoundly from psychotropic drugs in their mechanism and target of action (e.g., Neumann and Steinbeck, 1971). However, the frequently proposed use of these agents in the treatment of aggressive individuals, particularly sex offenders, warrants an examination of the evidence on which such proposals are based.

The data from studies with animals offer little, if any support for antiaggressive effects of antiandrogens. Cyproterone acetate and flutamide have been investigated in intact or castrated animals maintained on testosterone; cyproterone was injected daily for up to 5 weeks to mature animals or was given in the period shortly after birth when the presence of testosterone leads to masculinization. None of these treatments altered the level of aggressive behavior in mice, rats, or gerbils significantly, although several indices of gonadal activity were decreased (Edwards, 1970; Sayler, 1970; Brain *et al.*, 1974, 1976; Poole and Brain, 1975; Heilman *et al.*, 1976; Clark and Nowell, 1980; Prasad and Sheard, 1981). However, in a few experiments with mice, significant antiaggressive effects were observed after daily injections of either 3 or 5 mg cyproterone acetate (Kurischko and Oettel, 1977; Oettel and Kurischko, 1978;

Matte and Fabian, 1978). In addition, when a resident mouse confronted an intruding mouse treated with cyproterone acetate, fewer attacks were directed toward the treated animal. These findings may suggest that androgen-dependent pheromones are important in the provocation of murine aggression (Nowell and Wouters, 1973). It is also possible to reduce the incidence of displacement, or to supplant, so-called dominance behaviors in male red-winged blackbirds by subcutaneous implants of capsules that contain flutamide (Searcy and Wingfield, 1980).

An alternative view to the androgen dependency of aggressive behavior holds that aromatization of testosterone to estrogen is required for this behavior to develop and to be maintained (e.g., Beatty, 1979). If testosterone is an intermediate, then it is less surprising that blockade of androgen receptors often has little effect on aggressive behavior. In support of the critical role of estrogens in the display of aggressive behavior are the observations that antiestrogens such as CI-628 block testosterone-maintained aggressive behavior in castrated mice (Luttge, 1979; Clark and Nowell, 1979; Bowden and Brain, 1978).

The clinical data with antiandrogens, mostly gathered in European trials, are surprisingly limited (e.g., Sheard, 1979*b*; Whitehead, 1981; Berner *et al.*, 1983; Itil, 1981). Medroxyprogesterone acetate and cyproterone acetate have been reported to reduce so-called *sexual* aggressive behavior in several male patients (Blumer, 1971; Blumer and Migeon, 1975; Cooper *et al.*, 1972; Hoffet, 1968; Laschet and Laschet, 1967). Medroxyprogesterone also was found to improve significantly the behavior of episodic violent individuals with temporal lobe epilepsy (Blumer and Migeon, 1975). However, others found very short-lived, if any improvement in several imprisoned sexual offenders (Whitehead, 1981). Curiously, no double-blind, controlled study on the effects of antiandrogens on direct objective behavioral measures or verbal reports of aggression have been conducted. Considering the poor relationship between testosterone levels and human aggression and the ineffectiveness of antiandrogens in decreasing aggression, neither castration, nor treatment with antiandrogens, appear indicated in the treatment of pathologically aggressive or hostile individuals (e.g., Benton, 1983).

3.1.8. Summary

Current preclinical and clinical data indicate that none of the current therapeutically used drugs decreases aggressive behavior without affecting some other behavioral, sensory, or physiological function. Moreover, many drugs that are currently used, at least in part, for their antiaggressive effects, such as the benzodiazepines, antidepressants, or beta blockers, actually can increase certain aggressive responses under some conditions.

Various therapeutic drugs produce their antiaggressive effects in distinctively different ways. The recent emphasis on detailed quantitative ethological analysis of aggressive behavior patterns has begun to delineate the nature of the behavioral change brought about by the chemically diverse group of substances that are therapeutically employed, at least in part, for their antiaggressive properties.

Detailed behavioral analyses delineate a spectrum of behaviors that are labeled *aggressive*, each presumably based on distinct neural mechanisms. The term *antiaggressive* rarely encompasses the decrease in one specific aggressive behavior but rather a range of different aggressive behaviors. This is most apparent in preclinical tests for so-called antiaggressive drug effects, because the repertoire of aggressive behavior varies with situations of conflict. Although so-called antiaggressive drugs have been tried in patient populations with various diagnoses, it is apparent that the most beneficial use of beta blockers, lithium, benzodiazepines, or antipsychotics is limited to individuals with differential behavioral histories in defined environmental and social circumstances. Similarly, the currently known therapeutic agents act on neural receptors that are distributed throughout the neural axis in discrete pools, that constantly change in sensitivity and number, and that modulate many biogenic amines, peptides, and steroids directly or indirectly. Increasing insights into the mechanisms of action of the major therapeutic drugs and into the determinants and patterns of aggressive behavior will prompt the development of agents that act very specifically at behavioral and biochemical levels. The alternative to this utopian view is the present situation with pervasively acting substances that alter aggressive behavior along with many other types of behavior.

3.2. Drugs of Abuse and Aggression

Labeling a substance a *drug of abuse* depends largely on current societal conventions and laws. Many so-called therapeutic drugs may be abused and, conversely, many so-called abused substances have therapeutic effects. The presently adopted selection reflects currently prevailing conventions rather than a classification derived from mode or mechanisms of action.

3.2.1. Alcohol

Alcohol is the drug most often linked to heightened aggressive behavior. Yet, most research with experimental animal preparations fails to detect the aggression-heightening effects of alcohol, but rather the sedative effects are detected. It is not surprising that the literature on alcohol and human aggression is considerably more voluminous than that on animal aggression (e.g., Brain, 1986). In spite of the magnitude of alcohol's effects on aggressive behavior, their deleterious consequences, and the societal and clinical concerns with these changes, information on the determinants and mechanisms for the alcohol–aggression link is very limited.

3.2.1a. Research with Animals. Experimental studies on alcohol and aggression began with unusual species and situations in the late 1960s. For example, large doses of alcohol (e.g., 2.4 g/kg, p.o. and higher) eliminated avoidance and aggressive behavior by cocks and hens toward 1-day-old chicks and, instead, induced maternal behavior (Kovach, 1967; Tammie, 1968). Highly aggressive pit gamecocks were transiently prevented from fighting by very large alcohol doses but resumed fighting after recovering from the profound depression (Meinecke and Cherkin, 1972). Experiments in fish provided the first systematic evidence for a *biphasic dose–effect* relationship between alcohol and aggression; that is, low doses increase aggressive responses and higher doses decrease them (e.g., Peeke and Figler, 1981). When resident Siamese fighting fish or convict cichlids are placed in aquaria that contain a low concentration of alcohol or its congeners, they threaten and attack a mirror image or an intruder more frequently and for longer periods of time; higher alcohol concentrations suppress these aggressive responses without impairing feeding or swimming (Raynes *et al.*, 1968; Raynes and Ryback, 1970; Ellman *et al.*, 1972; Peeke *et al.*, 1973, 1975; Figler and Peeke, 1978, 1981). Alcohol also maintained high levels of attack when convict cichlids or leopard frogs were repeatedly provoked by an appropriate stimulus and slowed the habituation of the predatory attack or territorial defense (Peeke *et al.*, 1975; Ingle, 1973).

Table 7 summarizes the effects of alcohol on aggressive and defensive responses as produced by traditional test procedures. Alcohol *decreases* defensive biting and defensive postures by mice, rats, and monkeys exposed to electric shock, attack behavior by isolated mice toward a stimulus mouse, and mouse-killing behavior by rats. The latter effect was also seen when predatory killing was evoked by electrical stimulation of the lateral hypothalamus in cats; alcohol lengthened the latencies of attack (MacDonnell and Ehmer, 1969). The fact that high doses of alcohol are often necessary to decrease aggressive behavior points to the nonspecific nature of these behavioral changes.

Several earlier studies suggested that alcohol may increase aggressive behavior. When alcohol (5%) was placed in their drinking fluid for several weeks, isolation-reared rhesus monkeys began to engage in self-biting in reaction to threat (Chamove and Harlow, 1970); similarly, aggressive responses increased in singly housed pigtail macaques during an 8-week

TABLE 7
Doses of Alcohol for Modulating Aggression and Nonaggressive Motor Activity[a]

Aggression		Nonaggressive motor activity	Reference
Increases	Decreases		
Isolation-induced aggression			
In mice			
0.5 i.p.	None	>0.5 i.p.	Chance et al., 1973
None	4, 12 i.p.	N/S	Bertilson et al., 1977
None	>1, 1.5 i.p.	>1, 1.5 i.p.	Lagerspetz and Ekqvist, 1978
None	1 i.p.	1 i.p.	Smoothy et al., 1982
None	1, 2 i.p.	1, 2 i.p.	Smoothy and Berry, 1983
Pain-induced aggression			
In mice			
None	1.2–4.8 p.o.	2.4–4.8 p.o.	Irwin et al., 1971
None	1, 2 i.p.	N/S	Smoothy and Berry, 1984
In rats			
0.6 i.p.	1.8 i.p.	N/S	Weitz, 1974
None	2.0 i.p.	2.0 i.p.	Bammer and Eichelman, 1983
None	>0.6, 1.2 i.p.	N/S	Tramill et al., 1980
1.97, 3.9/d	5.9/day i.p.	N/S	Tramill et al., 1981
1.97/d, 15 d	1.97 i.p.	N/S	Tramill et al., 1983
In squirrel monkeys			
None	0.125–1.2 i.p.	0.125–1.2 i.p.	Emley and Hutchinson, 1983
Brain stimulation-induced affective defense			
In cats			
0.79–2.37 i.v.	None	N/S	Masserman and Jacobson, 1940
0.37 i.v.	1.5 i.v.	N/S	MacDonnell and Ehmer, 1969
Mouse killing			
In rats			
None	1.5, 2 i.p.	1.5, 2 i.p.	Bammer and Eichelman, 1983

[a] All doses are expressed in g/kg; N/S = data not specified.

period of alcohol (5%) drinking (Kamback, 1973). Occasionally, alcohol doses were selected that were lower than is common in behavioral experiments (less than 1 g/kg, p.o.), and an increased incidence of aggressive and defensive responses was seen at selected single low alcohol doses (e.g., Chance et al., 1973; Weitz, 1974; MacDonnell et al., 1971; see Table 7). Aggressive behavior by subordinate dogs in competitive situations was enhanced by an acute low alcohol dose (James, 1949; Pettijohn, 1979). However, this potentiation of aggressive behavior at low alcohol doses is not readily seen under all experimental conditions (e.g., Smoothy and Berry, 1983; Smoothy et al., 1982).

Recently, several efforts address such problems as (1) defining the critical pharmacological, behavioral, and environmental variables under which alcohol increases aggressive behavior, (2) investigating the neuroendocrine mechanisms by which alcohol may produce changes in aggressive behavior, (3) tracing the developmental and genetic origins for the aggression-heightening effects of alcohol, and (4) determining the past and present social and drug experiences of an individual that increase the sensitivity to the aggression-heightening effects of alcohol.

Detailed analyses of interactions between socially experienced rats, mice, and stumptail macaques showed primarily how increasing doses of alcohol began to compromise certain movements and postures and, ultimately, to induce ataxia (Krsiak and Borgesova, 1973; Crowley et al., 1974; Smoothy and Berry, 1983); for example, a nonataxic alcohol dose (1.2 g/kg, p.o.) reduced social interactions in pairs of rats, whereas nondominant group members of a stumptail macaque colony engaged in more heterosexual behavior and playful mounting without affecting dominance–submission relationships.

The marked sensitivity of certain elements of social behavior to alcohol is illustrated in several experimental series in mice and rats (Krsiak, 1975a, 1976; Miczek and Barry, 1977). Low doses of alcohol increased elements of aggressive behavior in isolated aggressive and timid mice (0.4 and 0.8 g/kg, p.o.) and dominant rats (0.5 g/kg, i.p.), whereas two to three times as high doses were necessary to decrease a large number of aggressive postures and movements (>1.6 g/kg, p.o. in mice, >1.5 g/kg, i.p. in rats); a further twofold increment in dose level produced sedation. The biphasic alcohol dose–effect relationship for attack and threat behavior was also seen in resident mice confronting intruders in their home cage (Miczek and O'Donnell, 1980; Yoshimura and Ogawa, 1983). When a resident mouse's attack behavior is established for several weeks and occurs at a relatively high rate, acute injections of low alcohol doses leave aggressive behavior largely unaltered; however, when the same mouse is subjected to conditions that lower its aggressive behavior, such as an unfamiliar environment, low alcohol doses (0.15, 0.3 g/kg, p.o.) increase attack and threat behavior two- to threefold (Miczek and O'Donnell, 1980). Several important clues on environmental and behavioral determinants of the aggression-modulating effects of alcohol emerged from these observations: Past history of attack or, alternatively, submissive behavior as well as familiarity with the environmental locale appears to determine whether low alcohol doses increase aggressive behavior and how sensitive the animal is to the aggression-decreasing, sedative, and ataxic effects of alcohol. The determinants for alcohol's effects on aggression and those that apply to the benzodiazepines and barbiturates appear to be closely similar. In fact, these three classes of drugs have additive and, possibly potentiating effects in their aggression-increasing as well as -decreasing effects (e.g., Miczek and O'Donnell, 1980; Miczek, 1985).

Recent experiments in monkeys and mice suggest that neuroendocrine events modulate alcohol effects on aggressive behavior. These neuroendocrine processes, in turn, depend on the history and context of social interactions. One characteristic feature of dominant squirrel monkeys living in established social groups is their very high level of testosterone in blood (*ca.* 150–300 ng/ml), which is six to ten times higher than that in subordinate monkeys. Dominant squirrel monkeys engage more frequently in low-intensity aggressive behavior toward other group members at low alcohol doses, whereas no "disinhibitory" effects of alcohol are evident in the low level of agonistic behavior characteristic of subordinate monkeys (Fig. 6; Winslow and Miczek, 1985). This aggression-increasing effect of alcohol in dominant monkeys is, however, seen only during the mating season, when testosterone levels are eight to ten times higher than those in the nonmating period (Winslow *et al.*, 1985). Daily subcutaneous injections of testosterone in subordinate group members produced blood levels comparable to those of dominant monkeys; low doses of alcohol increased levels of threat and aggressive displays in testosterone-maintained subordinates (Winslow *et al.*, 1986). Further experiments in castrated mice provide a direct test of the interaction between alcohol and testosterone on aggression (DeBold and Miczek, 1985). Male mice, after being castrated, were given either very small or very large amounts of testosterone or no testosterone in subcutaneously implanted capsules. Castrates maintained at high levels of testosterone attacked and threatened an opponent intruding into their home cage twice as often as did castrates maintained at low levels of testosterone or testosterone-free castrates. Low to intermediate doses of alcohol increased the rate of attack behavior of mice maintained at high testosterone levels even further, and very large alcohol doses (up to 5.6 g/kg, p.o.) were necessary to decrease their aggressive behavior (Fig. 6). These and further experiments suggest that alcohol's aggression-modulating effects may be mediated by the action of alcohol an androgen-sensitive neural mechanism (e.g., Miczek and DeBold, 1983; Lisciotto *et al.*, in press).

An important effect of alcohol on social interactions and aggressive behavior extends to the individual who interacts with the alcohol-treated partner or opponent (e.g., Miczek and Krsiak, 1979; Miczek and Thompson, 1983). The prerequisite for the detection of such effects is the concurrent measurement of all salient elements of social, aggressive, defensive, and flight behavior exhibited by both opponents during an aggressive interaction. This allows assessment not only of alcohol effects on the behavior pattern the drug recipient engages in, but also of the indirect effects on the behavior shown by the animal interacting with the drug recipient. When socially inexperienced rats are injected with alcohol (1.0, 1.5 g/kg, i.p.), they are attacked more often by an opponent (Miczek and Barry, 1977). Similar increases in aggressive behavior by alcohol-free mice, rats, and squirrel monkeys were seen when these animals confronted an alcohol-treated opponent (Miczek and O'Donnell, 1980; Sbor-

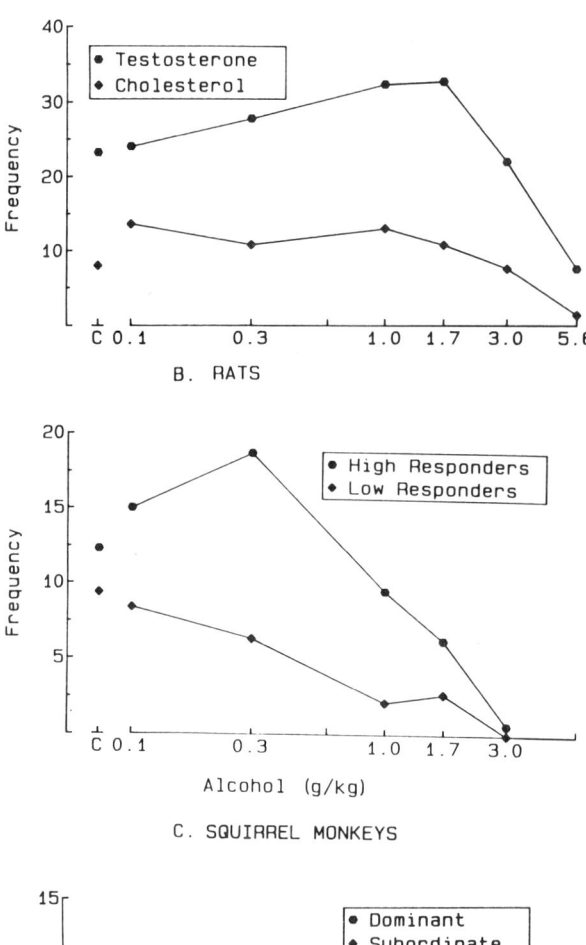

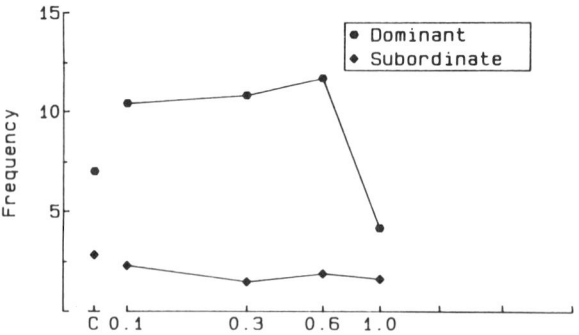

FIG. 6. Effects of acute alcohol doses (p.o.) on attack bites by resident mice (A) or rats (B) toward intruders, or aggressive displays by dominant squirrel monkeys (C) toward other group members. The mice were castrated and subsequently implanted subcutaneously with a capsule that contained testosterone or cholesterol as control. (Data from DeBold and Miczek 1985; Winslow and Miczek, 1985; and Miczek et al., unpublished observations.)

done *et al.*, 1981; Yoshimura and Ogawa, 1983; Miczek *et al.*, 1984c). It will be important to identify the critical behavioral and physical features that are changed by alcohol and that provoke more frequent attacks by an opponent.

Long-term exposure to alcohol and its effects on aggressive behavior have received little experimental attention. Marked changes in aggressive and escape behavior in mice result from prenatal alcohol exposure; after mothers have been given alcohol during pregnancy and/or lactation, their male offspring are more active and attack opponents more often or, alternatively, show more flight responses in adulthood (Krsiak *et al.*, 1977; Ewart and Cutler, 1979). When exposed to alcohol via the mother's milk, male mouse offspring engage in less predatory killing and in less fighting behavior in adulthood (Yanai and Ginsburg, 1976, 1977). Alcohol in the drinking fluid for 7 or 10 days altered aggressive and flight behavior of male mice insignificantly but increased social and sexual investigations (Cutler *et al.*, 1975a; Cutler, 1976). These initial investigations suggest large, long-lasting effects of alcohol, when it was given repeatedly during critical developmental stages. These first results should prompt systematic investigations that include parametric manipulations of alcohol concentration, duration, and developmental time period of exposure and that clearly delineate the processes that are altered by chronic alcohol drinking. It would be equally interesting to determine how past experiences with aggressive behavior or defeat alter the consumption of alcohol (e.g., Lagerspetz, 1964).

3.2.1b. Human Data. What has been known in the Western World from folklore (e.g., "Dutch courage") and legends (e.g., St. Martin's grape vines in the bones of a bird, lion, and donkey) for centuries is now documented by a large number of correlational statistical analyses, namely, that alcohol consumption and human violence are probabilistically linked. This statistical link between alcohol and aggression has been "explained" by several theories. The most enduring and popular postulates release from inhibitory control. After summarizing the retrospective, epidemiological studies that find a statistical association between measures of alcohol consumption and acts of violence and aggression, it will be important to critically evaluate these statistics.

One of the most serious statistics relates alcohol intoxication to *homicide*. Starting with examinations of police records for the involvement of alcohol in criminal homicides (e.g., Wolfgang and Strohm, 1956; Shupe, 1954), a series of studies covering different localities in many countries confirmed this association (e.g., MacDonald, 1961; McGeorge, 1963; Virkkunen, 1974; Tinklenberg, 1973; Goodwin, 1973; Mayfield, 1976; Gerson and Preston, 1979; Lester, 1980; Abel and Zeidenberg, 1985). Some samples found that up to 83% of murderers had consumed alcohol before their deadly assault. Sometimes alcohol intoxication leads to self-directed injury, culminating in suicide (e.g., Frankel *et al.*, 1976). High rates of alcohol consumption have been associated with *physical assaults* as assessed in juvenile delinquents, adult prisoners, or psychiatric patients (e.g., Guze *et al.*, 1962; Bach-Y-Rita *et al.*, 1971; Yarvis, 1972; Nicol *et al.*, 1973; Tinklenberg *et al.*, 1974, 1976, 1977; Mayfield, 1976; Simonds and Kashani, 1979; Roslund and Larson, 1979; Gerson and Preston, 1979; Spieker and Sarver, 1978; Hemphill and Fisher, 1980; Heather, 1981; Myers, 1982). Repeated criminal violence appears to be even more prevalent in alcoholics (e.g., Guze *et al.*, 1962; Schuckit, 1973; McCord, 1981; Coid, 1982; Lewis *et al.*, 1983a). Since alcohol is most often consumed in the company of acquaintances and family members in familiar surroundings, much of the violent and aggressive behavior by inebriated individuals is unreported. Yet, during the past decade some data on alcohol use and *family violence* have become available (e.g., Gayford, 1975; Hanks and Rosenbaum, 1977; Byles, 1978; Gerson, 1978; Corenblum, 1983; Leonard *et al.*, 1985). The probability of *sexual assaults,* particularly rapes, although poorly documented, being committed by individuals who have consumed alcohol is high (e.g., 50%, Rada, 1975; 72%, Johnson *et al.*, 1978; 63%, McCaldon, 1967).

These statistics, although highlighting important problems, are limited (e.g., Evans, 1986): (1) They represent only a small subset of cases. Most violent activities are not reported and thus are not prosecuted. (2) Inebriated individuals are apprehended more readily because of the poor planning and execution of the crime and the unsuccessful evasion of the consequences. (3) The presence of alcohol in the blood is rarely verified by actual measurements, and when verified, it is some time after the violent act. (4) Plea bargaining often allows lesser charges to be recorded, to avoid the more serious consequences for a violent crime such as rape. (5) It is difficult to determine whether an inebriated individual engaged in injurious activities "accidentally" or "aggressively." Recently, many more fatal traffic accidents have been prosecuted as vehicular homicide.

The most problematic aspect of the alcohol–aggression–violence–crime statistics concerns the frequent lack of data from *matched control* groups. It would be important to learn about the association of specific points in the ascending or descending portion of the blood alcohol curve with the probability of violent activities in individuals of matched background variables in matched circumstances. Moreover, a significant statistical association between alcohol use and physical assaults on family members or alcohol use and homicide has been lacking in some studies (e.g., Zacker and Bard, 1977; Abel *et al.*, 1985). A further significant confounding issue is the high incidence of *alcohol in the targets* and ultimate victims of physical assaults and homicides (e.g., Marek *et al.*, 1974; Oppenheim, 1977). Depending on selection criteria, sources, and localities, one-third to four-fifths of all victims of violent death had consumed alcohol either acutely or as part of their alcoholism (e.g., Spain *et al.*, 1951; le Roux and Smith, 1964; Haberman and Baden, 1974; Choi, 1975; Combs-Orme *et al.*, 1983). It is difficult to determine in retrospect to what degree and how the alcohol-consuming crime victim instigated or escalated the violent interaction (e.g., Tinklenberg, 1973).

An alternative approach to the study of alcohol and human aggression relies on experimental protocols with paid or volunteer subjects in laboratory settings (e.g., Taylor, 1983; Pihl, 1983; Cherek and Steinberg, 1986). To avoid the problems attending correlational statistics, social–psychological methodologies have been developed that operationally define aggressive behavior as administering an aversive stimulus to a fictitious competitor in a laboratory task. The experimental subject selects the intensity of the aversive stimulus (e.g., electric shock, white noise, subtraction of prize money) and presses a button for the delivery of the aversive stimulus. The experimental protocol may be arranged so that the fictitious competitor provokes and retaliates by delivering aversive stimuli to the experimental subject.

Although an early experiment failed to find any reliable effect of alcoholic drinks on a subject's selection of shock intensities and administration of these shocks to another individual (Bennett *et al.*, 1969), large and consistent effects of alcohol were seen in subsequent research with modified methodologies. Acute drinks containing 0.8, 0.9, or 2.5 ml/kg of 50% alcohol (vodka) or 1.32 ml/kg of 95% alcohol led to the selection of higher shock intensities and to the administration of longer-lasting shocks (Shuntich and Taylor, 1972; Taylor and Gammon, 1975, 1976; Taylor *et al.*, 1976, 1979; Zeichner and Pihl, 1978, 1980; Zeichner *et al.*, 1982); distilled beverages were more effective than beer (Pihl *et al.*, 1984). Full alcohol dose–effect curves for individual subjects showed lower alcohol doses to be most effective in increasing these types of aggressive responses (Fig. 7; Cherek *et al.*, 1984, 1985). The alcohol effect on selection of higher shock intensities and the application of longer-duration shocks was particularly large when the subject was provoked (e.g., Taylor *et al.*, 1979; Cherek *et al.*, 1985; Wilkinson, 1985), was unmodified by pain reactions from the fictitious competitor (Schmutte and Taylor, 1980; Zeichner and Pihl, 1978, 1980), but was modified by social interventions (Taylor and Gammon, 1976; Jeavons and Taylor, 1985). When a subject who was given a nonalcoholic drink *expected* an alcoholic beverage, he also selected a higher shock intensity and gave longer shocks to the competitor (Lang *et al.*, 1975; Pihl *et al.*, 1981; but see also Gustafson, 1985). This expectancy effect, presumably socially conditioned, appears to agree with the earlier conclusion of Carpenter and Armenti (1972) that the circumstances of drinking more effectively change behavior than the pharmacological properties of alcohol.

The methodological features of the social–psychological experiments

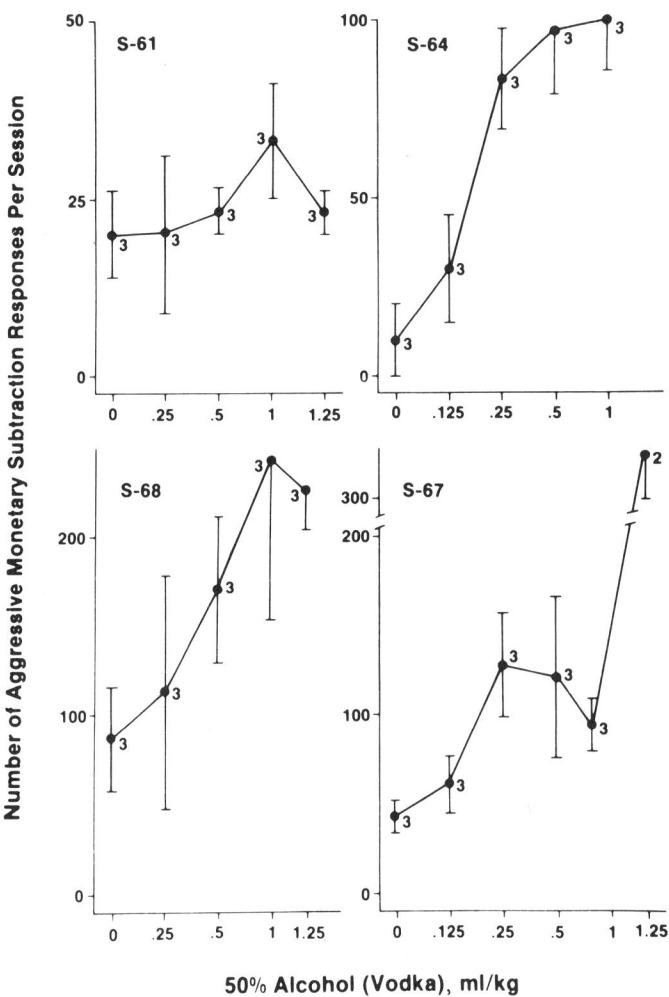

FIG. 7. The number of aggressive monetary subtraction responses per session for all subjects following the administration of placebo or 0.125, 0.25, 0.5, 1, and 1.25 ml/kg of 50% alcohol (vodka). Data points represent the means; vertical lines are ±SEM. The number near data points represent the number of sessions under each condition. (From Cherek et al., 1984.)

are superior to the earlier-mentioned correlational analyses in terms of adequate selection of subjects, control over the administration of alcohol, and the operational definition and quantification of the behavior. However, whether these laboratory measurements validly represent the violent and aggressive behavior that is of societal and health concern remains to be established. To increase the face validity of the aggressive behavior, controlled observations of experimental social settings or barrooms showed that the enhancement of aggressive behavior by alcohol depends on a host of situational, social, and personal variables, in addition to the type and amount of the alcoholic beverage (e.g., Boyatzis, 1974, 1975; Graham *et al.*, 1980).

The inquiry into the mechanism by which alcohol modulates human aggression has been pursued variously, ranging from action on hypothetical control processes to biochemical mechanisms (e.g., Pernanen, 1976; Babor *et al.*, 1983). Since aggression is a major symptom of primary antisocial syndromes (e.g., Cloninger, 1983), the genetic component in the antisocial personalities as well as in the tendency to abuse alcohol has been investigated (e.g., Bohman, 1978; Stabenau, 1984; Cadoret *et al.*, 1985; Lewis *et al.*, 1985). Adoption studies suggest a genetic component for the development of antisocial behavior as well as alcoholism; however, the covariation and interaction between these two syndromes is weak, if at all significant. Violent offenders with explosive or antisocial personalities who also abused alcohol showed lower acid metabolites of monoamines, particularly 5-hydroxyindolacetic acid, in CSF than passive-aggressive patients (Linnoila *et al.*, 1983). However, this change in serotonin metabolism may be specific neither to violent behavior nor to alcohol abuse but rather reflect dietary changes or mark "impulsivity."

Changes in endocrine activity may mediate the effects of alcohol on human aggression (e.g., Mendelson and Mello, 1974; Mendelson, 1977). Yet, the relationship between androgens, alcohol, and aggression appears to be complex. The initial attraction of this proposal was based on observations that alcohol modulates aggressive behavior as well as steroidogenesis, secretion, and metabolism of testosterone. However, the dependence of many kinds of human aggressive behavior on androgens appears tenuous and often nonexistent (e.g., Dotson *et al.*, 1975; see also Section 3.1.7). Alcohol also affects levels of luteinizing hormone, and it is this action that may provide clues for a potential mechanism of the effects of alcohol on aggressive behavior (Mendelson *et al.*, 1978, 1982). It is possible that luteinizing-releasing hormone or catecholamines and endogenous opioid peptides that modulate LH secretion are the behaviorally relevant changes.

3.2.2. Opiates

The sedative, sleep-inducing properties of opiates gave rise to the names of *morphine* as the prototypic drug and *narcotic* for its class, and these effects appear to have been the basis for the early treatment of violent individuals with these drugs. Recent interest in the psychopharmacology of opiates was spurred by the discoveries of three families of endogenous opioid peptides and several types of opioid receptors in the brain and other organs (e.g., Miller, 1984; Goldstein and James, 1984).

The functional significance of these endogenous substances, particularly in the mechanisms mediating aggression, flight, and social behavior as well as tolerance and dependence, has only begun to be investigated.

3.2.2a. Research with Animals. There are three distinct areas of research with opiates and aggressive behavior. The first concern was to document the effects of morphine in several traditional research protocols for the study of aggressive behavior in animals. Second, during the past decade, the opioid receptors and the endogenous opioid peptides have been investigated as potential mechanisms for the effects of opiate drugs on a multitude of functions, including aggression. Intriguing possibilities have arisen, since the performance of specific aggressive, submissive, and social behaviors themselves appears to modulate the activity of opioid peptides and receptors, and consequently, the actions of exogenous opiates. Third, the profound changes in aggressive and social behavior during chronic exposure to opiates and particularly during withdrawal from opiates are a continuing focus of research; the determinants, nature, and mechanisms of these behavioral changes remain poorly understood.

Early observations on Siamese fighting fish suggested a facilitation of attack and threat behavior toward an opponent or toward their own mirror image when the fish were placed in a water with a low morphine concentration (Walaszek and Abood, 1956; Braud and Weibel, 1969). However, most subsequent research with traditional research protocols in mice, rats, cats, and monkeys found *decreases* in aggressive and defensive behavior after morphine doses that were closely similar to those that *sedated* the animals. Specifically, morphine and other opiates suppressed aggressive behavior in isolated mice (Janssen *et al.*, 1960; Cook and Weidley, 1960; DaVanzo *et al.*, 1966); biting in reaction to electric shock stimuli in restrained squirrel monkeys (Emley and Hutchinson, 1972); aggressive and defensive behavior in reaction to electric foot shock (Irwin *et al.*, 1971); hissing vocalizations and ragelike reactions in cats electrically stimulated in the posterior hypothalamus or central gray area (Kido *et al.*, 1967); isolated acts, postures, and vocalizations of an aggressive or defensive nature induced by treatment with large doses of either DL-dopa, carbachol, or apomorphine (Yen *et al.*, 1970; Gianutsos and Lal, 1975; Krstic *et al.*, 1982), as well as mouse killing by rats (Janssen *et al.*, 1962). The behaviorally nonspecific nature of the suppressive effects of opiates on the various aggressive and defensive behaviors as assessed with traditional test protocols for animal aggression failed to indicate any special significance of these drugs either in aggression research or in antiaggressive therapy.

Ethologically oriented research explored the effects of opiates on aggressive behavior and other social behavior as seen in resident–intruder confrontations and during interactions between members of stable social groups. These procedures attempt to avoid the potentially confounding influences of restraint, electric shock, or treatment with toxic drug doses, all of which are known to interact with the effects of opiates. Morphine and fentanyl reduced the frequency of attacks by resident mice or convict cichlids confronting an intruder in the absence of significant alterations in other behaviors (Poshivalov, 1974, 1982; Avis and Peeke, 1975; Sieber *et al.*, 1982). Social interactions of a nonagonistic nature in established groups of pigtail macaques or in pairs of rats were also reduced by morphine or methadone (Crowley *et al.*, 1974, 1975; Meyerson, 1981, 1982; Plonsky and Freeman, 1982). In unfamiliar situations, however, intramygdaloid injections of morphine increased social interactions in pairs of rats and systemic morphine decreased distress vocalizations in infant guinea pigs and increased affiliative behavior in juvenile squirrel monkeys (Herman and Panksepp, 1978; File and Rodgers, 1979; Miczek *et al.*, 1981). These opiate effects are seen at doses well below those producing sedation or impairing motoric capacities, and these effects appear to be specific to social and aggressive behavior.

The discovery of endogenous opioid peptides prompted investigations into the role of these substances in processes that mediate aggressive, defensive, and social behavior. Mainly, three strategies have been pursued so far: (1) activation or blockade of opioid receptors, (2) correlation of some marker of endogenous opioid peptide activity with aggressive or social behavior, and (3) activation of opioid peptides by specific behavioral experiences that modulate opioid-mediated functions.

Inferences about the involvement of endogenous opioid peptides in aggressive and social behavior on the basis of naloxone or naltrexone effects remain preliminary, particularly when higher doses of these antagonists are used. Although antagonism by naloxone may be a necessary criterion for postulating mediation by endogenous opioid peptides, it does not constitute sufficient proof, since naloxone exerts pharmacological effects that are unrelated to opioid receptor blockade (e.g., Sawynok *et al.*, 1979). Naloxone has been found to alter defensive postures and movements by pairs of rats in reaction to electric foot shock in a complex way: A very low dose (0.1 mg/kg, i.p.) increased these responses (Rodgers, 1982), higher doses (2–4 mg/kg, i.p.) also may increase foot shock-induced defensive responses, but only transiently (Fanselow *et al.*, 1980; Gorelick *et al.*, 1981; Fanselow and Sigmundi, 1982; Tazi *et al.*, 1983), and even higher doses (4–10 mg/kg, i.p.) decrease this behavior (McGivern *et al.*, 1981; Rodgers, 1982). An increase in shock-induced aggressive-defensive responses at low naloxone doses is seen in mice of the C57B1/6 strain, but not in DBA/2 mice (Puglisi-Allegra and Oliverio, 1981). In guinea pigs, naloxone markedly increases distress vocalizations (Herman and Panksepp, 1978, 1981).

The earlier evidence on the aggression-decreasing effects of opiates may have suggested changes in the opposite direction with opioid receptor blockers. Yet, low doses of naloxone and naltrexone actually decrease aggressive behavior in certain strains of mice confronting an opponent (Puglisi-Allegra *et al.*, 1982; Olivier and van Dalen, 1982; Lynch *et al.*, 1983; Benton, 1984); moderate naloxone doses often have small or negligible effects on aggressive behavior in mice and rats confronting an opponent; and high doses are necessary to detect antiaggressive effects (Olivier and van Dalen, 1982; Rodgers and Hendrie, 1983; Miczek *et al.*, unpublished observations). In certain phases of the circadian rhythm, or after saline intake, naloxone may increase aggressive behavior of mice confronting intruders (Poshivalov, 1982; Paterson and Vickers, 1984).

In primates, naloxone and naltrexone do not alter the incidence of aggressive acts, postures, and displays (Meller *et al.*, 1980; Fabre-Nys *et al.*, 1982; Winslow *et al.*, 1983; Crowley *et al.*, 1985; Smith *et al.*, unpublished observations). These findings contrast with the increase in associative behaviors in talapoin monkeys and stumptail macaques after naltrexone treatment (Fabre-Nys *et al.*, 1982; Smith *et al.*, unpublished observations), whereas no significant changes in these types of behaviors are seen in rhesus or bonnet macaques or squirrel monkeys until very high naltrexone doses are reached (Abbott *et al.*, 1984; Crowley *et al.*, 1985; Winslow *et al.*, 1983). Social interactions may also be suppressed by naloxone in pairs of rats or mice (File, 1980; File and Rodgers, 1979; Vickers and Paterson, 1985). The evidence for opioid receptor blockade suggests increases in defensive and distress-type behaviors, no change or decreases in attack and threat behavior, and species-dependent changes in associative behavior.

Opioid peptides and agonists that react with specific opioid receptor types affect social and aggressive behaviors in various ways. The ultimate site of action of systemically administered peptides is uncertain (e.g., Banks and Kastin, 1985). When injected directly into cerebral ventricles, β-endorphin decreases sexual, social, and exploratory behavior in rats (Meyerson, 1981, 1982) but increases social interactions when injected subcutaneously; this latter effect is reversed by naltrexone pretreatment (van Ree and Niesink, 1983). Metenkephalin and related peptides, given intraventricularly, decreased attacks and threats by isolated mice and increased behavioral elements of social and motoric activity (Poshivalov, 1982). A naloxone-reversible impairment of foot shock-induced aggressive–defensive reactions in pairs of rats was seen when subcutaneous β-endorphin was given after the daily behavioral sessions (Tazi *et al.*, 1983, 1985). Synthetic agonists of kappa receptors have revealed complex effects: U50488 decreased aggressive behavior by isolated resident mice and increased nonsocial behavior; tifluadom, however, did not affect aggressive behavior, but rather this kappa agonist increased defensive reactions in isolated mice (Benton, 1985; Benton *et al.*, 1985; Brain *et al.*,

1985). These recent studies show potent effects of opioid peptides and synthetic opioid receptor agonists on aggressive and defensive behavior. However, dose dependency, routes of administration, and the nature of aggressive and defensive behaviors need to be explored more systematically before any conclusions about the role of these peptides and receptors in the control of aggressive behavior can be reached.

Social conflict results in profound opioid-mediated physiological and behavioral changes. Most intriguing is the observation that animals after defeat in a social confrontation markedly reduce their response to pain. Mice that intrude into the home cage of a resident and eventually are defeated by the resident show a large, long-lasting analgesia as assessed by different pain measurement techniques (e.g., Miczek et al., 1982, 1985; Miczek and Thompson, 1984; Rodgers and Hendrie, 1983; Rodgers and Randall, 1985; Teskey et al., 1984; Kavaliers and Hirst, 1985). This analgesic response is characteristic of the defeated animal, whether mouse or rat, and appears to be independent of the peripheral physiolological stress response to fighting (e.g., Rodgers et al., 1983; Miczek et al., 1986; Thompson et al., in press). Analgesia has also been seen in mouse-killing rats (Kromer and Dum, 1980). Naloxone or naltrexone, but not the quaternary forms of these opioid antagonists, block the analgesic response as well as the increased food intake in socially defeated mice (Miczek et al., 1982; Rodgers and Hendrie, 1983; Rodgers and Randall, 1985; Teskey et al., 1984). When injected into either the arcuate region of the hypothalamus or the periventricular gray area, naloxone effectively prevents the development of the analgesia in defeated mice, even in adrenalectomized mice (Fig. 8; Miczek et al., 1985). Naloxone also blocks the characteristic behavioral posture of a defeated mouse when given 24 hr after the initial experience and shortly before a test with a nonaggressive partner (Siegfried et al., 1982).

After repeated defeat experiences mice recover their response to pain, but show tolerance to morphine analgesia (Fig. 9; Miczek et al., 1982; Miczek and Winslow, in press; Rodgers and Randall, 1985). The shift to the right in morphine dose–effect curve may be seen after as little as a single defeat experience, although it appears to be functionally limited to the analgesic effects of morphine and such kappa agonists as ethylketocyclazocine, tifluadom, U50488 (Miczek, 1986). In vivo binding of [^{3}H]diprenorphine is greatly reduced and β-endorphin levels are increased in the brain stem of mice that are defeated for the first time and exhibit analgesia, but these changes in binding and endorphin levels reverse after 3–5 days of defeat experiences, when tolerance begins to appear (Thompson et al., 1986). Also, in coexisting pairs of dominant and subordinate gerbils β-endorphin and metenkephalin are increased in the amygdala of defeated gerbils, compared to their victorious opponents (Raab et al., 1985). Adaptation to social conflict, especially in the defeated

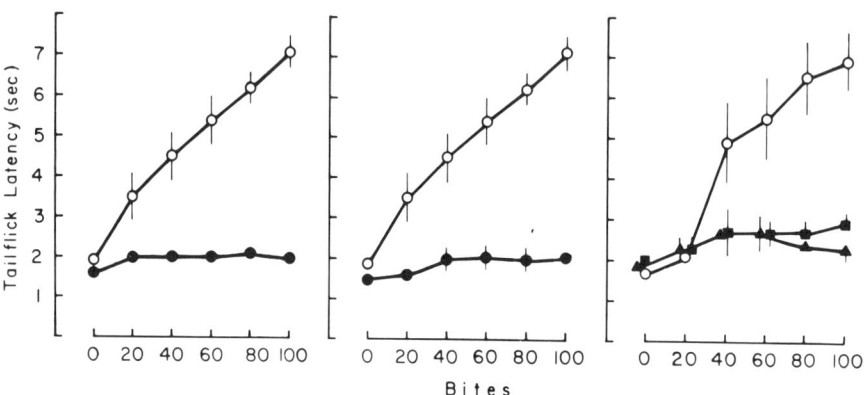

FIG. 8. The latency to flick the tail away from the heat stimulus (in seconds) as a function of exposure to attack bites from a stimulus animal. (Left) Saline (O—O) or 10 μg naloxone (●—●) was injected in a volume of 0.5 μl into the periaqueductal gray area. (Center) Saline (O—O) or 10 μg naloxone (●—●) was injected in a volume of 0.5 μl into the region of the arcuate nucleus. (Right) Saline (O—O), 1 μg naloxone (▲—▲), or 10 μg naloxone (■—■) in a volume of 0.25 μl was injected into the periaqueductal gray area. Vertical lines in data points, ±SEM. The heat stimulus was automatically terminated at 8 sec if no flick occurred. (From Miczek et al., 1985.)

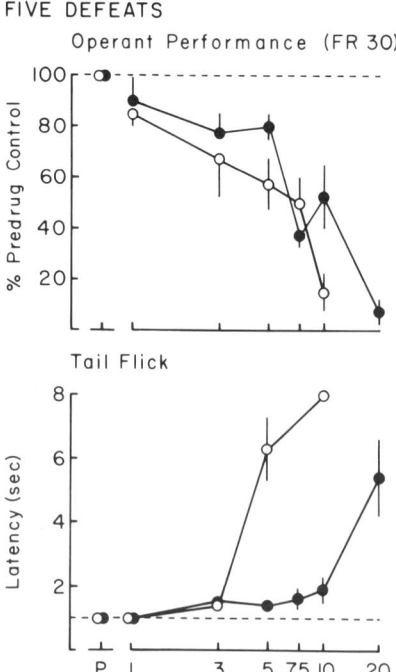

FIG. 9. Effects of morphine on operant performance under a fixed ratio 30 schedule of reinforcement (top) and on the latency to flick the tail from a heat stimulus (bottom) in mice before (O) and after (●) social defeat. The level of operant responding is expressed as percent of predrug control. Vertical lines at data points are ±SEM. The horizontal axis indicates the morphine doses; the values in "P" indicate the data from saline control sessions before each morphine dose. (From Miczek and Winslow, 1987b.)

individual, has important physiological and pharmacological consequences. It will be important to examine the generality of these phenomena beyond mice, opioid peptides, opiates, and analgesia and to delineate the mechanisms for the functionally specific tolerance to opiates.

Withdrawal from prolonged exposure to morphine leads to a syndrome of autonomic, somatic, and behavioral changes that also profoundly alters aggressive and defensive behavior (see p. 197). The magnitude and time course of the various withdrawal symptoms are determined by a range of variables such as opiate dose, duration of exposure, continuous or discrete administration, and precipitating event, as well as previous drug and behavioral experiences, age, sex, housing conditions, and species (e.g., Martin *et al.*, 1963; Wei *et al.*, 1973; Bläsig *et al.*, 1973). When withdrawal occurs in the presence of other animals, several elements of aggressive and defensive behavior are displayed. In rats, audible vocalizations, upright postures facing each other, leaps, and bites directed at forelimbs and snout are seen that resemble elements of defensive behavior (e.g., Boshka *et al.*, 1966; Thor and Teel, 1968; Thor *et al.*, 1970; Borgen *et al.*, 1970; Davis and Khalsa, 1971*a,b*; Lal, 1975*b*); in hamsters, offensive and defensive behaviors are exhibited (Avis and Peeke, 1979*a*); in mice, attack bites and threat responses increase (Kantak and Miczek, in press); in rhesus monkeys, aggressive and submissive responses alternate (e.g., Kreiskott, 1966). The previous and current social experiences, as well as environmental stimuli associated with morphine, determine the direction of the ensuing behavioral change during morphine withdrawal (Miksic *et al.*, 1976; Gellert and Sparber, 1979; Kantak and Miczek, in press). Aggressive and defensive behavior in morphine-withdrawn rats emerges at a time when autonomic and somatic symptoms of withdrawal have peaked and are declining; moreover, heightened aggressive and defensive behavior may be detected even weeks after exposure to morphine, particularly when pairs of withdrawn rats are given foot shocks electrically (e.g., Lal, 1975*b*; Florea and Thor, 1968; Davis and Khalsa, 1971*b*; Stolerman *et al.*, 1975). In mice, the time course of heightened aggressive behavior and somatic as well as autonomic symptoms of withdrawal are similar; for example, heightened attack and threat behavior may be seen during the time withdrawal jumps are evident; this occurs, for most mice, within 24 hr of the removal of 75-mg morphine pellet (Miczek, unpublished observations). The complex time course for the various symptoms and the range of symptoms of opiate withdrawal suggest participation of many neurotransmitters and neuromodulators in opiate withdrawal.

Increased sensitivity of striatal dopamine receptors has been proposed as a critical event that may be responsible for aggressive behavior in morphine-withdrawn rats (Lal, 1975*a*; Gianutsos and Lal, 1976*b*, 1978). Starting with the observations that *d*- or *l*-amphetamine intensified defensive responses in opiate-withdrawn rats (Florea and Thor, 1968; Thor, 1971; Lal *et al.*, 1971; Lal and Puri, 1972; Puri and Lal, 1973, 1974; Carlini and Gonzalez, 1972; Singh, 1975), several experimental manipulations of brain dopamine were found to modulate aggressive behavior in morphine withdrawal. Low doses of apomorphine, L-dopa, and methylphenidate potentiate and drugs or electrolytic brain lesions that block dopamine synthesis or receptors reduce aggressive and defensive behavior during morphine withdrawal (Kreiskott, 1966; Lal and Puri, 1972; Puri and Lal, 1973; Gianutsos *et al.*, 1974*b*; Kantak and Miczek, 1982). In addition to drugs that act preferentially on some aspects of dopaminergic neurotransmission, manipulations of brain acetylcholine, serotonin, and norepinephrine substantially alter defensive responses during morphine withdrawal (Gianutsos and Lal, 1976*a*). Particularly puzzling are the observations with clonidine: This α-adrenergic receptor agonist increases the defensive responses in morphine-withdrawn rats (Gianutsos *et al.*, 1975) but potently decreases attack and threat behavior of morphine-withdrawn mice (Kantak and Miczek, 1982). Similarly, THC intensifies aggressive behavior in morphine-withdrawn rats (Carlini and Gonzalez, 1972), but in the same dose range, THC blocks naloxone-precipitated withdrawal symptoms in morphine-dependent rats (Hine *et al.*, 1975*a*). Especially noteworthy are the so-called paradoxical observations that naloxone precipitates effectively autonomic and somatic withdrawal symptoms but fails to produce heightened aggressive and defensive responses in morphine-dependent mice and rats (Gianutsos *et al.*, 1975; Kantak and Miczek, in press). Of course, as described earlier, opioid receptor antagonists may have socially disruptive effects even in opiate-naive animals. To delineate the possible mechanisms, it appears necessary to differentiate specific changes in the regulation of several neurotransmitters and receptors that are linked to specific symptoms of opiate withdrawal, including heightened aggression.

3.2.2b. Human Data. The evidence on opiates and human aggression ranges from the earlier practice of using acute morphine as an antiaggressive drug to the increasing concern with the high incidence of aggression and criminal behavior in narcotic addicts (e.g., Brill, 1969; McGlothlin, 1979). Because of the high abuse liability, the nonspecific nature of the pacifying or antiaggressive properties, and the marked side effects on many physiological functions, opiates are not considered a useful treatment for violent individuals (e.g., Itil, 1981).

Aggressive behavior, hostility, and violent and assaultive acts are thought to increase during withdrawal from opiates (e.g., Itil, 1981). Actual data from drug abuse treatment programs are quite variable: Some researchers find increased aggressive behavior and hostile attitudes during methadone maintenance (Woody *et al.*, 1983); others see similar changes during the actual detoxification phase (Gossop and Roy, 1976;

Teasdale and Dip, 1972); and others do not see significant changes during detoxification but do see decreased social interactions during heroin acquisition (Babor *et al.*, 1976). Correlational statistics consistently associate narcotic addiction with high crime rates (e.g., Ball *et al.*, 1983; Nurco *et al.*, 1985, 1986). Studies on the career histories of narcotic addicts, longitudinal studies covering periods of active and nonactive addiction, as well as evaluative studies of methadone maintenance programs, show that active narcotic addiction is linked to high criminal activities. Acquisitive crimes committed during withdrawal from narcotics (mostly heroin) generate income to support the drug habit, and sometimes, although infrequently, narcotic addicts self-report and are arrested for crimes of violence (e.g., McGlothlin, 1979; Simonds and Kashani, 1979; Nurco *et al.*, 1985, 1986). It appears that individuals with antisocial personalities have higher rates of alcoholism and narcotic use; antisocial personalities may actually be antecedent to opiate abuse (e.g., Lewis *et al.*, 1983b; Lewis, 1984; Sutker and Archer, 1984). Although these correlational statistics identify a significant problem, the causal relationships remain to be elucidated.

It is surprising that the effects of acute and chronic opiates on aggressive and violent behavior in humans have not been directly assessed in controlled experiments. It appears that the development of opioid receptor antagonists offers new therapeutic tools in the treatment of aggressive behavior during opiate withdrawal.

3.2.3. Hallucinogens

Folklore, religious beliefs, and political propaganda have often focused on sensational instances that linked hallucinogens to unpredictable episodes of violent behavior. Chemically diverse substances—some similar to indoleamines, others similar to phenylethylamines or acetylcholine, others without any amino group—comprise the class of drugs that may induce hallucinations and may also engender symptoms that mimic psychosis; the action on brain serotonin by many of these substances as a potential mechanism of their hallucinogenic properties continues to be an intensively researched topic (e.g., Green, 1985; Jacobs and Gelperin, 1981; Freedman, 1986). Since the available evidence pertains mostly to the effects of lysergic acid diethylamide (LSD), mescaline, phencyclidine (PCP), and cannabis on aggressive behavior, these drugs are selected for illustrative discussion. The association of psychomotor stimulants, another group of potentially psychotomimetic drugs, with aggression will be addressed in Section 3.2.4.

3.2.3a. Research with Animals.

i. LSD. The first experimental preparations in behavioral pharmacology included those with LSD and fish behavior. When immersed in water containing LSD, Siamese fighting fish and green sunfish, as well as newts, engaged in more frequent aggressive displays and bites (Abramson and Evans, 1954; Evans et al., 1958; Evans and Abramson, 1958; McDonald and Heimstra, 1964); at higher doses (0.1–0.3 mg/kg, i.m.), LSD decreased aggressive displays in tropical fish (Saxena et al., 1962). Small, acute doses of LSD increased the frequency of aggressive, submissive, sexual, investigative behaviors in pairs of rats, depending upon the social context (Silverman, 1966a). However, increased aggressive behavior at low doses of LSD has *not* reliably been seen in most species. As a matter of fact, aggressive behavior in isolated mice is either not reliably altered over a wide range of LSD doses (up to 1 mg/kg, p.o.; Krsiak, 1979; Rewerski et al., 1971, 1973; Valzelli et al., 1967) or is actually decreased (Uyeno and Benson, 1965; Uyeno, 1966b; Banerjee, 1971b; Rewerski et al., 1971, 1973). Similarly, competitive behavior in pairs of rats, as well as social interactions in large groups of ants, mice, pigeons, and tropical fish, declined after acute doses of LSD (Siegel and Poole, 1969; Siegel, 1971; Uyeno, 1966a, 1967a,b; Kostowski and Tarchalska, 1972). Over a wide dose range, LSD also failed to alter predatory killing in rats or stimulation-evoked affective reactions in cats (Karli, 1959b; Baxter, 1964a; Rewerski et al., 1971).

Even low doses of LSD intensify defensive reactions and flight reactions (e.g., Silverman, 1966a). When isolated mice showed so-called timid behavior instead of aggressive behavior, LSD increased their flight reactions (Krsiak et al., 1971; Krsiak, 1975b). Also, defensive postures in reaction to electric foot shock were increased by LSD but not by other indole hallucinogens (Brunaud and Siou, 1959; Kostowski, 1966; Sbordone and Carder, 1974; Sheard et al., 1977; Walters et al., 1978). Increased submissive gestures were seen in stumptail macaques after the hallucinogen 5-methoxy *N,N*-dimethyltryptamine was administered; this effect is antagonized by dopamine receptor antagonists but not by serotonergic antagonists (Schlemmer and Davis, 1981). Siegel (1971) suggested that hallucinogens led to social dispersal and reduced social interactions by causing hypersensitivity to social and environmental stimuli. Whether the actions of LSD on serotonin-containing neurons in the raphe nuclei and the drug's effects on aggressive, submissive, flight, and social behavior are related remains to be explored.

ii. *Mescaline.* Early studies established that mescaline, like LSD, mostly reduces aggressive behavior in isolated mice and tropical fish, and competitive behavior in rats (e.g., Saxena et al., 1962; Uyeno, 1966a,b, 1967b; Rewerski et al., 1971; Poshivalov, 1980), although lower doses were usually ineffective (e.g., Valzelli et al., 1967). Unfortunately, it is unknown how these mescaline effects are related to aggressive behavior.

The term *pathological aggression* has been applied to the behavior that is exhibited by mescaline-treated rats exposed to repeated electric foot shocks (Sbordone et al., 1981). Mescaline, whether given to one or both members of a pair of rats, produced injurious and near-lethal biting attacks that persisted even when electric foot shock deliveries were terminated (Sbordone and Carder, 1974; Carder and Sbordone, 1975; Sbordone et al., 1978, 1979, Sbordone and Garcia, 1977). Mescaline, more than other hallucinogens, engendered this unusually intense, long-lasting pattern of biting attacks in reaction to electric foot shocks (Sbordone et al., 1979). The generality and validity of these observations need to be established.

iii. Phencyclidine. This synthetic drug (PCP) was introduced as anesthetic in the late 1950s and quickly withdrawn because of its psychotomimetic properties. The streetnames "angel dust" or "peace pill" versus "killer weed" or "rocket fuel" convey the opposing effects on mood and behavior associated with this drug. Only a few studies have been conducted on PCP-induced aggression in animals, and they have yielded inconsistent results. Increases or decreases in aggressive behavior were seen at selected doses in isolated mice; REM-sleep-deprived rats; mice, rats, and monkeys exposed to electric shock deliveries; and mice confronted with an intruder (Rewerski et al., 1971; Burkhalter and Balster, 1979; Cleary et al., 1981; Musty and Consroe, 1982; Tyler and Miczek, 1982; Emley and Hutchinson, 1983a; Jarvis et al., 1985). In mice or rats placed for the first time in an aggression-provoking situation, without previous drug experience, low PCP doses may increase aggressive behavior (Russell et al., 1984; Boyko-Wilmot and Vander Wende, 1981). The highly varied nature of PCP effects in individual subjects may be related to previous drug and behavioral experiences. The available data do not reveal systematic dose–effect curves other than those for the sedative effects of the drug, nor are there clues as to the potential mechanisms for these spurious effects.

The most consistent finding with PCP and aggression appears to be the increased aggressive behavior exhibited toward PCP-treated subjects: these mice, rats, and monkeys are attacked significantly more often (Miller et al., 1973; Tyler and Miczek, 1982; Russell et al., 1984). Apparently phencyclidine profoundly alters the sending and receiving of communicative signals that are significant in social and aggressive interactions.

iv. Cannabis. Up to 300 million people may be using cannabis, mostly in social settings. Yet, the effects of cannabis on social and aggressive behavior, even at the animal level, as well as the mechanisms of action for these effects remain poorly understood (e.g., Carlini, 1974; Abel, 1975, 1977; Miczek, 1976a; Miczek and Thompson, 1983; Frischknecht, 1984). Table 8 summarizes the effects of cannabis extracts or Δ-9-tetrahydrocannabinol (THC), the major psychoactive ingredient of cannabis, on aggressive behavior in animals as determined in traditional testing protocols: Δ-9-Tetrahydrocannabinol or cannabis extracts consistently

TABLE 8
Acute Doses of Cannabis Extract or THC for Modulating Aggression and Nonaggressive Motor Activity[a]

| Aggression | | Nonaggressive | |
Increases	Decreases	motor activity	Reference
Isolation-induced aggression			
In mice			
None	100–400 extr. i.p.	>400 i.p.	Garattini, 1965
None	2.5–4 extr. i.p.	80 i.p.	Santos et al., 1966
None	ED50 4.25 i.p.	ED50 18.75 i.p.	Carlini and Santos, 1970
None	ED50 4.0 i.p.	ED50 62.1 i.p.	Dubinsky et al., 1973
None	2.5, 5.0 i.p.	>5.0 i.p.	ten Ham and de Jong, 1975
None	1.25, 2.5 i.p.	5–20 i.p.	Dorr and Steinberg, 1976
None	2–4 i.p.	2–4 i.p.	Miczek, 1978
Pain-induced aggression			
In mice			
None	ED50 22.0 i.p.	ED50 62.1 i.p.	Dubinsky et al., 1973
In rats			
0.12–0.5	1, 2	N/S	Carder and Olson, 1972
None	>6.4 i.p.	4 i.p.	Manning and Elsmore, 1972
None	ED50 14.9 i.p.	N/S	Dubinsky et al., 1973
None	5–30 i.p.	N/S	Pradhan et al., 1980
Extinction- or schedule-induced aggression			
In pigeons			
None	0.125–1.0 i.m.	0.5, 1.0 i.m.	Cherek and Thompson, 1972
None	0.125–1.0 i.m.	0.5, 1.0 i.m.	Cherek et al., 1972
In rats			
None	1–4 i.p.	2, 4 i.p.	Miczek and Barry, 1974
Brain stimulation-induced affective defense			
In cats			
None	10, 20 i.p.	10, 20 i.p.	Dubinsky et al., 1973
Morphine withdrawal aggression			
In rats			
5 i.p.	N/S	N/S	Carlini and Gonzalez, 1972
Killing			
By rats			
None	6.4 i.p.	N/S	McDonough et al., 1972
None	20 extr. i.p.	N/S	Alves and Carlini, 1973
None	1, 2 i.v.	>2 i.v.	Kilbey et al., 1973a
None	0.25–2.5 i.v.	N/S	Kilbey et al., 1973b
None	5 i.p.	ED50 62.1 i.p.	Dubinsky et al., 1973a
None	10–40 i.p.	4 i.p.	Miczek, 1976b
None	1.25 i.v.	N/S	Kilbey et al., 1977

[a] All doses are expressed in mg/kg; extr. = cannabis extract; N/S = data not specified.

decreased isolation-induced aggression in mice at doses that are lower than those impairing motor activity; the degree of behavioral specificity for the antiaggressive effects depended on the sensitivity of the method by which motor activity was measured. Pairs of mice or rats that were exposed to electric foot shock or cats stimulated at hypothalamic sites exhibited fewer defensive reactions with acute doses of THC; that very high doses were required indicated behaviorally nonspecific suppression and possibly analgesic effects of THC. Also, relatively high doses of THC, unless given intravenously, often are necessary to decrease a rat's killing response to various prey animals. Conversely, low doses of THC decreased aggressive behavior, induced by extinction conditions or as an adjunct to operant behavior under control of schedules of reinforcement, in rats or pigeons. Occasional exceptions to this general pattern of results may be attributed to the effects of unusual drug vehicles (e.g., Matte, 1975; Dorr and Steinberg, 1976), injection–test intervals (e.g., Pradhan et al., 1980), or lack of familiarity with the testing environment or drug (e.g., Carder and Olson, 1972).

Drug effects on competitive behavior are often studied with the tacit implication that the hypothetical concepts of "dominance" and "aggressiveness" are the targets of drug action. It is not unexpected that cannabis extracts and THC have inconsistent effects on competitive behavior in rodents and monkeys, since performance in different dominance tests is poorly correlated (e.g., Masur et al., 1971, 1972, 1974; Miczek and Barry, 1974, 1975; Giono-Barber et al., 1974; Jones et al., 1974; Uyeno, 1976; Sieber et al., 1981). Laboratory tests for "dominance" still have limited predictive value (e.g., Syme et al., 1974; Bernstein, 1981).

Detailed ethological analysis of aggressive, defensive, submissive, and flight behavior in animals confronting an opponent in the absence of isolated housing, electric shocks, or food deprivation revealed two prominent effects of cannabis extracts and THC: specific antiaggressive effects and an increase in flight and submission (e.g., Frischknecht, 1984). In territorial resident mice or in group-living dominant mice, rats, and monkeys, acute low doses of THC or cannabis extracts decreased attack, threat, and pursuit directed toward an intruder (e.g., Fig. 10; Ely et al., 1975; Miczek, 1978; Sieber, 1982; Sieber et al., 1982); sometimes, however, this effect was accompanied by signs of sedation, depending on dose, drug vehicle, route of administration, and species (e.g., Sieber et al., 1980; Olivier et al., 1984). At higher doses, a second major effect of acute THC doses was the promotion of immobility, submissive postures, and escape (Siegel and Poole, 1969; Siegel, 1971; Miczek and Barry, 1974; Cutler et al., 1975a,b; Cutler and Mackintosh, 1975; Dorr and Steinberg, 1976; Sieber et al., 1980, 1982; Olivier et al., 1984); this latter THC effect is most often seen in animals without a history of aggressive behavior and in those that are actually the target of social initiatives or aggressive behavior. That

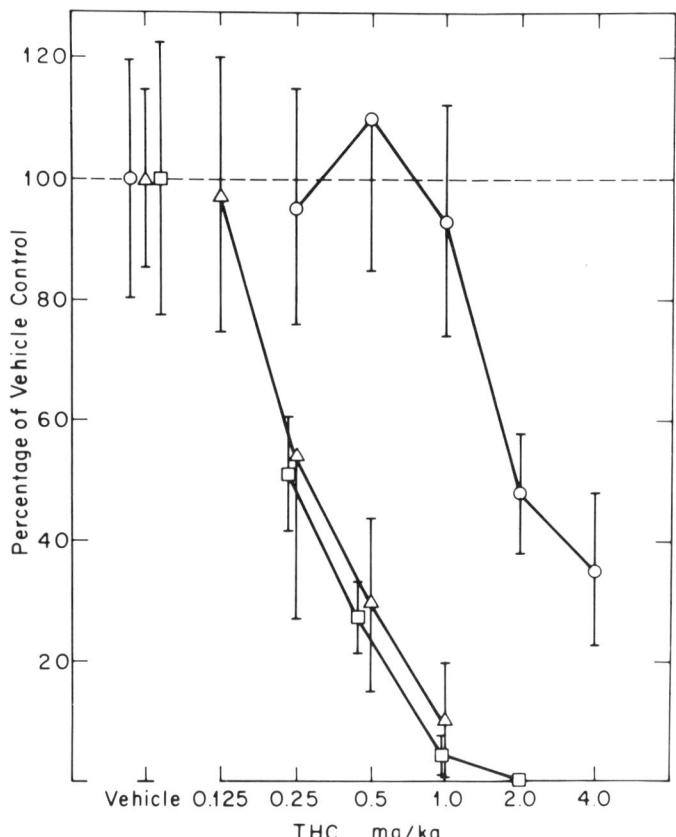

FIG. 10. Effects of THC on attack frequency by resident mice (○), rats (△), and squirrel monkeys (□) toward an intruder, expressed as percentage of vehicle control. The 100% level refers to the attack frequency during vehicle control tests. (From Miczek, 1978.)

drug-free animals substantially alter their aggressive behavior when interacting with THC-treated opponents or partners has been noted (Miczek and Barry, 1974; Miczek, 1977; Sieber *et al.*, 1980, 1982). The differential action of THC on attack and threat as well as on submissive and flight reactions, in addition to indirect alterations in aggressive behavior, highlights the significance of examining drug action on individually treated subjects in different social contexts.

The effects of THC and cannabis extracts appear to extend to many different kind of agonistic and social behaviors, impairing also reproductive behaviors (e.g., Frischknecht, 1984). Of particular interest are the effects of THC on conditioning and memory processes that surround aggressive behavior. For example, mice that are reinforced with the opportunity to engage in attack behavior in a discrimination task will continue to perform under satisfactory stimulus control, but they will decrease their aggressive behavior when given THC (0.6–2.5 mg/kg, i.p.; Kilbey et al., 1972). Recently, a cannabis extract was found to reduce the retention of the defeat response 24 hr after the first display of this behavior (Frischknecht et al., 1985). Considering the pervasive nature of the behavioral effects of THC and the many potential explanations for the effects on attack and threat behavior as well as on defeat, it is not surprising that the mechanisms for these behavioral effects are still unknown. Up to now, no specific neurotransmitter process appears to be unequivocally implicated in the actions of THC doses that profoundly affect behavioral and physiological events (e.g., Paton, 1975; Pertwee, 1985).

Chronic or repeated administration of cannabis extracts and THC has produced a complex and controversial set of findings; some of the initial studies on cannabis and aggressive behavior involved daily administration of extracts or THC to rats that were also exposed periodically to electric foot shock and a food deprivation regimen (e.g., Carlini and Masur, 1969, 1970; Carlini et al., 1972). Hypoglycemia, acidosis, or undernourishment did not appear to be the relevant determinants for the prolonged upright postures and sometimes mutilating biting exhibited by cannabis-treated rats. Low environmental temperature, inhibition of tryptophan hydroxylase, pretreatment with DL-dopa or intraventricular 6-OHDA, morphine withdrawal, estradiol treatment, and classification as highly emotional rats were among the variables that facilitated the bizarre social behavior engendered by chronic cannabis or THC treatment (Carlini and Gonzalez, 1972; Palermo Neto and Carlini, 1972; Palermo Neto and Carvalho, 1973; Palermo Neto et al., 1975; Fujiwara et al., 1984). Inhaled THC, over a prolonged time, may induce in a certain proportion of female rats bizarre mixtures of isolated elements of aggressive and defensive postures (e.g., Rosenkrantz and Braude, 1974). These observations are most often interpreted as evidence for a special interaction between stress and cannabis that gives rise to unusual forms of aggressive and defensive reactions (e.g., Carlini et al., 1976; Frischknecht, 1984).

Many questions about the cannabis–stress interactions need to be resolved; the intensity, duration, or potential adaptations to the stressful conditions that may be the prerequisite for the aggression-provoking effects of cannabis have not been explored. It is noteworthy that THC itself increases plasma corticosterone to levels at which only partial tolerance develops; moreover, the aggressive and defensive behavior is accompanied by large elevations in corticosterone, which return to resting levels at a rate that depends on the outcome of the conflict. It is not clear whether the cannabis–aggression phenomenon is mainly limited to laboratory rats; thus, the behavioral significance of the cannabis-induced elements of aggressive and defensive behavior need to be investigated.

In contrast to these findings, a complete, enduring suppression of aggressive behavior occurred with chronic administration of THC or cannabis extract to isolated mice, hamsters, rats, and pigeons (ten Ham and van Noordwijk, 1973; ten Ham and de Jong, 1974; Miczek, 1979a; Cherek et al., 1980). In none of these studies was any tolerance development to the antiaggressive effects of THC detected, although concurrent impairment of motoric functions or thermoregulation showed tolerance. Others again found evidence for tolerance to the antiaggressive effects of cannabis extracts or THC in mice, monkeys, and fish (Carlini, 1968; Gonzalez et al., 1971; Sassenrath and Chapman, 1975; Sieber et al., 1981). No consistent changes in aggressive behavior, as exhibited by socially living monkeys toward the members of their group, is evident after chronic cannabis or THC administration (Levett et al., 1977; Burgess et al., 1980); in certain groups of macaque monkeys, THC-treated subordinate members may engage in "irritable aggression" after several weeks of drug administration (Sassenrath and Chapman, 1975). The determinants for the antiaggressive effects of THC and its time course during chronic drug exposure need to be explored further.

The ability of THC or cannabis to induce certain aggressive and killing responses in laboratory rats that have not shown these behaviors previously has attracted attention. In rats deprived of rapid-eye-moment (REM) sleep, acute administration of THC or cannabis extract increases irritability and indiscriminate biting and induces aggressive and defensive postures in paired animals (Alves et al., 1973; Carlini and Lindsey, 1974; Carlini, 1977). Blockade of dopaminergic and noradrenergic receptors attenuates THC-induced aggressive behavior in REM-deprived rats, and intraventricular 6-OHDA intensifies the cannabis response (Carlini and Lindsey, 1974; Musty et al., 1976; Carlini et al., 1976, 1977). A second type of response, which is often concurrent with increased irritability, that may be induced by cannabis extracts and THC is mouse killing in so-called nonkiller rats. In rats of different strains, food deprived or not, THC or cannabis extracts, given chronically, induce mouse killing in up to 70% of the animals (Ueki et al., 1972a; Alves and Carlini, 1973; Miczek, 1976a, 1979a, Miczek and Dixit, 1980); under some conditions, even a single injection of THC may induce mouse killing (Yoshimura et al., 1974; Fujiwara and Ueki, 1978, 1979; Fujiwara et al., 1980, 1984). These cannabis-induced forms of aggressive–defensive and killing response may be related to a complex interaction between sleep or food deprivation, single housing, large dose of THC, genetic factors, and prior experience with aggressive behavior.

The most robust observation in research with animals is THC's potent antiaggressive effect when given at low, acute doses, as well as its property to facilitate submissive, defensive, and flight behavior. Although actions on neuronal pathways that release serotonin, catecholamines, acetylcholine, or GABA have been explored as potential mechanisms for THC's behavioral effects (Pertwee, 1985), none appear critically related to the drug's effects on aggressive behavior. The chronic effects of THC, particularly the conditions for tolerance development, and the interaction with environmental and pharmacological stressors need to be investigated further.

3.2.3b. Research with Humans. The association of hallucinogens with violent aggressive behavior dates back to historic times (e.g., Lewin, 1920; Siegel, 1980). Dramatic episodes of seemingly inexplicable violent behavior in hallucinogen-using individuals have led to frequent allegations that these drugs provoke violence. In fact, the empirical evidence is mostly limited to statistics from apprehended delinquents, clients of drug abuse clinics, case reports, or uncontrolled, open trials (e.g., Cherek and Steinberg, 1986). A severe limitation in evaluating the reports on hallucinogens and violent behavior derives from the fact that the subjects are routinely polydrug users.

In spite of marked differences in molecular structure and pharmacological profile, LSD and PCP are linked to violent, often bizarre accidents, suicides, and homicides (e.g., Sheard, 1983; Siegel, 1980). Case reports of violent aggressive behavior, including homicides and rapes, by LSD users highlight the often abrupt, unpredictable, repetitive, prolonged nature of such crimes of violence (e.g., Fink *et al.*, 1966; Knudsen, 1967; Barter and Reite, 1969; Williams, 1969; Malmquist, 1971; Reich and Heffs, 1972; Klepfisz and Racy, 1973; Itil and Seaman, 1978). In 30 long-term polydrug users, LSD increased hostility, which was more related to personality predispositions than to the drug itself (Edwards *et al.*, 1969). Whether LSD increased hostile social interactions in four-person groups depended on previous drug use and previous aggressive behavior (Cheek and Holstein, 1971). In a large South African sample of male offenders, LSD was rarely associated with violence (Hemphill and Fisher, 1980). The sporadic link of PCP with hostile and aggressive behavior parallels the pattern seen with LSD, although PCP violence is said to be more frequent and longer lasting (Siegel, 1980). The overall incidence of psychosis and violent behavior with PCP intoxication varies from very rare to frequent, depending on locality (e.g., Fauman *et al.*, 1976; Feldman *et al.*, 1976; but see Luisada, 1978; Hollister, 1984). Most disconcerting are the accounts of 37 of 45 criminals in southern California who committed violent aggressive behavior while intoxicated with PCP (Siegel, 1980). Similarly, 12 of 16 chronic PCP users reported violent behavior during PCP intoxication (Fauman and Fauman, 1979, 1980). Even during withdrawal from PCP, one-third of the users reported memory loss, violent behavior, and poor impulse control as the most unwanted symptoms (Rawson *et al.*, 1982).

Intoxication with PCP, as well as LSD, particularly chronically, may lead to aggressive outbursts as the result of intense reactions to real or imagined frustrations, poor judgment of long-term consequences of behavior, panic reactions (Siegel, 1978; Tinklenberg, 1973; Sheard, 1983). Most clinicians emphasize that an individual's prior history with violent behavior is of paramount importance in determining the behavioral effects of PCP or LSD (e.g., Luisada, 1978; Hollister, 1984; Siegel, 1978, 1980). At present, the literature with neither animal nor human subjects offers any promising clue about the potential mechanisms by which LSD or PCP may produce intense outbursts of violent behavior in certain individuals.

One of the most controversial topics in the psychopharmacological literature on aggression concerns the effects of such cannabis preparations as marihuana or hashish (e.g., Abel, 1977). A frequently cited historic episode, also recounted by Marco Polo, attributes murderous violence, which was sometimes directed toward Crusaders, to followers of an Ismaili sect, led by Sheik Hassan, who regularly drank a cannabis-containing beverage (e.g., Lewin, 1920). The term *hashish* has been traced to this sect, called the Assassins (*hashshashin* in Arabic). The violent activities of the Assassins were probably motivated by political and religious goals and separated in time from their consumption of cannabis. The association between cannabis and violence continues to be alleged, as in the movie *Reefer Madness*, produced in the 1930s by the U.S. government.

The main conclusion from several retrospective case reports and correlational statistical reports is that cannabis users engage in delinquent behavior, including acts of violence (e.g., Fossier, 1931; Gardikas, 1950; Bernhardson and Gunne, 1972; Simonds and Kashani, 1979); others again report a weak or no statistical correlation between criminal behavior and cannabis use (e.g., Chopra *et al.*, 1942; Bromberg and Rodgers, 1946; Moraes Andrade, 1964; Grupp, 1971; Soueif, 1971; Fisher and Steckler, 1974; Hemphill and Fisher, 1980). Extensive interviews with incarcerated juveniles at a California reformatory institution showed that marihuana was underrepresented in serious sexual or assaultive crimes, and the youths indicated that they expect marihuana to be the least likely drug to incite them to violence (Tinklenberg and Woodrow, 1974; Tinklenberg *et al.*, 1974, 1977). Yet, these reports fail to establish any direct causal relationship between cannabis consumption and subsequent violent behavior (e.g., Abel, 1977).

Attempts to study the effects of cannabis on aggressive behavior in humans experimentally have resorted to a social–psychological competition task or to staged group settings. In either situation, THC, administered either in a drink or in a cigarette, slightly, but reliably, decreased such experimental indices of aggression as verbal hostility or punitive actions against a competitor (Taylor *et al.*, 1976; Salzman *et al.*, 1976). In an experimental social setting, moderate marihuana users engaged in fewer social interactions when given marihuana cigarettes, acutely or chronically; heavy marihuana users failed to show any significant change in social behavior in this experimental setting, which suggests behavioral tolerance (Babor *et al.*, 1978a,b).

Although strong opinions on the issue of cannabis and aggression in humans are held, there is actually very little reliable empirical evidence, and the available data suggest a reduction in angry feelings and interpersonal aggressive behavior. Most retrospective and case studies suffer from the same limitations of inadequate sampling, design, and recording methods, as outlined earlier for the much stronger statistical association between alcohol and aggression. In order to predict the extraordinary behavioral changes in relatively rare individuals, considerably more information on the mechanisms of action of cannabis and on the neurobiological basis of aggressive behavior is required.

3.2.4. Psychomotor Stimulants

One may consider the early investigations of the effects of amphetamines on fatigue and endurance in humans (e.g., Laties and Weiss, 1981) as indirectly relevant to these drugs' effects on aggression, particularly in view of the high use of these drugs by military personnel and competitive athletes. In the area of drug abuse, the "speed–violence–crime nexus" has been of considerable psychiatric and societal concern. The most often reiterated opinion on amphetamines and aggression is that these drugs increase aggressive and violent behavior ("Speed kills," e.g., Allen *et al.*, 1975; Ellinwood, 1972). It is actually possible to adduce a substantial amount of experimental evidence to support this generalization (e.g., Eichelman *et al.*, 1981; Sheard, 1983), if one ignores an equally impressive array of data that shows disruption of aggressive and social interactions as a result of amphetamine use (e.g., Schiøring, 1981). It will be useful to examine how and under which circumstances psychomotor stimulants can cause extreme changes in social and aggressive behavior in animal and human studies.

3.2.4a. Research with Animals. Most work has focused on amphetamines that are prototypic for the class of psychomotor stimulants; comparatively little is known about the effects of methylphenidate, cocaine, and the methylxanthines on aggressive behavior in animals. Amphetamines have complex effects that depend on stimulus situation, species, previous behavioral experience, and, most important, dosage. Table 9 summarizes the evidence obtained with traditional experimental protocols; at intermediate to higher doses, amphetamine as well as other psychomotor stimulants decrease isolation- and extinction-induced aggressive behavior in mice, rats, and pigeons and most often increase concurrently nonaggressive motor activity (Table 9; Miczek and O'Donnell, 1978; Moore and Thompson, 1978; Valzelli and Bernasconi, 1973; Holloway and Thor, 1984, 1985). Selected single low doses of amphetamine may occasionally increase aggressive behavior by isolated mice. More consistent is the increase in pain-induced aggressive–defensive reactions by amphetamine, cocaine, and caffeine in mice, rats, and squirrel monkeys (Table 9; Brunaud and Siou, 1959; Hadfield et al., 1982; Traversa et al., 1985).

Similar to the often-studied blocking effects on a rat's mouse-killing response by antidepressant drugs, amphetamines reliably decrease this behavior at comparatively low doses (Table 9; Kulkarni and Plotnikoff,

TABLE 9
Doses of Amphetamines for Modulating Aggression and Nonaggressive Motor Activity[a]

Aggression		Nonaggressive	
Increases	Decreases	motor activity	Reference
Isolation-induced aggression			
In mice			
None	10.0 i.p.	10.0 i.p.	Melander, 1960
None	ED50 > 3 i.p.	ED50 3 i.p.	DaVanzo et al., 1966
None	5.0 i.p.	N/S	Valzelli, 1967
2.0 i.p.	>2.0 i.p.	>2.0 i.p.	Charpentier, 1969
None	4.0 i.p.	4.0 i.p.	Le Douarec and Broussy, 1969
2.0 i.p.	6.0 i.p.	N/S	Welch and Welch, 1969
None	10.0 i.p.	N/S	Scott et al., 1971
4.0 i.p.	8.0 i.p.	4.0, 8.0 i.p.	Hodge and Butcher, 1975
None	8.0 i.p.	8.0 i.p.	Miczek and O'Donnell, 1978
None	0.25–1 p.o.	>1.0 p.o.	Krsiak, 1979
None	5 i.p.	N/S	Essman and Valzelli, 1984
Pain-induced aggression			
In mice			
8.4 p.o.	None	9.3 p.o.	Stille et al., 1963
0.1 i.p.	None	N/S	Kostowski, 1966
0.5 p.o.	None	>0.5 p.o.	Hoffmeister and Wuttke, 1969
None	5.0 p.o.	2.5 p.o.	Tedeschi et al., 1969
In rats			
None	3.0 i.p.	N/S	Lal et al., 1968
0.25–1 i.p.	4.0 i.p.	N/S	Crowley, 1972
1.0 i.p.	3.0 i.p.	N/S	Powell et al., 1973
3.48 i.p.	N/S	N/S	Mukherjee and Pradhan, 1976a
None	>2.5 i.p.	N/S	Sheard, 1979a
In squirrel monkeys			
None	0.3, 1 i.m.	0.03–1 i.m.	DeWeese, 1977
0.125–1 s.c.	2.0 s.c.	>2 s.c.	Hutchinson et al., 1977
0.125–1 s.c.	2.0 s.c.	>2 s.c.	Emley and Hutchinson, 1972, 1983b

(continued)

TABLE 9
(*Continued*)

| Aggression | | Nonaggressive | |
Increases	Decreases	motor activity	Reference
Extinction-induced aggression			
In rats			
0.1 i.m.	0.5, 1.0 i.m.	0.1–1.0 i.m.	Miczek, 1974
Brain stimulation-induced aggression			
In rats			
None	2.0 i.p.	2.0 i.p.	Panksepp, 1971a
In cats			
5–7.5/cat i.p.	10/cat i.p.	N/S	Sheard, 1967
None	>4 i.p.	N/S	Baxter, 1968b
None	0.3, 0.8 i.p.	N/S	MacDonnell and Fessock, 1972
0.125–0.5 i.p.	1–1.5 i.p.	N/S	Marini et al., 1979b
0.5–3 i.p.	N/S	N/S	Maeda et al., 1985
Drug-induced aggression			
In mice			
L-dopa			
2.0 i.p.	N/S	N/S	Lal et al., 1970
In rats			
Withdrawal from opiates			
2.0 i.p.	N/S	N/S	Florea and Thor, 1968
ca. 3–11/day p.o.	N/S	N/S	Thor, 1971
1–4 i.p.	N/S	N/S	Lal et al., 1971
2.0 i.p.	N/S	N/S	Carlini and Gonzalez, 1972
2.0 i.p.	N/S	N/S	Puri and Lal, 1973
2.0 i.p.	N/S	N/S	Gianutsos et al., 1975
Mouse killing			
In rats			
None	2–15 i.p.	4–5 i.p.	Karli, 1958
None	ED50 1.5 i.p.	ED50 6.6 i.p.	Horovitz et al., 1965, 1966
None	ED50 0.8 i.p.	ED50 4.2 i.p.	Sofia, 1969a
None	0.5–2 i.p.	>2 i.p.	Kulkarni, 1968
None	ED50 1.8 i.p.	1–3 i.p.	Salama and Goldberg, 1970, 1973
None	5.0 i.p.	N/S	Valzelli and Bernasconi, 1971
None	ED50 0.18 i.p.	>0.18 i.p.	Malick, 1975
None	ED50 0.6 i.p.	N/S	Malick, 1976
None	1.5 i.p.	N/S	Gay et al., 1975
None	ED50 0.6 i.p.	N/S	Malick, 1976
None	0.75–3 i.p.	N/S	Gay and Cole, 1976
None	2.0 s.c.	N/S	Posner et al., 1976
None	2 i.p.	N/S	Barr et al., 1976
None	ED50 1.15 i.p.	N/S	Barr et al., 1977
None	0.5–2 i.p.	N/S	Barr et al., 1979
None	1–3 i.p.	2–3 i.p.	Russell et al., 1983

[a]All doses are expressed in mg/kg; N/S = data not specified. (From Abbot et al., 1984.)

1978). This effect can also be obtained by microinjecting amphetamines directly into discrete sites within the amygdala or hypothalamus; it appears to be anatomically dissociated from amphetamine anorexia (e.g., Leaf et al., 1969; Yoshimura and Miczek, 1983). However, when the predatory killing response is evoked by electrical brain stimulation, amphetamines shorten the latency to attack and to kill at low doses and increase it at higher doses (Table 9; Sheard, 1967; Panksepp, 1971a).

The induction of aggressive responses in otherwise placid laboratory mice or rats after treatment with amphetamines (see "Toxin and Drug-Induced Aggression," Section 2.2.3) is of primarily pharmacological interest. For example, when near-toxic doses of amphetamine, usually more than 10 mg/kg, are given a group of mice, episodes of rapid running, audible vocalizations, upright postures, biting, and, eventually, increased lethality are seen (e.g., Chance, 1946a,b; Randrup and Munkvad, 1969a,b). The so-called amphetamine *rage* response includes isolated elements of the repertoire of agonistic behavior, and these fragmentary elements are embedded in stereotyped motor activities (e.g., Hasselager et al., 1972). Like motor stereotypies, amphetamine aggressiveness appears to critically depend on the nigrostriatal dopamine system (e.g., Randrup and Munkvad, 1969a,b; Fog et al., 1970; Hasselager et al., 1972; Rolinski, 1973). It may be that the heightened aggressive behavior during morphine withdrawal or after REM sleep deprivation, which is even further increased by amphetamine, indicates increased sensitivity or up-regulation of dopamine receptors (Table 8; Lal, 1975b; Carlini et al., 1974; Kantak and Miczek, 1982). Whether heightened sensitivity to amphetamine toxicity is linked to aggressiveness in isolated mice or to some other consequence of isolated housing remains to be determined (e.g., Consolo et al., 1965a,b; Welch and Welch, 1966, 1973; Lagerspetz and Lagerspetz, 1971).

The utility of the amphetamine-aggressiveness phenomenon for identifying drugs with antipsychotic or antidepressant properties has been explored by combining high doses of amphetamine with tricyclics, monoamine oxidase inhibitors, or dopamine receptor blockers (e.g., Schrold, 1970; Hine et al., 1975b; Hasselager et al., 1972); pharmacological enhancement or blockade of amphetamine-induced behaviors, however, does not appear to be limited to those elements that are labeled *aggressive*. Another effort to model a major symptom of physiological disorders, such as the Lesch–Nyhan syndrome, the de Lange syndrome, and Tourette syndrome, is directed to induce self-injurious behavior by CNS stimulant drugs. High doses of pemoline or repeated administration of amphetamine or caffeine induces self-directed biting in rats that produces long-lasting injuries (e.g., Genovese et al., 1969; Mueller and Nyhan, 1982, 1983; Mueller et al., 1982). Dopamine agonists induce self-mutilating behavior to a larger extent when dopaminergic fibers have been destroyed neonatally by the neurotoxin 6-OHDA (e.g., Breese et al., 1984a,b). Similar self-multilating effects and mouse killing are induced by the repeated administration of theophylline; this is possibly related to elevated 5-HT and 5-HIAA in the amygdala (Sakata and Fuchimoto, 1973a,b; Sakata et al., 1975). The relationship of stimulant-induced aggressiveness and self-mutilation to functionally more understood aggressive behavior patterns needs to be explored at the behavioral and biochemical level.

Results with traditional methodologies suggest that amphetamine, cocaine, and other psychomotor stimulant drugs may increase or decrease aggressive responses or leave them unaltered (e.g., Table 9). This pattern of complex, often inconsistent findings is usually rationalized in terms of different methodologies engendering different responses that are collectively referred to as *aggression*. Although convenient, such conclusions are neither entirely satisfactory nor productive. The behavioral analysis of amphetamine's effects on aggression has been markedly furthered by a focus on biologically valid test situations; more detailed records of the characteristic repertoire of agonistic and nonagonistic elements of behavior; and attempts to analyze the interactional, sequential, and temporal features of aggressive behavior (e.g., Olivier et al., 1984; Miczek and Winslow, 1987a). Ethologically oriented studies demonstrated the following:

The *prevalent aggressive behavior pattern* of the individual is an important determinant of the subsequent effects of psychomotor stimulants on aggressive behavior. Amphetamines differentially modulate the pattern of attack and threat behavior versus defensive and flight reactions.

A second major determinant of amphetamine effects on aggressive behavior is the *dose*. Amphetamines modulate aggressive behavior in a dose-dependent biphasic manner. For example, low amphetamine doses often increase the incidence of attack and threat toward a conspecific opponent in fish and rats, whereas intermediate to higher doses decrease these responses and increase defensive and flight reactions (e.g., Weischer, 1966; Keller and Poster, 1970; Chance and Silverman, 1964; Silverman, 1966a; Miczek, 1974; Krsiak, 1975b, 1979; Zwirner et al., 1975; Poshivalov, 1980, 1981; Sieber et al., 1982). The differential effects of psychomotor stimulants are most apparent when drug effects on a resident's attack behavior are compared with those on an intruder's defense and flight (e.g., Hoffmeister and Wuttke, 1969; Miczek and O'Donnell, 1978; Miczek, 1979b). These findings may resolve the seemingly contradictory results that are obtained with psychomotor stimulants in the traditional tests of isolation-induced aggression in mice and pain-induced aggression in rats, since the former protocol primarily engenders attack behavior, and the latter protocol defensive reactions. Important further determinants for the aggression-modulating effects of psychomotor stimulants have been identified.

A comparison of isolated mice that attacked an opponent four to five times a minute with those that showed a near-zero level *baseline of attack behavior* revealed not only quantitative but even qualitatively different drug effects (e.g., Krsiak *et al.,* 1981, 1984). The catecholamine neurotoxin 6-hydroxydopamine increased attack behavior only in those mice that failed to attack before drug treatment, but it was also without notice-

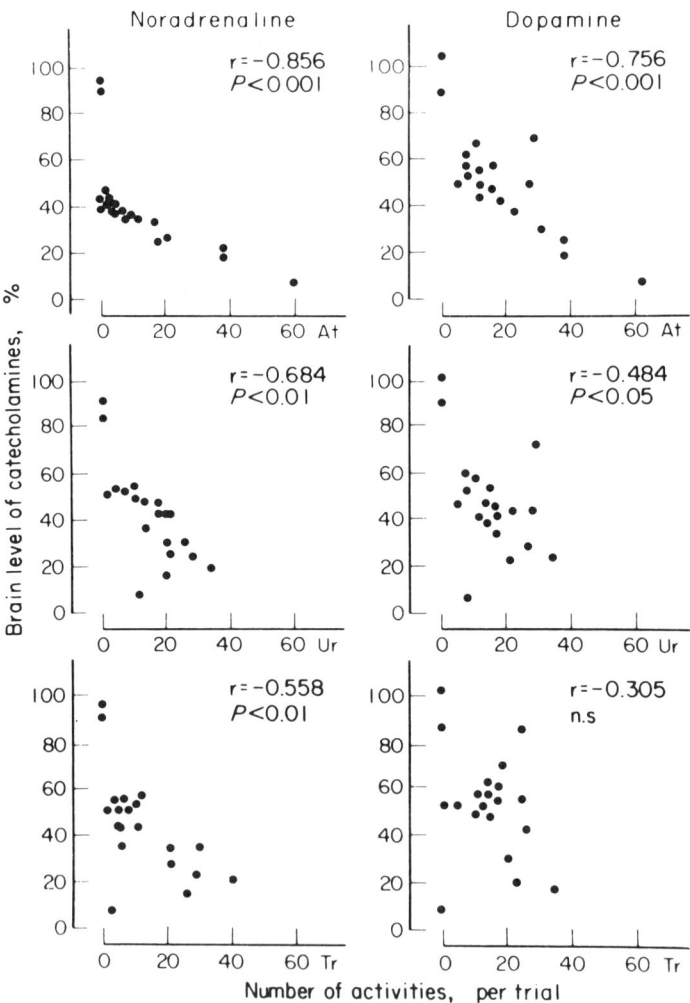

FIG. 11. Correlation between stimulation of aggressive activities and depletion of brain catecholamines produced by 50 µg 6-OHDA in initially nonaggressive, singly housed mice. (Abscissa) Individual level of norepinephrine and dopamine expressed as percentage of mean level of respective catecholamines in vehicle-treated animals. (Ordinate) Individual increase in the number of attacks (At), aggressive unrests (Ur), and tail rattles (Tr), compared with the pretreatment interaction. Spearman rank correlation coefficients (r) are given. (From Pöschlova *et al.,* 1976.)

able effects in mice with a high rate of attack behavior (Fig. 11; Pöschlova et al., 1976). Similarly, the same doses of (+)-amphetamine decreased aggressive elements of behavior in mice with high rates of these responses, whereas the opposite effect was seen in nonaggressive isolated mice (Krsiak, 1975b, 1979). The same animal may show different rates of attack behavior depending on the environmental situation and behavioral experiences. Eight times higher doses of amphetamine were required to decrease high rates of attack behavior in isolated mice studied in their home cage than when the same animals were tested in unfamiliar surroundings where they exhibited markedly lower rates of aggressive behavior (Miczek and O'Donnell, 1978). When a resident mouse confronts an intruder repeatedly, the rate of the resident's attacks declines exponentially in the course of consecutive encounters. Low to intermediate doses of d-amphetamine and apomorphine do not affect the initial high rates of attack behavior but do increase the low rates of attack behavior seen in later confrontations (Fig. 12; Winslow and Miczek, 1983). It appears that amphetamines increase low rates of aggressive behavior and decrease high rates. Contrary to this general pattern, amphetamine increases even further the already high rate of attack behavior in morphine-withdrawn mice and does not alter the lower rate of attack behavior in placebo-treated mice (Kantak and Miczek, 1982). Clearly, the rate-dependency of amphetamine's effects on aggressive behavior needs to be explored more systematically.

In socially organized animals, such as groups of primates, success and failure in dyadic interactions during social upheaval leads to a *social stratification of the group*. Dominant animals differ from subordinate animals not only in terms of their characteristic behavior pattern but also in terms of endocrine and neurochemical processes that are involved in amphetamine action. Amphetamines may increase submissive displays in high-ranking stumptail macaques (Schlemmer and Davis, 1981) or in subordinate rhesus monkeys (Haber et al., 1981); amphetamines may also increase aggressive and threat displays in dominant rhesus monkeys (Haber et al., 1981) or disrupt this behavior in dominant squirrel monkeys (Miczek and Gold, 1983a) or pigtail macaques (Crowley et al., 1974). Social status-dependent amphetamine effects are not limited to agonistic behavior; amphetamine increased locomotion in subordinate squirrel monkeys, but decreased this form of motor activity in the alpha member of the group (Miczek and Gold, 1983a). Even short-term experiences with agonistic behavior profoundly alter the subsequent effects of amphetamine. In mice without any history of aggressive behavior, low doses of amphetamine increase their attack behavior only during the initial confrontation with an intruding opponent but not after repeated fighting experiences (Noda et al., 1985). These effects parallel those obtained with drug administration during schedule-controlled behavior that depend on the conditioning history of the animal (e.g., McKearney, 1979).

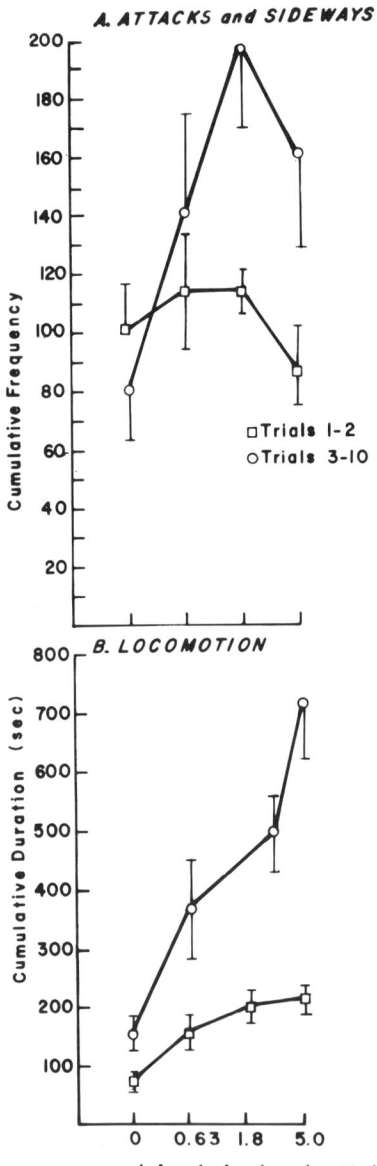

FIG. 12. Frequency of attacks and sideways threats (A) and duration of locomotion (B) during early and late phases of the habituation process. Data represent the effects of d-amphetamine injected 5 min before the first of 10 repeated confrontations. (From Winslow and Miczek, 1983.)

Amphetamine may induce changes in one combatant that alter *the aggressive behavior of the nondrugged combatant.* In addition to modulating the behavior of the drug recipient directly, large and systematic changes in aggressive behavior are seen in individuals who interact with amphetamine-treated opponents (indirect drug effects). For example, amphetamine-treated subordinate rats, monkeys, or intruder mice are attacked more frequently by their drug-free opponents; this effect is systematically related to the amphetamine dose in the victim (Miczek, 1974, 1977; Miczek and O'Donnell, 1978; Sheard, 1973; Crowley et al., 1974). The nature of the aggression-provoking stimuli induced in the amphetamine-treated combatant has not been identified.

The *time interval between consecutive administrations of amphetamine*, as well as the magnitude and duration of the individual amphetamine effects, greatly influence the behavioral effects of the drug (e.g., Garver et al., 1975; Segal et al., 1980). Daily administration of increasing doses of methamphetamine decreased aggressive behavior in seven mouse strains and genera, but not in *Onychomys* (Richardson et al., 1972). In spite of evidence for an augmented stereotypic response, tolerance or augmentation in the aggression-decreasing effects of amphetamine and cocaine after 2 or 4 weeks of daily stimulant administration was not observed (O'Donnell and Miczek, 1980). However, when rats living in large unisexual colonies are implanted with subcutaneous amphetamine pellets, they will initially exhibit hyperactivity and social withdrawal and eventually an unusually high incidence of startle, threat, and defensive reactions (Ellison et al., 1978a; Eison et al., 1978), at a phase of drug action when neurotoxic effects of amphetamine in striatal dopamine fibers are detected (Ellison et al., 1978b). In social colonies of macaques or marmosets, chronic administration of amphetamine led to stereotyped movements and progressive social withdrawal, but *not* increased defense and threat (Garver et al., 1975; Schlemmer et al., 1976; Ridley et al., 1979). The marked differences between discrete injections and continuous amphetamine exposure at behavioral and biochemical level need to be explored.

The seventh determinant of amphetamine effects is the *species*. The disruptive effects of this drug on patterns of aggressive behavior are readily seen in every species, from birds to primates (e.g., Moore and Thompson, 1978; Crowley et al., 1974; Miczek et al., 1981; Miczek and Gold, 1983a,b). Yet, systematic and reliable increases in aggression after low amphetamine doses are seen only in resident rats (e.g., Miczek, 1974, 1979b) and selected members of established groups of macaques (Smith and Byrd, 1984; Bellarosa et al., 1980; Haber et al., 1981). In hyperactive, uncontrollable dogs, amphetamine and other psychomotor stimulants have a so-called paradoxical calming effect that has been likened to the effects seen in children with an attention deficit disorder (e.g., Corson et al., 1976; Campbell, 1973).

The neurochemical mechanisms for amphetamine's effects on aggression and social behavior have not been identified. Although amphetamine increased motor activity and stereotyped repetitive motor routines critically depend on nigrostriatal and mesolimbic dopamine systems (e.g., Iversen, 1977), neither the sites nor substrates for the drug's aggression-modulating effects is known. Direct neurochemical data are usually obtained from animals that have just exhibited some aggressive behavior or, alternatively, from animals under conditions in which aggressive behavior is likely to occur. Early neurochemical studies indicated that catecholamines are involved in the process leading up to an aggressive act, as well as its consequences (e.g., Reis *et al.,* 1967; Eleftheriou and Church, 1968; Goldberg and Salama, 1969; Welch and Welch, 1971). During the past decade, analysis of discrete brain regions has supplanted whole brain measures; indices of synthetic and metabolic enzymes (e.g., tyrosine hydroxylase, dopamine-β-hydroxylase, PNMT, MAO), metabolites (e.g., DOPAC, HVA), and turnover as well as uptake have been obtained in aggressive versus nonaggressive animals (e.g., Hendley *et al.,* 1973; Ciaranello *et al.,* 1974; Lamprecht *et al.,* 1972; Maengwyn-Davies *et al.,* 1973). Substantial neurochemical and adrenal changes in aggressive animals were found, but the direction of these changes varied with the experimental preparation (e.g., Mos and van Valkenburg, 1979; Tizabi *et al.,* 1980*a,b*; Hadfield, 1983; Dantzer *et al.,* 1984). Since most of these studies employed such aversive conditions as isolated housing or the application of electric shock or the delivery of near-toxic doses of drugs (e.g., L-dopa, apomorphine, 6-OHDA) to induce aggressive behavior in otherwise placid laboratory animals, many neurochemical and hormonal measures were obscured. It is not clear which of the neurochemical changes are specific to aggression or defeat and which are relevant to the effects of psychomotor stimulants on these behaviors.

It has not been possible to antagonize the disruptive effects of amphetamine or cocaine on aggressive and social behavior with dopaminergic, noradrenergic, or serotonergic receptor blockers. The effects of amphetamine on a resident mouse's attack and threat behavior toward an intruder or on play fighting by juvenile rats was not blocked by haloperidol, propranolol, prazosin, phenoxybenzamine, or methysergide (Miczek, 1981, 1983, unpublished observations; Beatty *et al.,* 1984). Similarly, neither pimozide, haloperidol, nor chlorpromazine counteracted the socially disruptive effects of amphetamine in marmosets, macaques, vervets, or squirrel monkeys (Kjellberg and Randrup, 1971; Schiøring, 1977; Ridley *et al.,* 1979; Schlemmer and Davis, 1983; Miczek and Yoshimura, 1982).

Important clues about the potential neurobiological mechanisms by which amphetamines alter aggressive and social behavior patterns may be obtained from a more detailed moment-to-moment analysis of aggressive interactions (e.g., Miczek, 1983*b*; Poshivalov and Khodko, 1984). Several initial attempts revealed that amphetamine and other dopamine agonists alter the characteristic temporal patterns and sequences of aggressive behavioral elements in mice and ferrets at doses that are severalfold lower than those necessary for altering the total incidence of aggressive behavior (Krsiak and Pribik, 1978; Schmidt, 1984; Poshivalov and Khodko, 1982, 1984; Miczek *et al.,* 1983*a,b*). It appears that a primary effect of psychomotor stimulants is the disorganization of complex sequences and patterns of social and aggressive interactions and an increase in the repetition rate in a limited number of elements in the repertoire of agonistic behavior.

3.2.4b. Human Data. Although excessively aggressive children, adolescents, and even adults may be calmed by treatment with psychomotor stimulants, the same drugs may also induce extreme aggressive outbursts, which may even be homicidal (e.g., Allen *et al.*, 1975; Leventhal and Brodie, 1981; Campbell *et al.*, 1982; Cherek and Steinberg, 1986). These divergent changes in aggressive behavior appear most often in individuals who are diagnosed as either paranoid psychotics or hyperkinetics; increased aggressive behavior is associated with the paranoid psychotic state of amphetamine abuse, and decreased aggression may be seen after psychomotor stimulant treatment in children and adolescent who are considered to be suffering from attention deficit disorder or minimal brain dysfunction.

Opinions on the incidence of stimulant abuse and heightened aggressive behavior differ sharply. For example, Ellinwood (1971) reviewed in detail 13 cases of intense aggressive acts during intoxication with high amphetamine doses and determined that the drug state also induced paranoid and frightening delusions. These and similar clinical observations suggest that amphetamine-related aggression may be secondary to the psychotic paranoid state primarily induced by the intravenous use of high doses of the drug (e.g., Rickman *et al.*, 1961; Kramer, 1969; Carey and Mandel, 1969; Smith, 1969; Hampton, 1961; Angrist and Gershon, 1969). Ellinwood (1972) postulated that amphetamine use was more likely to lead to violence than any other drug. The seriousness of this conclusion is further underscored by the high correlation between patients who displayed violent episodes, often criminal in nature, and who were also taking amphetamines chronically (Siomopoulos, 1981; Bach-Y-Rita *et al.*, 1971). Amphetamine abusers were reported as showing symptoms of increased hostility and assaultive behavior (Kalant, 1966; Rawlin, 1968; Cockett and Marks, 1969; Angrist and Gershon, 1976). Conversely, a significant proportion of 109 adolescent delinquents were amphetamine and cocaine users or abusers, although a higher proportion had records of alcohol and marihuana abuse (Simonds and Kashani, 1979). It should be noted that none of the aforementioned data are based on comparisons of systematically matched samples, and all rely on retrospective verbal reports. Studies on institutionalized individuals involve a selected subject pool that may or may not distort the magnitude and severity of the problem of amphetamine-related aggression.

Low to moderate doses of amphetamine, however, were observed to increase verbal and motor activity as well as "friendliness and euphoria" (Nathanson, 1937; Laties, 1961; Cameron *et al.*, 1965; Griffiths *et al.*,

1977). When amphetamines were used to treat sleep or eating disorders, heightened aggressive behavior was not a problematic side effect (e.g., Leventhal and Brodie, 1981; Allen *et al.*, 1975). As a matter of fact, occasional case reports indicated a reduction in aggressive outbursts in "psychopaths" and dyscontrol patients (Shorvon, 1947; Hill, 1947; Richmond *et al.*, 1978). In systematic investigations of drug use patterns among incarcerated adolescent delinquents in California, Tinklenberg and associates found that less than 5% of the sample populations had been using amphetamine or cocaine at the time the violent criminal acts were committed (Tinklenberg and Woodrow, 1974; Tinklenberg *et al.*, 1974, 1977). Similarly, in a British sample of 53 individuals treated at a drug dependence unit, amphetamine abusers were the least hostile group, compared to narcotic and barbiturate abusers (Gossop and Roy, 1976). These and similar conflicting observations are difficult to reconcile; significant insights are to be expected from detailed analysis of an individual's behavioral and pharmacological history; predisposing biochemical processes; and interactions between drug, behavior, and environment.

Psychomotor stimulants are used therapeutically in pediatric psychiatry to reduce heightened aggressive behavior in children and adolescents. How exactly the violent outbursts and destructive and uncontrolled episodes of aggression are related to hyperkinesis, minimal brain dysfunction, or an attention deficit disorder is unclear; these diagnostic categories remain "controversial," "ill defined," "imprecise," and "soft" (e.g., Fish, 1971; Itil and Mukhopadhyay, 1978; Lion, 1975; Leventhal and Brodie, 1981). It is also not understood whether the increase in frequency and intensity in aggressive behavior is limited to the early developmental periods or continues in adulthood (e.g., Allen *et al.*, 1975; Campbell *et al.*, 1982; Cherek and Steinberg, 1986). Bradley (1937) was among the first to give amphetamine to the children he described as hyperactive, irritable, aggressive, and destructive; he found them to be more "placid and easygoing" after drug administration. Several subsequent open uncontrolled clinical trials confirmed the therapeutic potential of amphetamines in decreasing aggressive behavior in children with varying diagnoses or in delinquent adolescents (e.g., Bender and Cottington, 1942; Korey, 1944; Eisenberg *et al.*, 1963).

During the past 25 years, a series of placebo-controlled and often double-blind studies has investigated amphetamines and methylphenidate in aggressive children who were diagnosed as hyperkinetic, autistic, explosive, unsocialized, or emotionally disturbed; 10–40 mg/day of *d*- or *l*-amphetamine, given to 5- to 14-year-old boys or girls significantly reduced aggressive behavior and improved social behavior as assessed most often by ratings from teachers, parents, or clinical professionals (Conners, 1969, 1972; Winsberg *et al.*, 1972, 1974; Arnold *et al.*, 1973; Maletzky, 1974; Campbell *et al.*, 1976). Similarly, about 15–50 mg/day of methylphenidate improved learning, lengthened attention span, and lowered ratings for aggressivity and hyperactivity (Sprague *et al.*, 1970; Sprague and Sleator, 1977; Satterfield *et al.*, 1972; Rapoport *et al.*, 1974; Allen *et al.*, 1975; Werry and Aman, 1975; Garfinkel *et al.*, 1975; Loney *et al.*, 1978; Winsberg *et al.*, 1982; Pelham *et al.*, 1985). However, in several large samples of delinquent boys and hyperkinetic children, aggressive behavior and conduct problems persisted after amphetamine or methylphenidate treatment (e.g., Conners *et al.*, 1971; Saletu *et al.*, 1975) or even led, in some cases, to adverse effects (Lucas and Weiss, 1971).

Evidence for a separation of hyperaggressivity from such other symptoms as hyperactivity, attention deficits, and learning disorders comes from different sources (e.g., Fish, 1971). Symptoms of hyperaggressive behavior load on a factor that differs from those that describe learning, attention, and motoric activity (Conners, 1969). In follow-up studies, hyperactivity markedly decreased as the children grew older, while aggressivity scores improved less, suggesting a persistence of aggressive behavior into young adulthood (e.g., Minde *et al.*, 1972; Mendelson *et al.*, 1971). Occasionally, adults with a history of an attention deficit disorder in their childhood showed significantly less aggressive behavior when treated with amphetamine or methylphenidate (Stringer and Josef, 1983; Arnold *et al.*, 1972). In spite of the frequent reports of beneficial treatment effects with psychomotor stimulants, it is not clear under which conditions and in whom these drugs will act as antiaggressives. Separate dose–effect functions and time courses for the antiaggressive effects of psychomotor stimulants, compared to the effects on hyperactivity and cognitive functions, suggest different mechanisms for this array of symptoms.

A recent series of experiments attempted to deal with one of the critical issues in human aggression research, namely, the development and implementation of accurate, objective, and reliable measurement of aggressive behavior under controlled conditions (Cherek, 1981). When human subjects are engaged in an experimental competitive task and are provoked by losses in prize money, they will deliver blasts of noise and subtract prize money from their competitor. Amphetamine increased these aggressive responses at the 5- and 10-mg doses, whereas 20 mg of amphetamine, or caffeine, decreased these responses (Cherek *et al.*, 1983; Cherek and Steinberg, 1986). It will be interesting to explore this experimental measure of aggressive behavior further with clinically significant populations who are either prone to develop aggressive behavior after psychomotor stimulants or who are in need of treatment for their hyperaggressive behavior.

3.2.5. Summary

Alcohol, opiates, LSD, PCP, cannabis, and psychomotor stimulants have all been associated with increased aggressive behavior. The extent and significance of this association varies enormously with the drug, which precludes generalizations across these drugs. The large variability and, often, rarity of the link between these classes of drugs and heightened aggressive behavior point to complex and multiple determinants of this relationship. It appears that these drugs alter aggressive behavior differently; their aggression-increasing as well as aggression-decreasing effects suggest at least two separate mechanisms for two portions of the dose–effect curves. As has been discussed in detail for the psychomotor stimulants, not only such important pharmacological parameters as dosage and chronicity of treatment, but also such behavioral variables as previous social experience, current aggressive and defensive behavior, the baseline of aggressive behavior, and the drug state of the opponent are among the most critical determinants of drug effects on aggressive behavior.

Aggressive and defensive behavior may alter neuroendocrine and neurotransmitter functions and thus determine how these drugs affect aggression. This feedback relationship between behavior and brain function is seen in the profound changes in opioid peptides produced during certain social experiences, such as social defeat or social separation. Moreover, the tolerancelike changes seen after distinctive social and aggressive experiences appear to be functionally specific, which may provide new insights into the mechanisms mediating tolerance. The clinical implications of these recent observations have not been realized; the marked individual differences in drug effects on aggressive behavior may, at least in part, be based on neurochemical and physiological changes engendered by distinct social experiences.

Alcohol's effects on aggression resemble those produced by barbiturates and benzodiazepines, which blurs the distinction between therapeutic drugs and drugs of abuse. Curiously, the statistical and experimental data on alcohol in humans are considerably more numerous than those on alcohol in animals. It has been difficult to reproduce under controlled laboratory conditions the most socially relevant alcohol-aggression phenomena, although recent investigations into endocrine mechanisms may provide clues as to the mechanism for the effects of alcohol on aggression. No workable preparation exists for the study of the interrelationship between alcohol self-administration at intoxicating dose levels on social and aggressive behavior.

The identification of distinctive genetic and environmental factors and their mutual interactions may enhance the predictability of vehement aggressive and violent acts by the rare individual under the influence of psychotomimetic drugs. Research in animals and in humans highlights important interactions between stressful environmental conditions and antisocial personalities and the behavioral effects of hallucinogens and narcotics. The discovery of regulatory enzymes and receptors for neuropeptides, neuroamines, and steroids, as well as for drugs, promises to increase our understanding of the neurobiological mechanisms of aggression, to replace the current trial-and-error approach to the psychopharmacology of aggression.

ACKNOWLEDGMENTS

The preparation of this review and the experimental work from our own laboratory have been supported by research grants from the United States Public Health Service, National Institute on Drug Abuse (DA02632), and National Institute on Alcohol Abuse and Alcoholism (AA05122). I thank my colleagues Drs. J. F. DeBold, K. Noda, and J. P. Scott for their constructive comments, and Mr. J. T. Sopko for his expert assistance in assembling the computerized bibliographic database.

4. REFERENCES

ABBOTT, D. H., HOLMAN, S. D., BERMAN, M., NEFF, D. A., and GOY, R. W., 1984, Effects of opiate antagonists on hormones and behavior of male and female rhesus monkeys, *Arch. Sexual Behav.* **13**:1–25.

ABEL, E. L., 1975, Cannabis and aggression in animals, *Behav. Biol.* **14**:1–20.

ABEL, E. L., 1977, The relationship between cannabis and violence: A review, *Psychol. Bull.* **84**:193–211.

ABEL, E. L., and ZEIDENBERG, P., 1985, Age, alcohol and violent death: A postmortem study, *J. Stud. Alcohol* **46**:228–231.

ABEL, E. L., STRASBURGER, E. L., and ZEIDENBERG, P., 1985, Seasonal, monthly, and day-of-week trends in homicide as affected by alcohol and race, *Alcoholism Clin. Exp. Res.* **9**:281–283.

ABRAMSON, H. A., and EVANS, L. T., 1954, Lysergic acid diethylamide (LSD 25). II. Psychobiological effects on the Siamese fighting fish, *Science* **120**:990–991.

ADAMEC, R. E., and STARK-ADAMEC, C., 1983, Partial kindling and emotional bias in the cat: Lasting aftereffects of partial kindling of the ventral hippocampus. I. Behavioral changes, *Behav. Neural Biol.* **38**:205–222.

ALBERT, D. J., and WALSH, M. L., 1982, The inhibitory modulation of agonistic behavior in the rat brain: A review, *Neurosci. Biobehav. Rev.* **6**:125–143.

ALBERT, D. J., and WALSH, M. L., 1984, Neural systems and the inhibitory modulation of agonistic behavior: A comparison of mammalian species, *Neurosci. Biobehav. Rev.* **8**:5–24.

ALDERTON, H. R., and HODDINOTT, B. A., 1964, A controlled study of the use of thioridazine in the treatment of hyperactive and aggressive children in a children's psychiatric hospital, *Can. Psychiatr. J.* **9**:239–247.

ALEXANDRIS, A., and LUNDELL, F. W., 1968, Effect of thioridazine, amphetamine and placebo on the hyperkinetic syndrome and cognitive area in mentally deficient children, *Can. Med. Assoc. J.* **98**:92–96.

ALLEN, R. P., SAFER, D., and COVI, L., 1975, Effects of psychostimulants on aggression, *J. Nerv. Ment. Dis.* **160**:138–145.

ALLIKMETS, L. H. (1974) Cholinergic mechanisms in aggressive behaviour, *Med. Biol.* **52**:19–30.

ALLIKMETS, L. H., and LAPIN, I. P., 1967, Influence of lesions of the amygdaloid complex on behaviour and on effects of antidepressants in rats, *Int. J. Neuropharmacol.* **6**:99–108.

ALLIKMETS, L. H., DELGADO, J. M. R., and RICHARDS, S. A., 1968, Intra-mesencephalic injection of imipramine, promazine and chlorprothixene in awake monkeys, *Int. J. Neuropharmacol.* **7:**185–193.

ALLIKMETS, L. H., VAHING, V. A., and LAPIN, I. P., 1969, Dissimilar influences of imipramine, benactyzine and promazine on effects of micro-injections of noradrenaline, acetylcholine and serotonin into the amygdala in the cat, *Psychopharmacologia* **15:**392–403.

ALLIKMETS, L. H., STANLEY, M., and GERSHON, S., 1979, The effect of lithium on chronic haloperidol enhanced apomorphine aggression in rats, *Life Sci.* **25:**165–167.

ALTMANN, S. A., 1962, A field study of the sociobiology of rhesus monkeys, *Ann. NY Acad. Sci.* **102:**338–435.

ALTSHULER, K. Z., ABDULLAH, S., and RAINER, J. D., 1977, Lithium and aggressive behavior in patients with early total deafness, *Dis. Nerv. System* **38:**521–524.

ALVES, C. N., and CARLINI, E. A., 1973, Effects of acute and chronic administration of cannabis sativa extract on the mouse-killing behavior of rats, *Life Sci.* **13:**75–85.

ALVES, C. N., GOYOS, A. C., and CARLINI, E. A., 1973, Aggressiveness induced by marihuana and other psychotropic drugs in REM sleep deprived rats, *Pharmacol. Biochem. Behav.* **1:**183–189.

ANAND, M., GUPTA, G. P., and BHARGAVA, K. P., 1977, Modification of electroshock fighting by drugs known to interact with dopaminergic and noradrenergic neurons in normal and brain lesioned rats, *J. Pharm. Pharmacol.* **29:**437–439.

ANGRIST, B., and GERSHON, S., 1976, Clinical effects of amphetamine and L-dopa on sexuality and aggression, *Compr. Psychiatry* **17:**715–722.

ANGRIST, B. M., and GERSHON, S., 1969, Amphetamine abuse in New York City—1966–1968, *Semin. Psychiatry* **1:**195–207.

ANNELL, A. L., 1969, Lithium in the treatment of children and adolescents, *Acta Psychiatr. Scand.* (Suppl. 207):19–33.

ANTON, A. H., SCHWARTZ, R. P., and KRAMER, S., 1968, Catecholamines and behavior in isolated and grouped mice, *J. Psychiatr. Res.* **6:**211–220.

APFELBACH, R., 1976, Erhöhung der Beutefang-Effektivität durch Librium, *Naturwissenschaften* **63:**581.

APFELBACH, R., 1978, Instinctive predatory behavior of the ferret *(Putorius putorius furo* L.) modified by chlordiazepoxide hydrochloride (Librium), *Psychopharmacology* **59:**179–182.

APFELBACH, R., and DELGADO, J. M. R., 1974, Social hierarchy in monkeys *(Macaca mulatta)* modified by chlordiazepoxide hydrochloride, *Neuropharmacology* **13:**11–20.

APPLEGATE, C. D., 1980, 5,7-Dihydroxytryptamine-induced mouse killing and behavioral reversal with ventricular administration of serotonin in rats, *Behav. Neural Biol.* **30:**178–190.

ARNOLD, L. E., STROBL, D., and WEISENBERG, A., 1972, Hyperkinetic adult: Study of the "paradoxical" amphetamine response, *JAMA* **222:**693–694.

ARNOLD, L. E., KIRILCUK, V., CORSON, S. A., and CORSON, E. O., 1973, Levoamphetamine and dextroamphetamine: Differential effect on aggression and hyperkinesis in children and dogs, *Am. J. Psychiatry* **130:**165–170.

ASBERG, M., THOREN, P., TRASKMAN, L., BERTILSSON, L., and RINGBERGER, V., 1976, "Serotonin depression"—A biochemical subgroup within the affective disorders? *Science* **191:**478–480.

AVIS, H. H., 1974, The neuropharmacology of aggression: A critical review, *Psychol. Bull.* **81:**47–63.

AVIS, H. H., and PEEKE, H. V. S., 1975, Differentiation by morphine of two types of aggressive behavior in the convict cichlid *(Cichlasoma nigrofasciatum), Psychopharmacologia* **43:**287–288.

AVIS, H. H., and Peeke, H. V. S., 1979a, Morphine withdrawal induced behavior in the Syrian hamster *(Mesocricetus auratus), Pharmacol. Biochem. Behav.* **11:**11–15.

Avis, H. H., and Peeke, H. V. S., 1979b, The effects of pargyline, scopolamine, and imipramine on territorial aggression in the convict cichlid *(Cichlasoma nigrofasciatum), Psychopharmacolgy* **66:**1-2.
Azcarate, C. L., 1975, Minor tranquilizers in the treatment of aggression, *J. Nerv. Ment. Dis.* **160:**100-107.
Azrin, N. H., Hutchinson, R. R., and Hake, D. F., 1966, Extinction-induced aggression, *J. Exp. Anal. Behav.* **9:**191-204.
Babor, T. F., Meyer, R. E., Mirin, S. M., McNamee, H. B., and Davies, M., 1976, Behavioral and social effects of heroin self-administration and withdrawal, *Arch. Gen. Psychiatry* **33:**363-367.
Babor, T. F., Mendelson, J. H., Gallant, D., and Kuehnle, J. C., 1978a, Interpersonal behavior in group discussion during marijuana intoxication, *Int. J. Addictions* **13:**89-102.
Babor, T. F., Mendelson, J. H., Uhly, B., and Kuelnle, J. C., 1978b, Social effects of marijuana use in a recreational setting, *Int. J. Addictions* **13:**947-959.
Babor, T. F., Berglas, S., Mendelson, J. H., Ellingboe, J., and Miller, K., 1983, Alcohol affect, and the disinhibition of verbal behavior, *Psychopharmacology* **80:**53-60.
Bach-Y-Rita, G., Lion, J. R., Climent, C. E., and Ervin, F. R., 1971, Episodic dyscontrol: A study of 130 violent patients, *Am. J. Psychiatry* **127:**1473-1478.
Bainbridge, J. G., and Greenwood D. T., 1971, Tranquillizing effects of propranolol demonstrated in rats, *Neuropharmacology* **10:**453-458.
Ball, J. C., Rosen, L., Flueck, J. A., and Nurco, D. N., 1983, Lifetime criminality of heroin addicts, in: *Alcohol, Drug Abuse and Aggression* (E. Gottheil, K. A. Druley, T. E. Skolada, and H. M. Waxman, eds.), Charles C. Thomas, Springfield, IL, pp. 26-40.
Bammer, G., and Eichelman, B., 1983, Ethanol effects on shock-induced fighting and muricide by rats, *Aggressive Behav.* **9:**175-181.
Bandler, R., 1982a, Identification of neuronal cell bodies mediating components of biting attack behaviour in the cat: Induction of jaw opening following microinjections of glutamate into hypothalamus, *Brain Res.* **245:**192-197.
Bandler, R., 1982b, Neural control of aggressive behaviour, *Trends Neurosci.* **5:**390-394.
Bandler, R. J., 1970, Cholinergic synapses in the lateral hypothalamus for the control of predatory aggression in the rat, *Brain Res.* **20:**409-424.
Bandura, A., 1973, *Aggression: A Social Learning Analysis,* Prentice-Hall, Englewood Cliffs, NJ.
Banerjee, U., 1971a, An inquiry into the genesis of aggression in mice induced by isolation, *Behaviour* **90:**86-99.
Banerjee, U., 1971b, Influence of some hormones and drugs on isolation induced aggression in male mice, *Commun. Behav. Biol.* **6:**163-170.
Banks, W. A., and Kastin, A. J., 1985, Permeability of the blood-brain barrier to neuropeptides: The case for penetration, *Psychoneuroendocrinology* **10:**385-399.
Barkov, N. K., 1973, Effect of neuroleptics on aggressive behavior, *Neurosci. Behav. Physiol.* **6:**119-121. Translated from Russion in: *Zhurnal Nueropatologi i Psikhiatri,* 1972, **72:**108-111.
Barnes, H. W., Cunningham, B. L., Penberthy, C., and Gogerty, J. H., 1967, Effects of various CNS-active substances and CNS-modifying influences on mouse-killing behaviour of rats (abstr.), *Pharmacologist* **9:**200.
Barnett, A., Taber, R. I., and Roth, F. E., 1969, Activity of antihistamines in laboratory antidepressant tests, *Int. J. Neuropharmacol.* **8:**73-79.
Barnett, A., Taber, R. I., and Steiner, S. S., 1974, The behavioral pharmacology of Sch 12679, a new psychoactive agent, *Psychopharmacologia* **36:**281-290.
Barnett, S. A., 1975, *The Rat. A Study in Behavior,* University of Chicago Press, Chicago.
Barr, G. A., Gibbons, J. L., and Bridger, W. H., 1976, Neuropharmacological regulation of mouse killing by rats, *Behav. Biol.* **17:**143-159.

BARR, G. A., GIBBONS, J. L., and BRIDGER, W. H., 1977, Inhibition of rat predatory aggression by acute and chronic d- and l-amphetamine, *Brain Res.* **124**:565–570.

BARR, G. A., GIBBONS, J. L., and BRIDGER, W. H., 1979, A comparison of the effects of acute and subacute administration of beta-phenylethylamine and d-amphetamine on mouse killing behavior of rats, *Pharmacol. Biochem. Behav.* **11**:419–422.

BARTER, J. T., and REITE, M., 1969, Crime and LSD: The insanity plea, *Am. J. Psychiatry* **126**:113–119.

BAUEN, A., and POSSANZA, G. J., 1970, The mink as a psychopharmacological model, *Arch. Int. Pharmacodyn. Ther.* **186**:133–136.

BAXTER, B. L., 1964a, Lack of effect of LSD 25 on the hissing response elicited by electrical stimulation of the cat hypothalamus, *Fed. Proc.* **23**:147.

BAXTER, B. L., 1964b, The effect of chlordiazepoxide on the hissing response elicited via hypothalamic stimulation, *Life Sci.*, **3**:531–537.

BAXTER, B. L., 1968a, Elicitation of emotional behavior by electrical or chemical stimulation applied at the same loci in cat mesencephalon, *Exp. Neurol.* **21**:1–10.

BAXTER, B. L., 1968b, The effect of selected drugs on the "emotional" behavior elicited via hypothalamic stimulation, *Int. J. Neuropharmacol.* **7**:47–54.

BEATTY, W. W., 1979, Gonadal hormones and sex differences in nonreproductive behaviors in rodents: Organizational and activational influences, *Hormones Behav.* **12**:112–163.

BEATTY, W. W., COSTELLO, K. B., and BERRY, S. L., 1984, Suppression of play fighting by amphetamine: Effects of catecholamine antagonists, agonists and synthesis inhibitors, *Pharmacol. Biochem. Behav.* **20**: 747–755.

BECK, C. H. M., and COOPER, S. J., 1987, β-Carboline FG 7142-reduced aggression in male rats: Reversed by the benzodiazepine receptor antagonist, Ro15-1788. *Pharmacol. Biochem. Behav.* (in press).

BELLAROSA, A., BEDFORD, J. A., and WILSON, M. C., 1980, Sociopharmacology of d-amphetamine in *Macaca arctoides*, *Pharmacol. Biochem. Behav.* **13**:221–228.

BENDER, L., and COTTINGTON, F., 1942, The use of amphetamine sulfate (benzedrine) in child psychiatry, *Am. J. Psychiatry* **99**:116–121.

BENNETT, R. M., BUSS, A. H., and CARPENTER, J. A., 1969, Alcohol and human physical aggression, *Q. J. Stud. Alcohol* **30**:870–876.

BENTON, D., 1983, Do animal studies tell us anything about the relationship between testosterone and human aggression? in: *Animal Models of Human Behavior* (G. C. L. Davey, ed.), Wiley, New York, pp. 281–298.

BENTON, D., 1984, The long-term effects of naloxone, dibutyryl cyclic CMP, and chlorpromazine on aggression in mice monitored by an automated device, *Aggressive Behav.* **10**:79–89.

BENTON, D., 1985, Mu and kappa opiate receptor involvement in agonistic behaviour in mice, *Pharmacol. Biochem. Behav.* **23**:871–876.

BENTON, D., SMOOTHY, R., and BRAIN, P. F., 1985, Comparisons of the influence of morphine sulphate, morphine-3-glucuronide and tifluadom on social encounters in mice, *Physiol. Behav.* **35**:689–693.

BERKOWITZ, L., 1983, Aversively stimulated aggression: Some parallels and differences in research with animals and humans, *Am. Psychologist* **38**:1135–1144.

BERNER, W., BROWNSTONE, G., and SLUGA, W., 1983, The cyproteronacetat treatment of sexual offenders, *Neurosci. Biobehav. Rev.* **7**:441–443.

BERNHARDSON, G., and GUNNE, L-M, 1972, Forty-six cases of psychosis in cannabis abusers, *Int. J. Addictions* **7**:9–16.

BERNSTEIN, I. S., 1981, Dominance: The baby and the bathwater, *Behav. Brain Sci.* **4**:419–457.

BERNSTON, G. G., and LEIBOWITZ, S. F., 1973, Biting attack in cats: Evidence for central muscarinic mediation, *Brain Res.* **51**:366–370.

BERNTSON, G. G., BEATTIE, M. S., and WALKER, J. M., 1976, Effects of nicotine and muscarinic compounds on biting attack in the cat, *Pharmacol. Biochem. Behav.* **5:**235–239.

BERTILSON, H. S., MEAD, J. D., MORGRET, M. K., and DENGERIMK, H. A., 1977, Measurement of mouse squeals for 23 hours as evidence of long-term effects of alcohol on aggression in pairs of mice, *Psychol. Rep.* **41:**247–250.

BISBEE, D. S., and CAHOON, D. D., 1973, The effects of induced nausea upon shock-elicited aggression, *Bull. Psychonom. Soc.* **1:**19–21.

BLANCHARD, D. C., and BLANCHARD, R. J., 1984, Inadequacy of pain–aggression hypothesis revealed in naturalistic settings, *Aggressive Behav.* **10:**33–46.

BLANCHARD, R. J., FUKUNAGA, K., BLANCHARD, D. C., and KELLEY, M. J., 1975, Conspecific aggression in the laboratory rat, *J. Comp. Physiol. Psychol.* **80:**1204–1209.

BLANCHARD, R. J., BLANCHARD, D. C., and TAKAHASHI, L. K., 1978, Pain and aggression in the rat, *Behav. Biol.* **23:**291–305.

BLÄSIG, J., HERZ, A., REINHOLD, K., and ZIEGLGANSBERGER, S., 1973, Development of physical dependence on morphine in respect to time and dosage and quantification of the precipitated withdrawal syndrome in rats, *Psychopharmacologia* **33:**19–38.

BLUMER, D., 1971, Das Sexualverhalten der Schlafenlappenepileptiker vor und nach chirurgischer Behandlung, *J. Neuro-Visceral Relations* (Suppl. 10):469–476.

BLUMER, D., and MIGEON, C., 1975, Hormone and hormonal agents in the treatment of aggression, *J. Nerv. Ment. Dis.* **160** (2)**:**127–137.

BLUMER, D. P., WILLIAMS, H. W., and MARK, V. H., 1974, The study and treatment, on a neurological ward, of abnormally aggressive patients with focal brain disease, *Confinia Neurol.* **36:**125–176.

BOHMAN, M., 1978, Some genetic aspects of alcoholism and criminality, *Arch. Gen. Psychiatry* **35:**269–276.

BOISSIER, J. R., GRASSET, S., and SIMON, P., 1968, Effect of some psychotropic drugs on mice from a spontaneously aggressive strain, *J. Pharm. Pharmacol.* **20:**972–973.

BOND, A., and LADER, M., 1979, Benzodiazepines and aggression, in: *Psychopharmacology of Aggression* (M. Sandler, ed.), Raven Press, New York, pp. 173–182.

BORGEN, L. A., KHALSA, J. H., KING, W. T., and DAVIS, M., 1970, Strain differences in morphine-withdrawal-induced aggression in rats, *Psychonom. Sci.* **21:**35–36.

BOSHKA, S. C., WEISMAN, H. M., and THOR, D. H., 1966, A technique for inducing aggression in rats utilizing morphine withdrawal, *Psychol. Rec.* **16:**541–543.

BOWDEN, N. J., and BRAIN, P. F., 1978, Blockade of testosterone-maintained intermale fighting in albino laboratory mice by an aromatization inhibitor, *Physiol. Behav.* **20:**543–546.

BOYATZIS, R. E., 1974, The effect of alcohol consumption on the aggressive behavior of males in a stressful setting, *Q. J. Stud. Alcohol* **35:**959–972.

BOYATZIS, R. E., 1975, The predisposition toward alcohol-related interpersonal aggression in men, *J. Stud. Alcohol* **36:**1196–1326.

BOYKO-WILMOT, C., and VANDER WENDE, C., 1981, Phencyclidine increases the intensity and spontaneity of fighting in isolated mice, *Neurosci. Abstr.* **7:**261.

BOYLE, D., and TOBIN, J. M., 1961, Pharmaceutical management of behavior disorders, *J. Med. Soc. NJ* **58:**427–429.

BRADFORD, D. L., OLIVIER, B., VAN DALEN, D., and SCHIPPER, J., 1984, Serenics: The pharmacology of fluprazine and DU 28412, in *Ethopharmacological Aggression Research* (K. A. Miczek, M. R. Kruk, and B. Olivier, eds.), Liss, New York, pp. 191–207.

BRADLEY, C., 1937, The behavior of children receiving benzedrine, *Am. J. Psychiatry* **94:**577–585.

BRADY, J. V., and NAUTA, W. J. H., 1953, Subcortical mechanisms in emotional behavior: Affective changes following septal forebrain lesion in the albino rat, *J. Comp. Physiol. Psychol.* **46:**339–346.

BRAESTRUP, C., and SQUIRES, R. F., 1977, Brain specific benzodiazepine receptors in rats characterized by high affinity ³H-diazepam binding, *Proc. Natl. Acad. Sci. USA* **74**:3805.
BRAIN, P. F., 1972, Oral lithium chloride, endocrine function and isolation-induced agonistic behaviour in male albino mice, *J. Endocrinol.* **55**:1–2.
BRAIN, P. F., 1975, What does individual housing mean to a mouse? *Life Sci.* **16**:187–200.
BRAIN, P. F., 1981, Differentiating types of attack and defense in rodents, in: *Multidisciplinary Approaches to Aggression Research* (P. F. Brain and D. Benton, eds.), Elsevier, Amsterdam, pp. 53–78.
BRAIN, P. F., 1986, *Alcohol and Aggression*, Croom Helm, London.
BRAIN, P. F., and AL-MALIKI, S., 1979, Effects of lithium chloride injections on rank-related fighting, maternal aggression and locust-killing responses in naive and experienced "TO" strain mice, *Pharmacol. Biochem. Behav.* **10**:663–669.
BRAIN, P. F., and NOWELL, N. W., 1970, Some observations on intermale aggression testing in albino mice, *Commun. Behav. Biol.* **5**:7–17.
BRAIN, P. F., and POOLE, A. E., 1976, The role of endocrines in isolation-induced intermale fighting in albino laboratory mice. II. Sex steroid influences in aggressive mice, *Aggressive Behav.* **2**:55–76.
BRAIN, P. F., EVANS, C. M., and POOLE, A. E., 1974, Studies on the effects of cyproterone acetate administered in adulthood or in early life on subsequent endocrine function and agonistic behaviour in male albino laboratory mice, *J. Endocrinol.* **61**:22–23.
BRAIN, P. F., BENTON, D., GOLDSMITH, J. F., and BOWDEN, N. J., 1976, Influences of cyproterone acetate and ethamoxytriphetol on fighting behaviour and sex accessory weights of castrated, testosterone-implanted or sham-implanted "aggressive" mice, *J. Endocrinol.* **69**:16.
BRAIN, P. F., AL-MALIKI, S., and BENTON, D., 1981a, Attempts to determine the status of electroshock-induced attack in male laboratory mice, *Behav. Proc.* **6**:171–189.
BRAIN, P. F., BENTON, D., CHILDS, G., and PARMIGIANI, S., 1981b, The effect of the type of opponent in tests of murine aggression, *Behav. Proc.* **6**:319–327.
BRAIN, P. F., JONES, S. E., BRAIN, S., and BENTON, D., 1984, Sequence analysis of social behavior illustrating the actions of two antagonists of endogenous opioids, in: *Ethopharmacological Aggression Research* (K. A. Miczek, M. R. Kruk, and B. Olivier, eds.), Liss, New York, pp. 43–58.
BRAIN, P. F., SMOOTHY, R., and BENTON, D., 1985, An ethological analysis of the effects of tifluadom on social encounters in male albino mice, *Pharmacol. Biochem. Behav.* **23**:979–985.
BRAUD, W. G., and WEIBEL, J. E., 1969, Acquired stimulus control of drug-induced changes in aggressive display in *Betta splendens*, *J. Exp. Analy. Behav.* **12**:773–777.
BREESE, G. R., BAUMEISTER, A. A., MCCOWN, T. J., EMERICK, S. G., FRYE, G. D., CROTTY, K., and MUELLER, R. A., 1984a, Behavioral differences between neonatal and adult 6-hydroxydopamine treated rats to dopamine agonists: Relevance to neurological symptoms in clinical syndromes with reduced brain dopamine, *J. Pharmacol. Exp. Ther.* **231**:343–354.
BREESE, G. R., BAUMEISTER, A. A., MCCOWN, T. J., EMERICK, S. G., FRYE, G. D., and MUELLER, R. A., 1984b, Neonatal-6-hydroxydopamine treatment: Model of susceptability for self-mutilation in the Lesch–Nyhan syndrome, *Pharmacol. Biochem. Behav.* **21**:459–461.
BRILL, H., 1969, Drugs and aggression, *Med. Counterpoint* **1**(9):33–38.
BROMBERG, W., and RODGERS, T. C., 1946, Marihuana and aggressive crime, *Am. J. Psychiatry* **102**:825–827.
BROWN, C. R., 1978, The use of benzodiazepines in prison populations, *J. Clin. Psychiatry* **38**:219–222.
BRUNAUD, M., and SIOU, G., 1959, Action de substances psychotropes, chez le rat, sur un etat d'aggressivite provoquee, in: *Neuro-Psychopharmacology* (P. B. Bradley, P. Deniker, and C. Radouco-Thomas, eds.), Elsevier, Amsterdam, pp. 282–286.

BURGESS, J. W., WITT, P. N., PHOEBUS, E., and WEISBARD, C, 1980, The spacing of rhesus monkey troops changes when a few group members receive delta-9THC or d-amphetamine, *Pharmacol. Biochem. Behav.* **13:**121-124.
BURKHALTER, J. E., and BALSTER, R. L., 1979, The effects of phencyclidine on isolation-induced aggression in mice, *Psychol. Rep.* **45:**571-576.
BUSS, A. H., 1961, *The Psychology of Aggression*, Wiley, New York.
BYLES, J. A., 1978, Violence, alcohol problems and other problems in disintegrating families, *J. Stud. Alcohol* **39:**551-553.
CADE, J. F. J., 1949, Lithium salts in the treatment of psychotic excitement, *Med. J. Aust.* **2:**349-352.
CADORET, R. J., O'GORMAN, T. W., TROUGHTON, E., and HEYWOOD, E., 1985, Alcoholism and antisocial personality, *Arch. Gen. Psychiatry* **42:**161-167.
CAIN, D. P., 1974, Olfactory bulbectomy: Neural structures involved in irritability and aggression in the male rat, *J. Comp. Physiol. Psychol.* **86:**213-220.
CAIRNS, R. B., and NAKELSKI, J. S., 1971, On fighting in mice: Ontogenetic and experiential determinants, *J. Comp. Physiol. Psychol.* **74:**354-364.
CAIRNS, R. B., and SCHOLZ, S. D., 1973, Fighting in mice: Dyadic escalation and what is learned, *J. Comp. Physiol. Psychol.* **85:**540-550.
CAIRNS, R. B., HOOD, K. E., and MIDLAM, J., 1985, On fighting in mice: Is there a sensitive period for isolation effects? *Animal Behav.* **33:**166-180.
CAMERON, J. S., SPECHT, P. G., and WENDT, G. R., 1965, Effects of amphetamines on moods, emotions, and motivations, *J. Psychol.* **61:**93-121.
CAMPBELL, M., FISH, B., KOREIN, J., SHAPIRO, T., COLLINS, P., and KOH, C., 1972, Lithium and chlorpromazine: A controlled crossover study of hyperactive severely disturbed young children, *J. Autism Child. Schizophrenia* **2:**234-263.
CAMPBELL, M., SMALL, A. M., COLLINS, P. J., FREIDMAN, E., DAVID, R., and GENIESER, N., 1976, Levodopa and levoamphetamine: A crossover study in young schizphrenic children, *Curr. Ther. Res.* **19:**70-86.
CAMPBELL, M., COHEN, I. L., and SMALL, A. M., 1982, Drugs in aggressive behavior, *J. Am. Acad. Child Psychiatry* **21:**107-117.
CAMPBELL, W. E., 1973, Behavioral modification of hyperkinetic dogs, *Mod. Vet. Pract.* **54:**49-52.
CARDER, B., and OLSON, J., 1972, Marihuana and shock induced aggression in rats, *Physiol. Behav.* **8:**599-602.
CARDER, B., and SBORDONE, R., 1975, Mescaline treated rats attack immobile targets, *Pharmacol. Biochem. Behav.* **3:**923-925.
CAREY, J. T., and MANDEL, J., 1969, The bay area "speed scene," *J. Psychedelic Drugs* **2:**189-209.
CARLINI, E. A., 1968, Tolerance to chronic administration of *Cannabis sativa* (marihuana) in rats, *Pharmacology* **1:**135-142.
CARLINI, E. A., 1974, *Cannabis sativa* and aggressive behavior in laboratory animals, *Arch. Invest. Med.* **5:**161-172.
CARLINI, E. A., 1977, Further studies of the aggressive behavior induced by delta-9-tetrahydrocannabinol in REM sleep-deprived rats, *Psychopharmacology* **53:**135-145.
CARLINI, E. A., and GONZALEZ, C., 1972, Aggressive behaviour induced by marihuana compounds and amphetamine in rats previously made dependent on morphine, *Experientia* **28:**542-544.
CARLINI, E. A., and LINDSEY, C. J., 1974, Pharmacological manipulations of brain catecholamines and the aggressive behavior induced by marihuana in REM-sleep-deprived rats, *Aggressive Behav.* **1:**81-99.
CARLINI, E. A., and MASUR, J., 1969, Development of aggressive behavior in rats by chronic administration of cannabis sativa (marihuana), *Life Sci.* **8:**607-620.

CARLINI, E. A., and MASUR, J., 1970, Development of fighting behavior in starved rats by chronic administration of (−) delta-9-tetrahydocannabinol and cannabis extracts, *Commun. Behav. Biol.* **5:**57–81.

CARLINI, E. A., and SANTOS, M., 1970, Structure activity relationship of four tetrahydrocannabinols and the pharmacological activity of five semi-purified extracts of *Cannabis sativa*, *Psychopharmacologia* **18:**82–93.

CARLINI, E. A., HAMAOUI, A., and MARTZ, R. M. W., 1972, Factors influencing the aggressiveness elicited by marihuana in food-deprived rats, *Br. J. Pharmacol.* **44:**794–804.

CARLINI, E. A., MASUR, J., CZERESNIA, S., and SKITNEVSKY, H., 1974, Brain amine levels and competitive behavior between rats in a straight runaway, *Pharmacol. Biochem. Behav.* **2:**55–62.

CARLINI, E. A., LINDSEY, C. J., and TUFIK, S., 1976, Environmental and drug interference with effects of marihuana, *Ann. NY Acad. Sci.* **281:**229–242.

CARLINI, E. A., LINDSEY, C. J., and TUFIK, S., 1977, Cannabis, catecholamines, rapid eye movement sleep and aggressive behavior, *Br. J. Pharmacol.* **61:**371–379.

CARPENTER, J. A., and ARMENTI, N. P., 1972, Some effects of ethanol on human sexual and aggressive behavior, in: *The Biology of Alcoholism: Physiology and Behavior* (B. Kissin and H. Begleiter, eds.), Plenum, New York, pp. 509–543.

CHAMOVE, A. S., and HARLOW, H. F., 1970, Exaggeration of self-aggression following alcohol ingestion in rhesus monkeys, *J. Abnorm. Psychol.* **75:**207–209.

CHANCE, M. R. A., 1946a, A peculiar form of social behavior induced in mice by amphetamine, *Behaviour* **1:**60–70.

CHANCE, M. R. A., 1946b, Aggregation as a factor influencing the toxicity of sympathomimetic amines in mice, *J. Pharmacol. Exp. Ther.* **87:**214–219.

CHANCE, M. R. A., 1968, Ethology and psychopharmacology, in: *Psychopharmacology* (C. Joyce, ed.), Tavistock, London, pp. 283–318.

CHANCE, M. R. A., and SILVERMAN, A. P., 1964, The structure of social behaviour and drug action, in: *Animal Behaviour and Drug Action* (H. Steinberg and A. V. S. de Reuck, eds.), Churchill, London, pp. 65–79.

CHANCE, M. R. A., MACKINTOSH, J. H., and DIXON, A. K., 1973, The effects of ethyl alcohol on social encounters between mice, *J. Alcoholism* **8:**90–93.

CHARPENTIER, J., 1969, Analysis and measurement of aggressive behaviour in mice, in: *Aggressive Behaviour* (S. Garattini and E. B. Sigg, eds.), Exerpta Medica Foundation, Amsterdam, pp. 86–100.

CHEEK, F. E., and HOLSTEIN, C. M., 1971, Lysergic acid diethylamide tartrate (LSD-25) dosage levels, group differences, and social interaction, *J. Nerv. Ment. Dis.* **153:**133–147.

CHEN, G., BOHNER, B., and BRATTON, A. C., 1963, The influence of certain central depressants on fighting behavior of mice, *Arch. Int. Pharmacodyn. Ther.* **142:**30–34.

CHEREK, D. R., 1981, Effects of smoking different doses of nicotine on human aggressive behavior, *Psychopharmacology* **75:**339–345.

CHEREK, D. R., and STEINBERG, J. L., 1986, Effects of drugs on human aggression, in: *Advances in Human Psychopharmacology* (G. D. Burrows and J. S. Werry, eds.), JAI Press, Greenwich, CT (in press).

CHEREK, D. R., and THOMPSON, T., 1972, Schedule-induced aggression: Effects of delta-9-hydrocannabinol, Proceedings, 80th Annual Convention, American Psychiatric Association, pp. 847–848.

CHEREK, D. R., THOMPSON, T., and HEISTAD, G. T., 1972, Effects of delta-1-tetrahydrocannabinol and food deprivation level on responding maintained by the opportunity to attack, *Physiol. Behav.* **9:**795–800.

CHEREK, D. R., THOMPSON, T., and HEISTAD, G. T., 1973, Responding maintained by the opportunity to attack during an interval food reinforcement schedule, *J. Exp. Anal. Behav.* **19:**113–123.

CHEREK, D. R., THOMPSON, T., and KELLY, T., 1980, Chronic delta-9-tetrahydrocannabinol administration and schedule-induced aggression, *Pharmacol. Biochem. Behav.* **12**:305–309.
CHEREK, D. R., STEINBERG, J. L., and BRAUCHI, J. T., 1983, Effects of caffeine on human aggressive behavior, *Psychiatry Res.* **8**:137–145.
CHEREK, D. R., STEINBERG, J. L., and BRAUCHI, J. T., 1984, Regular or decaffeinated coffee and subsequent human aggressive behavior, *Psychiatry Res.* **11**:251–258.
CHEREK, D. R., STEINBERG, J. L., and MANNO, B. R., 1985, Effects of alcohol on human aggressive behavior, *J. Stud. Alcohol* **46**:321–328.
CHOI, S. Y., 1975, Death in young alcoholics, *J. Stud. Alcohol* **36**:1224–1229.
CHOPRA, R. M., CHOPRA, G. S., and CHOPRA, I. C., 1942, *Cannabis sativa* in relation to mental disease and crime in India, *Ind. J. Med. Res.* **30**:155–171.
CHRISTMAS, A. J., and MAXWELL, D. R., 1970, A comparison of the effects of some benzodiazepines and other drugs on aggressive and exploratory behaviour in mice and rats, *Neuropharmacology* **9**:17–29.
CIARANELLO, R. D., LIPSKY, A., and AXELROD, J., 1974, Association between fighting behavior and catecholamine biosynthetic enzyme activity in two inbred mouse sublines, *Proc. Natl. Acad. Sci. USA* **71**:3006–3008.
CLARK, C. R., and NOWELL, N. W., 1979, The effect of the antiestrogen Cl-628 on androgen-induced aggressive behavior in castrated male mice, *Hormones Behav.* **12**:205–210.
CLARK, C. R., and NOWELL, N. W., 1980, The effect of the non-steroidal antiandrogen flutamide on neural receptor binding of testosterone and intermale aggressive behavior in mice, *Psychoneuroendocrinology* **5**:39–45.
CLEARY, J., HERAKOVIC, J., and POLING, A., 1981, Effects of phencyclidine on shock-induced aggression in rats, *Pharmacol. Biochem. Behav.* **15**:813–818.
CLONINGER, C. R., 1983, Antisocial behavior, in: *Psychopharmacology 1* (H. Hippius and G. Winokur, eds.), Elsevier, Amsterdam, pp. 353–370.
COCKETT, R., and MARKS, V., 1969, Amphetamine taking among young offenders, *Br. J. Psychiatry* **115**:1203–1204.
COHEN, M., OAKS, G., FREEDMAN, N., ENGELHARDT, D. M., and MARGOLIS, R. A., 1968, Family interaction patterns, drug treatment, and change in social aggression, *Arch. Gen. Psychiatry* **19**:50–56.
COID, J., 1982, Alcoholism and violence, *Drug Alcohol Depend.* **9**:1–13.
COLE, H. F., and WOLF, H. H., 1966, The effects of some psychotropic drugs on conditioned avoidance and aggressive behaviors *Psychopharmacologia* **8**:389–396.
COLE, H. F., and WOLF, H. H., 1970, Laboratory evaluation of aggressive behavior of the grasshopper mouse *(Onychomys), J. Pharm. Sci.* **59**:969–971.
COMBS-ORME, T., TAYLOR, J. R., SCOTT, E. B., and HOLMES, S. J., 1983, Violent deaths among alcoholics: A descriptive study, *J. Stud. Alcohol* **44**:938–949.
CONNER, R. L., and LEVINE, S., 1969, Hormonal influences on aggressive behavior, in: *Aggressive Behaviour* (S. Garattini and E. B. Sigg, eds.), Wiley, New York, pp. 150–163.
CONNERS, C. K., 1969, A teacher rating scale for use in drug studies with children, *Am. J. Psychiatry* **126**:152–156.
CONNERS, C. K., 1972, Psychological effects of stimulant drugs in children with minimal brain dysfunction, *Pediatrics* **49**:702–708.
CONNERS, C. K., KRAMER, R., ROTHSCHILD, G. H., SCHWARTZ, L., and STONE, A., 1971, Treatment of young delinquent boys with diphenylhydantoin sodium and methyphenidate, *Arch. Gen. Psychiatry* **24**:156–160.
CONNOLLY, J. R., 1968, Behavioral disorders in mental retardates, *Pennsylvania Med.* **71**:67–69.
CONSOLO, S., GARATTINI, S., GHIELMETTI, R., and VALZELLI, L., 1965a, Concentrations of amphetamine in the brain in normal or aggressive mice, *J. Pharm. Pharmacol.* **17**:666.

Consolo, S., Garattini, S., and Valzelli, L., 1965b, Amphetamine toxicity in aggressive mice, *J. Pharm. Pharmacol.* **17**:53–54.

Cook, L., and Weidley, E., 1957, Behavioral effects of some psychopharmacological agents, *Ann. NY Acad. Sci.* **66**:740–752.

Cook, L., and Weidley, E., 1960, Effects of a series of psychopharmacological agents on isolation induced attack behavior in mice, *Fed. Proc.* **19**:22.

Cooper, A. J., Ismail, A. A. A., Phanjoo, A. L., and Love, D. L., 1972, Antiandrogen (cyproterone acetate) therapy in deviant hypersexuality, *Br. J. Psychiatry* **120**:59–63.

Corenblum, B., 1983, Reactions to alcohol-related marital violence: Effects of one's own abuse experience and alcohol problems on causal attributions, *J. Stud. Alcohol* **44**(4):665–674.

Corson, S. A., Corson, E. O.'L., Arnold, L. E., and Knopp, W., 1976, Animal models of violence and hyperkinesis, in: *Animal Models in Human Psychobiology* (G. Serban and A. Kling, eds.), Plenum, New York, pp. 111–139.

Coscina, D. V., Seggie, J., Godse, D. D., and Stancer, H. C., 1973, Induction of rage in rats by central injection of 6-hydroxydopamine, *Pharmacol. Biochem. Behav.* **1**:1–6.

Courvoisier, S., Fournel, J., Ducrot, J., Kolsky, M., and Koetschet, P., 1953, Proprietes pharmacodynamiques du chlorhydrate de chloro-3(dimethylamino-3'propyl)-10 phenothiazine (4.560 R.P.), *Arch. Int. Pharmacodyn. Ther.* **92**:305–361.

Coutinho, C. B., King, M., Carbone, J. J., Manning, J. E., Boff, E., and Crews, T., 1971, Chlordiazepoxide metabolism as related to the reduction in the aggressive behaviour of cynomolgus primates, *Xenobiotica* **1**:287–301.

Covi, L., and Uhlenhuth, E. H., 1969, Methodological problems in the psychopharmacological study of the dangerous anti-social personality, in: *Aggressive Behavior* (S. Garattini and E. R. Sigg, eds.), Wiley Interscience, New York, pp. 326–335.

Crawley, J. N., 1985, Exploratory behavior models of anxiety in mice, *Neurosci. Biobehav. Rev.* **9**:37–44.

Crawley, J. N., Schleidt, W. M., and Contrera, J. F., 1975, Does social environment decrease propensity to fight in male mice? *Behav. Biol.* **15**:73–83.

Crowley, T. J., 1972, Dose-dependent facilitation or suppression of rat fighting by methamphetamine, phenobarbital, or imipramine, *Psychopharmacologia* **27**:213–222.

Crowley, T. J., 1983, Substance abuse research in monkey social groups, in: *Ethopharmacology: Primate Models of Neuropsychiatric Disorder* (K. A. Miczek, ed.), Liss, New York, pp. 255–275.

Crowley, T. J., and Rutledge, C. O., 1974, Chronic methamphetamine, imipramine and phenobarbital effects on shock-induced aggression in rats, in: *Drug Addiction. Neurobiology and Influences on Behavior* (J. M. Singh and H. Lal, eds.), Symposia Specialists, Miami, pp. 65–80.

Crowley, T. J., Stynes, A. J., Hydinger, M., and Kaufman, I. C., 1974, Ethanol, methamphetamine, pentobarbital, morphine, and monkey social behavior, *Arch. Gen. Psychiatry* **31**:829–838.

Crowley, T. J., Hydinger, M., Stynes, A. J., and Feiger, A., 1975, Monkey motor stimulation and altered social behavior during chronic methadone administration, *Psychopharmacologia* **43**:135–144.

Crowley, T. J., Macdonald, M. J., and Zerbe, G., 1985, Naltrexone: No effect on simian social and motor behavior, *Psychopharmacology* **87**:250–251.

Cunningham, M. A., Pillai, V., and Blachford, Rogers, W. J., 1968, Haloperidol in the treatment of children with severe behaviour disorders, *Br. J. Psychiatry* **114**:845–854.

Cutler, M. G., 1976, Changes in the social behaviour of laboratory mice during administration and on withdrawal from non-ataxic doses of ethyl alcohol, *Neuropharmacology* **15**:495–498.

Cutler, M. G., and Mackintosh, J. H., 1975, Effects of delta-9-tetrahydrocannabinol on social behaviour in the laboratory mouse and rat, *Psychopharmacologia* **44**:287–289.

CUTLER, M. G., MACKINTOSH, J. H., and CHANCE, M. R. A., 1975a, Effects of the environment on the behavioural response of mice to non-ataxic doses of ethyl alcohol, *Neuropharmacology* **14:**841–846.

CUTLER, M. G., MACKINTOSH, J. H., and CHANCE, M. R. A., 1975b, Effects of cannabis resin on social behaviour in the laboratory mouse, *Psychopharmacologia* **41:**271–276.

CUTLER, N., and HEISER, J. F., 1978, Retrospective diagnosis of hypomania following successful treatment of episodic violence with lithium: A case report, *Am. J. Psychiatry* **135**(6):753–754.

DALE, P. G., 1980, Lithium therapy in aggressive mentally subnormal patients, *Br. J. Psychiatry* **137:**469–474.

DALY, R. J., and KANE, F. J., JR., 1965, Two severe reactions to benzodiazepine compounds, *Am. J. Psychiatry* **122:**577–578.

DANTZER, R., ARNONE, M., and MORMEDE, P., 1980, Effects of frustration on behaviour and plasma corticosteroid levels in pigs, *Physiol. Behav.* **24:**1–4.

DANTZER, R., GUILLONEAU, D., MORMEDE, P., HERMAN, J. P., and LEMOAL, M., 1984, Influence of shock-induced fighting and social factors on dopamine turnover in cortical and limbic areas in the rat, *Pharmacol. Biochem. Behav.* **20:**331–335.

DARUNA, J. H., 1978, Patterns of brain monoamine activity and aggressive behavior, *Neurosci. Biobehav. Rev.* **2:**101–113.

DAS, N. N., DASGUPTA, S. R., and WERNER, G., 1954, Changes of behaviour and electroencephalogram in rhesus monkeys caused by chlorpromazine, *Arch. Int. Pharmacol. Ther.* **99:**451–457.

DAVANZO, J. P., and SYDOW, M., 1979, Inhibition of isolation-induced aggressive behavior with GABA transaminase inhibitors, *Psychopharmacology* **62:**23–27.

DAVANZO, J. P., DAUGHERTY, M., RUCKART, R., and KANG, L., 1966, Pharmacological and biochemical studies in isolation-induced fighting mice, *Psychopharmacologia* **9:**210–219.

DAVIS, W. M., and KHALSA, J. H., 1971a, Increased shock induced aggression during morphine withdrawal, *Life Sci.* **10:**1321–1327.

DAVIS, W. M., and KHALSA, J. H., 1971b, Some determinants of aggressive behavior induced by morphine withdrawal, *Psychonom. Sci.* **24:**13–15.

DEBOLD, J. F., and MICZEK, K. A., 1981, Sexual dimorphisms in the hormonal control of aggressive behavior of rats, *Pharmacol. Biochem. Behav.* **14**(Suppl. 1):89–93.

DEBOLD, J. F., and MICZEK, K. A., 1984, Aggression persists after ovariectomy in female rats, *Hormone Behav.* **18:**177–190.

DEBOLD, J. F., and MICZEK, K. A., 1984, Aggression persists after ovariectomy in female rats, *Hormones Behav.* **18:**177–190.

DEBOLD, J. F., and MICZEK, K. A., 1985, Testosterone modulates the effects of ethanol on male mouse aggression, *Psychopharmacology* **86:**286–290.

DECUYPER, H., VAN PRAAG, H. M., and VERSTRAETEN, D., 1985a, The effect of milenperone on the aggressive behavior of psychogeriatric patients, *Neuropsychobiology* **13:**1–16.

DECUYPER, H., VAN PRAAG, H. M., and VERSTRAETEN, D., 1985b, The effect of milenperone on the aggressive behavior of oligophrenic patients, *Neuropsychobiology* **13:**101–105.

DELGADO, J. M. R., 1963, Cerebral heterostimulation in a monkey colony, *Science* **141:**161–163.

DELGADO, J. M. R., 1973, Antiaggressive effects of chlordiazepoxide, in: *The Benzodiazepines* (S. Garattini, E. Mussini, and L. O. Randall, eds.), Raven Press, New York, pp. 419–432.

DELGADO, J. M. R., GRAU, C., DELGADO-GARCIA, J. M., and RODERO, J. M., 1976, Effects of diazepam related to social hierarchy in rhesus monkeys, *Neuropharmacology* **15:**409–414.

DELINI-STULA, A., and VASSOUT, A., 1978, Influence of baclofen and GABA-mimetic agents of spontaneous and olfactory-bulb-ablation-induced muricidal behaviour in the rat, *Arzneim.-Forsch. Drug Res.* **28:**1508–1509.

DELINI-STULA, A., and VASSOUT, A., 1979, Differential effects of psychoactive drugs on aggressive responses in mice and rats, in: *Psychopharmacology of Aggression* (M. Sandler, ed.), Raven Press, New York, pp. 41–60.

DELINI-STULA, A., and VASSOUT, A., 1981, The effects of antidepressants on aggressiveness induced by social deprivation in mice, *Pharmacol. Biochem. Behav.* **14**:33–41.

DENENBERG, V. H., GAULIN-KREMER, E., GANDELMAN, R., and ZARROW, M. X., 1973, The development of standard stimulus animals for mouse *(Mus musculus)* aggression testing by means of olfactory bulbectomy, *Animal Behav.* **21**:590–598.

DEPAULIS, A., 1983, A microcomputer method for behavioural data acquisition and subsequent analysis, *Pharmacol. Biochem. Behav.* **19**:729–732.

DEPAULIS, A., and VERGNES, M., 1983, Induction of mouse-killing in the rat by intraventricular injection of a GABA-agonist, *Physiol. Behav.* **30**:383–388.

DEPAULIS, A., and VERGNES, M., 1984, Gabaergic modulation of mouse-killing in the rat, *Psychopharmacology* **83**:367–372.

DEPAULIS, A., and VERGNES, M., 1985, Elicitation of conspecific attack or defense in the male rat by intraventricular injection of a GABA agonist or antagonist, *Physiol. Behav.* **35**:447–453.

DEWEESE, J., 1977, Schedule-induced biting under fixed-interval schedules of food or electric-shock presentation, *J. Exp. Anal. Behav.* **27**:419–431.

DIDIERGEORGES, F., VERGNES, M., and KARLI, P., 1968, Sur le mode d'action d'une influence inhibitrice d'origine olfactive s'exercant sur l'aggressivite interspecifique du Rat, *C. Re. Seances Soc. Biol.* **62**:267–270.

DIMASCIO, A., 1973, The effects of benzodiazepines on aggression: Reduced or increased: in: *The Benzodiazepines* (S. Garattini, E. Mussini, and R. O. Randall, eds.), Raven Press, New York, pp. 433–440.

DIMASCIO, A., SHADER, R. I., and HARMATZ, J., 1969, Psychotropic drugs and induced hostility, *Psychosomatics* **10**:46–47.

DIXON, A. K., 1982, A possible olfactory component in the effects of diazepam on social behavior of mice, *Psychopharmacology* **77**:246–252.

DLABAC, A., 1973, Apomorphine-induced aggressivity in rats and its alterations, *Activitas Nerv. Superior* **15**:133.

DOLLARD, J., DOBB, L., MILLER, N., MOWRER, O., and SEARS, R., 1939, *Frustration and Aggression,* Yale University Press, New Haven, CT.

DORR, M., and STEINBERG, H., 1976, Effects of delta-9-tetrahydrocannabinol on social behavior in mice, *Psychopharmacology* **47**:87–91.

DOSTAL, T., and ZVOLTSKY, P., 1970, Antiaggressive effect of lithium salts in severely mentally retarded adolescents, *Int. Pharmacopsychiatry* **5**:203–207.

DOTSON, L. E., ROBERTSON, L. S., and TUCHFELD, B., 1975, Plasma alcohol, smoking, hormone concentrations and self-reported aggression, *J. Stud. Alcohol* **36**:578–586.

DUBINSKY, B., and GOLDBERG, M. E., 1971, The effect of imipramine and selected drugs on attack elicited by hypothalamic stimulation in the cat, *Neuropharmacology* **10**:537–545.

DUBINSKY, B., KARPOWICZ, J. K., and GOLDBERG, M. E., 1973a, Effects of tricyclic antidepressants on attack elicited by hypothalamic stimulation: Relation to brain biogenic amines, *J. Pharmacol. Exp. Ther.* **187**:550–557.

DUBINSKY, B., ROBICHAUD, R. C., and GOLDBERG, M. E., 1973b, Effects of (−)delta 9-trans-tetrahydrocannabinol and its selectivity in several models of aggressive behavior, *Pharmacology* **9**:204–216.

DYER, R. S., WALSH, T. J., WONDERLIN, W. F., and BERCEGEAY, M., 1982, The trimethyltin syndrome in rats, *Neurobehav. Toxicol. Teratol.* **4**:127–133.

EDWARDS, A. E., BLOOM, M. H., and COHEN, S., 1969, The psychedelics: Love or hostility potion? *Psychol. Rep.* **24**:843–846.

EDWARDS, D. A., 1970, Effects of cyproterone acetate on aggressive behaviour and the seminal vesicles of male mice, *J. Endocrinol.* **46**:477–481.

EIBL-EIBESFELDT, I., 1961, The fighting behavior of animals, *Sci. Am.* **203**:112–120.

EICHELMAN, B., 1977, Pharmacological treatment of aggressive disturbances, in: *Psycho-*

pharmacology: From Theory to Practice (J., Barchas, R. Berger, R., Ciaranello, and G. Elliott, eds.), Oxford University Press, New York, pp. 260-269.

EICHELMAN, B., 1978, Animal models: Their role in the study of aggressive behavior in humans, *Progr. Neuro-Psychopharmacol.* **2**:633-643.

EICHELMAN, B., 1979, Role of biogenic amines in aggressive behavior, in: *Psychopharmacology of Aggression* (M. Sandler, ed.), Raven Press, New York, pp. 61-93.

EICHELMAN, B., 1983, The limbic system and aggression in humans, *Neurosci. Biobehav. Rev.* **7**:391-394.

EICHELMAN, B., and BARCHAS, J., 1975, Facilitated shock-induced aggression following antidepressive medication in the rat, *Pharmacol. Biochem. Behav.* **3**:601-604.

EICHELMAN, B., THOA, N. B., and PEREZ-CRUET, J., 1973, Alkali metal cations: Effects on aggression and adrenal enzymes, *Pharmacol. Biochem. Behav.* **1**:121-123.

EICHELMAN, B., ELLIOTT, G. R., and BARCHAS, J. D., 1981, Biochemical, pharmacological, and genetic aspects of aggression, in: *Biobehavioral Aspects of Aggression* (D. A. Hamburg and M. B. Trudeau, eds.), Liss, New York, pp. 51-84.

EISENBERG, L, LACHMAN, R., MOLLING, P. A., LOCKNER, A., MIZELLE, J. D., and CONNERS, C. K., 1963, A psychopharmacologic experiment in a training school for delinquent boys: Methods, problems, findings, *Am. J. Orthopsychiatry* **33**:431-447.

EISENSTEIN, N., IORIO, L. C., and CLODY, D. E., 1982, Role of serotonin in the blockade of muricidal behavior by tricyclic antidepressants, *Pharmacol. Biochem. Behav.* **17**:847-849.

EISON, M. S., WILSON, W. J., and ELLISON, G., 1978, A refillable system for continuous amphetamine administration: Effects upon social behavior in rat colonies, *Commun. Psychopharmacol.* **2**:151-157.

ELEFTHERIOU, B. E., and CHURCH, R. L., 1968, Brain levels of serotonin and norepinephrine in mice after exposure to aggression and defeat, *Physiol. Behav.* **3**:977-980.

ELIE, R., LANGLOIS, Y., COOPER, S. F., GRAVEL, G., and ALBERT, J., 1980, Comparison of SCH-12679 and thioridazine in aggressive mental retardates, *Can. J. Psychiatry* **25**:484-491.

ELLINWOOD, E. H., JR., 1971, Assault and homicide associated with amphetamine abuse, *Am. J. Psychiatry* **127**:90-95.

ELLINWOOD, E. H., 1972, Amphetamine psychosis: Individuals, settings, and sequences, in: *Current Concepts on Amphetamine Abuse* (E. H. Ellinwood and S. Cohen, eds.), NIMH, Rockville, MD, pp. 143-157.

ELLIOTT, F. A., 1977, Propanolol for the control of belligerent behavior following acute brain damage, *Ann. Neurol.* **1**:489-491.

ELLISON, G., EISON, M. S., and HUBERMAN, H. S., 1978a, Stages of constant amphetamine intoxication: Delayed appearance of abnormal social behaviors in rat colonies, *Psychopharmacology* **56**:293-299.

ELLISON, G., EISON, M. S., HUBERMAN, H. S., and DANIEL, F., 1978b, Long-term changes in dopaminergic innervation of caudate nucleus after continuous amphetamine administration, *Science* **201**:276-278.

ELLMAN, G. L., HERZ, M. J., and PEEKE, H. V. S., 1972, Ethanol in a cichlid fish: Blood levels and aggressive behavior, *Proc. Western Pharmacol. Soc.* **15**:92-95.

ELY, D., HENRY, J. P., and JAROSZ, C. J., 1975, Effects of marihuana (delta-9-THC) on behavior patterns and social roles in colonies of CBA mice, *Behav. Biol.* **13**:263-276.

EMLEY, G. S., and HUTCHINSON, R. R., 1972, Basis of behavioral influence of chlorpromazine, *Life Sci.* **11**:43-47.

EMLEY, G. S., and HUTCHINSON, R. R., 1983a, Effects of phencyclidine on aggressive behavior in squirrel monkeys, *Pharmacol. Biochem. Behav.* **18**:163-166.

EMLEY, G. S., and HUTCHINSON, R. R., 1983b, Unique influences of ten drugs upon postshock biting attack and pre-shock manual responding, *Pharmacol. Biochem. Behav.* **19**:5-12.

ERSKINE, M. S., DENENBERG, V. H., and GOLDMAN, B. D., 1978, Aggression in the lactating rat: Effects of intruder age and test arena, *Behav. Biol.* **23**:52-66.

ESSMAN, E. J., and VALZELLI, L., 1984, Regional brain serotonin receptor changes in differentially housed mice: Effects of amphetamine, *Pharmacol. Res. Commun.* **16**:401–408.

ESSMAN, W. B., 1978, Benzodiazepines and aggressive behavior, in: *Modern Problems of Pharmacopsychiatry* (L. Valzelli, ed.), Karger, Basel, pp. 13–28.

EVANS, C. M., 1986, Alcohol and violence: Problems relating to methodology, statistics and causation, in: *Alcohol and Aggression* (P. F. Brain, ed.), Croom Helm, London, pp. 138–160.

EVANS, L. T., and ABRAMSON, H. A., 1958, Lysergic acid diethylamide (LSD-25): XXV. Effect on social order of newts, *Triturus V. viridescens* (RAF), *J. Psychol.* **45**:153–169.

EVANS, L. T., ABRAMSON, H. A., and FREMONT-SMITH, N., 1958, Lysergic acid diethylamide (LSD-25): XXVI. Effect on social order of the fighting fish, *Betta splendens*, *J. Psychol.* **45**:263–273.

EWART, F. G., and CUTLER, M. G., 1979, Effects of ethyl alcohol on development and social behavior in the offspring of laboratory mice, *Psychopharmacology* **62**:247–251.

FABRE-NYS, C., MELLER, R. E., and KEVERNE, E. B., 1982, Opiate antagonists stimulate affiliative behaviour in monkeys, *Pharmacol. Biochem. Behav.* **16**:653–659.

FALK, J. L., 1977, The origin and functions of adjunctive behavior, *Animal Learning Behav.* **5**:325–335.

FANSELOW, M. S., and SIGMUNDI, R. A., 1982, The enhancement and reduction of defensive fighting by naloxone pretreatment, *Physiol. Psychol.* **10**(3):313–316.

FANSELOW, M. S., SIGMUNDI, R. A., and BOLLES, R. C., 1980, Naloxone pretreatment enhances shock-elicited aggression, *Physiol. Psychol.* **8**:369–371.

FARETRA, G., DOOHER, L., and DOWLING, J., 1970, Comparison of haloperidol and fluphenazine in disturbed children, *Am. J. Psychiatry* **126**:1670–1673.

FAUMAN, B., ALDINGER, G., FAUMAN, M., and ROSEN, P., 1976, Psychiatric sequelae of phencyclidine abuse, *Clin. Toxicol.* **9**:529–538.

FAUMAN, M. A., and FAUMAN, B. J., 1979, Violence associated with phencyclidine abuse, *Am. J. Psychiatry* **136**:1584–1586.

FAUMAN, M. A., and FAUMAN, B. J., 1980, Chronic phencyclidine (PCP) abuse: A psychiatric perspective. Part I: General aspects and violence, *Psychopharmacol. Bull.* **16**:70–72.

FELDMAN, P. E., 1962, An analysis of efficacy of diazepam, *J. Neuropsychiatry* **3**:S62–S67.

FELDMAN, W. W., AGAR, M. H., and BESCHNER, G. M., 1979, *Angel Dust: An Ethnographic Study of PCP Users*, Lexington Books, Lexington, MA.

FIGLER, M. H., and PEEKE, H. V. S., 1978, Alcohol and the prior residence effect in male convict cichlids *(Cichlasoma nigrofasciatum)*, *Aggressive Behav.* **4**:125–132.

FILE, S. E., 1980, Naxolone reduces social and exploratory activity in the rat, *Psychopharmacology* **71**:41–44.

FILE, S. E., 1982, Colony aggression: Effects of benzodiazepines on intruder behavior, *Physiol. Psychol.* **10**:413–416.

FILE, S. E., 1984, The stress of intruding: Reduction by chlordiazepoxide, *Physiol. Behav.* **33**:345–347.

FILE, S. E., 1985, What can be learned from the effects of benzodiazepines on exploratory behavior? *Neurosci. Biobehav. Rev.* **9**:45–54.

FILE, S. E., and PELLOW, S., 1985, The anxiogenic action of RO 5-4864 in the social interaction test: Effect of chlordiazepoxide, RO 15-1788 and CGS 8216, *Naunyn-Schmiedeberg's Arch. Pharmacol.* **328**:225–228.

FILE, S. E., and PELLOW, S., 1986, Intrinsic actions of the benzodiazepine receptor antagonist Ro 15-1788, *Psychopharmacology* **88**:1–11.

FILE, S. E., and RODGERS, R. J., 1979, Partial anxiolytic action of morphine sulphate following microinjection into the central nucleus of the amygdala in rats, *Pharmacol. Biochem. Behav.* **11**:313–318.

FILE, S. E., and TUCKER, J. C., 1983, Lorazepam treatment in the neonatal rat alters submissive behavior in adulthood, *Neurobehav. Toxicol. Teratol.* **5**:289–294.

FINK, M., SIMEON, J., HAQUE, W., and ITIL, T., 1966, Prolonged adverse reactions to LSD in psychotic subjects, *Arch. Gen. Psychiatry* **15**:450–454.
FISH, B., 1971, The "one child, one drug" myth of stimulants in hyperkinesis, *Arch. Gen. Psychiatry* **25**:193–203.
FISHER, G., and STECKLER, A., 1974, Psychological effects, personality and behavioral changes attributed to marihuana use, *Int. J. Addictions* **9**:101–126.
FLOODY, O. R., 1983, Hormones and aggression in female mammals, in: *Hormones and Aggressive Behavior* (B. B. Svare, ed.), Plenum Press, New York, pp. 39–90.
FLOREA, J., and THOR, D. H., 1968, Drug withdrawal and fighting in rats, *Psychonom. Sci.* **12**:33.
FLYNN, J. P., SMITH, D., COLEMAN, K., and OPSAHL, C. A., 1979, Anatomical pathways for attack behavior in cats, in: *Human Ethology. Claims and Limits of a New Discipline* (M. von Cranach, K. Foppa, W. Lepenies, and D. Ploog, eds.), Cambridge University Press, Cambridge, pp. 301–315.
FOG, R., 1969, Rage reactions produced in rats by a combination of thymoleptics and monoamine oxidase inhibitors, *Pharmacol. Res. Commun.* **1**:79–83.
FOG, R., RANDRUP, A., and PAKKENBERG, H., 1970, Lesions in corpus striatum and cortex of rat brains and the effect on pharmacologically induced stereotyped, aggressive and cataleptic behaviour, *Psychopharmacologia* **18**:364–356.
FOSSIER, A. E., 1931, The mariahuana menace, *New Orleans Med. Surg. J.* **44**:247–252.
FOX, K. A., and SNYDER, R. L., 1969, Effect of sustained low doses of diazepam on aggresion and mortality in grouped male mice, *J. Compa. Physiol. Psychol.* **69**:663–666.
FOX, K. A., TOCKOSH, J. R., and WILCOX, A. H., 1970, Increased aggression among grouped male mice fed chlordiazepoxide, *Eur. J. Pharmacol.* **11**:119–121.
FRANKEL, B. G., FERRENCE, R. G., JOHNSON, F. G., and WHITEHEAD, P. C., 1976, Drinking and self-injury: Toward untangling the dynamics, *Br. J. Addiction* **71**:299–306.
FREEDMAN, D. X., 1986, Hallucinogenic drug research: If so, so what? (Symposium summary and commentary), *Pharmacol. Biochem. Behav.* **24**:407–415.
FREYHAN, F., 1959, Therapeutic implications of differential effects of new phenothiazine compounds, *Am. J. Psychiatry* **115**:577–585.
FRISCHKNECHT, H. R., 1984, Effects of cannabis drugs on social behaviour of laboratory rodents, *Prog. Neurobiol.* **22**:39–58.
FRISCHKNECHT, H. R., SIEGFRIED, B., SCHILLER, M., and WASER, P. G., 1985, Hashish extract impairs retention of defeat-induced submissive behavior in mice, *Psychopharmacology* **86**:270–273.
FUJIWARA, M., and UEKI, S., 1978, Muricide induced by single injection of delta-9-tetrahydrocannabinol, *Physiol. Behav.* **21**:581–585.
FUJIWARA, M., and UEKI, S., 1979, The course of aggressive behavior induced by a single injection of delta-9-tetrahydrocannabinol and its characteristics, *Physiol. Behav.* **22**:535–539.
FUJIWARA, M., IBII, N., KATAOKA, Y., and UEKI, S., 1980, Effects of psychotropic drugs on delta-9-tetrahydrocannabinol induced long-lasting muricide, *Psychopharmacology* **68**:7–13.
FUJIWARA, M., KATAOKA, Y., HORI, Y., and UEKI, S., 1984, Irritable aggression induced by delta-9-tetrahydrocannabinol in rats pretreated with 6-hydroxydopamine, *Pharmacol. Biochem. Behav.* **20**:457–462.
FUKUDA, T., and TSUMAGARI, T., 1983, Effects of psychotropic drugs on the rage responses induced by electrical stimualtion of the medial hypothalamus in cats, *Jpn. J. Pharmacol.* **33**:885–890.
FUNDERBURK, W. H., FOXWELL, M. H., and HAKALA, M. W., 1970, Effects of psychotherapeutic drugs on hypothalamic-induced hissing in cats, *Neuropharmacology* **9**:1–7.
GANDELMAN, R., 1972, Mice: Postpartum aggression elicited by the presence of an intruder, *Hormones Behav.* **3**:23–28.
GARATTINI, S., 1965, Effects of a cannabis extract on gross behaviour, in: *Hashish: Its Chem-*

istry and Pharmacology (G. E. W. Wolstenholme and J. Knight, eds.), J. and A. Churchill, London, pp. 70–94.

GARATTINI, S., and VALZELLI, L., 1981, Is the isolated animal a possible model for phobia and anxiety? *Prog. Neuro-Psychopharmacol.* **5**:159–165.

GARDIKAS, C. G., 1950, Hashish and crime, *Enkephalos* **2**:201–211.

GARDOS, G., DIMASCIO, A., SALZMAN, C., and SHADER, R. I., 1968, Differential actions of chlordiazepoxide and oxazepam on hostility, *Arch. Gen. Psychiatry* **18**:757–760.

GARFINKEL, B. D., WEBSTER, C. D., and SLOMAN, L., 1975, Methylphenidate and caffeine in the treatment of children with minimal brain dysfunction, *Am. J. Psychiatry* **132**:723–728.

GARVER, D. L., SCHLEMMER, R. F., JR., MAAS, J. W., and DAVIS, J. M., 1975, A schizophreniform behavioral psychosis mediated by dopamine, *Am. J. Psychiatry* **132**:33–38.

GAY, P. E., and CLARK, L. D., 1976, Effects of some physiological and pharmacological manipulations on shock-facilitated mouse killing by *Onychomys leucogaster* (Northern grasshopper mouse), *Aggressive Behav.* **2**:107–121.

GAY, P. E., and COLE, S. O., 1976, Interactions of amygdala lesions with effects of pilocarpine and *d*-amphetamine on mouse killing, feeding, and drinking in rats, *J. Comp. Physiol. Psychol.* **90**:630–642.

GAY, P. E., LEAF, R. C., and ARBLE, F. B., 1975, Inhibitory effects of pre- and posttest drugs on mouse-killing by rats, *Pharmacol. Biochem. Behav.* **3**:33–45.

GAYFORD, J. J., 1975, Wife battering: A preliminary survey of 100 cases, *Br. Med. J.* **1**:194–197.

GELLERT, V. F., and SPARBER, S. B., 1979, Effects of morphine withdrawal on food competition hierarchies and fighting behavior in rats, *Psychopharmacology* **60**:165–172.

GENOVESE, E., NAPOLI, P. A., and BOLEGO-ZONTA, N., 1969, Selfaggressiveness: A new type of behavioral change induced by pemoline, *Life Sci.* **8**:513–515.

GERSHON, S., 1968, Use of lithium salts in psychiatric disorders, *Dis. Nerv. System* **29**:51–55.

GERSON, L. W., 1978, Alcohol-related acts of violence: Who was drinking and where the acts occurred, *J. Stud. Alcohol* **39**:1294–1296.

GERSON, L. W., and PRESTON, D. A., 1979, Alcohol consumption and the incidence of violent crime, *J. Stud. Alcohol* **40**:307–312.

GIANUTSOS, G., and LAL, H., 1975, Aggression in mice after para-chloroamphetamine, *Res. Commun. Chem. Pathol. Pharmacol.* **10**:379–382.

GIANUTSOS, G., and LAL, H., 1976a, Drug-induced aggression, in: *Current Developments in Psychopharmacology* (W. Essman and L. Valzelli, eds.), Plenum Press, New York, pp. 198–220.

GIANUTSOS, G., and LAL, H., 1976b, Blockade of apomorphine-induced aggression by morphine or neuroleptics: Differential alteration by antimuscarinics and naloxone, *Pharmacol. Biochem. Behav.* **4**:639–642.

GIANUTSOS, G., and LAL, H., 1978, Narcotic analgesics and aggression, in: *Modern Problems of Pharmacopsychiatry: Psychopharmacology of Aggression* (L. Valzelli, T. Ban, F. A. Freyhan, and P. Pichot, eds.), Karger, New York, pp. 114–138.

GIANUTSOS, G., DRAWBAUGH, R. B., HYNES, M. D., and LAL, H., 1974a, Behavioral evidence for dopaminergic supersensitivity and chronic haloperidol, *Life Sci.* **14**:887–898.

GIANUTSOS, G., HYNES, M. D., PURI, S. K., DRAWBURGH, R. B., and LAL, H., 1974b, Effect of apomorphine and nigrostriatal lesions on aggression and striatal dopamine turnover during morphine withdrawal: Evidence for dopaminergic supersensitivity in protracted abstinence, *Psychopharmacologia* **34**:37–44.

GIANUTSOS, G., HYNES, M. D., DRAWBURGH, R. B., and LAL, H., 1975, Paradoxical absence of aggression during naloxone-precipitated morphine withdrawal, *Psychopharmacologia* **43**:43–46.

GIBBONS, J. L., BARR, G. A., and BRIDGER, W. H., 1978, Effects of para-chlorophenylalanine and 5-hydroxytryptophan on mouse killing behavior in killer rats, *Pharmacol. Biochem. Behav.* **9:**91–98.

GIBBONS, J. L., BARR, G. A., BRIDGER, W. H., and LEIBOWITZ, S. F., 1979, Manipulations of dietary tryptophan: Effects on mouse killing and brain serotonin in the rat, *Brain Res.* **169:**139–153.

GINSBURG, B., and ALLEE, W. C., 1942, Some effects of conditioning on social dominance and subordination in inbred strains of mice, *Physiol. Zool.* **15:**485–506.

GIONO-BARBER, P., PARIS, M., BERTULETTI, G., and GIONO-BARBER, H., 1974, Cannabis effects on dominance behavior in the Cynocephale monkey, *J. Pharmacol.* **5:**591–602.

GLERSER, G. C., GOTTSCHALK, L. A., FOX, R., and LIPPERT, W., 1965, Immediate changes in affect with chlordiazepoxide, *Arch. Gen. Psychiatry* **13:**291–295.

GODDARD, P., and LOKARE, V. G., 1970, Diazepam in the management of epilepsy, *Br. J. Psychiatry* **117:**213–214.

GOETZL, U., GRUNBERG, F., and BERKOWITZ, B., 1977, Lithium carbonate in the management of hyperactive aggressive behavior of the mentally retarded, *Comp. Psychiatry* **18(6):**599–606.

GOLDBERG, M. E., 1970, Pharmacologic activity of a new class of agents which selectively inhibit aggressive behavior in rats, *Arch. Int. Pharmacodyn. Ther.* **186:**287–297.

GOLDBERG, M. E., and SALAMA, A. I., 1969, Norepinephrine turnover and brain monoamine levels in aggressive mouse-killing rats, *Biochem. Pharmacol.* **18:**532–534.

GOLDBERG, M. E., SLEDGE, K., DUBINSKY, B., and ROBICHAUD, R. C., 1973, The influence of SKF-525A on the acute pharmacological properties of chlordiazepoxide, *Arch. Int. Pharmacodyn. Ther.* **204:**12–19.

GOLDSMITH, J. F., BRAIN, P. F., and BENTON, D., 1976, Effects of age at differential housing and the duration of individual housing/group on intermale fighting behavior and adrenocortical activity in TO strain mice, *Aggressive Behav.* **2:**307–323.

GOLDSTEIN, A., and JAMES, I. F., 1984, Multiple opioid receptors. Criteria for identification and classification, *Trends Pharmacol. Sci.* **5:**503–505.

GONZALEZ, S. C., MATSUDO, V. K. R., and CARLINI, E. A., 1971, Effects of marihuana compounds on the fighting behavior of Siamese fighting fish *(Betta splendens), Pharmacology* **6:**186–190.

GOODWIN, D. W., 1973, Alcohol in suicide and homicide, *Q. J. Stud. Alcohol* **34:**144–156.

GORELICK, D. A., ELLIOTT, M. L., and SBORDONE, R. J., 1981, Naloxone increases shock-elicited aggression in rats, *Res. Commun. Substances Abuse* **2:**419–422.

GOSSOP, M. R., and ROY, A., 1976, Hostility in drug dependent individuals: Its relation to specific drugs, and oral or intravenous use, *Br. J. Psychiatry* **128:**188–193.

GOTTSCHALK, L. A., and COHN, J. B., 1978, The relationship of diazepam and ketazolam blood levels to anxiety and hostility in chronic alcoholics, *Psychopharmacol. Bull.* **14:**39–43.

GRAHAM, K., LA ROCQUE, L., YETMAN, R., ROSS, T. J., and GUISTRA, E., 1980, Aggression and barroom environments, *J. Stud. Alcohol* **41:**277–292.

GRANT, E. C., and MACKINTOSH, J. H., 1963, A comparison of the social postures of some common laboratory rodents, *Behaviour* **21:**246–259.

GRANT, S. J., GALLOWAY, M. P., MAYOR, R., FENERTY, J. P., FINKELSTEIN, M. F., ROTH, R. H., and REDMOND, D. E., JR., 1985, Precipitated diazepam withdrawal elevates noradrenergic metabolism in primate brain, *Eur. J. Pharmacol.* **107:**127–132.

GRAY, W. D., OSTERBERG, A. C., and RAUH, C. E., 1961, Neuropharmacological actions of mephenoxalone, *Arch. Int. Pharmacodyn. Ther.* **84:**198–215.

GREEN, R. A., 1985, *Neuropharmacology of Serotonin*, Oxford University Press, New York.

GREENBLATT, D. J., SHADER, R. I., and KOCH-WESER, J., 1975, Flurazepam hydrochloride *Clin. Pharmacol. Ther.* **17:**1–14.

GREENDYKE, R. M., SCHUSTER, D. B., and WOOTON, J. A., 1984, Propranolol in the treatment of assaultive patients with organic brain disease, *J. Clin. Psychopharmacol.* **4:**282–285.

GRIFFITHS, R. R., STITZER, M., CORKER, K., BIGELOW, G., and LIEBSON, I., 1977, Drug-produced changes in human social behavior: Facilitation by *d*-amphetamine, *Pharmacol. Biochem. Behav.* **7**:365–372.

GRUPP, S. E., 1971, Prior criminal record and adult marihuana arrest dispositions, *J. Criminal Law, Criminology Police Sci.* **62**:74–79.

GUAITANI, A., MARCUCCI, F., and GARATTINI, S., 1971, Increased aggression and toxicity in grouped male mice treated with tranquilizing benzodiazepines, *Psychopharmacologia* **19**:241–245.

GULDENPFENNIG, W. M., 1973, Clinical experience with a new benzodiazepine in the treatment of epilepsy, *S. Afr. Med. J.* **47**:998–1000.

GUSTAFSON, R., 1985, Alcohol and aggression: Pharmacological versus expectancy effects, *Psychol. Rep.* **57**:955–966.

GUSTAVSON, C. R., GARCIA, J., HANKINS, W. G., and RUSINIAK, K. W., 1974, Coyote predation control by aversive conditioning, *Science* **184**:581–583.

GUZE, S. B., TUASON, V. B., GATFIELD, P. D., STEWART, M. A., and PICKEN, B., 1962, Psychiatric illness and crime with particular reference to alcoholism; studies of 233 criminals, *J. Nerv. Ment. Dis.* **134**:512–521.

HABER, S., BARCHAS, P. R., and BARCHAS, J. D., 1981, A primate analogue of amphetamine-induced behaviors in humans, *Biol. Psychiatry* **16**:181–195.

HABERMAN, P. W., and BADEN, M. M., 1974, Alcoholism and violent death, *Q. J. Stud. Alcohol* **35**:221–231.

HACKE, W., 1980, Die pharmakologische Beeinflussung aggressiven und autoaggressiven Verhaltens bei Geistigbehinderten mit Melperone, *Pharmakopsychiatr. Neuro-psychopharmakol.* **13**:20–24.

HADFIELD, H. G., 1983, Dopamine: Mesocortical vs nigrostriatal uptake in isolated fighting mice and control, *Behav. Brain Res.* **7**:269–281.

HADFIELD, M. G., 1982, Cocaine: Peak time of action on isolation-induced fighting, *Neuropharmacology* **21**:711–713.

HADFIELD, M. G., NUGENT, E. A., and MOTT, D. E., 1982, Cocaine increases isolation-induced fighting in mice, *Pharmacol. Biochem. Behav.* **16**:359–360.

HAEFELY, W., 1984, Actions and interactions of benzodiazepine agonists and antagonists at GABAergic synapses, in: *Actions and Interactions of GABA and Benzodiazepines* (N. G. Bowery, ed.), Raven Press, New York, pp. 263–285.

HAHN, R. A., HYNES, M. D., and FULLER, R. W., 1982, Apomorphine-induced aggression in rats chronically treated with oral clonidine: Modulation by central serotonergic mechanisms, *J. Pharmacol. Exp. Ther.* **220**:389–393.

HALL, R. C. W., and ZISOOK, S., 1981, Paradoxical reactions to benzodiazepines, *Br. J. Clin. Pharmacol.* **11**:99S–104S.

HAMPTON, W. H., 1961, Observed psychiatric reactions following use of amphetamine and amphetamine-like substances, *Bull. NY Acad. Sci.* **37**:167–175.

HANKS, S. E., and ROSENBAUM, C. P., 1977, Battered women: A study of women who live with violent alcohol-abusing men, *Am. J. Orthopsychiatry* **47**:291–306.

HARA, C., WATANABE, S., and UEKI, S., 1983, Effects of psychotropic drugs microinjected into the hypothalmus on muricide, catalepsy and cortical EEG in OB rats, *Pharmacol. Biochem. Behav.* **18**:423–431.

HARA, C., WATANABE, S., and UEKI, S., 1984, Anti-muricide mechanisms of chlorpromazine and imipramine in OB rats: Adrenoceptors and hypothalamic functions, *Pharmacol. Biochem. Behav.* **21**:267–272.

HASSELAGER, E., ROLINSKI, Z., and RANDRUP, A., 1972, Specific antagonism by dopamine inhibitors of items of amphetamine induced aggressive behaviour, *Psychopharmacologia* **24**:485–495.

HEATHER, N., 1981, Relationships between delinquency and drunkenness among Scottish young offenders, *Br. J. Alcohol Alcoholism* **16**:50–61.

HEGSTRAND, L. R., and EICHELMAN, B., 1983, Increased shock-induced fighting with supersensitive beta-adrenergic receptors, *Pharmacol. Biochem. Behav.* **19:**313–320.

HEILMAN, R. D., BRUGMANS, M., GREENSLADE, F. C., and DAVANZO, J. P., 1976, Resistance of androgen-mediated aggressive behavior in mice to flutamide, an antiandrogen, *Psychopharmacology* **47:**75–80.

HEISE, G. A., and BOFF, E., 1961, Taming action of chlordiazepoxide, *Fed. Proc.* **20:**393.

HELLER, K. E., 1984, Effects of repeated exposure to electric footshock on subsequent agonistic behaviour and adrenocortical secretion in male mice of different androgen status, *Behav. Proc.* **9:**61–72.

HEMPHILL, R. E., and FISHER, W., 1980, Drugs, alcohol and violence in 604 male offenders referred for inpatient psychiatric assessment, *S. Afr. Med. J.* **57:**243–247.

HENDLEY, E. D., MOISSET, B., and WELCH, B. L., 1973, Catecholamine uptake in cerebral cortex: Adaptive change induced by fighting, *Science* **180:**1050–1052.

HENDRIE, C. A., and BENNETT, S., 1983, A microcomputer technique for the detailed analysis of animal behavior, *Physiol. Behav.* **30:**233–235.

HERMAN, B., and PANKSEPP, J., 1978, Effect of morphine and naloxone on separation distress and approach attachment: Evidence for opiate mediation of social affect, *Pharmacol. Biochem. Behav.* **9:**213–220.

HERMAN, B. H., and PANKSEPP, J., 1981, Ascending endorphin inhibition of distress vocalization, *Science* **211:**1060–1062.

Hess, W. R., 1928, Stammganglien-Reizversuche, *Berichte Ges. Physiol.* **47:**554.

HESS, W. R., 1948, *Das Zwischenhirn. Syndrome, Lokalisationen, Funktionen,* Benno Schwabe and Co., Basel.

HESS, W. R., and BRÜGGER, M., 1943, Das subkortikale Zentrum der affektiven Abwehrreaktion, *Helv. Physiol. Acta* **1:**33–52.

HEUSCHELE, W. P., 1961, Chlordiazepoxide for calming zoo animals, *J. Am. Vet. Med. Assoc.* **139:**996–998.

HILL, D., 1947, Amphetamine in psychopathic states, *Br. J. Addiction* **44:**50–54.

HINDE, R. A., 1983, *Primate Social Relationships,* Sinauer Associates, Inc., Sunderland, MA.

HINE, B., FRIEDMAN, E., TORRELIO, M., and GERSHON, S., 1975a, Morphine-dependent rats: Blockade of precipitated abstinence by tetrahydrocannabinol, *Science* **187:**443–445.

HINE, B., WALLACH, M. B., and GERSHON, S., 1975b, Involvement of biogenic amines in drug-induced aggressive pecking in chicks, *Psychopharmacologia,* **43:**215–221.

HODGE, G. K., and BUTCHER, L. L., 1975, Catecholamine correlates of isolation-induced aggression in mice, *Eur. J. Pharmacol.* **31:**81–93.

HOFFET, H., 1968, On the application of the testosterone blocker cyproterone acetate (SH 714) in sex deviants and psychiatric patients in institutions, *Praxis* **7:**221–230.

HOFFMEISTER, F., and WUTTKE, W., 1969, On the actions of psychotropic drugs on the attack- and aggressive-defensive behaviour of mice and cats, in: *Aggressive Behaviour* (S. Garattini and E. B. Sigg, eds.), Excerpta Medica Foundation, Amsterdam, pp. 273–280.

HOLLISTER, L. E., 1984, Effects of hallucinogens in humans, in: *Hallucinogens: Neurochemical, Behavioral, and Clinical Perspectives* (B. L. Jacobs, ed.), Raven Press, New York, pp. 19–33.

HOLLOWAY, W. R., and THOR, D. H., 1984, Acute and chronic caffeine exposure effects on play fighting in the juvenile rat, *Neurobehav. Toxicol. Teratol.* **6:**85–91.

HOLLOWAY, W. R., JR., and THOR, D. H., 1985, Interactive effects of caffeine, 2-chloroadenosine and haloperidol on activity, social investigation and play fighting of juvenile rats, *Pharmacol. Biochem. Behav.* **22:**421–426.

HOOD, K. E., 1984, Aggression among female rats during the estrus cycle, in: *Biological Perspectives on Aggression* (K. J. Flannelly, R. J. Blanchard, and D. C. Blanchard, eds.), Liss, New York, pp. 181–188.

Hopf, S., Hartmann-Wiesner, E., Kühlmorgen, B., and Mayer, S., 1974, The behavioral repertoire of the squirrel monkey (Saimiri), *Folia Primatol.* **21:**225–249.

Horovitz, Z. P., Furgiuele, A. R., Brannick, L. J., Burke, J. C., and Craver, B. N., 1963, A new chemical structure with specific depressant effects on the amygdala and on the hyper-irritability of the "septal rat," *Nature* **200:**369–370.

Horovitz, Z. P., Ragozzino, P. W., and Leaf, R. C., 1965, Selective block of rat mouse-killing by antidepressants, *Life Sci.* **4:**1909–1912.

Horovitz, Z. P., Piala, J. J., High, J. P., Burke, J. C., and Leaf, R. C., 1966, Effects of drugs on the mouse-killing (muricide) test and its relationship to amygdaloid function, *Int. J. Neuropharmacol.* **5:**405–411.

Howard, J. L., Soroko, F. E., and Cooper, B. R., 1981, Empirical behavioral models of depression, with emphasis on tetrabenazine antagonism, in: *Antidepressants: Neurochemical, Behavioral, and Clinical Perspectives* (S. J. Enna, J. B. Malick, and E. Richelson, eds.), Raven Press, New York, pp. 107–120.

Huntingford, F. A., 1976, The relationship between inter- and intra-specific aggression, *Animal Behav.* **24:**485–497.

Hutchinson, R. R., 1983, The pain-aggression relationship and its expression in naturalistic settings, *Aggressive Behav.* **9:**229–242.

Hutchinson, R. R., Azrin, N. H., and Hake, D. F., 1966, An automatic method for the study of aggression in squirrel monkeys, *J. Exp. Anal. Behav.* **9:**233–237.

Hutchinson, R. R., Azrin, N. H., and Renfrew, J. W., 1968, Effects of shock intensity and duration on the frequency of biting attack by squirrel monkeys, *J. Exp. Anal. Behav.* **11:**83–88.

Hutchinson, R. R., Emley, G. S., and Krasnegor, N. A., 1977, The effects of cocaine on the aggressive behavior of mice, pigeons and squirrel monkeys, in: *Cocaine and Other Stimulants* (E. H. Ellinwood, Jr., and M. M. Kilbey, eds.), Plenum Press, New York, pp. 457–480.

Ieni, J. R., and Thurmond, J. B., 1985, Maternal aggression in mice: Effects of treatments with PCPA, 5-HTP and 5-HT receptor antagonists, *Eur. J. Pharmacol.* **111:**211–220.

Ingle, D., 1973, Reduction of habituation of prey-catching activity by alcohol intoxication in the frog, *Behav. Biol.* **8:**123–129.

Ingram, I. M., and Timbury, G. C., 1960, Side-effects of librium, *Lancet* **2:**766.

Irwin, S., Kinohi, R., Van Sloten, M., and Workman, M. P., 1971, Drug effects on distress-evoked behavior in mice: Methodology and drug class comparisons, *Psychopharmacologia* **20:**172–185.

Itil, T. M., 1981, Drug therapy in the management of aggression, in: *Multidisciplinary Approaches to Aggression Research* (P. F. Brain and D. Benton, eds.), Elsevier/North-Holland, New York, pp. 489–501.

Itil, T. M., and Mukhopadhyay, S., 1978, Pharmacological management of human violence, in: *Psychopharmacology of Aggression, Modern Problems of Pharmacopsychiatry* (L. Valzelli, T. A. Ban, F. A. Freyhan, and P. Pichot, eds.), Karger, Basel, pp. 139–158.

Itil, T. M., and Seaman, P., 1978, Drug treatment of human aggression, *Prog. Neuropsychopharmacol.* **2:**659–669.

Itil, T. M., and Wadud, A., 1975, Treatment of human aggression with major tranquilizers, antidepressants, and newer psychotropic drugs, *J. Nerv. Ment. Dis.* **160:**83–99.

Itil, T. M., Rizzo, A. E., and Shapiro, D. M., 1967, Study of behavior and EEG correlation during treatment of disturbed children, *Dis. Nerv. System* **28:**731–736.

Iversen, S. D., 1977, Brain dopamine systems and behavior, in: *Handbook of Psychopharmacology: Drugs, Neurotransmitters and Behavior* (L. L. Iversen, S. D. Iversen, and S. H. Snyder, eds.), Plenum Press, New York, pp. 333–384.

Jacobs, B. L., and Gelperin, A., 1981, *Serotonin Neurotransmission and Behavior*, MIT Press, Cambridge, MA.

JAMES, W. T., 1949, Dominant and submissive behavior in puppies as indicated by food intake, *J. Gen. Psychol.* **75**:33–45.

JANSSEN, P. A. J., JAGENEAU, A. H., and NIEMEGEERS, J. E., 1960, Effects of various drugs on isolation-induced fighting behavior of male mice, *J. Pharmacol. Exp. Ther.* **129**:471–475.

JANSSEN, P. A. J., NIEMEGEERS, C. J. E., and VERBRUGGEN, F. J., 1962, A propos d'une methode d'investigation de substances susceptibles de modifier le comportement agressif inne du rat blanc vis-a-vis de la souris blanche, *Psychopharmacologia* **3**:114–123.

JARVIS, M. F., KRIEGER, M., COHEN, G., and WAGNER, G. C., 1985, The effects of phencyclidine and chlordiazepoxide on target biting of confined male mice, *Aggressive Behav.* **11**:201–205.

JEAVONS, C. M., and TAYLOR, S. P., 1985, The control of alcohol-related aggression: Redirecting the inebriate's attention to socially appropriate conduct, *Aggressive Behav.* **11**:93–101.

JEFFERSON, J. W., 1982, The use of lithium in childhood and adolescence: An overview, *J. Clin. Psychiatry* **43**:174–177.

JOHNSON, S. D., GIBSON, L., and LINDEN, R., 1978, Alcohol and rape in Winnipeg, 1966–1975, *J. Stud. Alcohol* **39**:1887–1894.

JONES, B. C., CLARK, D. L., CONSROE, P. F., and SMITH, H. J., 1974, Effects of (−) delta-9 trans-tetrahydrocannabinol on social behavior of squirrel monkey dyads in water competition situations, *Psychopharmacologia* **37**:37–43.

JONES, S. E., and BRAIN, P. F., 1985, An illustration of simple sequence analysis with reference to the agonistic behaviour of four strains of laboratory mouse, *Behav. Proc.* **11**:365–388.

KALANT, O. J., 1966, *The Amphetamines—Toxicity and Addiction,* University of Toronto Press, Toronto.

KALINA, R. K., 1964, Diazepam: Its role in a prison setting, *Dis. Nerv. System* **25**:101–107.

KAMBACK, M. C., 1973, The hippocampus and motivation: A re-examination, *J. Gen. Psychol.* **89**:313–324.

KAMPOV-POLEVOI, A. B., 1978, Effect of drugs on domination–subordination relationships in pairs of rats, *Byull. Eksp. Biol. Med.* **86**:306–308.

KANTAK, K. M., and MICZEK, K. A., 1982, Pharmacological separation of aggression from other symptoms of morphine withdrawal, *Neurosci. Abstr.* **8**:592.

KANTAK, K. M., and MICZEK, K. A., 1987, Aggression during morphine withdrawal: Effects of method of withdrawal, fighting experience and social role, *Psychopharmacology* (in press).

KARCZMAR, A. G., RICHARDSON, D. L., and KINDEL, G., 1978, Neuropharmacological and related aspects of animal aggression, *Prog. Neuro-Psychopharmacol.* **2**:611–631.

KARLI, P., 1956, The Norway rat's killing response to the white mouse: An experimental analysis, *Behaviour* **10**:81–103.

KARLI, P., 1958, Action de l'amphetamine et de la chlorpromazine sur l'aggressivite interspecifique Rat-Souris, *C. R. Soc. Biol.* **152**:1796–1798.

KARLI, P., 1959a, Action de substances dites "tranquillisantes" sur l'agressivite interspecifique Rat-Souris, *C. R. Soc. Biol.* **153**:467–469.

KARLI, P., 1959b, Recherches pharmacologiques sur le comportement d'agression Rat-Souris, *C. R. Soc. Biol.* **153**:497–498.

KARLI, P., 1961, Action du methaminodiazepoxide ("Librium") sur l'agressivite interspecifique Rat-Souris, *C. R. Soc. Biol.* **155**:625–627.

KARLI, P., 1981, Conceptual and methodological problems associated with the study of brain mechanisms underlying aggressive behavior, in: *The Biology of Aggression* (P. F. Brain, and D. Benton, eds.), Sijthoff and Noordhoff, Rockville, MD, pp. 322–361.

KATZ, R. J., 1980, Role of serotonergic mechanisms in animal models of predation, *Prog. Neuro-Psychopharmacol.* **4:**219–231.

KAVALIERS, M., and HIRST, M., 1985, Fmrfamide, a putative endogenous opiate antagonist: Evidence from suppression of defeat-induced analgesia and feeding in mice, *Neuropeptides* **6:**485–494.

KELLEHER, R. T., and MORSE, W. H., 1968, Determinants of the specificity of behavioral effects of drugs, *Ergebnisse Physiol. Biol. Chem. Exp. Pharmakol.* **60:**1–56.

KELLER, D. E., and POSTER, D. S., 1970, Effects of psychoactive drugs on stereotyped aggressive behavior of *Betta splendens*, *Am. Zool.* **10:**288.

KELLY, D. D., 1974, The experimental imperative: Laboratory analyses of aggressive behaviors, in: *Aggression. Research Publications Association for Research in Nervous and Mental Diseases* (S. H. Frazier, ed.), Williams & Wilkins, Baltimore, pp. 21–41.

KELLY, J. T., KOCH, M., and BUEGEL, D., 1976, Lithium carbonate in juvenile manic-depressive illness, *Dis. Nerv. System* **37:**90–92.

KERR, W. C., 1976, Lithium salts in the management of a child batterer, *Med. J. Aust.* **2:**414–415.

KIDO, R., HIROSE, K., YAMAMOTO, K-I., and MATSUSHITA, A., 1967, Effects of some drugs on aggressive behaviour and the electrical activity of the limbic system, in: *Progress in Brain Research. Symposium on the Structure and Function of the Limbic System* (W. R. Adley, P. Tokizane, eds.), Elsevier, Amsterdam, pp. 365–387.

KILBEY, M. M., FRITCHIE, G. E., MCLENDON, D. M., and JOHNSON, K. M., 1972, Attack behavior in mice inhibited by delta-9-tetrahydrocannabinol, *Nature* **238:**463–465.

KILBEY, M. M., MOORE, J. W., and HALL, M., 1973a, Delta-9-Tetrahydrocannabinol induced inhibition of predatory aggression in the rat, *Psychopharmacologia* **31:**157–166.

KILBEY, M. M., MOORE, J. W., JR., and HARRIS, R. T., 1973b, Effects of delta-9-tetrahydrocannabinol on appetitive and aggressive-rewarded maze performance in the rat, *Physiol. Psychol.* **1:**174–176.

KILBEY, M. M., JOHNSON, K. M., and MCLENDON, D. M., 1977, Time course of delta-9-tetrahydrocannabinol inhibition of predatory aggression, *Pharmacol. Biochem. Behav.* **7:**117–120.

KIMBREL, G. McA., 1969, Relationship of the upright agonistic posture in the foot shock situation to dominance-submission in male C57BL/6 mice, *Psychonom. Sci.* **16:**167–168.

KJELLBERG, B., and RANDRUP, A., 1971, The effects of amphetamine and pimozide, a neuroleptic, on the social behaviour of vervet monkeys *(Cercopithecus* sp.), in: *Advances in Neuro-psychopharmacology* (O. Vinar, Z. Votaya, and P. B. Bradley, eds.), North Holland Publishing Co., Amsterdam-London, pp. 305–310.

KLEPFISZ, A., and RACY, J., 1973, Homicide and LSD, *JAMA* **223:**429–430.

KLETZTIN, M., 1969, An experimental analysis of aggressive-defensive behavior in mice, in: *Aggressive Behavior* (S. Garattini and E. B. Sigg, eds.), Excerpta Medica Foundation, Amsterdam, pp. 253–262.

KLIGMAN, D., and GOLDBERG, D. A., 1975, Temporal lobe epilepsy and aggression, *J. Nerv. Ment. Dis.* **160:**324–341.

KNIGHT, W. R., HOLTZ, J. R., and SPROGIS, G. R., 1963, Acetophenazine and fighting behavior in mice, *Science* **141:**830–831.

KNUDSEN, K., 1967, Homicide after treatment with lysergic acid diethylamide, *Acta Psychiatr. Scand.* **40:**389–395.

KNUTSON, J. F., 1970, Aggression during the fixed-ratio and extinction components of a mutliple schedule of reinforcement, *J. Exp. Anal. Behav.* **13:**221–231.

KOCHANSKY, G. E., SALZMAN, C., SHADER, R. I., HARMATZ, J. S., and OGELTREE, A. M., 1975, The differential effects of chlordiazepoxide and oxazepam on hostility in a small group setting, *Am. J. Psychiatry* **132:**861–863.

KOOLHAAS, J. M., 1978, Hypothalamically induced intraspecific aggressive behaviour in the rat, *Exp. Brain Res.* **32:**365–375.
KOREY, S. R., 1944, The effects of benzedrine sulfate on the behavior of psychopathic and neurotic juvenile delinquents, *Psychiatry Q.* **18:**127–137.
KORF, J., and KUIPER, H. E., 1971, Induction of bizarre behaviour in rats by *p*-chloroamphetamine, a serotonin depletor, after repeated drug administration, *Psychopharmacologia* **21:**328–337.
KOSTOWSKI, W., 1966, A note on the effects of some psychotropic drugs on the aggressive behaviour in the ant, *Formica rufa, J. Pharm. Pharmacol.* **18:**747–749.
KOSTOWSKI, W., and TARCHALSKA, B., 1972, The effects of some drugs affecting brain 5-HT on the aggressive behaviour and spontaneous electrical activity of the central nervous system of the ant, *Formica rufa, Brain Res.* **38:**143–149.
KOSTOWSKI, W., VALZELLI, L., and KOZAK, W., 1983, Chlordiazepoxide antagonizes locus coeruleus-mediated suppression of muricidal aggression, *Eur. J. Pharmacol.* **91:**329–330.
KOVACH, J. K., 1967, Maternal behavior in the domestic cock under the influence of alcohol, *Science* **15:**835–837.
KOZAK, W., VALZELLI, L., and GARATTINI, S., 1984, Anxiolytic activity on locus coeruleus-mediated suppression of muricidal aggression, *Eur. J. Pharmacol.* **105:**323–326.
KRAEMER, G. E., 1985, The primate social environment, brain neurochemical changes and psychopathology, *Trends Neurosci.* **8:**339–340.
KRAMER, J. C., 1969, Introduction to amphetamine abuse, *J. Psychedelic Drugs* **2:**1–16.
KRAMES, L., MILGRAM, N. W., and CHRISTIE, D. P., 1973, Predatory aggression: Differential suppression of killing and feeding, *Behav. Biol.* **9:**641–647.
KREISKOTT, H., 1963, Zur Verhaltensforschung im Rahmen der Psychopharmakologie, *Med. Chem.* **7:**57–78.
KREISKOTT, H., 1966, Das Entzugssyndrom morphinsuechtiger Rhesusaffen—Modell einer pharmakogenen Psychose? *Arzneim.-Forsch. (Drug Res.)* **16:**219–220.
KREISKOTT, H., 1969, Some comments on the killing response behaviour of the rat, in: *Aggressive Behaviour* (S. Garattini and E. B. Sigg, eds.), Excerpta Medica Foundation, Amsterdam, pp. 56–58.
KROMER, W., and DUM, J. E., 1980, Mouse-killing in rats induces a naloxone-blockable increase in nociceptive threshold, *Eur. J. Pharmacol.* **63:**195–198.
KRSIAK, M., 1974*a*, Isolation-induced timidity in mice as a measure of anxiolytic activity of drugs, *Activ. Nerv. Superior* **16:**141–142.
KRSIAK, M., 1974*b*, Behavioral changes and aggressivity evoked by drugs in mice, *Res. Commun. Chem. Pathol. Pharmacol.* **7:**237–257.
KRSIAK, M., 1975*a*, Tail rattling in aggressive mice as a measure of tranquillizing activity of drugs, *Activ. Nerv. Superior* **17:**225–226.
KRSIAK, M., 1975*b*, Timid singly-housed mice: Their value in prediction of psychtropic activity of drugs, *Br. J. Pharmacol.* **55:**141–150.
KRSIAK, M., 1976, Effect of ethanol on aggression and timidity in mice, *Psychopharmacology* **51:**75–80.
KRSIAK, M., 1979, Effects of drugs on behaviour of aggressive mice, *Br. J. Pharmacol.* **65:**525–533.
KRSIAK, M., and BORGESOVA, M., 1973, Effect of alcohol on behaviour of pairs of rats. *Psychopharmacologia* **32:**201–209.
KRSIAK, M., PRIBIK, V., 1978, Effect of amphetamine on sequences of behavioural activities in mice. *Activ. Nerv. Superior* **20:**9–11.
KRSIAK, M., STEINBERG, H., 1969, Psychopharmacological aspects of aggression: A review of the literature and some new experiments, *J. Psychosom. Res.* **13:**243–252.

Krsiak, M., Borgesova, M., and Kadlecova, O., 1971, LSD-accentuated individual type of social behaviour in mice, *Activ. Nerv. Superior* **13**:211–212.

Krsiak, M., Elis, J., Poschlova, N., and Masek, K., 1977, Increased aggressiveness and lower brain serotonin levels in offspring of mice given alcohol during gestation, *J. Stud. Alcohol* **38**:1696–1704.

Krsiak, M., Sulcova, A., Tomasikova, Z., Dlohozkova, N., Kosar, E., and Masek, K., 1981, Drug effects on attack, defense and escape in mice, *Pharmacol. Biochem. Behav.* **14**:47–52.

Krsiak, M., Sulcova, A., Donat, P., Tomasikova, Z., Dlohozkova, N., Kosar, E., and Masek, K., 1984, Can social and agonistic interactions be used to detect anxiolytic activity of drugs? in: *Ethopharmacological Aggression Research* (K. A. Miczek, M. R. Kruk, and B. Olivier, eds.), Liss, New York, pp. 93–114.

Krstic, S. K., Stefanovic-Denic, K., and Beleslin, D. B., 1982, Effect of morphine and morphine-like drugs of carbachol-induced fighting in cats, *Pharmacol. Biochem. Behav.* **17**:371–373.

Kruk, M. R., van der Poel, A. M., and de Vos-Frerichs, T. P., 1979, The induction of aggressive behaviour by electrical stimulation in the hypothalamus of male rats, *Behaviour* **70**:292–321.

Kruk, M. R., van der Laan, C. E., Meelis, W., Phillips, R. E., Mos, J., and van der Poel, A. M., 1984, Brain-stimulation induced agonistic behaviour: A novel paradigm in ethopharmacological aggression research, in: *Ethopharmacological Aggression Research* (K. A. Miczek, M. R. Kruk, and B. Olivier, eds.), Liss, New York, pp. 157–177.

Kulkarni, A. S., 1968, Muricidal block produced by 5-hydroxytryptophan and various drugs, *Life Sci.* **7**:125–128.

Kulkarni, A. S., and Plotnikoff, N. P., 1978, Effects of central stimulants on aggressive behavior, in: *Psychopharmacology of Aggression. Modern Problems of Pharmacopsychiatry* (L. Valzelli, ed.), Karger, Basel, pp. 69–81.

Kurischko, A., and Oettel, M., 1977, Androgen-dependent fighting behaviour in male mice, *Endokrinologie* **70**:1–5.

Lagerspetz, K., 1964, Studies on the aggressive behaviour of mice, *Ann. Aca. Sci. Fennicae* **131**:1–131.

Lagerspetz, K. M. J., and Ekqvist, K., 1978, Failure to induce aggression in inhibited and in genetically non-aggressive mice through injections of ethyl alcohol, *Aggressive Behav.* **4**:105–113.

Lagerspetz, K. Y. H., and Lagerspetz, K. M. J., 1971, Amphetamine toxicity in genetically aggressive and non-aggressive mice, *J. Pharm. Pharmacol.* **23**:542–543.

Lal, H., 1975a, Narcotic dependence, narcotic action and dopamine receptors, *Life Sci.* **17**:483–496.

Lal, H., 1975b, Morphine-withdrawal aggression, in: *Methods in Narcotic Research* (S. Ehrenpreis and E. A. Neidel, eds.), Dekker, New York, pp. 149–171.

Lal, H., and Puri, S. K., 1972, Morphine-withdrawal aggression: Role of dopaminergic stimulation, in: *Drug Addiction: Experimental Pharmacology* (J. M. Singh and H. Lal, eds.), Futura, New York, pp. 301–310.

Lal, H., Defeo, J. J., and Thut, P., 1968, Effect of amphetamine on pain-induced aggression, *Commun. Behav. Biol.* **1**:333–336.

Lal, H., Nesson, B., and Smith, N., 1970, Amphetamine-induced aggression in mice pretreated with dihydroxyphenylalanine (dopa) and/or reserpine, *Biol. Psychiatry* **2**:299–301.

Lal, H., O'Brien, J., and Puri, S. K., 1971, Morphine-withdrawal aggression: Sensitization by amphetamines, *Psychopharmacologia* **22**:217–223.

Lammers, A. J. J. C., and van Rossum, J. M., 1968, Bizarre social behavior in rats induced by a combination of a peripheral decarboxylase inhibitor and DOPA, *Eur. J. Pharmacol.* **5:**103–106.

LAMPRECHT, F., EICHELMAN, B., THOA, N. B., WILLIAMS, R. B., and KOPIN, I. J., 1972, Rat fighting behavior: Serum dopamine-β-hydroxylase and hypothalamic tyrosine hydroxylase, *Science* **177:**1214–1215.

LANG, A. R., GOECKNER, D. J., ADESSO, V. J., and MARLATT, G. A., 1975, Effects of alcohol on aggression in male social drinkers, *J. Abnorm. Psychol.* **84:**508–518.

LANGFELDT, T., 1974, Diazepam-induced play behavior in cats during prey killing, *Psychopharmacologia* **36:**181–184.

LANGFELDT, T., and URSIN, H., 1971, Differential action of diazepam on flight and defense behavior in the cat, *Psychopharmacologia* **19:**61–66.

LANGLEY, W., 1981, Failure of food-aversion conditioning to suppress predatory attack of the grasshopper mouse, *Onychomys leucogaster*, *Behav. Neural Biol.* **33:**317–333.

LAPIN, I. P., 1962, Qualitative and quantitative relationships between the effects of imipramine and chlorpromazine on amphetamine group toxicity, *Psychopharmacologia* **3:**413–422.

LAPIN, I. P., 1967, Simple pharmacological procedures to differentiate antidepressants and cholinolytics in mice and rats, *Psychopharmacologia* **11:**79–87.

LASCHET, U., and LASCHET, L., 1967, Antiandrogentherapie der pathologisch gesteigerten und abartigen Sexualitat des Mannes, *Klin. Wochenschr.* **25:**324–325.

LATIES, V. G., 1961, Modification of affect, social behavior and performance by sleep deprivation and drugs, *J. Psychiatr. Res.* **1:**12–25.

LATIES, V. G., and WEISS, B., 1981, The amphetamine margin in sports, *Fed. Proc.* **40:**2689–2692.

LE DOUAREC, J. C., and BROUSSY, L., 1969, Dissociation of the aggressive behaviour in mice produced by certain drugs, in: *Aggressive Behaviour* (S. Garattini and E. B. Sigg, eds.), Excerpta Medica Foundation, Amsterdam, pp. 281–295.

LE ROUX, L. C., and SMITH, L. S., 1964, Violent deaths and alcoholic intoxication, *J. Forensic Med.* **11:**131–147.

LE VANN, L. J., 1971, Clinical comparison of haloperidol with chlorpromazine in mentally retarded children, *Am. J. Ment. Defic.* **6:**719–723.

LEAF, R. C., LERNER, L., and HOROVITZ, Z. P., 1969, The role of the amygdala in the pharmacological and endocrinological manipulation of aggression, in: *Aggressive Behavior* (S. Garattini and E. B. Sigg, eds.), Excerpta Medica Foundation, Amsterdam, pp. 120–131.

LEAF, R. C., WNEK, D. J., GAY, P. E., CORCIA, R. M., and LAMON, S., 1975, Chlordiazepoxide and diazepam induced mouse killing by rats, *Psychopharmacologia* **44:**23–28.

LEAF, R. C., WNEK, D. J., and LAMON, S., 1978, Despite various drugs, cats continue to kill mice, *Pharmacol. Biochem. Behav.* **9:**445–452.

LEFKOWITZ, M. M., 1969, Effects of diphenylhydantoin on disruptive behavior, *Arch. Gen. Psychiatry* **20:**643–651.

LEGRAND, R., and FIELDER, R., 1973, Role of dominance-submission relationships in shock-induced fighting of mice, *J. Comp. Physiol. Psychol.* **82:**501–506.

LEONARD, K. E., BROMET, E. J., PARKINSON, D. K., DAY, N. L., and RYAN, C. M., 1985, Patterns of alcohol use and physically aggressive behavior in men, *J. Stud. Alcohol* **46:**279–282.

LESTER, D., 1980, Alcohol and suicide and homicide, *J. Stud. Alcohol* **41:**1220–1223.

LEVENTHAL, B. L., and BRODIE, H. K. H., 1981, The pharmacology of violence, in: *Biobehavioral Aspects of Aggression* (D. A. Hamburg and M. B. Trudeau, eds.), Liss, New York, pp. 85–106.

LEVETT, A., SAAYMAN, G. S., and AMES, F., 1977, The effects of cannabis sativa on the behavior of adult female chacma baboons *(Papio ursinus)* in captivity, *Psychopharmacology* **53**:79–81.

LEWIN, L., 1920, *Die Gifte in der Weltgeschichte: Toxikologische allgemeinverstaendliche Untersuchungen der historischen Quellen*, Springer, Berlin.

LEWIS, C. E., 1984, Alcoholism, antisocial personality, narcotic addiction: An integrative approach, *Psychiatr. Dev.* **3**:223–235.

LEWIS, C. E., CLONINGER, C. R., and PAIS, J., 1983a, Alcoholism, antisocial personality and drug use in a criminal population, *Alcohol Alcoholism* **18**:53–60.

LEWIS, C. E., CROUGHAN, J. L., WHITMAN, B. Y., and MILLER, J. P., 1983b, Association of alcoholism and antisocial personality in a narcotic-dependent population: The Lexington addicts, *Psychiatry Res.* **10**:31–46.

LEWIS, C. E., ROBINS, L., and RICE, J., 1985, Association of alcoholism with antisocial personality in urban men, *J. Nerv. Ment. Dis.* **173**:166–174.

LEYHAUSEN, P., 1960, *Verhaltensstudien an Katzen*, 2nd ed., Paul Parey, Berlin.

LINNOILA, M., VIRKKUNEN, M., SCHEININ, M., NUUTILA, A., RIMON, R., and GOODWIN, F. K., 1983, Low cerebrospinal fluid 5-hydroxyindoleacetic acid concentration differentiates impulsive from nonimpulsive violent behavior, *Life Sci.* **33**:2609–2614.

LION, J. R., 1975, Conceptual issues in the use of drugs for the treatment of aggression in man, *J. Nerv. Ment. Dis.* **160**:76–82.

LION, J. R., 1979, Benzodiazepines in the treatment of aggressive patients, *J. Clin. Psychiatry* **40**:70–71.

LION, J. R., AZCARATE, C., and KOEPKE, H., 1975a, "Paradoxical rage reactions" during psychotropic medication, *Dis. Nerv. Syst.* **36**:557–558.

LION, J. R., HILL, J., and MADDEN, D. J., 1975b, Lithium carbonate and aggression: A case report, *Dis. Nerv. Syst.* **36**:97–98.

LISCIOTTO, C. A., DEBOLD, J. F., and MICZEK, K. A., 1987, Sexual differentiation and the effects of alcohol on aggressive behavior in mice, *Pharmacol. Biochem. Behav.* (in press)

LISTER, R. E., BEATTIE, I. A., and BERRY, P. A., 1971, Effects of drugs on the social behaviour of baboons, in: *Advances in Neuro-psychopharmacology* (O. Vinar, Z. Votava, and Bradley, P. B., eds.), North-Holland Publishing Co., Amsterdam-London, pp. 299–303.

LLORENTE, A. F., 1969, The management of behavior disorders with thioridazine in the mentally retarded, *J. Maine Med. Assoc.* **60**:229–231.

LOISELLE, R. H., and CAPPARELL, H. V., 1967, Effects of chlorpromazine HCl and chlordiazepoxide HCl on "instinctual" aggressive behavior in rats, *Psychiatr. Commun.* **9**:29–33.

LOIZZO, A., and MASSOTTI, M., 1973, Taming effect of nonnarcotic analgesics on the septal syndrome in rats, *Pharmacol. Biochem. Behav.* **1**:367–370.

LONEY, J., PRINZ, R. J., MISHALOW, J., and JOAD, J., 1978, Hyperkinetic/aggressive boys in treatment: Predictors of clinical response to methylphenidate, *Am. J. Psychiatry* **135**:1487–1491.

LOONEY, T. A., and COHEN, P. S., 1982, Aggression induced by intermittent positive reinforcement, *Biobehav. Rev.* **6**:15–37.

LUCAS, A. R., and WEISS, M., 1971, Methylphenidate hallucinosis, *JAMA* **217**:1079–1081.

LUISADA, P. V., 1978, The phencyclidine psychosis: Phenomenology and treatment, in: *Phencyclidine (PCP) Abuse: An Appraisal* (R. C. Petersen and R. C. Stillman, eds.), NIDA Research Monograph 21, Rockville, MD, pp. 241–253.

LUTTGE, W. G., 1979, Anti-estrogen inhibition of testosterone-stimulated aggression in mice, *Sep. Exp.* **35**:273.

LYNCH, W. C., LIBBY, L., and JOHNSON, H. F., 1983, Naloxone inhibits intermale aggression in isolated mice, *Psychopharmacology* **79**:370–371.

MACDONALD, J. M., 1961, *The Murderer and His Victim*, Thomas, Springfield, IL.

MACDONNELL, M. F., and EHMER, M., 1969, Some effects of ethanol on aggressive behavior in cats, *Q. J. Stud. Alcohol* **30:**312–319.

MACDONNELL, M. F., FESSOCK, L., and BROWN, S. H., 1971, Ethanol and the neural substrate for affective defense in the cat, *Q. J. Stud. Alcohol* **32:**406–419.

MACDONNELL, M. F., and FESSOCK, L., 1972, Some effects of ethanol, amphetamine, disulfiram and *p*-CPA on seizing of prey in feline predatory attack and on associated motor pathways, *Q. J. Stud. Alcohol* **33:**437–450.

MACKINTOSH, J. H., CHANCE, M. R. A., and SILVERMAN, A. P., 1977, The contribution of ethological techniques to the study of drug effects, in: *Handbook of Psychopharmacology Principles of Behavioral Pharmacology* (L. L. Iversen, S. D. Iversen, and S. H. Snyder, eds.), Plenum, New York, pp. 3–35.

MAEDA, H., SATO, T., and MAKI, S., 1985, Effects of dopamine agonists on hypothalamic defensive attack in cats, *Physiol. Behav.* **35:**89–92.

MAENGWYN-DAVIES, G. D., JOHNSON, D. G., THOA, N. B., WEISE, V. K., and KOPIN, I. J., 1973, Influence of isolation and of fighting on adrenal tyrosine hydroxylase and phenylethanolamine-*N*-methyltransferase activities in three strains of mice, *Psychopharmacologia* **28:**339–350.

MAIER, S. F., ANDERSON, C., and LIEBERMAN, D. A., 1972, Influence of control of shock on subsequent shock-elicited aggression, *J. Comp. Physiol. Psychol.* **81:**94–100.

MAJ, J., MOGILNICKA, E., and KORDECKA, A., 1979, Chronic treatment with antidepressant drugs: Potentiation of apomorphine-induced aggressive behaviour in rats, *Neurosci. Lett.* **13:**337–341.

MAJ, J., MOGILNICKA, E., and KORDECKA-MAGIERA, A., 1980, Effects of chronic administration of antidepressant drugs on aggressive behavior induced by clonidine in mice, *Pharmacol. Biochem. Behav.* **13:**153–154.

MAJ, J., ROGOZ, Z., SKUZA, G., and SOWINSKA, H., 1982, Effects of chronic treatment with antidepressants on aggressiveness induced by clonidine in mice, *J. Neural Transmission* **55:**19–25.

MALETZKY, B. M., 1973, The episodic dyscontrol syndrome, *Dis. Nerv. Syst.* **34:**178–185.

MALETZKY, B. M., 1974, *d*-Amphetamine and delinquency: Hyperkinesis persisting? *Dis. Nerv. Syst.* **35:**543–547.

MALETZKY, B. M., and KLOTTER, J., 1974, Episodic dyscontrol: A controlled replication, *Dis. Nerv. Syst.* **35:**175–179.

MALICK, J. B., 1970*a*, Effects of selected drugs on stimulus-bound emotional behavior elicited by hypothalamic stimulation in the cat, *Arch. Int. Pharmacodyn. Ther.* **186:**137–141.

MALICK, J. B., 1970*b*, A behavioral comparison of three lesion-induced models of aggression in the rat, *Physiol. Behav.* **5:**679–681.

MALICK, J. B., 1975, Differential effects of *d*- and *l*-amphetamine on mouse-killing behavior in rats, *Pharmacol. Biochem. Behav.* **3:**697–699.

MALICK, J. B., 1976, Pharmacological antagonism of mouse-killing behavior in the olfactory bulb lesion-induced killer rat, *Aggressive Behav.* **2:**123–130.

MALICK, J. B., 1978*a*, Selective antagonism of isolation-induced aggression in mice by diazepam following chronic administration, *Pharmacol. Biochem. Behav.* **8:**497–499.

MALICK, J. B., 1978*b*, Inhibition of fighting in isolated mice following repeated administration of lithium chloride, *Pharmacol. Biochem. Behav.* **8:**579–581.

MALICK, J. B., 1979, The pharmacology of isolation-induced aggressive behavior in mice, in: *Current Developments in Psychopharmacology* (W. B. Essman and L. Valzelli, eds.), SP Medical and Scientific Books, New York, pp. 1–27.

MALICK, J. B., SOFIA, R. D., and GOLDBERG, M. E., 1969, A comparative study of the effects of selected psychoactive agents upon three lesion-induced models of aggression in the rat, *Arch. Int. Pharmacodyn. Ther.* **181:**459–465.

MALMQUIST, C. P., 1971, Premonitory signs of homicidal aggression in juveniles, *Am. J. Psychiatry* **128**:461–465.

MANDEL, P., CIESIELSKI, L., MAITRE, M., SIMLER, S., KEMPF, E., and MACK, G., 1981, Inhibitory amino acids, aggressiveness, and convulsions, in: *Amino Acid Neurotransmitters* (F. V. DE Feudis, and P. Mandel, eds.), Raven Press, New York, pp. 1–9.

MANN, M., MICHAEL, S. D., and SVARE, B., 1980, Ergot drugs suppress plasma prolactin and lactation but not aggression in parturient mice, *Hormones Behav.* **14**:319–328.

MANNING, F. J., and ELSMORE, T. F., 1972, Shock-elicited fighting and delta-9-tetrahydrocannabinol, *Psychopharmacologia* **25**:218–228.

MAREK, Z., WIDACKI, J., and HANAUSEK, T., 1974, Alcohol as a victimogenic factor of robberies, *Forensic Sci.* **4**:119–123.

MARINI, J. L., and SHEARD, M. H., 1977, Antiaggressive effect of lithium ion in man, *Acta Psychiatr. Scand.* **55**:269–286.

MARINI, J. L., SHEARD, M. H., and KOSTEN, T., 1979a, Study of the role of serotonin in lithium action using shock-elicited fighting, *Commun. Psychopharmacol.* **3**:225–233.

MARINI, J. L., WALTERS, J. K., and SHEARD, M. H., 1979b, Effects of d- and l-amphetamine on hypothalamically-elicited movement and attack in the cat, *Aggressologie* **20**:155–160.

MARK, V. H., and ERVIN, F. R., 1970, *Violence and the Brain*, Harper and Row, New York.

MARKS, P. C., O'BRIEN, M., and PAXINOS, G., 1977, 5,7-DHT-induced muricide: Inhibition as a result of preoperative exposure of rats to mice, *Brain Res.* **135**:383–388.

MARKS, P. C., O'BRIEN, M., and PAXINOS, G., 1978, Chlorimipramine inhibition of muricide: The role of the ascending 5-HT projection, *Brain Res.* **149**:270–273.

MARLER, P., 1976, On animal aggression: The roles of strangeness and familiarity, *Am. Psychologist* **31**:239–246.

MARTIN, W. R., WIKLER, A., EADES, C. G., and PESCOR, F. T., 1963, Tolerance to and physical dependence on morphine in rats, *Psychopharmacologia* **4**:247–260.

MASSERMAN, J. H., and JACOBSON, L., 1940, Effects of ethyl alcohol on the cerebral cortex and the hypothalamus of the cat, *Arch. Neurol. Psychiatry* **43**:334–340.

MASUR, J., MARTZ, R. M. W., BIENIEK, D., and KORTE, F., 1971, Influence of (−) delta-9-trans-terahydrocannabinol and mescaline on the behavior of rats submitted to food competition situations, *Psychopharmacologia* **22**:187–194.

MASUR, J., KARNIOL, I. G., and PALERMO NETO, J., 1972, *Cannabis sativa* induces "winning" behaviour in previously "loser" rats, *J. Pharm. Pharmacol.* **24**:262.

MATTE, A. C., 1975, Effects of hashish on isolation induced aggression in wild mice, *Psychopharmacologia* **45**:125–128.

MATTE, A. C., and FABIAN, E., 1978, The effect of cyproterone acetate on motor activity, aggression, "emotionality," body weight and testes in wild mice, *Andrologia* **10**:155–162.

MAYFIELD, D., 1976, Alcoholism, alcohol, intoxication and assaultive behavior, *Dis. Nerv. Syst.* **37**:288–291.

MCCALDON, R. J., 1967, Rape, *Can. J. Criminol. Corrections* **9**:37–59.

MCCARTY, R. C., WHITESIDES, G. H., and TOMOSKY, T. K., 1976, Effects of para-chlorophenylalanine on the predatory behavior of *Onychomys torridus*, *Pharmacol. Biochem. Behav.* **4**:217–220.

MCCORD, J., 1981, Alcoholism and criminality, *J. Stud. Alcohol* **42**:739–748.

MCDONALD, A. L., and HEIMSTRA, N. W., 1964, Modification of aggressive behavior of green sunfish with dextra-lysergic acid diethylamide, *J. Psychol.* **57**:19–23.

MCDONALD, R. L., 1967, The effects of personality type on drug response, *Arch. Gen. Psychiatry* **17**:680–686.

MCDONOUGH, J. H., Jr., MANNING, F. J., and ELSMORE, T. F., 1972, Reduction of predatory aggression of rats following administration of Δ^9-tetrahydrocannabinol, *Life Sc.* **11**:103–111.

MCGEORGE, J., 1963, Alcohol and crime, *Med. Sci. Law* **3:**27–48.
MCGIVERN, R. F., LOBAUGH, N. J., and COLLIER, A. C., 1981, Effect of naloxone and housing conditions on shock-elicited reflexive fighting: Influence of immediate prior stress, *Physiol. Psychol.* **9:**251–256.
MCGLONE, J. J., RITTER, S., and KELLEY, K. W., 1980, The antiaggressive effect of lithium is abolished by area postrema lesion, *Physiol. Behav.* **24:**1095–1100.
MCGLOTHLIN, W. H., 1979, Drugs and crime, in: *Handbook on Drug Abuse* (R. I. Dupont, A. Goldstein, and J. O'Donnell, eds.), US Government Printing Office, Washington, DC, pp. 357–364.
MCINTYRE, D. C., 1978, Amygdala kindling and muricide in rats, *Physiol. Behav.* **21:**49–56.
MCKEARNEY, J. W., 1979, Interrelations among prior experience and current conditions in the determination of behavior and the effects of drugs, in: *Advances in Behavioral Pharmacology* (T. Thompson and P. B. Dews, eds.), Academic Press, New York, pp. 39–64.
MCKENZIE, G. M., 1971, Apomorphine-induced aggression in the rat, *Brain Res.* **34:**323–330.
MEINECKE, R. O., and CHERKIN, A., 1972, Failure of ethanol or pentobarbital to suppress fighting in the pit gamecock *(Gallus gallus)*, *Psychopharmacologia* **25:**189–194.
MELANDER, B., 1960, Psychopharmacodynamic effects of diethylpropion, *Acta Pharmacol. Toxicol.* **17:**182–190.
MELLER, R. E., KEVERNE, E. B., and HERBERT, J., 1980, Behavioural and endocrine effects of naltrexone in male talapoin monkeys, *Pharmacol. Biochem. Behav.* **13:**663–672.
MENDELSON, J. H., 1977, Endocrines and aggression, *Psychopharmacol. Bull.* **13:**22–23.
MENDELSON, J. H., and MELLO, N. K., 1974, Alcohol, aggression and androgens, in: *Aggression* (S. H. Frazier, ed.), Williams & Wilkins, Baltimore, pp. 225–247.
MENDELSON, J. H., MELLO, N. K., and ELLINGBOE, J., 1978, Effects of alcohol on pituitary-gonadal hormones, sexual function, and aggression in human males, in: *Psychopharmacology: A Generation of Progress* (M. A. Lipton, A. DiMascio, and K. F., Killam, eds.), Raven Press, New York, pp. 1677–1692.
MENDELSON, J. H., DIETZ, P. E., and ELLINGBOE, J., 1982, Postmortem plasma luteinizing hormone levels and antemortem violence, *Pharmacol. Biochem. Behav.* **17:**171–173.
MENDELSON, W., JOHNSON, N., and STEWART, M. A., 1971, Hyperactive children as teenagers: A follow-up study, *J. Nerv. Ment. Dis.* **153:**273–279.
MEYERSON, B. J., 1981, Comparison of the effects of beta-endorphin and morphine on exploratory and socio-sexual behaviour in the male rat, *Eur. J. Pharmacol.* **69:**453–463.
MEYERSON, B. J., 1982, Socio-sexual behaviours in rats after neonatal and adult beta- endorphin treatment, *Scand. J. Psychol.* (Suppl. 1):85–89.
MICZEK, K. A., 1974, Intraspecies aggression in rats: Effects of *d*-amphetamine and chlordiazepoxide, *Psychopharamcologia* **39:**275–301.
MICZEK, K. A., 1976a, Does THC induce aggression? Suppression and induction of aggressive reactions by chronic and acute delta-9-tetrahydrocannabinol treatment in laboratory rats, in: *Pharmacology of Marihuana* (M. Braude and S. Szara, eds.), Raven Press, New York, pp. 499–514.
MICZEK, K. A., 1976b, Mouse-killing and motor activity: Effects of chronic delta 9-tetrahydrocannabinol and pilocarpine, *Psychopharmacology* **47:**59–64.
MICZEK, K. A., 1977, A behavioral analysis of aggressive behaviors induced and modulated by delta 9-tetrahydrocannabinol, pilocarpine, *d*-amphetamine and *l*-dopa, *Activ. Nerv. Superior* **19:**224–225.
MICZEK, K. A., 1978, Delta-9-Tetrahydrocannabinol: Antiaggressive effects in mice, rats, and squirrel monkeys, *Science* **199:**1459–1461.
MICZEK, K. A., 1979a, Chronic delta-9-tetrahydrocannabinol in rats: Effect on social interactions, mouse killing, motor activity, consummatory behavior, and body temperature, *Psychopharmacology* **60:**137–146.

Miczek, K. A., 1979b, A new test for aggression in rats without aversive stimulation: Differential effects of d-amphetamine and cocaine, *Psychopharmacology* **60**:253–259.

Miczek, K. A., 1981, Differential antagonism of d-amphetamine effects on motor activity and agonistic behavior in mice, *Neurosci. Abstr.* **7**:343.

Miczek, K. A., 1982, Ethological analysis of drug action on aggression, defense and defeat, in: *Behavioral Models and the Analysis of Drug Action* (M. Y. Spiegelstein and A. Levy, eds.), Elsevier, Amsterdam, pp. 225–239.

Miczek, K. A., 1983a, Ethopharmacology of aggression, defense, and defeat, in: *Aggressive Behavior: Genetic and Neural Approaches* (E. C. Simmel, M. E. Hahn, and J. K. Walters, eds.), Lawrence Erlbaum Associates, Hillsdale, NJ, pp. 147–166.

Miczek, K. A., 1983b, Ethological analysis of drug action on aggression and defense, *Prog. Neuro-Psychopharmacol. Biol. Psychiatry* **7**:519–524.

Miczek, K. A., 1985, Alcohol and aggressive behavior in rats: Interaction with benzodiazepines, *Soc. Neurosci. Abstr.* **11**:1290.

Miczek, K. A., 1986, Functionally specific tolerance to opioid agonists after social defeat: Analgesia and operant performance, *Soc. Neurosc. Abstr.* (in press).

Miczek, K. A., 1987, Diazepam increases aggressive behavior and punishment-suppressed drinking: Antagonism by Ro15-1788, *Psychopharmacology* (in press).

Miczek, K. A., and Barry, H., III, 1974, Delta-9-Tetrahydrocannabinol and aggressive behavior in rats, *Behav. Biol.* **11**:261–267.

Miczek, K. A., and Barry, H., III, 1975, What does the tube test measure? *Behav. Biol.* **13**:537–539.

Miczek, K. A., and Barry, H., III, 1976, Pharmacology of sex and aggression, in: *Behavioral Pharmacology* (S. D. Glick and J. Goldfarb, eds.), Mosby, St. Louis, pp. 176–257.

Miczek, K. A., and Barry, H., III, 1977, Effects of alcohol on attack and defensive–submissive reactions in rats, *Psychopharmacology* **52**:231–237.

Miczek, K. A., and DeBold, J. F., 1983, Hormone-drug interactions and their influence on aggressive behavior, in: *Hormones and Aggressive Behavior* (B. B. Svare, ed.), Plenum Press, New York, pp. 313–347.

Miczek, K. A., and Dixit, B. N., 1980, Behavioral and biochemical effects of chronic delta 9-tetrahydrocannabinol in rats, *Psychopharmacology* **67**:195–202.

Miczek, K. A., and Gold, L. H., 1983a, Ethological analysis of amphetamine action on social behavior in squirrel monkeys *(Saimiri sciureus)*, in: *Ethopharmacology: Primate Models of Neuropsychiatric Disorders* (K. A. Miczek, ed.), Liss, New York, pp. 137–155.

Miczek, K. A., and Gold, L. H., 1983b, d-Amphetamine in squirrel monkeys of different social status: Effects on social and agonistic behavior, locomotion, and stereotypies, *Psychopharmacology* **81**:183–190.

Miczek, K. A., and Grossman, S. P., 1972, Effects of septal lesions on inter- and intraspecies aggression in rats, *J. Comp. Physiol. Psychol.* **79**:37–45.

Miczek, K. A., and Krsiak, M., 1979, Drug effects on agonistic behavior, in: *Advances in Behavioral Pharmacology* (T. Thompson and P. B. Dews, eds.), Academic Press, New York, pp. 87–162.

Miczek, K. A., and O'Donnell, J. M., 1978, Intruder-evoked aggression in isolated and nonisolated mice: Effects of psychomotor stimulants and l-dopa, *Psychopharmacology* **57**:47–55.

Miczek, K. A., and O'Donnell, J. M., 1980, Alcohol and chlordiazepoxide increase suppressed aggression in mice, *Psychopharmacology* **69**:39–44.

Miczek, K. A., and Thompson, M. L., 1983, Drugs of abuse and aggression: An ethopharmacological analysis, in: *Alcohol, Drug Abuse and Aggression* (E. Gottheil, K. A. Druley, T. E. Skoloda, and H. M. Waxman, eds.), Thomas, Springfield, IL, pp. 164–188.

Miczek, K. A., and Thompson, M. L., 1984, Analgesia resulting from defeat in a social confrontation: The role of endogenous opioids in brain, in: *Modulation of Sensorimotor*

Activity During Altered Behavioural States (R. Bandler, ed.), Liss, New York, pp. 431–456.

MICZEK, K. A., and WINSLOW, J. T., 1987a, Psychopharmacological research on aggressive behavior, in: *Experimental Psychopharmacology* (A. Greenshaw, and C. Dourish, eds.), Humana Press, New York.

MICZEK, K. A., and WINSLOW, J. T., 1987b, Response to pain and operant performance in socially defeated mice: Selective cross-tolerance to morphine and antagonism by naltrexone, *Psychopharmacology* (in press).

MICZEK, K. A., and YOSHIMURA, H., 1982, Disruption of primate social behavior by d-amphetamine and cocaine: Differential antagonism by antipsychotics, *Psychopharmacology* **76**:163–171.

MICZEK, K. A., ALTMAN, J. L., APPEL, J. B., and BOGGAN, W. O., 1975, Para-chlorophenylalanine, serotonin and killing behavior, *Pharmacol. Biochem. Behav.* **3**:355–361.

MICZEK, K. A., WOOLLEY, J., SCHLISSERMAN, S., and YOSHIMURA, H., 1981, Analysis of amphetamine effects on agonistic and affiliative behavior in squirrel monkeys *(Saimiri sciureus)*, *Pharmacol. Biochem. Behav.* **14**(Suppl.1):103–107.

MICZEK, K. A., THOMPSON, M. L., and SHUSTER, L., 1982, Opioid-like analgesia in defeated mice, *Science* **215**:1520–1522.

MICZEK, K. A., DEBOLD, J. F., and THOMPSON, M. L., 1984a, Pharmacological, hormonal, and behavioral manipulations in the analysis of aggressive behavior, in: *Ethopharmacological Aggression Research* (K. A. Miczek, M. R. Kruk, and B. Olivier, eds.), Alan R. Liss, New York, pp. 1–26.

MICZEK, K. A., KRUK, M. R., and OLIVIER, B., 1984b, *Ethopharmacological Aggression Research*, Liss, New York.

MICZEK, K. A., WINSLOW, J. T., and DEBOLD, J. F., 1984c, Heightened aggressive behavior by animals interacting with alcohol-treated conspecifics: Studies with mice, rats and squirrel monkeys, *Pharmacol. Biochem. Behav.* **20**:349–353.

MICZEK, K. A., THOMPSON, M. L., and SHUSTER, L., 1985, Naloxone injections into the periaqueductal grey area and arcuate nucleus block analgesia in defeated mice, *Psychopharmacology* **87**:39–42.

MIKSIC, S., SMITH, N., and LAL, H., 1976, Reduction of morphine-withdrawal aggression by conditional social stimuli, *Psychopharmacology* **48**:115–117.

MILLER, R., 1984, How do opiates act? *Trends Neurosci.* **7**:184–185.

MILLER, R. E., LEVINE, J. M., and MIRSKY, I. A., 1973, Effects of psychoactive drugs on nonverbal communication and group social behavior of monkeys, *J. Personality Soc. Psychol.* **28**:396–405.

MINDE, K., WEISS, G., and MENDELSON, N., 1972, A 5-year follow-up study of 91 hyperactive school children, *J. Am. Acad. Child Psychiatry* **11**:595–610.

MIRSKY, A. F., and HARMAN, N., 1974, On aggressive behavior and brain disease-some questions and possible relationships derived from the study of men and monkeys, in: *The Neuropsychology of Aggression* (R. F. Whalen, ed.), Plenum Press, New York, pp. 185–210.

MOGILNICKA, E., and PRZEWLOCKA, B., 1981, Facilitated shock-induced aggression after chronic treatment with antidepressant drugs in the rat, *Pharmacol. Biochem. Behav.* **14**:129–132.

MOGILNICKA, E., BOISSARD, C. G., WALDMEIER, P. C., and DELINI-STULA, A., 1983, The effects of single and repeated doses of maprotiline, oxaprotiline and its enantiomers on foot-shock induced fighting in rats, *Pharmacol. Biochem. Behav.* **19**:719–723.

MONROE, R. R., 1975, Anticonvulsants in the treatment of aggression, *J. Nerv. Ment. Dis.* **160**:119–126.

MONROE, R. R., 1978, *Brain Dysfunction in Aggressive Criminals,* Heath, Lexington, MA.

MONROE, R. R., and DALE, R., 1967, Chlordiazepoxide in the treatment of patients with "activated EEG's," *Dis. Nerv. Syst.* **28:**390–396.

MONROE, R. R., PASKEWITZ, D. A., BALIS, G. U., LION, J. R., and RUBIN, J. S., 1978, Response to anticonvulsant (primidone) medication, in: *Brain Dysfunction in Aggressive Criminals* (R. R. Monroe, ed.), Heath, Lexington, MA, pp. 149–160.

MONTGOMERY, S. A., and MONTGOMERY, D., 1982, Pharmacological prevention of suicidal behaviour, *J. Affective Disorders* **4:**291–298.

MOORE, M. S., and THOMPSON, D. M., 1978, Acute and chronic effects of cocaine on extinction-induced aggression, *J. Exp. Anal. Behav.* **29:**309–318.

MOORE, M. S., TYCHSON, R. L., and THOMPSON, D. M., 1976, Extinction-induced mirror responding as a baseline for studying drug effects on aggression, *Pharmacol. Biochem. Behav.* **4:**99–102.

MORAES ANDRADE, O., 1964, The criminogenic action of cannabis (marihuana) and narcotics, *Bull. Narcotics* **16:**23–28.

MORPURGO, C., 1968, Aggressive behavior induced by large doses of 2-(2,6-dichlorphenylamino)-2-imidazoline hydrochloride (ST 155) in mice, *Eur. J. Pharmacol.* **3:**374–377.

MORRISON, S. D., ERWIN, C. W., GIANTURCO, D. T., and GERBER, C. J., 1973, Effect of lithium on combative behavior in humans, *Dis. Nerv. Syst.* **34:**186–189.

MOS, J., and VAN VALKENBURG, C. F. M., 1979, Specific effect on social stress and aggression on regional dopamine metabolism in rat brain, *Neurosci. Lett.* **15:**325–327.

MUELLER, K., and NYHAN, W. L., 1982, Pharmacologic control of pemoline induced self-injurious behavior in rats, *Pharmacol. Biochem. Behav.* **16:**957–963.

MUELLER, K., and NYHAN, W. L., 1983, Clonidine potentiates drug induced self-injurious behavior in rats, *Pharmacol. Biochem. Behav.* **18:**891–894.

MUELLER, K., SABODA, S., PALMOUR, R., and NYHAN, W. L., 1982, Self-injurious behavior produced in rats by daily caffeine and continuous amphetamine, *Pharmacol. Biochem. Behav.* **17:**613–617.

MUKHERJEE, B. P., and PRADHAN, S. N., 1976a, Effects of lithium on foot shock-induced aggressive behavior in rats, *Arch. Int. Pharmacodyn. Ther.* **222:**125–131.

MUKHERJEE, B. P., and PRADHAN, S. N., 1976b, Effects of lithium on septal hyperexcitability and muricidal behavior in rats, *Res. Commun. Psychol. Psychiatry Behav.* **1:**241–247.

MÜLLER-OERLINGHAUSEN, B., 1985, Lithium long-term treatment—Does it act via serotonin? *Pharmacopsychiatry* **18:**214–217.

MURMANN, W., ALMIRANTE, L., and SACCANI-GUELFI, M., 1966, Central nervous system effects of four beta-adrenergic receptor blocking agents, *J. Pharm. Pharmacol.* **18:**317–318.

MURRAY, N., 1962, Covert effects of chlordiazepoxide therapy, *J. Neuropsychiatry* **3:**168–170.

MUSTY, R. E., and CONSROE, P. F., 1982, Phencyclidine produces aggressive behavior in rapid eye movement sleep-deprived rats, *Life Sci.* **30:**1733–1738.

MUSTY, R. E., LINDSEY, C. L., and CARLINI, E. A., 1976, 6-Hydroxydopamine and the aggressive behavior induced by marihuana in REM sleep-deprived rats, *Psychopharmacology* **48:**175–179.

MYERS, T., 1982, Alcohol and violent crime re-examined: Self-reports from two sub-groups of Scottish male prisoners, *Br. J. Addiction* **77:**399–413.

NAKAMURA, K., and THOENEN, H., 1972, Increased irritability: A permanent behavior change induced in the rat by intraventricular administration of 6-hydroxydopamine, *Psychopharmacologia* **24:**359–372.

NATHANSON, M., 1937, The central action of beta-aminopropylbenzene (benzedrine), *Clin. Invest.* **180:**528–531.

NEUMANN, F., and STEINBECK, H., 1971, Antiandrogene: Tierexperimentelle Grundlagen und klinische Anwendungsmöglichkeiten, *Internist* **12:**198–205.

NICOL, A. R., GUNN, J. C., GRISTWOOD, J., FOGGITT, R. H., and WATSON, J. P., 1973, The relationship of alcoholism to violent behaviour resulting in long-term imprisonment, *Br. J. Psychiatry* **123**:47–51.
NIEMEGEERS, C. J. E., VAN NUETEN, J. M., and JANSSEN, P. A. J., 1974, Azaperone, a sedative neuroleptic of the butyrophenone series with pronounced anti-aggressive and anti-shock activity in animals, *Arzneim.-Forsch. (Drug Res.)* **24**:1798–1806.
NIEMINEN, L., and MOTTONEN, M., 1975, The pain aggression induced by bronopol in the rat, *Acta Pharmacol. Toxicol.* **37**:237–241.
NODA, K., MICZEK, K. A., and KREAM, R., 1985, Regional monoamine activity, sensitivity to amphetamine and aggressive behavior in mice, *Soc. Neurosci. Abstr.* **11**:549.
NOWELL, N. W., and WOUTERS, A., 1973, The effects of cyproterone acetate upon aggressive behaviour in the laboratory mouse, *J. Endocrinol.* **57**:36–37.
NURCO, D. N., BALL, J. C., SHAFFER, J. W., and HANLON, T. E., 1985, The criminality of narcotic addicts, *J. Nerv. Ment. Dis.* **173**:94–102.
NURCO, D. N., SHAFFER, J. W., BALL, J. C., KINLOCK, T. W., and LANGROD, J., 1986, A comparison by ethnic group and city of the criminal activities of narcotic addicts, *J. Nerv. Ment. Dis.* **174**:112.
O'BOYLE, M., 1974, Rats and mice together: The predatory nature of the rats mouse-killing response, *Psychol. Bull.* **81**:261–269.
O'BOYLE, M., LOONEY, T. A., and COHEN, P. S., 1973, Suppression and recovery of mouse killing in rats following immediate lithium-chloride injections, *Bull. Psychonom. Soc.* **1**:250–252.
O'DONNELL, J. M., and MICZEK, K. A., 1980, No tolerance to antiaggressive effect of d-amphetamine in mice, *Psychopharmacology* **68**:191–196.
O'KELLY, L. I., and STECKLE, L. C., 1939, A note on long enduring emotional responses in the rat, *J. Psychol.* **8**:125–131.
OETTEL, V. M., and KURISCHIKO, A., 1978, Physiologisch-endokrinologische Studien zum Aggressionsverhalten von Mäuseböcken, *Zeitschr. Versuchstier Kunde* **20**:186–193.
OGAWA, S., and MAKINO, J., 1984, Aggressive behavior in inbred strains of mice during pregnancy, *Behav. Neural Biol.* **40**:195–204.
OJEDA, P. A., 1970, Treatment with thioridazine of emotionally disturbed children in a day hospital, *Michigan Med.* **69**:215–217.
OLIVIER, B., and VAN DALEN, D., 1982, Social behavior in rats and mice: An ethologically based model for differentiating psychoactive drugs, *Aggressive Behav.* **8**:163–168.
OLIVIER, B., MOS, J., VAN DER POEL, A. M., KRIJZER, F. N. C., and KRUK, M. R., 1984, Effects of a new psychoactive drug (DU 27716) on different models of rat agonistic behaviour and EEG, in: *Biological Perspectives on Aggression* (K. J. Flannelly, R. J. Blanchard, and D. C. Blanchard, eds.), Liss, New York, pp. 261–279.
OLIVIER, B., MOS, J., and VAN OORSCHOT, R., 1985, Maternal aggression in rats: Effects of chlordiazepoxide and fluprazine, *Psychopharmacology* **86**:68–76.
OLIVIER, B., MOS, J., and VAN OORSCHOT, R., 1986, Maternal aggression in rats: Lack of interaction between chlordiazepoxide and fluprazine, *Psychopharmacology* **88**:40–43.
ONODERA, K., OGURA, Y., and KISARA, K., 1981, Characteristics of muricide induced by thiamine deficiency and its suppression by antidepressants or intraventricular serotonin, *Physiol. Behav.* **27**:847–853.
OPPENHEIM, W. L., 1977, The "battered alcoholic syndrome," *J. Trauma* **17**:850–856.
OVERALL, J. E., HOLLISTER, L. E., MEYER, F., KIMBELL, I., and SHELTON, J., 1964, Imipramine and thioridazine in depressed and schizophrenic patients, *JAMA* **189**:605–608.
OWEN, R. T., 1980, YG-19-256, *Drugs Future* **5**:98–99.
OZAWA, H., MIYAUCHI, T., and SUGAWARA, K., 1975, Potentiating effect of lithium chloride on aggressive behaviour induced in mice by nialamide plus L-Dopa and by clonidine, *Euro. J. Pharmacol.* **34**:169–179.

PALERMO NETO, J., and CARLINI, E. A., 1972, Aggressive behaviour elicited in rats by cannabis sativa: Effects of p-chlorophenylalanine and DOPA, Eur. J. Pharmacol. 17:215–220.

PALERMO NETO, J., and CARVALHO, F. V., 1973, The effects of chronic cannabis treatment on the aggressive behavior and brain 5-hydroxytryptamine levels of rats with different temperaments, Psychopharmacologia 32:383–392.

PALERMO NETO, J., NUNES, J. F., and CARVALHO, F. V., 1975, The effects of chronic cannabis treatment upon brain 5-hydroxytryptamine, plasma corticosterone and aggressive behavior in female rats with different hormonal status, Psychopharmacologia 42:195–200.

PALLMEYER, T. P., and PETTI, T. A., 1979, Effects of imipramine on aggression and dejection in depressed children, Am. J. Psychiatry 136:1472–1473.

PANKSEPP, J., 1971a, Drugs and stimulus-bound attack, Physiol. Behav. 6:317–320.

PANKSEPP, J., 1971b, Aggression elicited by electrical stimulation of the hypothalamus in albino rats, Physiol. Behav. 6:321–329.

PANTER, B. M., 1977, Lithium in the treatment of a child abuser, Am. J. Psychiatry 134:1436–1437.

PARMIGIANI, S., and BRAIN, P. F., 1983, Effects of residence, aggressive experience and intruder familiarity on attack shown by male mice, Behav. Proc. 8:45–57.

PATERSON, A. T., and VICKERS, C., 1984, Saline drinking and naloxone: Lightcycle dependent effects on social behaviour in male mice, Pharmacol. Biochem. Behav. 21:495–499.

PATON, W. D. M., 1975, Pharmacology of marijuana, Annu. Rev. Pharmacol. 15:191–220.

PAUL, D. M., 1975, Drugs and aggression, Med. Sci. Law 15:16–21.

PAUL, L., MILEY, W. M., and BAENNINGER, R., 1971, Mouse killing by rats: Roles of hunger and thirst in its initiation and maintenance, J. Comp. Physiol. Psychol. 76:242–249.

PAYNE, A. P., and SWANSON, H. H., 1970, Agonistic behaviour between pairs of hamsters of the same and opposite sex in a neutral observation area, Behaviour 36:259–269.

PAYNE, A. P., ANDREWS, M. J., and WILSON, C. A., 1985, The effects of isolation, grouping and aggressive interactions on indole and catecholamine levels and apparent turnover in the hypothalamus and midbrain of the male golden hamster, Physiol. Behav. 34:911–916.

PEEKE, H. V. S., and FIGLER, M. H., 1981, Modulation of aggressive behavior in fish by alcohol and congeners, Pharmacol. Biochem. Behav. 14(Suppl. 1):79–84.

PEEKE, H. V. S., ELLMAN, G. E., HERZ, M. J., 1973, Dose dependent alcohol effects on the aggressive behavior of the conflict cichlid (Cichlasoma nigrofaciatum),Behav. Biol. 8:115–122.

PEEKE, H. V. S., PEEKE, S. C., AVIS, H. H., and ELLMAN, G., 1975, Alcohol, habituation and the patterning of aggressive responses in a cichlid fish, Pharmacol. Biochem. Behav. 3:1031–1036.

PELHAM, W. E., BENDER, M. E., CADDELL, J., BOOTH, S., and MOORER, S. H., 1985, Methylphenidate and children with attention deficit disorder, Arch. Gen. Psychiatry 42:948–952.

PENALOZA-ROJAS, J. H., BACH-Y-RITA, G., RUBIO-CHEVANNIER, H. F., and HERNANDEZ-PEON, R., 1961, Effects of imipramine on hypothalamic and amygdaloid excitability, Exp. Neurol. 4:205–213.

PERNANEN, K., 1976, Alcohol and crimes of violence, in: Social Aspects of Alcoholism (B. Kissin and H. Begleiter, eds.), Plenum Press, New York, pp. 351–444.

PERTWEE, R. G., 1985, Cannabis, in: Psychopharmacology 2. Preclinical Psychopharmacology (D. G. Grahame-Smith, ed.), Elsevier, Amsterdam, pp. 364–391.

PETRIE, W. A., and BAN, T. A., 1981, Propranolol in organic agitation, Lancet i:324.

PETTIJOHN, T. F., 1979, The effects of alcohol on agonistic behavior in the Telomian dog, Psychopharmacology 60:295–301.

PETTIJOHN, T. F., DAVIS, K. L., and SCOTT, J. P., 1980, Influence of living area space on agonistic interaction in Telomian dogs, *Behav. Neural Biol.* **28**:343–349.

PIHL, R. O., 1983, Alcohol and aggression: A psychological perspective, in: *Alcohol, Drug Abuse, and Aggression* (E. Gottheil, K. A. Druly, T. E. Skoloda, and H. M. Waxman, eds.), Thomas, Springfield, IL, pp. 292–313.

PIHL, R. O., ZEICHNER, A., NIAURA, R., NAGY, K., and ZACCHIA, C., 1981, Attribution and alcohol-mediated aggression, *J. Abnorm. Psychol.* **90**:468–475.

PIHL, R. O., SMITH, M., and FARRELL, B., 1984, Alcohol and aggression in men: A comparison of brewed and distilled beverages, *J. Stud. Alcohol* **45**:278–282.

PINEL, J. P. J., TREIT, D., and ROVNER, L. I., 1977, Temporal lobe aggression in rats, *Science* **197**:1088–1089.

PLONSKY, M., and FREEMAN, P. R., 1982, The effects of methadone on the social behavior and activity of the rat, *Pharmacol. Biochem. Behav.* **16**:569–571.

PODOBNIKAR, I. G., 1971, Implementation of psychotherapy by librium in a pioneering rural-industrial psychiatric practice, *Psychosomatics* **12**:205–209.

PÖLDINGER, W., 1981, Pharmakotherapie der Aggressivität, *Schweiz. Arch. Neurol. Neurochir. Psychiatr.* **129**:147–155.

POLSKY, R. H., 1975, Hunger, prey feeding, and predatory aggression, *Behav. Biol.* **13**:81–93.

POOLE, A. E., and BRAIN, P. F., 1975, Effects of neonatal cyproterone acetate administration on isolation-induced fighting behavior and mounting behavior in male and female TO strain albino mice, *Aggressive Behav.* **1**:165–176.

POOLE, T. B., 1973, Some studies on the influence of chlordiazepoxide on the social interaction of golden hamsters *(Mesocricetus auratus) Br. J. Pharmacol.* **48**:538–545.

PÖSCHLOVA, N., MASEK, K., and KRSIAK, M., 1976, Facilitated intermale aggression in the mouse after 6-hydroxydopamine administration, *Neuropharmacology* **15**:403–407.

POSHIVALOV, V. P., 1974, Pharmacological analysis of aggressive behaviour of mice induced by isolation, *J. Higher Nerv. Activ.* **24**:1079–1081.

POSHIVALOV, V. P., 1978, Ethological analysis of the action exerted by medazepam and diazepam on the zoosocial behavior of isolated mice, *Farmacol. Toksikol.* **41**:263–266.

POSHIVALOV, V. P., 1980, The integrity of the social hierarchy in mice following administration of psychotropic drugs, *Br. J. Pharmacol.* **70**:367–373.

POSHIVALOV, V. P., 1981, Pharmaco-ethological analysis of social behaviour of isolated mice, *Pharmacol. Biochem. Behav.* **14,S1**:53–59.

POSHIVALOV, V. P., 1982, Ethological analysis of neuropeptides and psychotropic drugs: Effects on intraspecies aggression and sociability of isolated mice, *Aggressive Behav.* **8**:355–369.

POSHIVALOV, V. P., and KHODKO, S. T., 1982, Mathematical description and experimental analysis of animals' intraspecific behaviour, *J. Higher Nerv. Activ.* **32**:1090–1095.

POSHIVALOV, V. P., and KHODKO, S. T., 1984, Mathematical description and experimental pharmaco-ethological analysis of animal intraspecific agonistic behavior, in: *Ethopharmacological Aggression Research* (K. A. Miczek, M. R. Kruk, and B. Olivier, eds.), Liss, New York, pp. 59–80.

POSHIVALOV, V. P., KHODKO, S. T., and BESOV, E. V., 1979, Ethograph: A computer system for the recording and analysis of zoosocial behavior, *J. Higher Nerv. Activ.* **29**:420–423.

POSNER, I., MILEY, W. M., and MAZZAGATTI, N. J., 1976, Effects of d-amphetamine and pilocarpine on the mouse-killing response of hungry and satiated rats, *Physiol. Psychol.* **4**:457–460.

POTEGAL, M., YOBURN, B., and GLUSMAN, M., 1983, Disinhibition of muricide and irritability by intraseptal muscimol, *Pharmacol. Biochem. Behav.* **19**:663–669.

POWELL, D. A., FRANCIS, J., and SCHNEIDERMAN, N., 1971, The effects of castration, neonatal injections of testosterone, and previous experience with fighting on shock-elicited aggression, *Commun. Behav. Biol.* **5**:371–377.

POWELL, D. A., WALTERS, K., DUNCAN, S., and HOLLEY, J. R., 1973, The effects of chlorpromazine and d-amphetamine upon shock-elicited aggression, *Psychopharmacologia* **30**:303–314.

PRADHAN, S. N., 1975, Aggression and central neurotransmitters, in: *International Review of Neurobiology* (C. C. Pfeiffer and J. M. Smythies, eds.), Academic Press, New York, p. 213.

PRADHAN, S. N., GHOSH, B., AULAKH, C. S., and BHATTACHARYYA, A. K., 1980, Effects of delta-9-tetrahydrocannabinol on foot shock-induced aggression in rats, *Commun. Psychopharmacol.* **4**:27–34.

PRASAD, V., and SHEARD, M., 1981, The effect of cyproterone acetate on shock elicited aggression in rats, *Pharmacol. Biochem. Behav.* **15**:691–694.

PRASAD, V., and SHEARD, M. H., 1982, Effect of lithium upon desipramine enhanced shock-elicited fighting in rats, *Pharmacol. Biochem. Behav.* **17**:337–378.

PRASAD, V., and SHEARD, M. H., 1983a, Time course of chronic desipramine on shock-elicited fighting in rats, *Aggressologie* **24**:15–17.

PRASAD, V., and SHEARD, M. H., 1983b, Synergistic effect of propranolol and quipazine on desipramine enhanced shock-elicited fighting in rats, *Pharmacol. Biochem. Behav.* **19**:419–421.

PUGLISI-ALLEGRA, S., and MANDEL, P., 1980, Effects of sodium n-dipropylacetate, muscimol hydrobromide and (R,S) nipecotic acid amide on isolation-induced aggressive behavior, *Psychopharmacology* **70**:287–290.

PUGLISI-ALLEGRA, S., and OLIVERIO, A., 1981, Naloxone potentiates shock-induced aggressive behavior in mice, *Pharmacol. Biochem. Behav.* **15**:513–514.

PUGLISI-ALLEGRA, S., and RENZI, P., 1977, A technique for the measurement of aggressive behavior in mice, *Behav. Res. Method. Instr.* **9**:503–504.

PUGLISI-ALLEGRA, S., and RENZI, P., 1980, An automated device for screening the effects of psychotropic drugs on aggression and motor activity in mice, *Pharmacol. Biochem. Behav.* **13**:287–290.

PUGLISI-ALLEGRA, S., OLIVERIO, A., and MANDEL, P., 1982, Effects of opiate antagonists on social and aggressive behavior of isolated mice, *Pharmacol. Biochem. Behav.* **17**:691–694.

PUIG-ANTICH, J., 1982, Major depression and conduct disorder in prepuberty, *J. Am. Acad. Child Psychiatry* **21**:118–128.

PURI, S. K., and LAL, H., 1973, Effect of dopaminergic stimulation or blockade on morphine-withdrawal aggression, *Psychopharmacology* **32**:113–120.

PURI, S. K., and LAL, H., 1974, Reduced threshold to pain induced aggression specifically related to morphine dependence, *Psychopharmacology* **35**:237–241.

QUENZER, L. F., and FELDMAN, R. S., 1975, The mechanism of anti-muricidal effects of chlordiazepoxide, *Pharmacol. Biochem. Behav.* **3**:567–571.

QUENZER, L. F., FELDMAN, R. S., and MOORE, J. W., 1974, Toward a mechanism of the anti-aggression effects of chlordiazepoxide in rats, *Psychopharmacologia* **34**:81–94.

RAAB, A., and OSWALD, R., 1980, Coping with social conflict: Impact on the activity of tyrosine hydroxylase in the limbic system and in the adrenals, *Physiol. Behav.* **24**:387–394.

RAAB, A., SEIZINGER, B. R., and HERZ, A., 1985, Continuous social defeat induces an increase of endogenous opioids in discrete brain areas of the Mongolian gerbil, *Peptides* **6**:387–391.

RADA, R. T., 1975, Alcoholism and forcible rape, *Am. J. Psychiatry* **132**:444–446.

RADA, R. T., and DONLON, P. T., 1972, Piperacetazine vs. thioridazine for the control of schizophrenia in outpatients, *Psychosomatics* **13**:373–376.

RALEIGH, M. J., MCGUIRE, M. T., BRAMMER, G. L., and YUWILER, A., 1984, Social and environmental influences on blood serotonin concentrations in monkeys, *Arch. Gen. Psychiatry* **41**:405–410.

RALEIGH, M. J., BRAMMER, G. L., MCGUIRE, M. T., and YUWILER, A., 1985, Dominant social status facilitates the behavioral effects of serotonergic agonists, *Brain Res.* **348**:274–282.

RAMPLING, D., 1978, Aggression: A paradoxical response to tricyclic antidepressants, *Am. J. Psychiatry* **135**:117–118.

RANDALL, L. O., SCHALLEK, W., HEISE, G. A., KEITH, E. F., and BAGDON, R. E., 1960, The psychosedative properties of methaminodiazepoxide, *J. Pharmacol. Exp. Ther.* **29**:163–171.

RANDRUP, A., and MUNKVAD, I., 1969a, Relation of brain catecholamines to aggressiveness and other forms of behavioral excitation, in: *Aggressive Behavior* (S. Garattini and E. B. Sigg, eds.), Excerpta Medica Foundation, Amsterdam, pp. 228–235.

RANDRUP, A., and MUNKVAD, I., 1969b, Pharmacological studies on the brain mechanisms underlying two forms of behavioral excitation: Stereotyped hyperactivity and "rage," *Ann. NY Acad. Sci.* **159**:928–938.

RAPOPORT, J. L., QUINN, P. O., BRADBARD, G., RIDDLE, K. D., and BROOKS, E., 1974, Imipramine and methylphenidate treatments of hyperactive boys, *Arch. Gen. Psychiatry* **30**:789–793.

RATEY, J. J., MORRILL, R., and OXENKRUG, G., 1983, Use of propranolol for provoked and unprovoked episodes of rage, *Am. J. Psychiatry* **140**:1356–1357.

RAWLIN, J. W., 1968, Street level abusage of amphetamines, in: *Amphetamine Abuse* (J. R. Russo, ed.), Thomas, Springfield, IL, pp. 51–65.

RAWSON, R. A., TENNANT, F. S., McCANN, P. H., and McCANN, M. A., 1982, Characteristics of 68 chronic phencyclidine abusers who sought treatment, in: *Problems of Drug Dependence 1981* (L. S. Harris, ed.), NIDA Research 41 Monograph Series, Rockville, MD, pp. 483–487.

RAYNES, A. E., and RYBACK, R. S., 1970, Effect of alcohol and congeners on aggressive response in *Betta splendens*, *Q. J. Stud. Alcohol* **5**:130–135.

RAYNES, A. E., RYBACK, R., and INGLE, D., 1968, The effect of alcohol on aggression in *Betta splendens*, *Commun. Behav. Biol.* **2**:141–146.

REDMOND, D. E., JR., HINRICHS, R. L., MAAS, J. W., and KLING, A., 1973, Behavior of free-ranging macaques after intraventricular 6-hydroxydopamine, *Science* **181**:1256–1258.

REICH, P., and HEFFS, R. B., 1972, Homicide during a psychosis induced by LSD, *JAMA* **219**:869–871.

REIS, D. J., 1974, The chemical coding of aggression in brain, in: *Neurohumoral Coding of Brain Function* (R. D. Myers and R. R. Drucker-Colin, eds.), Plenum Press, New York, pp. 125–150.

REIS, D. J., and FUXE, K., 1964, Brain norepinephrine: Evidence that neuronal release is essential for sham rage behavior following brainstem transection in cat, *Proc. Nat. Acad. Sci. USA* **64**:108–112.

REIS, D. J., MIURA, M., and WEINBREN, M., 1967, Brain catecholamines: Relation to defense reaction evoked by acute brainstem transection in cat, *Science* **156**:1768–1770.

REWERSKI, W., KOSTOWSKI, W., PIECHOCKI, T., and RYLSKI, M., 1971, The effects of some hallucinogens on aggressiveness of mice and rats. I, *Pharmacology* **5**:314–320.

REWERSKI, W. J., PIECHOCKI, T., and RYLSKI, M., 1973, Effects of hallucinogens on aggressiveness and thermoregulation in mice, in: *The Pharmacology of Thermoregulation* (E. Schonbaum and P. Lomax, eds.), Karger, New York, pp. 432–436.

RICHARDSON, D., KARCZMAR, A. G., and SCHUDDER, C. L., 1972, Intergeneric behavioral differences among methamphetamine treated mice, *Psychopharmacologia* **25**:347–375.

RICHMOND, J. S., YOUNG, J. R., and GROVES, J. E., 1978, Violent dyscontrol responsive to d-amphetamine, *Am. J. Psychiatry* **135**:365–366.

RICKELS, K., and DOWNING, R. W., 1974, Chlordiazepoxide and hostility in anxious outpatients, *Am. J. Psychiatry* **131**:442–444.

RICKMAN, E., WILLIAMS, E. Y., and BROWN, R. K., 1961, Acute toxic psychiatric reactions related to amphetamine medication, *Med. Ann. DC* **30**:209–212.

RIDLEY, R. M., BAKER, H. F., and SCRAGGS, P. R., 1979, The time course of the behavioral effects of amphetamine and their reversal by haloperidol in a primate species, *Biol. Psychiatry* **14**:753–765.

RIFKIN, A., QUITKIN, F., CARRILLO, C., BLUMBERG, A. G., and KLEIN, D. F., 1972, Lithium carbonate in emotionally unstable character disorder, *Arch. Gen. Psychiatry* **27**:519–523.

ROBICHAUD, R. C., GYLYS, J. A., SLEDGE, K. A., and HILLYARD, I. W., 1970, The pharmacology of prazepam, a new benzodiazepine derivative, *Arch. Int. Pharmacodyn. Ther.* **185**:213–227.

RODGERS, R. J., 1982, Differential effects of naloxone and diprenorphine on defensive behavior in rats, *Neuropharmacology* **21**:1291–1294.

RODGERS, R. J., and DEPAULIS, A., 1982, GABAergic influences on defensive fighting in rats, *Pharmacol. Biochem. Behav.* **17**:451–456.

RODGERS, R. J., and HENDRIE, C. A., 1983, Social conflict activates status-dependent endogenous analgesic or hyperalgesic mechanisms in male mice: Effects of naloxone on nociception and behavior, *Physiol. Behav.* **30**:775–780.

RODGERS, R. J., and RANDALL, J. I., 1985, Social conflict analgesia: Studies on naloxone antagonism and morphine cross-tolerance in male DBA/2 mice, *Pharmacol. Biochem. Behav.* **23**:883–887.

RODGERS, R. J., and WATERS, A. J., 1984, Effects of the benzodiazepine antagonist Ro 15-1788 on social and agonistic behaviour in male albino mice, *Physiol. Behav.* **33**:401–409.

RODGERS, R. J., and WATERS, A. J., 1985, Benzodiazepines and their antagonists: A pharmacoethological analysis with particular reference to effects on "aggression," *Neurosci. Biobehav. Rev.* **9**:21–35.

RODGERS, R. J., HENDRIE, C. A., and WATERS, A. J., 1983, Naloxone partially antagonizes post-encounter analgesia and enhances defensive responding in male rats exposed to attack from lactating conspecifics, *Physiol. Behav.* **30**:781–786.

ROLINSKI, Z., 1973, Analysis of aggressiveness-stereotype complex induced in mice by amphetamine or nialamide and L-dopa, *Polish J. Pharmacol. Pharm.* **25**:551–558.

ROLINSKI, Z., 1975, Interspecies aggressiveness of rats towards mice after the application of p-chlorophenylalanine, *Polish J. Pharmacol. Pharm.* **27**:223–229.

ROLINSKI, Z., and HERBUT, M., 1979, Determination of the role of serotonergic and cholinergic systems in apomorphine-induced aggressiveness in rats, *Polish J. Pharmacol. Pharm.* **31**:97–106.

ROLINSKI, Z., and KOZAK, W., 1979, The role of the catecholaminergic system in footshock-induced fighting in mice, *Psychopharmacology* **65**:285–290.

ROMANIUK, A., 1974, Neurochemical bases of defensive behavior in animals, *Acta Neurobiol. Exp.* **34**:205–214.

ROMANIUK, A., BRUDZYNSKI, S., and GRONSKA, J., 1973, The effect of chemical blockade of hypothalamus cholinergic system on defensive reactions in cats, *Acta Physiol. Polonia* **24**:809–816.

ROMANIUK, A., BRUDZYNSKI, S., and GRONSKA, J., 1974, The effects of intrahypothalamic injections of cholinergic and adrenergic agents on defensive behavior in cats, *Acta Physiol. Polonia* **25**:297–305.

ROSE, R. M., HOLADAY, J. W., and BERNSTEIN, I. S., 1971, Plasma testosterone, dominance rank and aggressive behavior in a group of male rhesus monkeys, *Nature* **231**:366–368.

ROSENKRANTZ, H., and BRAUDE, M. C., 1974, Acute, subacute and 23-day chronic marihuana inhalation toxicities in the rat, *Toxicol. Appl. Pharmacol.* **28**:428–441.

ROSLUND, B., and LARSON, C. A., 1979, Crimes of violence and alcohol abuse in Sweden, *Int. J. Addictions* **14**:1103–1115.

ROSS, S. B., and OGREN, S.-O., 1976, Anti-aggressive action of dopamine-beta-hydroxylase inhibitors in mice, *J. Pharm. Pharmacol.* **28**:590–592.

ROSSI, A. C., 1975, The "mouse-killing" rat: Ethological discussion on an experimental model of aggression, *Pharmacol. Res. Commun.* **7**:199–216.

Rush, J., and Mendels, J., 1975, Effects of lithium chloride on muricidal behavior in rats, *Pharmacol. Biochem. Behav.* **3:**795–797.

Russell, J. W., Singer, G., and Bowman, G., 1983, Effects of interactions between amphetamine and food deprivation on covariation of muricide, consummatory behaviour and activity, *Pharmacol. Biochem. Behav.* **18:**917–926.

Russell, J. W., Greenberg, B. D., and Segal, D. S., 1984, The effects of phencyclidine on spontaneous aggressive behavior in the rat, *Biol. Psychiatry* **19:**195–202.

Sade, D. S., 1967, Determinants of dominance in a group of free-ranging rhesus monkeys, in: *Social Communication among Primates* (S. A. Altmann, ed.), University of Chicago Press, Chicago, pp. 99–114.

Sakata, T., and Fuchimoto, H., 1973a, Stereotyped and aggressive behavior induced by sustained high dose of theophylline in rats, *Jpn. J. Pharmacol.* **23:**781–785.

Sakata, T., and Fuchimoto, H., 1973b, Further aspects of aggressive behavior induced by sustained high dose of theophylline in rats, *Jpn. J. Pharmacol.* **23:**787–792.

Sakata, T., Fuchimoto, H., Kodama, J., and Fukushima, M., 1975, Changes of brain serotonin and muricide behavior following chronic administration of theophylline in rats, *Physiol. Behav.* **15:**449–453.

Salama, A. I., and Goldberg, M. E., 1970, Neurochemical effects of imipramine and amphetamine in aggressive mouse-killing (muricidal) rats, *Biochem. Pharmacol.* **19:**2023–2032.

Salama, A. I., and Goldberg, M. E., 1973, Enhanced locomotor activity following amphetamine in mouse-killing rats, *Arch. Int. Pharmacodyn. Ther.* **204:**162–169.

Saletu, B., Saletu, M., Simeon, J., Viamontes, G., and Itil, T. M., 1975, Comparative symptomatological and evoked potential studies with *d*-amphetamine, thioridazine, and placebo in hyperkinetic children, *Biol. Psychiatry* **10:**253–275.

Salzman, C., DiMascio, A., Shader, R. I., and Harmatz, J. S., 1969, Chlordiazepoxide, expectation and hostility, *Psychopharmacologia* **14:**38–45.

Salzman, C., Kochansky, G. E., Shader, R. I., Porrino, L. J., Harmatz, J. S., and Swett, C. P., Jr., 1974, Chlordiazepoxide-induced hostility in a small group setting, *Arch. Gen. Psychiatry* **31:**401–405.

Salzman, C., Kochansky, G. E., Shader, R. I., Harmatz, J. S., and Ogletree, A. M., 1975, Is oxazepam associated with hostility? *Dis. Nerv. Syst.* **36:**30–32.

Salzman, C., Van Der Kolk, B. A., and Shader, R. I., 1976, Marijuana and hostility in a small-group setting, *Am. J. Psychiatry* **133:**1029–1033.

Santos, M., Sampaio, M. R. P., Fernandez, N. S., and Carlini, E. A., 1966, Effects of *Cannabis sativa* (marihuana) on fighting behavior of mice, *Psychopharmacologia* **8:**437–444.

Sapolsky, R. M., 1982, The endocrine stress-response and social status in the wild baboon, *Hormones Behav.* **16:**279–292.

Sassenrath, E. N., 1971, Increased adrenal responsiveness related to social stress in rhesus monkeys, *Hormones Behav.* **1:**283–298.

Sassenrath, E. N., and Chapman, L. F., 1975, Tetrahydrocannabinol-induced manifestations of the "marihuana syndrome" in group-living macaques, *Fed. Proc.* **34:**1666–1670.

Satterfield, J. H., Cantwell, D. P., Lesser, L. I., and Podosin, R. L., 1972, Physiological studies of the hyperkinetic child: I, *Am. J. Psychiatry* **128:**102–108.

Sawynok, J., Pinsky, C., and LaBella, F. S., 1979, Minireview on the specificity of naloxone as an opiate antagonist, *Life Sci.* **25:**1621–1632.

Saxena, A., Bhattacharya, B. K., and Mukerji, B., 1962, Behavioural studies in fish with mescaline, LSD, and thiopropazate and their interactions with serotonin and DOPA, *Arch. Int. Pharmacodyn. Ther.* **140:**327–335.

Sayler, A., 1970, The effect of anti-androgens on aggressive behavior in the gerbil, *Physiol. Behav.* **5:**667–671.

SBORDONE, R. J., and CARDER, B., 1974, Mescaline and shock induced aggression in rats, *Pharmacol. Biochem. Behav.* **2**:777–782.

SBORDONE, R. J., and GARCIA, J., 1977, Untreated rats develop "pathological" aggression when paired with a mescaline-treated rat in a shock-elicited aggression, *Behav. Biol.* **21**:451–461.

SBORDONE, R. J., WINGARD, J. A., ELLIOTT, M. L., and JERVEY, J., 1978, Mescaline produces pathological aggression in rats regardless of age or strain, *Pharmacol. Biochem. Behav.* **8**:543–546.

SBORDONE, R. J., WINGARD, J. A., GORELICK, D. A., and ELLIOTT, M. L., 1979, Severe aggression in rats induced by mescaline but not other hallucinogens, *Psychopharmacology* **66**:275–280.

SBORDONE, R. J., GORELICK, D. A., and ELLIOTT, M. L., 1981, An ethological analysis of drug-induced pathological aggression, in: *Multidisciplinary Approaches to Aggression Research* (P. F. Brain and D. Benton, eds.), Elsevier/North-Holland, Amsterdam, pp. 369–385.

SCHECKEL, C. L., and BOFF, E., 1966, Effects of drugs in aggressive behavior in monkeys, *Excerpta Med. Int.* **129**:789–795.

SCHEEL-KRÜGER, J., and RANDRUP, A., 1968, Aggressive behavior provoked by pargyline in rats pretreated with diethyldithiocarbamate, *J. Pharm. Pharmacol.* **20**:948–949.

SCHIØRRING, E., 1977, Changes in individual and social behavior induced by amphetamine related compounds in monkeys and man, in: *Cocaine and Other Stimulants* (E. H. Ellinwood and M. M. Kilbey, eds.), Plenum Press, New York, pp. 481–522.

SCHIØRRING, E., 1981, Psychopathology induced by "speed drugs," *Pharmacol. Biochem. Behav.* **14**(Suppl. 1):109–122.

SCHLEMMER, R. F., and DAVIS, J. M., 1981, Evidence for dopamine mediation of submissive gestures in the stumptail macaque monkey, *Pharmacol. Biochem. Behav.* **14**(Suppl. 1):95–102.

SCHLEMMER, R. F., and DAVIS, J. M., 1983, A comparison of three psychomimetic-induced models of psychosis in non-human primate social colonies, in: *Ethopharmacology: Primate Models of Neuropsychiatric Disorders* (K. A. Miczek, ed.), Liss, New York, pp. 33–78.

SCHLEMMER, R. F., JR., CASPER, R. C., SIEMSEN, F. K., GARVER, D. L., and DAVIS, J. M., 1976, Behavioral changes in a juvenile primate social colony with chronic administration of d-amphetamine, *Psychopharmacol. Commun.* **2**:49–59.

SCHMIDT, W., and APFELBACH, R., 1977, Psychopharmakologische Beeinflussung des Beutefangverhaltens beim Frettchen (*Putorius furo* L.), *Psychopharmacology* **51**:147–152.

SCHMIDT, W. J., 1979, Effects of d-amphetamine, maprotiline, L-dopa, and haloperidol on the components of the predatory behavior of the ferret, *Putorius furo* L, *Psychopharmacology* **64**:355–359.

SCHMIDT, W. J., 1980, Unlike rats, ferrets do kill under antidepressants, *Naturwissenschaften* **67**:262–263.

SCHMIDT, W. J., 1983, Involvement of dopaminergic neurotransmission in the control of goal-directed movements, *Psychopharmacology* **80**:360–364.

SCHMIDT, W. J., 1984, L-Dopa and apomorphine disrupt long- but not short-behavioural chains, *Physiol. Behav.* **33**:671–680.

SCHMIDT, W. J., and MEIERL, G., 1980, Antidepressants and the control of predatory behavior, *Physiol. Behav.* **25**:17–19.

SCHMUTTE, G. T., and TAYLOR, S. P., 1980, Physical aggression as a function of alcohol and pain feedback, *J. Soc. Psychol.* **110**:235–244.

SCHNEIDER, C., 1968, Behavioural effects of some morphine antagonists and hallucinogens in the rat, *Nature* **220**:586–587.

SCHREIER, H. A., 1979, Use of propranolol in the treatment of postencephalitic psychosis, *Am. J. Psychiatry* **136**:840–841.

SCHRØLD, J., 1970, Aggressive behaviour in chicks induced by tricyclic antidepressants, *Psychopharmacologia* **17**:225–233.
SCHUCKIT, M. A., 1973, Alcoholism and sociopathy—Diagnostic confusion, *Q. J. Stud. Alcohol* **34**:157–164.
SCHWEIKERT, W., 1971, Anxious-depressed adults and problem children treated with thioridazine in private practice, *Curr. Ther. Res. Clin. Exp.* **12**:162–168.
SCOTT, J. P., 1958, *Aggression,* The University of Chicago Press, Chicago.
SCOTT, J. P., 1966, Agonistic behavior of mice and rats: A review, *Am. Zoologist* **6**:683–701.
SCOTT, J. P., and FREDERICSON, E., 1951, The causes of fighting in mice and rats, *Physiol. Zool.* **24**:273–309.
SCOTT, J. P., LEE, C., and HO, J. E., 1971, Effects of fighting, genotype, and amphetamine sulfate on body temperature of mice, *J. Comp. Physiol. Psychol.* **76**:349–352.
SCRIABINE, A., and BLAKE, M., 1962, Evaluation of centrally acting drugs in mice with fighting behavior induced by isolation, *Psychopharmacologia* **2**:224–226.
SEARCY, W. A., and WINGFIELD, J. C., 1980, The effects of androgen and antiandrogen on dominance and aggressiveness in male red-winged blackbird, *Hormones Behav.* **14**:126–135.
SEGAL, D. S., WEINBERGER, S. B., CAHILL, J., and MCCUNNEY, S. J., 1980, Multiple daily amphetamine administration: Behavioral and neurochemical alterations, *Science* **207**:904–906.
SEIDEN, L. S., and VOSMER, G., 1984, Formation of 6-hydroxydopamine in caudate nucleus of the rat brain after a single large dose of methylamphetamine, *Pharmacol. Biochem. Behav.* **21**:29–31.
SENAULT, B., 1968, Syndrome aggressif induit par l'apomorphine chez le rat, *J. Physiol.* **60**:543–544.
SENAULT, B., 1970, Comportement d'agressivité intraspecifique induit par l'apomorphine chez la rat, *Psychopharmacologia* **18**:271–287.
SHADER, R. I., JACKSON, A. H., and DODES, L. M., 1974, The antiaggressive effects of lithium in man, *Psychopharmacologia* **40**:17–24.
SHAW, C. R., LOCKETT, H. J., LUCAS, A. R., LAMONTAGNE, C. H., and GRIMM, F., 1963, Tranquilizer drugs in the treatment of emotionally disturbed children: I. Inpatients in a residential treatment center, *J. Am. Acad. Child Psychiatry* **2**:725–742.
SHEARD, M. H., 1967, The effects of amphetamine on attack behavior in the cat, *Brain Res.* **5**:330–338.
SHEARD, M. H., 1969, The effect of *p*-chlorophenylalanine on behavior in rats: relation to brain serotonin and 5-hydroxyindoleacetic acid, *Brain Res.* **15**:524–528.
SHEARD, M. H., 1970*a,* Behavioral effects of *p*-chlorophenylalanine in rats: Inhibition by lithium, *Commun. Behav. Biol.* **5**:1–3.
SHEARD, M. H., 1970*b,* Effect of lithium on foot shock aggression in rats, *Nature* **228**:284–285.
SHEARD, M. H., 1971, Effect of lithium on human aggression, *Nature* **230**:113–114.
SHEARD, M. H., 1973, Aggressive behavior: Modification by amphetamine, *p*-chlorophenylalanine and lithium in rats, *Agressologie* **14**:323–326.
SHEARD, M. H., 1975, Lithium in the treatment of aggression, *J. Nerv. Ment. Dis.* **160**(2):108–118.
SHEARD, M. H., 1977, Animal models of aggressive behavior, in: *Animal Models in Psychiatry and Neurology* (I. Hanin, and E. Usdin, eds.), Pergamon Press, Oxford, pp. 247–257.
SHEARD, M. H., 1978, The effect of lithium and other ions on aggressive behavior in: *Psychopharmacology of Aggression. Modern Problems of Pharmacopsychiatry* (L. Valzelli, ed.), Karger, Basel, pp. 53–68.
SHEARD, M. H., 1979*a,* The role of drugs affecting catecholamines on shock-elicited fighting

in rats, in: *Catecholamines: Basic and Clinical Frontiers* (E. Usdin, I. Kopin, and J. Barchas, eds.), Pergamon, New York, pp. 1690–1692.
SHEARD, M. H., 1979b, Testosterone and aggression, in: *Psychopharmacology of Aggression* (M. Sandler, ed.), Raven Press, New York, pp. 111–121.
SHEARD, M. H., 1981, Shock-induced fighting (SIF): Psychopharmacology studies, *Aggressive Behav.* **7**:41–49.
SHEARD, M. H., 1983, Psychopharmacology of aggression, in: *Clinical Psychopharmacology* (H. Hippius and G. Winokur, eds.), Excerpta Medica, Amsterdam, pp. 188–201.
SHEARD, M. H., 1984, Clinical pharmacology of aggressive behavior, *Clin. Neuropharmacol.* **7**:173–183.
SHEARD, M. H., ASTRACHAN, D. I., and DAVIS, M., 1977, The effect of d-lysergic acid diethylamide (LSD) upon shock-elicited fighting in rats, *Life Sci.* **20**:427–430.
SHEARD, M. H., and MARINI, J. L., 1978, Treatment of human aggressive behavior: Four case studies of the effect of lithium, *Compr. Psychiatry* **19**:37–45.
SHEARD, M. H., MARINI, J. L., BRIDGES, C. I., and WAGNER, E., 1976, The effect of lithium on impulsive aggressive behavior in man, *Am. J. Psychiatry* **133**:1409–1413.
SHIBATA, S., WATANABE, S., LIOU, S. Y., and UEKI, S., 1983, Effects of adrenergic blockers on the inhibition of muricide by desipramine and noradrenaline injected into the amygdala in olfactory bulbectomized rats, *Pharmacol. Biochem. Behav.* **18**:203–207.
SHIBATA, S., NAKANISHI, H., WATANABE, S., and UEKI, S., 1984, Effects of chronic administration of antidepressants on mouse-killing behavior (muricide) in olfactory bulbectomized rats, *Pharmacol. Biochem. Behav.* **21**:225–230.
SHORVON, H. J., 1947, Benzedrine in psychopathy and behaviour disorders, *Br. J. Addiction* **44**:58–63.
SHUNTICH, R. J., and TAYLOR, S. P., 1972, The effects of alcohol on human physical aggression, *J. Exp. Res. Personality* **6**:34–38.
SHUPE, L. M., 1954, Alcohol and crime, A study of the urine alcohol concentration found in 882 persons arrested during or immediately after the commission of a felony, *J. Criminal Law Criminol. Police Sci.* **44**:661–664.
SIEBER, B., 1982, Influence of hashish extract on the social behavior of encountering male baboons *(Papio c. anubis)*, *Pharmacol. Biochem. Behav.* **17**:209–216.
SIEBER, B., FRISCHKNECHT, H.-R, and WASER, P. G., 1980, Behavioral effects of hashish in mice. I. Social interactions and nest-building behavior of males, *Psychopharmacology* **70**:149–154.
SIEBER, B., FRISCHKNECHT, H.-R., and WASER, P. G., 1981, Behavioral effects of hashish in mice, IV. Social dominance, food dominance, and sexual behavior within a group of males, *Psychopharmacology* **73**:142–146.
SIEBER, B., FRISCHKNECHT, H.-R., and WASER, P., 1982, Behavioural effects of hashish in mice in comparison with psychoactive drugs, *Gen. Pharmacol.* **13**:315–320.
SIEGEL, A., 1984, Anatomical and functional differentiation within the amygdala—Behavioral state modulation, in: *Modulation of Sensorimotor Activity during Alterations in Behavioral States* (R. Bandler, ed.), Liss, New York, NY, pp. 299–323.
SIEGEL, A., and EDINGER, H. M., 1983, Role of the limbic system in hypothalamically elicited attack behavior, *Neurosci. Biobehav. Rev.* **7**:395–407.
SIEGEL, H. I., GIORDANO, A. L., MALLAFRE, C. M., and ROSENBLATT, J. S., 1983, Maternal aggression in hamsters: Effects of stage of lactation, presence of pups, and repeated testing, *Hormones Behav.* **17**:86–93.
SIEGEL, R. K., 1971, Studies of hallucinogens in fish, birds, mice and men: The behavior of "psychedelic" populations, in: *Advances in Neuro-psychopharmacology* (O. Vinar, P. Votava, and P. B. Bradley, eds.), Czechoslovak Medical Press, London, pp. 311–318.

SIEGEL, R. K., 1978, Phencyclidine, criminal behavior, and the defense of diminished capacity, in: *Phencyclidine (PCP) Abuse: An Appraisal* (R. C. Peterson and R. C. Stillman, eds.), NIDA Research Monograph Series 21, Washington, DC, pp. 272–288.
SIEGEL, R. K., 1980, PCP and violent crime: The people vs. peace, *J. Psychedelic Drugs* **12**:317–330.
SIEGEL, R. K., and POOLE, J., 1969, Psychedelic-induced social behavior in mice: A preliminary report, *Psychol. Rep.* **25**:704–706.
SIEGFRIED, B., FRISCHKNECHT, H.-R., and WASER, P. G., 1982, A new learning model for submissive behavior in mice: Effects of naloxone, *Aggressive Behav.* **8**:112–115.
SILVERMAN, A. P., 1965a, Ethological and statistical analysis of drug effects on the social behaviour of laboratory rats, *Br. J. Pharmacol.* **24**:579–590.
SILVERMAN, A. P., 1965b, Social behaviour of rats and the action of chlorpromazine, *Neuropsychopharmacology* **4**:346–351.
SILVERMAN, A. P., 1966a, The social behaviour of laboratory rats and the action of chlorpromazine and other drugs, *Behaviour* **27**:1–38.
SILVERMAN, A. P., 1966b, Barbiturates, LSD, and the social behaviour of laboratory rats, *Psychopharmacologia* **10**:155–171.
SIMONDS, J. F., and KASHANI, J., 1979, Drug abuse and criminal behavior in delinquent boys committed to a training school, *Am. J. Psychiatry* **136**:1444–1448.
SINGH, J. M., 1975, Methadone-induced behavioral changes: Circular movements, aggression, and electrophysiological aspects, *Int. J. Addictions* **10**:659–673.
SIOMOPOULOS, V., 1981, Violence: The ugly face of amphetamine abuse, *Illinois Med. J.* **159**:375–377.
SKOLNICK, P., REED, G. F., and PAUL, S. M., 1985, Benzodiazepine-receptor mediated inhibition of isolation-induced aggression, *Pharmacol. Biochem. Behav.* **23**:17–20.
SMITH, D. E., KING, M. B., and HOEBEL, B. G., 1970, Lateral hypothalamic control of killing: Evidence for a cholinoceptive mechanism, *Science* **167**:900–901.
SMITH, D. F., 1985, Lithium, animal behavior and monoamines: Five questions and possible ways of answering them, *Acta Pharmacol. Toxicol.* **56**:198–202.
SMITH, E. O., and BYRD, L. D., 1983, Studying the behavioral effects of drugs in group-living nonhuman primates, in: *Ethopharmacology: Primate Models of Neuropsychiatric Disorders* (K. A. Miczek, ed.), Liss, New York, pp. 1–31.
SMITH, E. O., and BYRD, L. D., 1984, Contrasting effects of d-amphetamine on affiliation and aggression in monkeys, *Pharmacol. Biochem. Behav.* **20**:255–260.
SMITH, R. C., and CRIM, D., 1969, The world of the Haight Ashbury speed freak, *J. Psychedelic Drugs* **2**:172–188.
SMOOTHY, R., and BERRY, M. S., 1983, Effects of ethanol on behavior of aggressive mice from two different strains: A comparison of simple and complex behavioral assessments, *Pharmacol. Biochem. Behav.* **19**:645–653.
SMOOTHY, R., and BERRY, M. S., 1984, Effects of ethanol on murine aggression assessed by biting of an inanimate target, *Psychopharmacology* **83**:268–271.
SMOOTHY, R., BOWDEN, N. J., and BERRY, M. S., 1982, Ethanol and social behaviour in naive Swiss mice, *Aggressive Behav.* **8**:204–207.
SOFIA, R. D., 1969a, Structural relationship and potency of agents which selectively block mouse killing (muricide) behavior in rats, *Life Sci.* **8**:1201–1210.
SOFIA, R. D., 1969b, Effects of centrally active drugs on four models of experimentally-induced aggression in rodents, *Life Sci.* **8**:705–716.
SOUEIF, M. I., 1971, The use of cannabis in Egypt: A behavioural study, *Bull. Narcotics* **23**:17–21.
SPAIN, D., BRADESS, V., and EGGTON, A., 1951, Alcohol and violent death. A one year study of consecutive cases in a representative community, *JAMA* **146**:334–335.

SPIEKER, G., and SARVER, C. R., 1978, Alcohol and crime, *Br. J. Alcohol Alcoholism* **13:**184–189.
SPRAGUE, R. L., and SLEATOR, E. K., 1977, Methylphenidate in hyperkinetic children: Differences in dose effects on learning and social behavior *Science* **198:**1274–1276.
SPRAGUE, R. L., BARNES, K. R., and WERRY, J. S., 1970, Methylphenidate and thioridazine: Learning, reaction time, activity, and classroom behavior in disturbed children, *Am. J. Orthopsychiatry* **40:**615–628.
STABENAU, J. R., 1984, Implications of family history of alcoholism, antisocial personality, and sex differences in alcohol dependence, *Am. J. Psychiatry* **141:**1178–1182.
STEKLIS, H. D., BRAMMER, G. L., RALEIGH, M. J., and MCGUIRE, M. T., 1985, Serum testosterone, male dominance, and aggression in captive groups of Vervet monkeys *(Cercopithecus aethiops sabaeus)*, *Hormones Behav.* **19:**154–163.
STILLE, G., ACKERMANN, H., EICHENBERGER, E., and LAUENER, H., 1963, Vergleichende pharmakologische Untersuchung eines neuen zentralen Stimulans, 1-*p*-tolyl-1-oxo-2-pyrrolidino-*n*-pentan-HCl, *Arzneim. Forsch.* **13:**871–877.
STOLERMAN, I. P., JOHNSON, C. A., BUNKER, P., and JARVIK, M. P., 1975, Weight loss and shock-elicited aggression as indices of morphine abstinence in rats, *Psychopharmacologia* **45:**157–161.
STRICKLAND, J. A., and DAVANZO, J. P., 1986, Must antidepressants be anticholinergic to inhibit muricide? *Pharmacol. Biochem. Behav.* **24:**135–137.
STRINGER, A. Y., and JOSEF, N. C., 1983, Methylphenidate in the treatment of aggression in two patients with antisocial personality disorder, *Am. J. Psychiatry* **140:**1365–1366.
SULCOVA, A., 1985, Tranquilizing effects of alprazolam in animal model of agonistic behavior, *Activ. Nerv. Superior* **27:**310–311.
SULCOVA, A., and KRSIAK, M., 1980, Effect of piracetam on agonistic behaviour in mice, *Activ. Nerv. Superior* **22:**200–201.
SULCOVA, A., and KRSIAK, M., 1984, The benzodiazepine-receptor antagonist Ro 15-1788 antagonizes effects of diazepam on aggressive and timid behavior in mice, *Activ. Nerv. Superior* **26:**255–256.
SULCOVA, A., and KRSIAK, M., 1985, Effects of ethyl beta-carboline-3-carboxylate and diazepam on aggressive and timid behaviour in mice, *Activ. Nerv. Superior* **27:**308–310.
SULCOVA, A., KRSIAK, M., and MASEK, K., 1976, Effect of repeated administration of chlorpromazine and diazepam on isolation-induced timidity in mice, *Activ. Nerv. Superior* **18:**233–234.
SULCOVA, A., KRSIAK, M., and MASEK, K., 1978, Effects of baclofen on agonistic behaviour in mice, *Activ. Nerv. Superior* **20:**241–242.
SULCOVA, A., KRSIAK, M., MASEK, K., and OSTROVSKAYA, R. U., 1979, Bicuculline antagonized effects of diazepam on aggressive and timid behaviour in mice, *Activ. Nerv. Superior* **21:**179–180.
SULCOVA, A., KRSIAK, M., and MASEK, K., 1981, Effects of calcium valproate and aminooxyacetic acid on agonistic behaviour in mice, *Activ. Nerv. Superior* **23:**287–289.
SUTKER, P. B., and ARCHER, R. P., 1984, Opiate abuse and dependence disorders, in: *Comprehensive Handbook of Psychopathology* (H. E. Adams and P. B. Sutker, eds.), Plenum Publishing Corp., pp. 585–621.
SVARE, B., and GANDELMAN, R., 1976, Postpartum aggression in mice: The influence of suckling stimulation, *Hormones Behav.* **7:**407–416.
SVARE, B. B., and MANN, M. A., 1983, Hormonal influences on maternal aggression, in: *Hormones and Aggressive Behavior* (B. B. Svare, ed.), Plenum Press, New York, pp. 91–104.
SYME, G. J., POLLARD, J. S., SYME, L. A., and REID, R. M., 1974, An analysis of the limited access measure of social dominance in rats, *Animal Behav.* **22:**486–500.

TAMIMIE, H. S., 1968, Response of chicks to alcohol treated females, *Poultry Sci.* **47:**1634–1635.
TAYLOR, S. P., 1983, Alcohol and human aggression, in: *Alcohol, Drug Abuse and Aggression* (E. Gottheil, K. A. Druley, T. E. Skoloda, and H. M. Waxman, eds.), Thomas, Springfield, IL, pp. 280–291.
TAYLOR, S. P., and GAMMON, C. B., 1975, Effects of type and dose of alcohol on human physical aggression, *J. Personality Soc. Psychol.* **32:**169–175.
TAYLOR, S. P., and GAMMON, C. B., 1976, Aggressive behavior of intoxicated subjects: The effect of third party intervention, *J. Stud. Alcohol* **37:**917–930.
TAYLOR, S. P., VARDARIS, R. M., RAWTICH, A. B., GAMMON, C. B., CRANSTON, J. W., and LUBETKIN, A. I., 1976, The effects of alcohol and delta-9-tetrahydrocannabinol on human physical aggression, *Aggressive Behav.* **2:**153–161.
TAYLOR, S. P., SCHMUTTE, G. T., LEONARD, K. E., and CRANSTON, J. W., 1979, The effects of alcohol and extreme provocation on the use of a highly noxious electric shock, *Motivation Emotion* **3:**73–81.
TAZI, A., DANTZER, R., MORMEDE, P., and LE MOAL, M., 1983, Effects of post-trial administration of naloxone and beta-endorphin on shock-induced fighting in rats, *Behav. Neural Biol.* **39:**192–202.
TAZI, A., DANTZER, R., MORMEDE, P., and LE MOAL, M., 1985, Effects of post-trial injection of beta-endorphin on shock-induced fighting are dependent on baseline of fighting, *Behav. Neural Biol.* **43:**322–326.
TEASDALE, J., and DIP, M. A., 1972, The perceived effect of heroin on the interpersonal behavior of heroin-dependent patients, and a comparison with stimulant-dependent patients, *Int. Addictions* **7:**533–548.
TEDESCHI, D. H., FOWLER, P. J., MILLER, E. B., and MACKO, E., 1969, Pharmacological analysis of footshock-induced fighting behaviour, in: *Aggressive Behaviour* (S. Garattini and E. B. Sigg, eds.), Excerpta Medica Foundation, Amsterdam, pp. 245–252.
TEDESCHI, R. E., TEDESCHI, D. H., MUCHA, A., COOK, L., MATTIS, P. A., and FELLOWS, E. J., 1959, Effects of various centrally acting drugs on fighting behavior of mice, *J. Pharmacol. Exp. Ther.* **125:**28–34.
TEN HAM, M., and DE JONG, Y., 1974, Tolerance to the hypothermic and aggression-attenuating effect of delta-8 and delta-9-tetrahydrocannabinol in mice, *Eur. Pharmacol.* **28:**144–148.
TEN HAM, M., and DE JONG, Y., 1975, Absence of interaction between delta-9-tetrahydrocannabinol and cannabidiol (CBD) in aggression, muscle control and body temperature experiments in mice, *Psychopharmacologia* **41:**169–174.
TEN HAM, M., and VAN NOORDWIJK, J., 1973, Lack of tolerance to the effect of two tetrahydrocannabinols on aggressiveness, *Psychopharmacologia* **29:**171–176.
TESKEY, G. C., KAVALIERS, M., and HIRST, M., 1984, Social conflict activates opioid analgesic and ingestive behaviors in male mice, *Life Sci.* **35:**303–315.
THIESSEN, D. D., and UPCHURCH, M., 1981, Haloperidol and clonidine increase, and apomorphine decreases ultrasonic vocalizations by gerbils, *Psychopharmacology* **75:**287–290.
THOA, N. B., EICHELMAN, B., and NG, K. Y., 1972a, Aggression in rats treated with dopa and 6-hydroxydopamine, *J. Pharm. Pharmacol.* **24:**337–338.
THOA, N. B., EICHELMAN, B., and NG, L. K. Y., 1972b, Shock-induced aggression: Effects of 6-hydroxydopamine and other pharmacological agents. *Brain Res.* **43:**467–475.
THOA, N. B., EICHELMAN, B., RICHARDSON, J. S., and JACOBOWITZ, D., 1972c, 6-Hydroxydopa depletion of brain norepinephrine and the facilitation of aggressive behavior, *Science* **178:**75–77.

THOMPSON, M. L., BRUNNER, E., HOEFLER, H., HARTLEY, J., KUMAR, M. S. A., SHUSTER, L., and KREAM, R., 1986, Changes in opioid receptor binding and levels of opioid peptides in the brain following acute and chronic defeat in mice, *Soc. Neurosci. Abstr.*, **12**:411

THOMPSON, M. L., MICZEK, K. A., NODA, K., SCHUSTER, L., and KUMAR, M. S. A., 1987, Analgesia in defeated mice: Evidence for mediation via central rather than pituitary or adrenal endogenous opioid peptides, *Pharmacol. Biochem. Behav.* (in press).

THOMPSON, T., and BLOOM, W., 1966, Aggressive behavior and extinction-induced response-rate increase, *Psychonom. Sci.* **5**:335–336.

THOR, D. H., 1971, Amphetamine induced fighting during morphine withdrawal, *J. Gen. Psychol.* **84**:245–250.

THOR, D. H., and TEEL, B. G., 1968, Fighting of rats during post-morphine withdrawal: Effect of prewithdrawal dosage, *Am. J. Psychol.* **81**:439–442.

THOR, D. H., HOATS, D. L., and THOR, C. J., 1970, Morphine induced fighting and prior social experience, *Psychonom. Sci.* **18**:137–139.

THOR, D. H., GHISELLI, W. B., and LAMBELET, D. C., 1974, Sensory control of shock-elicited fighting in rats, *Physiol. Behav.* **13**:683–686.

THURMOND, J. B., 1975, Technique for producing and measuring territorial aggression using laboratory mice, *Physiol. Behav.* **14**:879–881.

TINBERGEN, N., 1968, On war and peace in animals and man: An ethologist's approach to the biology of aggression, *Science* **160**:1411–1418.

TINKLENBERG, J. R., 1973, Alcohol and violence, in: *Alcoholism: Progress in Research and Treatment* (P. G. Bourne and R. Fox, eds.), Academic Press, New York, pp. 195–210.

TINKLENBERG, J. R., and STILLMAN, R. C., 1970, Drug use and violence, in: *Violence and the Struggle for Existence* (D. N. Daniels, M. F. Gilula, and F. M. Ochberg, eds.), Little, Brown, Boston, pp. 327–365.

TINKLENBERG, J. R., and WOODROW, K. M., 1974, Drug use among youthful assaultive and sexual offenders, in: *Aggression* (S. H. Frazier, ed.), Research Publication Association for Research in Nervous and Mental Disease, Williams & Wilkens, Baltimore, pp. 209–224.

TINKLENBERG, J. R., MURPHY, P. L., MURPHY, P., DARLEY, C. F., ROTH, C. F., and KOPELL, B. S., 1974, Drug involvement in criminal assaults by adolescents, *Arch. Gen. Psychiatry* **30**:685–689.

TINKLENBERG, J. R., ROTH, W. T., KOPELL, B. S., and MURPHY, P., 1976, Cannabis and alcohol effects in assaultiveness in adolescent delinquents, *Ann. NY Acad. Sci.* **282**:85–94.

TINKLENBERG, J. R., ROTH, W. T., KOPELL, B. S., and MURPHY, P., 1977, Cannabis and alcohol effects on assaultiveness in adolescent delinquents, in: *Chronic Cannabis Use* (R. L. Dornbush, M. Fink, and A. M. Freedman, eds.), New York Academy of Science, New York, pp. 85–94.

TIZABI, Y., THOA, N. B., MAENGWYN-DAVIES, G. D., KOPIN, I. J., and JACOBOWITZ, D. M., 1979, Behavioral correlation of catecholamine concentration and turnover in discrete brain areas of three strains of mice, *Brain Res.* **166**:199–205.

TIZABI, Y., MASSARI, V. J., and JACOBOWITZ, D. M., 1980a, Isolation induced aggression and catecholamine variations in discrete brain areas of the mouse, *Brain Res. Bull.* **5**:81–86.

TIZABI, Y., O'DONOHUE, T. L., and JACOBOWITZ, D. M., 1980b, Variations in plasma and adrenal catecholamines and related enzymes in isolated-aggressive mice, *Commun. Psychopharmacol.* **4**:433–439.

TOBIN, J. M., and LEWIS, N. D. C., 1960, New psychotherapeutic agent, chlordiazepoxide. Use in treatment of anxiety states and related symptoms, *JAMA* **174**:1242–1249.

TRAMILL, J. L., TURNER, P. E., SISEMORE, D. A., and DAVIS, S. F., 1980, Hungry, drunk, and not real mad: The effects of alcohol injections on aggressive responding, *Bull. Psychonom. Soc.* **15**:339–341.

TRAMILL, J. L., WESLEY, A. L., and DAVIS, S. F., 1981, The effects of chronic ethanol challenges on aggressive responding in rats maintained on a semideprivation diet, *Bull. Psychonom. Soc.* **17:**51–52.

TRAMILL, J. L., GUSTAVSON, K., WEAVER, M. S., MOORE, S. A., and DAVIS, S. F., 1983, Shock-elicited aggression as a function of acute and chronic ethanol challenges, *J. Gen. Psychol.* **109:**53–58.

TRAVERSA, U., DeANGELIS, L., LOGGIA, R. D., BERTOLISSI, M., NARDINI, G., and VERTUA, R., 1985, Effects of caffeine and chlor-desmethyldiazepam on fighting behavior of mice with different reactivity baselines, *Pharmacol. Biochem. Behav.* **23:**237–241.

TUNKS, E. R., and DERMER, S. W., 1977, Carbamazepine in the dyscontrol syndrome associated with limbic system dysfunction, *J. Nerv. Ment. Dis.* **164:**56–63.

TUPIN, J. P., 1985, Psychopharmacology and Aggression, in: *Clinical Treatment of the Violent Person* (L. H. Roth, ed.), US Department of Health and Human Services, Rockville, MD, pp. 83–99.

TUPIN, J. P., SMITH, D. B., CLANON, T. L., KIM, L. I., NUGENT, A., and GROUPE, A., 1973, The long-term use of lithium in aggressive prisoners, *Compr. Psychiatry* **14:**311–317.

TYLER, C. B., and MICZEK, K. A., 1982, Effects of phencyclidine on aggressive behavior in mice, *Pharmacol. Biochem. Behav.* **17:**503–510.

TYRER, S. P., WALSH, A., EDWARDS, D. E., BERNEY, T. P., and STEPHENS, D. A., 1984, Factors associated with a good response to lithium in aggressive mentally handicapped subjects, *Prog. Neuro-psychopharmacol. Biol. Psychiatry* **8:**751–755.

UCER, E., and KREGER, K. C., 1969, A double-blind study comparing haloperidol with thioridazine in emotionally disturbed, mentally retarded children, *Curr. Ther. Res.* **11:**278–283.

UEKI, S., FUJIWARA, M., and OGAWA, N., 1972a, Mouse-killing behavior (muricide) induced by delta-9-tetrahydrocannabinol in the rat, *Physiol. Behav.* **9:**585–587.

UEKI, S., MURIMOTO, S., and OGAWA, N., 1972b, Effects of psychotropic drugs on emotional behavior in rats with limbic lesions, with special reference to olfactory bulb ablations, *Folia Psychiatr. Neurol. Jpn.* **26:**246–255.

ULRICH, R., 1966, Pain as a cause of aggression, *Am. Zoologist* **6:**643–662.

ULRICH, R. E., and AZRIN, N. H., 1962, Reflexive fighting in response to aversive stimulation, *J. Exp. Anal. Behav.* **5:**511–520.

ULRICH, R. E., HUTCHINSON, R. R., and AZRIN, N. H., 1965, Pain-elicited aggression, *Psychol. Rec.* **15:**111–126.

UPCHURCH, M., and SCHALLERT, T., 1982, Neuroleptic-sensitive posture and movement related to subordinate social status in Mongolian gerbils (*Meriones unguiculatus*), *Behav. Neural Biol.* **35:**308–314.

UYENO, E. T., 1966a, Effects of *d*-lysergic acid diethylamide and 2-brom-lysergic acid diethylamide on dominance behavior in the rat, *Int. J. Neuropharmacol.* **5:**317–322.

UYENO, E. T., 1966b, Inhibition of isolation-induced attack behavior of mice by drugs, *J. Pharmaceutical Sci.* **55:**215–216.

UYENO, E. T., 1967a, Lysergic acid diethylamide and dominance behavior of the squirrel monkey, *Arch. Int. Pharmacodyn. Ther.* **169:**66–69.

UYENO, E. T., 1967b, Lysergic acid diethylamide and sexual dominance behavior of the male rat, *Int. J. Neuropsychiatry* **3:**188–190.

UYENO, E. T., 1976, Effects of delta 9-tetrahydrocannabinol and 2,5-dimethoxy-4-methylamphetamine on rat sexual dominance behavior, *Proc. Western Pharmacol. Soc.* **19:**369–372.

UYENO, E. T., and BENSON, W. M., 1965, Effects of lysergic acid diethylamide on attack behaviour of male albino mice, *Psychopharmacologia* **7:**20–26.

VALENSTEIN, E. S., COX, V. C., and KAKOLEWSKI, J. W., 1970, Reexamination of the role of the hypothalamus in motivation, *Psychol. Rev.* **77:**16–31.

VALZELLI, L., 1967, Drugs and aggressiveness, *Adv. Pharmacol.* **5:**79–108.
VALZELLI, L., 1969, Aggressive behavior induced by isolation, in: *Aggressive Behavior* (S. Garattini and E. B. Sigg, eds.), Wiley, New York, pp. 70–76.
VALZELLI, L., 1973a, Activity of benzodiazepines on aggressive behavior in rats and mice, in: *The Benzodiazepines* (S. Garattini, E. Mussini, and L. O. Randall, eds.), Raven Press, New York, pp. 405–417.
VALZELLI, L., 1973b, The "isolation syndrome" in mice, *Psychopharmacologia* **31:**305–320.
VALZELLI, L., 1978, Human and animal studies on the neurophysiology of aggression, *Prog. Neuro-Psychopharmacol.* **2:**591–610.
VALZELLI, L., 1979, Effect of sedatives and anxiolytics on aggressivity, in: *Differential Psychopharmacology of Anxiolytics and Sedatives* (J. R. Boissier, ed.), Karger, Basel, pp. 143–156.
VALZELLI, L., and BERNASCONI, S., 1971, Differential activity of some psychotropic drugs as a function of emotional levels in animals, *Psychopharmacologia* **20:**91–96.
VALZELLI, L., and BERNASCONI, S., 1973, Behavioral and neurochemical effects of caffeine in normal and aggressive mice, *Pharmacol. Biochem. Behav.* **1:**251–254.
VALZELLI, L., and BERNASCONI, S., 1976, Psychoactive drug effect on behavioural changes induced by prolonged socio-environmental deprivation in rats, *Psychol. Med.* **6:**271–276.
VALZELLI, L., and GARATTINI, S., 1968, Behavioral changes and 5-hydroxytryptamine turnover in animals, *Adv. Pharmacol.* **6B:**249–260.
VALZELLI, L., GIACALONE, E., and GARATTINI, S., 1967, Pharmacological control of aggressive behavior in mice, *Eur. J. Pharmacol.* **2:**144–146.
VAN HEMEL, P. E., 1975, Rats and mice together: The aggressive nature of mouse killing rats, *Psychol. Bull.* **82:**456–459.
VAN PRAAG, H. M., 1982, Depression, suicide and the metabolism of serotonin in the brain, *J. Affective Disorders* **4:**275–290.
VAN PUTTEN, T., and SANDERS, D. G., 1975, Lithium in treatment failures, *J. Nerv. Ment. Dis.* **161:**255–264.
VANDENBERGH, J. G., 1971, The effects of gonadal hormones on the aggressive behaviour of adult golden hamsters *(Mesocricetus auratus)*, *Animal Behav.* **19:**589–594.
VAN REE, J. M., and NIESINK, R. J. M., 1983, Low doses of beta-endorphin increase social contacts of rats tested in dyadic encounters, *Life Sci.* **33**(Suppl. 1):611–614.
VASSOUT, A., and DELINI-STULA, A., 1977, Effets de β-bloqueurs (propranolol et oxprenolol) et du diazepam sur differents modeles d'agressivite chez le rat, *J. Pharmacol.* **8:**5–14.
VERGNES, M., 1980, Amygdaloid control over interspecies aggression in the rat, in: *Limbic Epilepsy and the Dyscontrol Syndrome* (M. Girgis and L. G. Kiloh, eds.), Elsevier/North-Holland, Amsterdam, pp. 85–91.
VERGNES, M., and KARLI, P., 1963, Declenchement on comportement d'agression interspecifique rat-souris par ablation bilaterale des bulbes olfactifs. Action de l'hydroxyzine sur cette agressivite provoquee, *C. R. Seances Soc. Biol.* **157:**1061–1063.
VERGNES, M., and KARLI, P., 1969, Effets de la stimulation de l'hypothalamus lateral, de l'amygdale et de l'hippocampe sur le comportement d'agression interspecifique rat-souris, *Physiol. Behav.* **4:**889–894.
VERGNES, M., and KARLI, P., 1970, Declenchement d'un comportement d'agression par stimulation electrique de l'hypothalamus median chez le rat, *Physiol. Behav.* **5:**1427–1430.
VERGNES, M., and KEMPF, E., 1981, Tryptophan deprivation: Effects on mouse-killing and reactivity in the rat, *Pharmacol. Biochem. Behav.* **14**(Suppl.1):19–23.
VERGNES, M., and KEMPF, E., 1982, Effect of hypothalamic injections of 5,7-dihydroxytryptamine on elicitation of mouse-killing in rats, *Behav. Brain Res.* **5:**387–397.
VERGNES, M., PENOT, C., KEMPF, E., and MACK, G., 1977, Lesion selective des neurones

serotonergiques du raphe par 5,7 dihydroxytryptamine: Effets sur le comportment d'aggression interspecifique du rat, *Brain Res.* **133:**167–171.

VETRO, A., SZENTISTVANYI, I., PALLAG, L., VARGHA, M., and SZILARD, J., 1985, Therapeutic experience with lithium in childhood aggression, *Pharmacopsychiatry* **14:**121–127.

VIALATTE, J., 1966, Troubles du comportement chez l'enfant interet du traitement symptomatique par un psycholeptique, *Ann. Pediatr.* **45:**733–735.

VICKERS, C., and PATERSON, A. T., 1985, Social behaviour in pairs of C57BL/6 mice of both sexes in the open field: Effects of saline drinking and of naloxone, *Pharmacol. Biochem. Behav.* **23:**905–909.

VIRKKUNEN, M., 1974, Alcohol as a factor precipitating aggression and conflict behaviour leading to homicide, *Br. J. Addiction* **69:**149–154.

VOGEL, J. R., and LEAF, R. C., 1972, Initiation of mouse killing in non-killer rats by repeated pilocarpine treatment, *Physiol. Behav.* **8:**421–424.

VOTAVA, Z., 1969, Aggressive behavior evoked by LSD-25 in rats pretreated with reserpine, in: *Aggressive Behavior* (S. Garattini and E. B. Sigg, eds.), Excerpta Medica Foundation, Amsterdam, pp. 236–237.

WAGNER, G. C., NABERT, D. R., and TOLBERT, R. K., 1983, The effects of tail shock on target-biting behavior of confined mice, *Aggressive Behav.* **9:**309–313.

WAIZER, J., HOFFMAN, S. P., POLIZOS, P., and ENGELHARDT, D. M., 1974, Outpatient treatment of hyperactive school children with imipramine, *Am. J. Psychiatry* **131:**587–591.

WALASZEK, E. J., and ABOOD, L. G., 1956, Effect of tranquilizing drugs on fighting response of Siamese fighting fish, *Science* **124:**440–441.

WALSH, L. L., 1982, Strain and sex differences in mouse killing by rats, *J. Comp. Physiol. Psychol.* **96:**278–283.

WALTERS, J. K., SHEARD, M. H., and DAVIS, M., 1978, Effects of N,N-dimethyltryptamine (DMT) and 5-methoxy-*N,N*-dimethyltryptamine (5-MeODMT) on shock elicited fighting in rats, *Pharmacol. Biochem. Behav.* **9:**87–90.

WASMAN, M., and FLYNN, J. P., 1962, Directed attack elicited from hypothalamus, *Arch. Neurol.* **6:**220–227.

WATANABE, S., INOUE, M., and UEKI, S., 1979, Effects of psychotropic drugs injected into the limbic structures on mouse-killing behavior in the rat with olfactory bulb ablations, *Jpn. J. Pharmacol.* **29:**493–496.

WEBBE, F. M., DEWEESE, J., and MALAGODI, E. F., 1974, Induced attack during multiple fixed-ratio, variable-ratio schedules of reinforcement, *J. Exp. Anal. Behav.* **22:**197–206.

WEI, E., LOH, H., and WAY, E. L., 1973, Quantitative aspects of precipitated abstinence in morphine-dependent rats, *J. Pharmacol. Exp. Ther.* **184:**398–403.

WEINSTOCK, M., and WEISS, C., 1980, Antagonism by propranolol of isolation-induced aggression in mice: Correlation with 5-hydroxytryptamine receptor blockade, *Neuropharmacology* **19:**653–656.

WEISCHER, M., 1969, Über die antiaggressive Wirkung von Lithium, *Psychopharmacologia* **15:**245–254.

WEISCHER, M.-L., 1966, Einfluss von Anorektika der Amphetamin-reihe auf das Verhalten des Siamesischen Kampffisches Betta Splendens, *Arzneim.-Forsch.* **16:**1310–1311.

WEISCHER, M.-L., and OPITZ, K., 1972, Einfluss von Fenfluramin, Chlorphentermine und verwandten Verbindungen auf das Verhalten von aggressiven Mäusen, *Arch. Int. Pharmacodyn. Ther.* **195:**252–259.

WEITZ, M. K., 1974, Effects of ethanol on shock-elicited fighting behavior in rats, *Q. J. Stud. Alcohol* **35:**953–958.

WELCH, A. S., and WELCH, B. L., 1971, Isolation, reactivity and aggression: Evidence for an involvement of brain catecholamines and serotonin, in: *Physiology of Aggression and Defeat* (B. E. Eleftheriou and J. P. Scott, eds.), Plenum Press, New York, pp. 91–142.

WELCH, B. L., and WELCH, A. S., 1966, Graded effect of social stimulation upon *d*-amphetamine toxicity, aggressiveness and heart and adrenal weight, *J. Pharmacol. Exp. Ther.* **151:**331–338.

WELCH, B. L., and WELCH, A. S., 1968, Rapid modification of isolation-induced aggressive behavior and elevation of brain catecholamines and serotonin by the quick-acting monoamine-oxidase inhibitor pargyline, *Commun. Behav. Biol.* **1:**347–351.

WELCH, B. L., and WELCH, A. S., 1969, Aggression and the biogenic amine neurohumors, in: *Aggressive Behavior* (S. Garattini and E. B. Sigg, eds.), Excerpta Medica Foundation, Amsterdam, pp. 188–202.

WELCH, B. L., and WELCH, A. S., 1973, Chronic social stimulation and tolerance to amphetamine: Interacting effects of amphetamine and natural nervous stimulation upon brain amines and behavior, in: *Current Concepts in Amphetamine Abuse* (E. H. Ellinwood and S. Cohen, eds.), US Government Printing Office, Washington, DC, pp. 107–115.

WERRY, J. S., and AMAN, M. G., 1975, Methylphenidate and haloperidol in children, *Arch. Gen. Psychiatry* **32:**790–795.

WHITEHEAD, T., 1981, Sex hormone treatment of prisoners, in: *Multidisciplinary Approaches to Aggression Research* (P. F. Brain and D. Benton, eds.), Elsevier/North-Holland, Amsterdam, pp. 503–511.

WILKINSON, C. J., 1985, Effects of diazepam (Valium) and trait anxiety on human physical aggression and emotional state, *J. Behav. Med.* **8:**101–114.

WILLIAMS, D. T., MEHL, R., YUDOFSKY, S., ADAMS, D., and ROSEMAN, B., 1982, The effect of propranolol on uncontrolled rage outbursts in children and adolescents with organic brain dysfunction, *J. Am. Acad. Child Psychiatry* **21:**129–135.

WILLIAMS, L. N., 1969, LSD and manslaughter, *Lancet* **9:**332.

WILLNER, P., THEODOROU, A., and MONTGOMERY, A., 1981, Subchronic treatment with the tricyclic antidepressant DMI increases isolation-induced fighting in rats, *Pharmacol. Biochem. Behav.* **14:**475–479.

WILSON, E. O., 1975, *Sociobiology,* Belknap Press, Cambridge.

WINSBERG, B. G., BIALER, I., KUPIETZ, S., and TOBIAS, J., 1972, Effects of imipramine and dextroamphetamine on behavior of neuropsychiatrically impaired children, *Am. J. Psychiatry* **128:**1425–1431.

WINSBERG, B. G., PRESS, M., BIALER, I., and KUPIETZ, S., 1974, Dextroamphetamine and methylphenidate in the treatment of hyperactive/aggressive children, *Pediatrics* **53:**236–241.

WINSBERG, B. G., KUPIETZ, S. S., SVERD, J., HUNGUND, B. L., and YOUNG, N. L., 1982, Methylphenidate oral dose plasma concentrations and behavioral response in children, *Psychopharmacology* **76:**329–332.

WINSLOW, J. T., and MICZEK, K. A., 1983, Habituation of aggression in mice: Pharmacological evidence of catecholaminergic and serotonergic mediation, *Psychopharmacology* **81:**286–291.

WINSLOW, J. T., and MICZEK, K. A., 1985, Social status as determinant of alcohol effects on aggressive behavior in squirrel monkeys *(Saimiri sciureus), Psychopharmacology* **85:**167–172.

WINSLOW, J. T., KOZAK, A., and MICZEK, K. A., 1983, The effects of naloxone and amphetamine on squirrel monkey behavior in groups, *Neurosci. Abstr.* **9:**120.

WINSLOW, J. T., MICZEK, K. A., and ELLINGBOE, J., 1985, Seasonal variation of the effects of alcohol on aggressive behavior and gonadal hormones in high-status squirrel monkeys, *Neurosci. Abstr.* **11:**294.

WINSLOW, J. T., MICZEK, K. A., and ELLINGBOE, J., 1986, Testosterone–alcohol interactions and aggressive behavior in subordinate squirrel monkeys, *Neurosci. Abstr.* **12** (pt.1):288.

WISE, D. A., 1974, Aggression in the female golden hamster: Effects of reproductive state and social isolation, *Hormones Behav.* **5:**235–250.

WISE, D. A., and PRYOR, T. L., 1977, Effects of ergocornine and prolactin on aggression in the postpartum golden hamster, *Hormones Behav.* **8:**30–39.

WOLFGANG, M. E., and STROHM, R. B., 1956, The relationship between alcohol and criminal homicide, *Q. J. Stud. Alcohol* **17**:411–425.
WOODWORTH, C. H., 1971, Attack elicited in rats by electrical stimulation of the lateral hypothalamus, *Physiol. Behav.* **6**:345–353.
WOODY, G. E., PERSKY, H., MCLELLAN, A. T., O'BRIEN, C. P., and ARNDT, I., 1983, Psychoendocrine correlates of hostility and anxiety in addicts, in: *Alcohol, Drug Abuse and Aggression* (E. Gottheil, K. A. Druley, T. E. Skoloda, and H. M. Waxman, eds.), Thomas, Springfield, IL, pp. 227–244.
WORRALL, E. P., MOODY, J. P., and NAYLOR, G. J., 1975, Lithium in non-manic-depressives: Antiaggressive effect and red blood cell lithium values, *Br. J. Psychiatry* **126**:464–468.
YAMAMOTO, T., and UEKI, S., 1978, Effects of drugs on hyperactivity and aggression induced by raphe lesions in rats, *Pharmacol. Biochem. Behav.* **9**:821–826.
YANAI, J., and GINSBURG, B. E., 1976, Long-term effects of early ethanol on predatory behavior in inbred mice, *Physiol. Psychol.* **4**:409–411.
YANAI, J., and GINSBURG, B. E., 1977, Long term reduction of male agonistic behavior in mice following early exposure to ethanol, *Psychopharmacology* **52**:31–34.
YARVIS, R. M., 1972, Psychiatric pathology and social deviance in 25 incarcerated offenders, *Arch. Gen. Psychiatry* **26**:79–84.
YARYURA-TOBIAS, J. A., and NEZIROGLU, F. A., 1975, Violent behavior, brain dysrhythmia, and glucose dysfunction: A new function, *J. Orthomol. Psychiatry* **4**:182–188.
YEN, C. Y., STANGER, R. L., and MILLMAN, N., 1959, Ataractic suppression of isolation-induced aggressive behavior, *Arch. Int. Pharmacodyn. Ther.* **123**:179–185.
YEN, H. C. Y., KATZ, M. H., and KROP, S., 1970, Effects of various drugs on 3,4-dihydroxyphenylalanine (D1-DOPA)-induced excitation (aggressive behavior) in mice, *Toxicol. Appl. Pharmacol.* **17**:597–604.
YEPES, L. E., BALKA, E. B., WINSBERG, B. G., and BIALER, I., 1977, Amitriptyline and methylphenidate treatment of behaviorally disordered children, *J. Child Psychol. Psychiatry* **18**:39–52.
YESAVAGE, J. A., 1982, Inpatient violence and the schizophrenic patient: An inverse correlation between danger-related events and neuroleptic levels, *Biol. Psychiatry* **17**:1331–1337.
YOSHIMURA, H., and MICZEK, K. A., 1983, Separate neural sites for *d*-amphetamine suppression of mouse killing and feeding behavior in rats, *Aggressive Behav.* **9**:353–363.
YOSHIMURA, H., and OGAWA, N., 1983, Pharmaco-ethological analysis of agonistic behavior between resident and intruder mice: Effects of ethylalcohol, *Folia Pharmacol. Jpn.* **81**:135–141.
YOSHIMURA, H., and OGAWA, N., 1984, Pharmaco-ethological analysis of agonistic behavior between resident and intruder mice: Effects of psychotropic drugs, *Folia Pharmacol. Jpn.* **84**:221–228.
YOSHIMURA, H., and OGAWA, N., 1985, Pharmaco-ethological analysis of agonistic behavior between resident and intruder mice: Effects of adrenergic β-blockers, *Jpn. J. Psychopharmacol.* **5**:223–229.
YOSHIMURA, H., FUJIWARA, M., and UEKI, S., 1974, Biochemical correlates in mouse-killing behavior of the rat: Brain acetylcholine and acetylcholinesterase after administration of delta-9-tetrahydrocannabinol, *Brain Res.* **81**:567–570.
YUDOFSKY, S., WILLIAMS, D., and GORMAN, J., 1981, Propranolol in the treatment of rage and violent behavior in patients with chronic brain syndromes, *Am. J. Psychiatry* **138**:218–220.
YUDOFSKY, S. C., STEVENS, L., SILVER, J., BARSA, J., and WILLIAMS, D., 1984, Propranolol in the treatment of rage and violent behavior associated with Korsakoffs' psychosis, *Am. J. Psychiat.* **141**:114–115.
ZACKER, J., and BARD, M., 1977, Further findings on assaultiveness and alcohol use in interpersonal disputes, *Am. J. Commun. Psychol.* **5**:373–383.

ZEICHNER, A., and PIHL, R. O., 1978, Effects of alcohol and behavior contingencies on human aggression, *J. Abnorm. Psychol.* **88**:153–160.

ZEICHNER, A., and PIHL, R. O., 1980, Effects of alcohol and instigator intent on human aggression, *J. Stud. Alcohol* **41**:265–276.

ZEICHNER, A., PIHL, R. O., NIAURA, R., and ZACCHIA, C., 1982, Attentional processes in alcohol-mediated aggression, *J. Stud. Alcohol* **43**:714–724.

ZETLER, G., and HAUER, B., 1975, Pharmacological dissociation between vocalization and biting produced in rats by the combination of imipramine and isocarboxazid, *Psychopharmacologia* **45**:73–77.

ZETLER, G., and OTTEN, U., 1969, Aggressivität der Ratte nach kombinierter Behandlung mit Monoaminoxydase-Inhibitoren und anderen psychotropen Pharmaka, insbesondere Thymoleptica, *Naunyn-Schmiedeberg's Arch. Exp. Pathol. Pharmakol.* **264**:32–54.

ZWIRNER, P. P., PORSOLT, R. D., and LOEW, D. M., 1975, Inter-group aggression in mice. A new method for testing the effects of centrally active drugs, *Psychopharmacologia* **45**:133–138.

5

THE ELECTROPHYSIOLOGICAL AND BIOCHEMICAL PHARMACOLOGY OF THE MESOLIMBIC AND MESOCORTICAL DOPAMINE NEURONS

Michael J. Bannon, Arthur S. Freeman, Louis A. Chiodo, Benjamin S. Bunney, and Robert H. Roth

1. INTRODUCTION

Since the early pioneering anatomical studies of Dahlström and Fuxe (1964), it has been known that midbrain dopamine (DA)-containing neurons project to and innervate not only the striatum but also various limbic regions. These observations and those of Ungerstedt (1971) led to the functional organization of midbrain DA neurons into the nigrostriatal and mesolimbic DA systems. However, in 1973, Thierry and colleagues presented biochemical evidence for the existence of DA in the cerebral cortex, independent of that normally present within the norepinephrine-con-

---

Michael J. Bannon, Arthur S. Freeman, Louis A. Chiodo, Benjamin S. Bunney, and Robert H. Roth • Departments of Psychiatry and Pharmacology, Yale University School of Medicine and the Abraham Ribicoff Research Facilities, Connecticut Mental Health Center, New Haven, Connecticut 06508.   Present address for Drs. Bannon, Freeman, and Chiodo: Center for Cell Biology, Sinai Hospital of Detroit, Detroit, Michigan 48235.

taining neurons (Thierry *et al.*, 1973*a,b*). Other work demonstrated that a DA-sensitive adenylate cyclase was present in the cortex (von Hungen and Roberts, 1973). Subsequent anatomical studies, which employed more sensitive fluorescence histochemical techniques, confirmed the presence of a mesocortical DA system (Berger *et al.*, 1974, 1976; Hökfelt *et al.*, 1974; Lindvall *et al.*, 1977, 1978; Lindvall and Björklund, 1978*a,b*). During the last 10 years, much basic electrophysiological, pharmacological, and biochemical research has been directed toward providing a more detailed understanding of the functioning of these midbrain DA systems. The following review is an overview of those studies. The anatomy of these systems will also be discussed, as will the possible roles these systems play in conditioned and unconditioned behaviors. Although it is not within the scope of this discussion to review the nigrostriatal DA system exhaustively, reference will be made to studies of these neurons in order to assess similarities and differences among the midbrain DA pathways. Biochemical, behavioral, and anatomical aspects of the midbrain DA systems have been the topics of reviews in previous volumes of this *Handbook* (Sedvall, 1975; Iversen, 1977*a*; Lindvall and Björklund, 1978*b*).

2. ANATOMY OF MIDBRAIN DOPAMINE SYSTEMS

2.1. The Nigrostriatal DA System

For many years, the investigation of midbrain DA neurons was centered on those cells located in the zona compacta region of the substantia nigra (area A9 of Dahlström and Fuxe, 1964). The A9 area forms a thin layer just dorsal to the zona reticulata region of this nucleus. A large portion of A9 DA cells project to the caudate nucleus or putamen, thus giving rise to the nigrostriatal DA pathway (Hökfelt *et al.*, 1974; Lindvall and Björklund, 1978*a,b*; Lindvall, 1979). Anatomical studies demonstrate tight reciprocal connections between the substantia nigra and the striatum, and a series of supportive electrophysiological experiments have demonstrated that A9 neurons are regulated, at least in part, by a striatonigral feedback loop (Bunney and Aghajanian, 1976, 1978; also see Section 6).

2.2. Mesolimbic and Mesocortical DA Systems

As stated earlier, in addition to nigrostriatal DA neurons there are numerous other DA cells in the midbrain which do not innervate the striatum, but rather project to limbic or cortical areas. Many of these DA cells belong to the A10 cell group of Dahlström and Fuxe (1964). The cell bodies of most of these neurons are located in the ventral tegmental area (VTA), which occupies the region medial to the substantia nigra, dorsolateral to the interpeduncular nucleus and ventral to the red nucleus (Hökfelt et al., 1973; Ungerstedt, 1971). The total number of A10 DA neurons equals or exceeds the number of A9 DA cells (Swanson, 1982). Another organizational distinction is that, to some extent, the DA neurons of A9 and A10 seem to innervate different target tissues, although their projections do overlap in several terminal areas.

Identification of the terminal fields of A10 DA neurons has been made using techniques of retrograde tracing and fluorescence histochemistry. Injection of the retrograde tracer horseradish peroxidase (HRP) into the nucleus accumbens results in the labeling of neurons in the A10 area (Nauta, 1978; Phillipson, 1979). However, prior destruction of dopaminergic axons by injection of the catecholamine neurotoxin 6-hydroxydopamine (6-OHDA) into the medial forebrain bundle prevents most of the A10 labeling by HRP (Wang, 1981a). Thus, it appears that the projection from A10 to the nucleus accumbens is largely dopaminergic. This finding is supported by fluorescent retrograde tracing combined with tyrosine hydroxylase immunohistochemistry (Swanson, 1982). Similarly, the great majority of A10 cells innervating the lateral septum are dopaminergic (Swanson, 1982). In contrast to the A10 projections to the nucleus accumbens and lateral septum, approximately half of the A10 cells terminating in the amygdala and entorhinal cortex are dopaminergic, whereas DA cells comprise only about one-third of the cells of the A10-prefrontal cortex and A10-cingulate cortex pathways (Swanson, 1982). The A10 DA neurons project largely to limbic (e.g., nucleus accumbens, olfactory tubercle, central nucleus of the amygdala, septum) and cortical (e.g., prefrontal, cingulate, piriform, entorhinal) regions of the forebrain, thereby forming the mesolimbic and mesocortical DA pathways, respectively (Berger et al., 1974, 1976; Berger, 1977; Lindvall et al., 1977; Lindvall and Björklund, 1978a,b; Lindvall, 1979; Swanson, 1982). We will employ this terminology when referring to the DA pathways emanating from the A10 area (also see Section 3.2).

It should be mentioned that a modified terminology for subdivisions of the mesencephalic DA system has recently been introduced on the basis of new insights into the organization of the basal forebrain (see Björklund and Lindvall, 1985). In this classification, certain limbic areas (nucleus accumbens, olfactory tubercle, bed nucleus of the stria terminalis), as well as the caudate putamen, constitute the entire striatal complex and represent projection sites of the mesostriatal DA system. The mesolimbocortical DA system corresponds, in this classification, to projections to the septum, amygdala, habenula and cortical areas.

The A8 cell group is generally considered to be a caudal extension of areas A9 and A10. Neurons in A8 project to a number of limbic and cortical sites as well as to the striatum (Lenard and Nauta, 1979; Deutch *et al.*, 1984). Several of these projections have recently been shown to include dopaminergic components (Deutch *et al.*, 1984). The position and extent of the A8 projections, as well as the behavioral effects of 6-OHDA lesions of A8 suggest that this cell group may exert an influence on the A9 and A10 DA neuronal systems (Deutch, 1982; Deutch *et al.*, 1984).

3. DISTINGUISHING BETWEEN A9 AND A10 DOPAMINE SYSTEMS

3.1. Behavioral Studies

Because of the relationship of the striatum to central nervous system motor circuitry and the presence of projections from the nucleus accumbens to the globus pallidus and substantia nigra, as well as to the VTA and the limbic/hypothalamic axis (Nauta, 1978), midbrain DA pathways are favorably positioned to affect motor output. As has been reviewed (Iversen, 1977a; Beninger, 1983), severe forebrain DA depletions result in deficits in the performance of conditioned (learned) and unconditioned motor acts. Such deficits are apparently the result of an impairment in the initiation of sequences of purposeful behavior. Selective lesioning techniques have helped to identify functional differences among the DA systems with respect to their effects on motor behavior, although it is becoming evident that distinctions among the systems are subtler than was once imagined. Thus, both the nigrostriatal and mesolimbic DA systems are involved in some aspect of behavioral arousal, the nigrostriatal system appearing to play a major role in the facilitation of sensorimotor integration, whereas the mesolimbic system may modulate affective responses to environmental (e.g., presence of a conspecific) or interoceptive (e.g., hunger) stimuli (Iversen, 1977b). Thus, together, the A9 and A10 DA systems may provide the circuitry for influencing the selection and execution of particular acts. Selective catecholamine lesions (6-OHDA) of the VTA, which presumably destroy the mesolimbic and mesocortical DA systems, result in an irreversible syndrome that is marked by difficulties in suppressing previously learned responses, locomotor hyperactivity, and disturbances in organized behavior (LeMoal *et al.*, 1969; Galey *et al.*, 1977; Tassin *et al.*, 1978). A good correlation was found between the increases in locomotor activity and decreases in frontal cortical DA resulting from these lesions (Tassin *et al.*, 1978). Loss of frontal cortical DA after 6-OHDA lesion of the VTA is also associated with the expression of inappropriate behaviors, heightened distractibility by environmental stimuli, and impairment of delayed alternation performance (Simon et al., 1980); local depletion of DA by injection of 6-OHDA into the prefrontal cortex produces similar hyperactivity (Carter and Pycock, 1980; Pycock et al., 1980). Lesions primarily affecting the mesocortical DA system also result in cognitive deficits such as impaired performance of delayed alternation tasks in monkeys (Brozoski et al., 1979).

In humans, diminished influence of A9 DA cells in the striatum is associated with the extrapyramidal movement disorders of Parkinson's disease, as well as the parkinsonism and dyskinesias induced by antipsychotic drugs (neuroleptics), which block DA receptors. Dysfunction of limbic and cortical DA projections has been implicated in affective and cognitive disorders, and these pathways may be functionally hyperactive in schizophrenia (Snyder, 1972; Matthysse, 1973; Stevens, 1973; Hökfelt et al., 1974; Snyder et al., 1974; Glowinski, 1975; Meltzer and Stahl, 1976). Thus, characterization of those DA cells originating in A10 may be more relevant to the testing of the DA hypothesis of schizophrenia than is the study of the nigrostriatal DA cells. For this reason, studies of the electrophysiology and biochemistry of A10 DA neurons have been undertaken with the hope of unraveling the mechanisms of action of drugs found to be useful in the treatment of psychosis (see Section 5.2). Detailed knowledge of how drugs interact with A10 DA neurons will possibly advance our understanding of the neuronal substrates of psychoses.

3.2. Anatomical Considerations

For the investigator seeking to elucidate functional differences between A9 and A10 DA cell populations, the fact that A10 DA cells project to a variety of limbic and cortical regions, and a small percentage of them (located mainly anteroventrally) to striatal sites, presents a problem. Also problematical are the results of a recent study that demonstrate that some A9 neurons innervate limbic and cortical areas and a small percentage of the cells in A9 collateralize to innervate more than one forebrain region (Loughlin and Fallon, 1984). However, this study employed only HRP tracing techniques, which do not allow for the distinction between DA and non-DA neurons. Anatomical studies have established that the overwhelming majority of A10 neurons do not collateralize, and thus, a given A10 cell generally does not innervate more than one terminal field (Fallon, 1981; Loughlin and Fallon, 1984). This finding has been shown to hold for A10 cells immunohistochemically identified as dopaminergic (Swanson, 1982). Electrophysiological evidence supports the anatomical findings in that only a very low percentage of A10 DA cells can be antidromically activated by electrical stimulation of more than one forebrain area (Deneau et al., 1980; Chiodo and Bunney, unpublished data). The latter fact is extremely important, since it provides a basis on which the classification of DA neurons may be made. For example, the electrophysiological characteristics of DA neurons antidromically activated from a particular target area may be compared with other similarly identified subpopulations of DA cells. Since biochemical studies of DA neurons usually sample tissue containing DA nerve terminals, it is possible to study the DA biochemistry of a specific region without considering the precise anatomical localization of the respective cell bodies. Biochemical changes occurring in the terminal fields of DA cells shown to originate in A10 can be assessed using well-established indices of DA function such as DA turnover, the concentrations of DA and DA metabolites, and tyrosine hydroxylase activity. Therefore, both electrophysiological and biochemical techniques allow the electrophysiological characteristics of identified DA neurons that project to a specific forebrain site to be compared with biochemical measures of the activity at dopaminergic synapses. For the purposes of this discussion, the mesolimbic and mesocortical DA pathways will be thought of as originating primarily in A10 and the mesostriatal DA pathway in A9 (i.e., the nigrostriatal DA pathway). However, the importance of identifying the projection sites of all the DA cells in a given electrophysiological study cannot be overstated, especially when one is attempting to characterize distinct midbrain DA pathways in order to formulate hypotheses regarding the effects of drugs on the different systems.

4. IDENTIFICATION AND CHARACTERIZATION

Electrophysiological recordings from putative DA cells located in the A9 and A10 regions of the midbrain were first obtained in 1973 with the use of extracellular single-unit recording techniques (Bunney et al., 1973a). The tentative identification of these cells as dopaminergic was based on several findings. L-Dopa was iontophoresed from the recording micropipette into the neuropil surrounding the putative DA cell being recorded. After the brains of these animals were processed for catecholamine histochemistry, neurons in the vicinity of the pipette tip showed a more intense DA fluorescence than other cells in the zona compacta because DA neurons in proximity to the electrode tip took up the L-dopa and converted it to DA, which resulted in an increase in the intracellular concentrations of the neurotransmitter. In another series of experiments, DA neurons were destroyed unilaterally with 6-OHDA. No neurons possessing the electrophysiological characteristics attributed to tentatively identified DA cells (see the discussion below) were found on the lesioned side, whereas cells with such characteristics were found in abundance on the nonlesioned side. This evidence, as well as the response of these neurons to DA agonists and antagonists, permitted the identification of DA neurons on the basis of a specific, extracellularly recorded action potential and firing pattern. These cells exhibit slow firing rates (1–10/sec) and have long-duration (2–5 msec) biphasic action potentials, with the initial positive component often displaying a prominent "notch" corresponding to a break between the initial segment and somatodendritic components of the action potential (Grace and Bunney, 1983). Action potentials may occur in a single spike pattern or in a bursting mode characterized by decreasing spike amplitude within a burst (Fig. 1). Additionally, all cells with the above characteristics have slow conduction velocities (approximately 0.5 m/sec) (Guyenet and Aghajanian, 1978; Grace and Bunney, 1980; German *et al.*, 1980; Wang, 1981*a*; Chiodo and Bunney, 1983; White and Wang, 1984*a*; Chiodo *et al.*, 1984), in accordance with the unmyelinated nature of their axons (Hökfelt *et al.*, 1973). However, all this evidence was indirect proof that the cells being recorded were dopaminergic. Direct proof was provided by intracellular recording and subsequent visualization of the heightened histofluorescence resulting from intracellular injection of L-dopa, tetrahydrobiopterin (a cofactor for tyro-

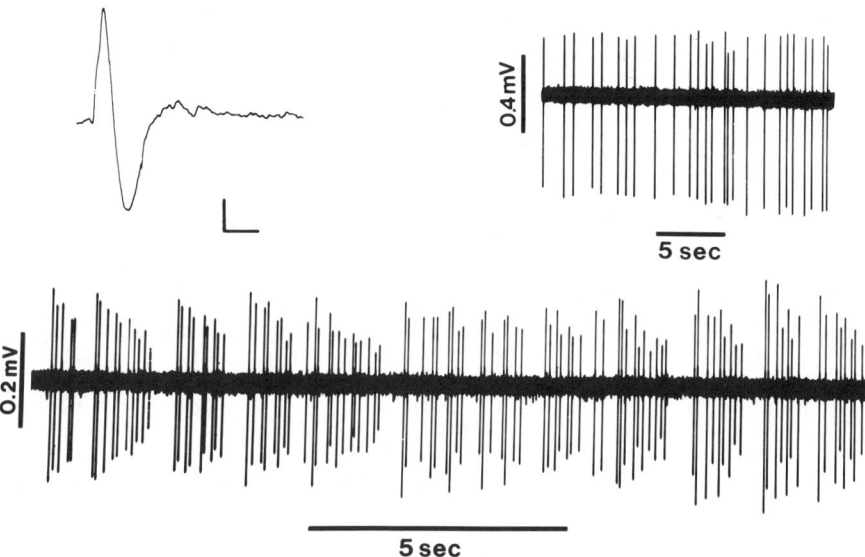

FIG. 1. Upper left, an individual action potential of a DA neuron. Calibration = 100 μV, 2 msec. Oscillograph recordings show the single spike (upper right) and bursting (lower) firing patterns exhibited by DA cells. (Waveform, from Chiodo and Bunney, 1983; burst recording, from Bunney *et al.*, 1973*a*.)

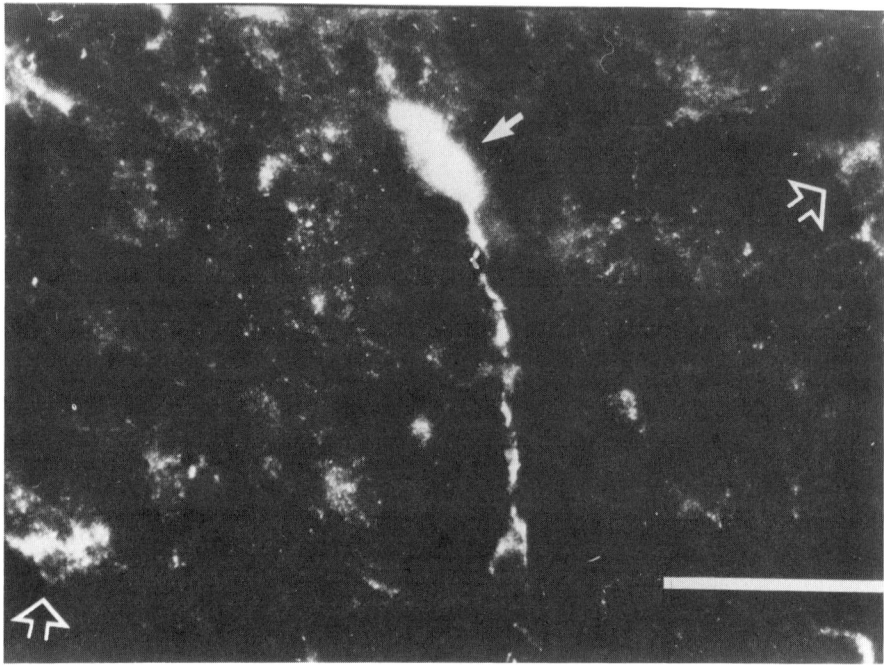

FIG. 2. Fluorescence photomicrograph of the ventral tegmental area. An individual, antidromically identified mesoprefrontal DA neuron is shown to be intensely fluorescent (closed arrow) following intracellular injection of colchicine. The injected cell is seen to be surrounded by less bright (open arrows), normally fluorescent noninjected DA neurons. Scale bar: 25 μm. (From Chiodo et al., 1984.)

sine hydroxylase), or colchicine (which blocks axoplasmic transport and results in the buildup of DA in the cell body) from the recording pipette (Fig. 2) (Grace and Bunney, 1980, 1983; Chiodo et al., 1984). These directly identified DA cells were found to have electrophysiological characteristics identical in every respect to those attributed to DA cells identified by indirect methods.

In recent years, the technique of single-unit recording in freely moving animals has been applied to the study of DA neurons. The extracellularly recorded firing properties of presumed A9 and A10 DA neurons in unrestrained rats have been found to be similar to those of conclusively identified DA cells (see above), including the ability to fire in single spike and bursting patterns (Freeman and Bunney, 1987; Freeman et al., 1985). In these studies, an overwhelming percentage (>90%) of neurons were observed to display at least some degree of burst firing. Other investigators have also found that the firing characteristics of presumed DA cells in unrestrained rats (Miller et al., 1983) and cats (Steinfels et al., 1981; Trulson et al., 1981; Trulson and Preussler, 1984) resemble those of identified DA neurons.

The terminal fields of DA neurons are easily identified and are studied with standard techniques to measure DA, DA metabolites, and DA-metabolizing enzymes (Moore and Kelly, 1978; Thierry et al., 1978; Cooper et al., 1982). The biochemical characteristics of the DA innervation of the limbic areas and cortical areas have recently been reviewed in depth (Bannon and Roth, 1983).

5. DOPAMINE NEURON FUNCTION REGULATION

The regulation of the activity of central neurons may be accomplished through the combined influence of several distinct mechanisms. For example, some of the cells that are innervated by the neurons in question can establish feedback pathways capable of modulating the activity of their afferent inputs. Through the influence of feedback pathways, the activity of a neuron may be adjusted so as not to fall below or to exceed certain normal limits. A feedback loop of this sort has been shown to participate in the control of the nigrostriatal DA pathway (see Aghajanian and Bunney, 1974a). Although it is likely that this mode of regulation may be operative in A10 DA systems, anatomical studies have not demonstrated a well-defined pathway such as that from the striatum to the substantia nigra (see Section 6.1).

A second way in which the activity of a neuron may be altered is by the action of inputs not associated with feedback loops. These inputs may produce inhibitory or excitatory effects that do not depend on the level of activity of the affected target cell (see Section 6).

Another mode of regulation occurs when the neuron has the capacity to adjust its activity as manifested by changes in impulse flow and biochemical activity. This form of regulation is possible in neurons that are responsive to their own transmitter. Receptors on the cell surface that specifically recognize the released transmitter are termed *autoreceptors* (Carlsson, 1975). Pharmacological, biochemical, and electrophysiological evidence provides support for the existence of central regulatory DA autoreceptors (Aghajanian and Bunney, 1973, 1977; Bunney and Aghajanian, 1975a; Groves et al., 1975; see reviews by Nowycky and Roth, 1978; Roth, 1979, 1984; Meltzer, 1980). The level of autoreceptor stimulation determines the magnitude of changes in cellular processes determining the biochemical and physiological state of the neuron. Nerve terminal autoreceptors influence the release and synthesis of DA. Autoreceptors on the cell body and dendrites (somatodendritic) can influence DA neuronal discharge activity, which, in turn, would influence both the synthesis and release of DA (Roth, 1979). Until very recently, most of the information regarding the existence and function of DA autoreceptors came from the study of the nigrostriatal DA pathway.

Dopamine receptors in the CNS can thus be divided anatomically into two general categories: DA receptors located on the DA neuron (autoreceptors) and postsynaptic DA receptors on other cell types. In A9, there is substantial evidence for feedback regulation of DA neuronal function involving the action of DA at both classes of these receptors. In recent years, it has become evident that autoreceptor regulation of A10 DA neurons also occurs.

5.1. Effects of DA Agonists on A10 DA Neuron Activity

The effects of DA agonists on the firing rate of DA neurons have been studied by several laboratories (see reviews by Bunney, 1979; Wang et al., 1984). Both directly and indirectly acting agonists decrease the activity of most A10 DA neurons. For example, depression of firing results from the systemic administration of d-amphetamine, methylphenidate, apomorphine, or L-dopa (Fig. 3) (Bunney et al., 1973a,b; Bunney, 1979; Browder et al., 1981; Wang 1981c). Microiontophoretically ejected apomorphine and DA have powerful inhibitory effects on the firing of A10 DA cells, similar to the electrophysiological effects of systemically administered DA agonists (Aghajanian and Bunney, 1973). The inhibition is accompanied by an increased amplitude of the extracellularly recorded action potentials, suggesting that the neuron is hyperpolarized by these treatments. Recently, in vivo intracellular recording has confirmed that A9 DA cells undergo hyperpolarization (approximately 8 mV) in association with DA agonist-induced depression of firing (Grace and Bunney, 1983). In a further analogy to the effects of systemically administered apomorphine on A10 DA cell firing, the inhibitory effects of iontophoretically applied DA can be antagonized by intravenous or iontophoretic administration of a DA receptor blocker (Aghajanian and Bunney, 1974a, 1977); in the 1977 study, the pharmacological specificity of the DA-induced inhibition was demonstrated by the inability of the α-antagonist piperoxane or the β-antagonist sotalol to block the depressant effects of DA. The DA autoreceptors that mediate the inhibitory effects of iontophoretically applied DA agonists on DA cells have the pharmacological characteristics of the D-2 subtype of DA receptors (White and Wang, 1984a).

Beart and McDonald (1980) demonstrated stimulation-induced release of exogenous [^{3}H]-DA from VTA slices that was indistinguishable from the release observed in slices of substantia nigra. Wang (1981b) provided evidence that local release of endogenous DA from mesolimbic DA

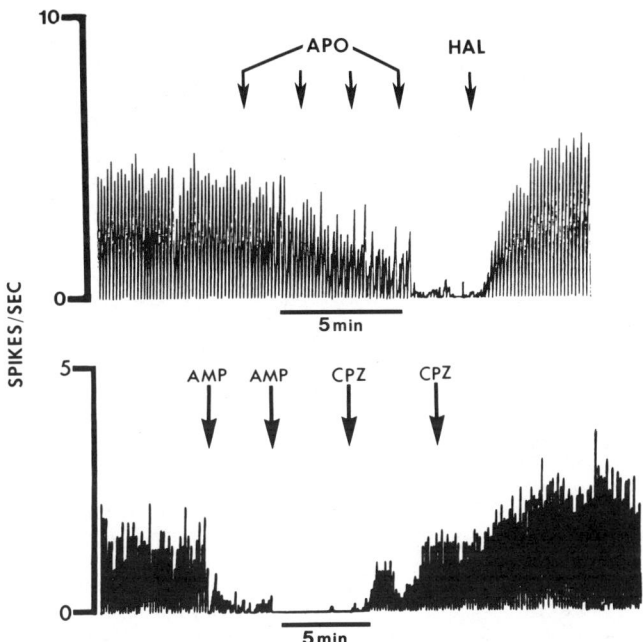

FIG. 3. Top, antagonism by haloperidol (HAL) of apomorphine (APO)-induced slowing of A10 DA cell. Apomorphine (2.5, 5, 10, 20 μg/kg, i.v.) led to total inhibition of firing, which was reversed to above basal rate by haloperidol (0.1 mg/kg) (Freeman and Bunney, unpublished data). Bottom, antagonism by chlorpromazine (CPZ) of d-amphetamine (AMP)-induced slowing of DA cell. d-Amphetamine (0.25 mg/kg, i.v.) significantly decreased firing rate. An additional 0.5 mg/kg produced total inhibition of firing. Chlorpromazine reversed the inhibition and increased firing above the basal rate. (From Bunney et al., 1973a.)

neurons has an inhibitory effect on DA cell firing. In this study, the nucleus accumbens was electrically stimulated to antidromically activate A10 DA neurons. Current levels high enough to evoke antidromic spikes depressed the spontaneous activity of the recorded A10 DA neuron. Similar results were obtained by German et al. (1980). The depressant effects were postulated to be the result of the release of DA at dendrodendritic and/or axon collateral inhibitory synapses, since they were blocked by the intravenous or iontophoretic administration of DA antagonists (Wang, 1981b). Additionally, this autoregulatory system may be the site of action for the inhibitory effect of intravenously administered d-amphetamine on A10 DA cell activity, since diencephalic transections did not alter the depressant effect of d-amphetamine on the firing of A10 DA cells. However, pretreatment with α-methyl-p-tyrosine (AMT) reduced the potency of d-amphetamine, and combined pretreatment with AMT and reserpine prevented the effect of d-amphetamine on neuronal firing (Wang, 1981c). These results were interpreted as evidence that d-amphetamine acts within

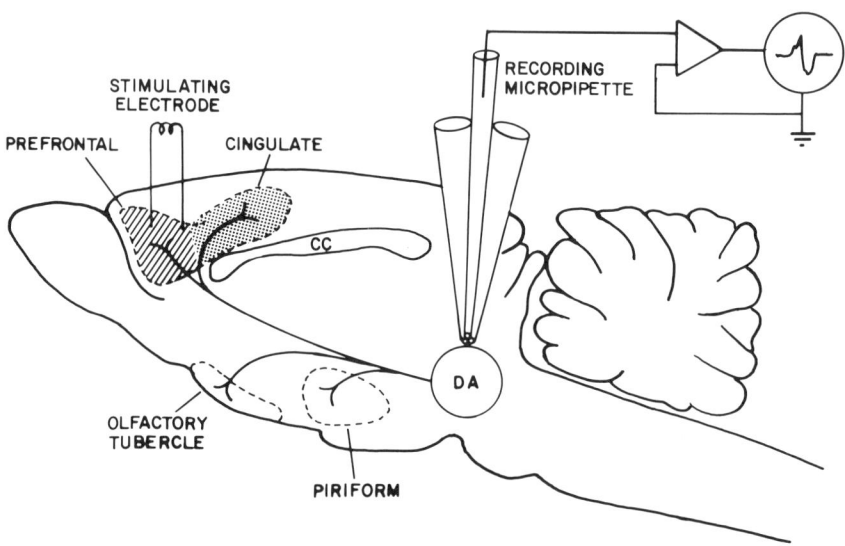

FIG. 4. Schematic representation of various DA systems in rat brain. Projections of midbrain DA neurons to the piriform, cingulate, and prefrontal cortices and to the olfactory tubercle are shown. Also shown is the experimental setup for antidromic activation. The stimulating electrode is shown in the prefrontal cortex while the glass pipette recording electrode is positioned in the midbrain region containing DA cell bodies. Only if the recorded DA cell projects to the prefrontal cortex will an antidromic spike be recorded when the prefrontal cortex is selectively stimulated.

the A10 region to release newly synthesized as well as stored DA, which may then inhibit cell firing by stimulating somatodendritic autoreceptors. This differs from the primary mode of inhibitory action of d-amphetamine on A9 DA neurons: d-Amphetamine is believed to release DA from nigrostriatal nerve terminals and to block its reuptake into the presynaptic terminal, thus increasing synaptic DA levels. The resulting stimulation of postsynaptic DA receptors activates a feedback loop to inhibit A9 DA neuronal activity (Bunney et al., 1973a; Rebec and Groves, 1975; Bunney and Aghajanian, 1976, 1978; Bunney and Grace, 1978). The local effect of d-amphetamine within the substantia nigra (Groves et al., 1975) appears to be manifest only with high doses of the drug (Bunney and Aghajanian, 1978; Bunney, 1979).

In attempting to understand the effects of DA agonists on A10 DA cell activity, it is important to consider inherent differences in the autoregulatory properties of the various DA subgroups. The electrophysiology and biochemistry of the DA neurons projecting to various regions of the cortex (e.g., prefrontal, cingulate, and piriform) have been studied in detail (Bannon et al., 1983a; Chiodo et al., 1984). Mesocortical as well as nigrostriatal DA neurons were antidromically activated from their respective projection sites (Fig. 4), and the firing rates of cells of the various mesocortical pathways were found to differ. The mean firing rates for mesoprefrontal, mesocingulate, and mesopiriform DA neurons were 9.3, 5.9, and 4.3 spikes/sec, respectively, whereas nigrostriatal DA cells fired at an average rate of 3.1/sec. In addition to having significantly faster firing rates, mesoprefrontal and mesocingulate DA cells also burst fire significantly more than those innervating the piriform cortex or the caudate. In mesoprefrontal and mesocingulate DA neurons, approximately 50% of the total number of action potentials occur in bursts or doublets, compared to only 8% and 2% for mesopiriform and nigrostriatal DA cells, respectively. The increased firing rate and bursting pattern of mesoprefrontal and mesocingulate DA cells agree with biochemical studies that demonstrate higher DOPAC/DA ratios and higher turnover rates in these cells, compared to mesopiriform, mesolimbic, and nigrostriatal DA neurons (Fig. 5) (for a review, see Bannon and Roth, 1983).

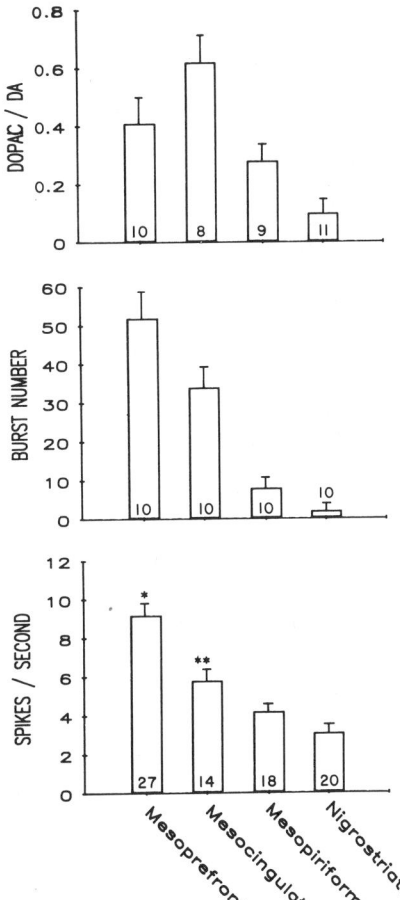

FIG. 5. Electrophysiological (firing rate, degree of bursting) and biochemical (DA turnover) characteristics of different antidromically identified mesocortical DA neurons are illustrated along with those of the nigrostriatal DA pathway. Vertical bars represent the means (±SEM) of the indicated measurement; DOPAC, dihydroxyphenylacetic acid. Numbers within the bars represent the number of separate experiments (DOPAC/DA determinations) or the number of cells studied (burst number, firing rate). Burst number equals the percentage of action potentials occurring within bursts. The burst numbers of all the groups differed significantly from each other at $p < .01$; analysis of variance and *post hoc* Scheffè comparison. *$p < .01$ relative to mesopiriform and nigrostriatal; **$p < .01$ relative to mesoprefrontal and $p < .05$ relative to mesopiriform and nigrostriatal; analysis of variance and *post hoc* Scheffè comparison.

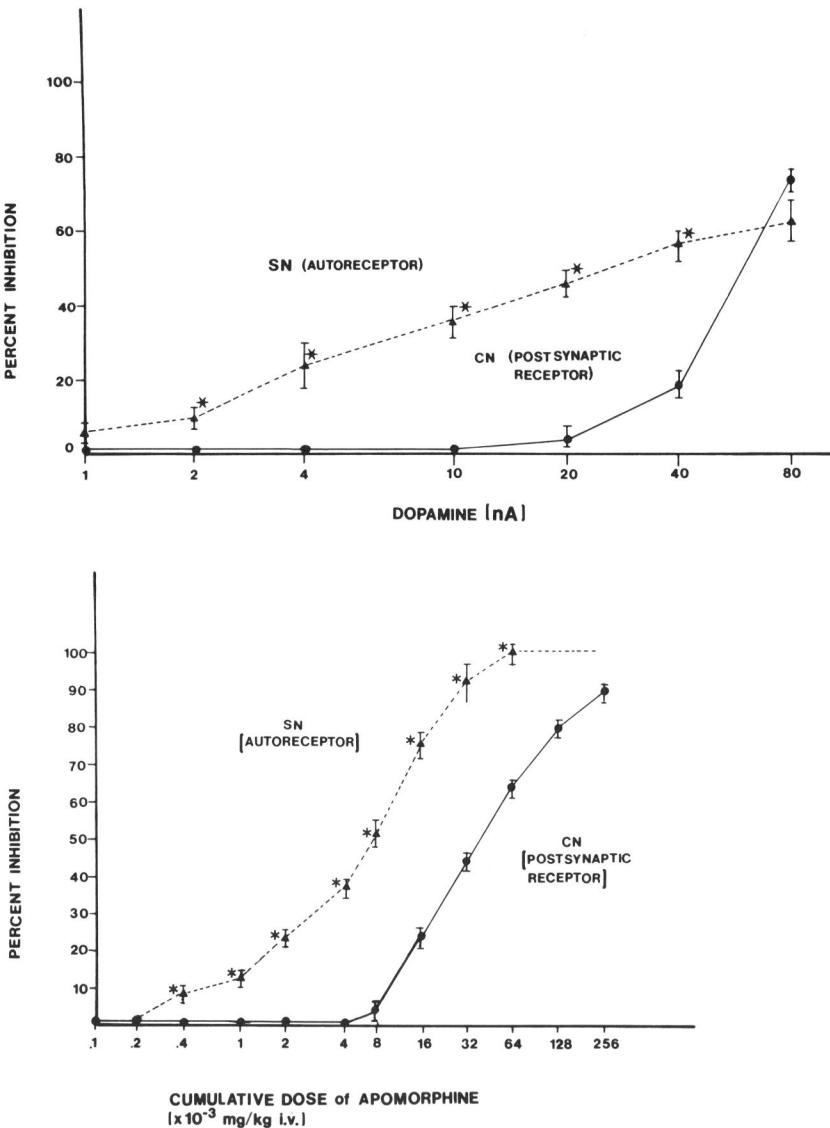

FIG. 6. Top, log dose–response curves for inhibition of firing rate of spontaneously active neurons in the substantia nigra zona compacta (SN) and caudate nucleus (CN) in response to iontophoretically applied DA (0.1 M, pH 4). Each point represents the mean ($\pm$SEM, n = 10) inhibition obtained with a given ejection current of DA. Bottom, cumulative log dose–response curves for inhibition of firing rate of cells of the SN and CN in response to i.v. apomorphine. Each point represents the mean ($\pm$SEM, n = 10) inhibition obtained at a given cumulative dose. (From Skirboll et al., 1979.)

Since it would be expected that firing rate and firing pattern would be influenced by the presence or absence of impulse-regulating DA autoreceptors, the existence of somatodendritic autoreceptors was determined by testing the ability of low doses of apomorphine [which have been shown to be specific for autoreceptors; Skirboll *et al.*, 1979 (Fig. 6)] and microiontophoretically applied DA to inhibit neuronal firing. Nigrostriatal and mesopiriform neurons were inhibited by autoreceptor-specific doses of apomorphine (ED_{50} = 8 and 15 µg/kg, respectively), but DA cells projecting to the prefrontal and cingulate cortices were either insensitive to or only weakly inhibited by the drug (less than 25% inhibition at 128 µg/kg). Furthermore, all DA cells antidromically activated from either the piriform cortex or the caudate could be inhibited by microiontophoretic application of DA (1 min, 10–40 nA), whereas all mesoprefrontal and mesocingulate DA cells were totally unresponsive to even prolonged, high-current microiontophoretic application of DA (Chiodo *et al.*, 1984). These results have been confirmed by White and Wang (1984b) (Fig. 7).

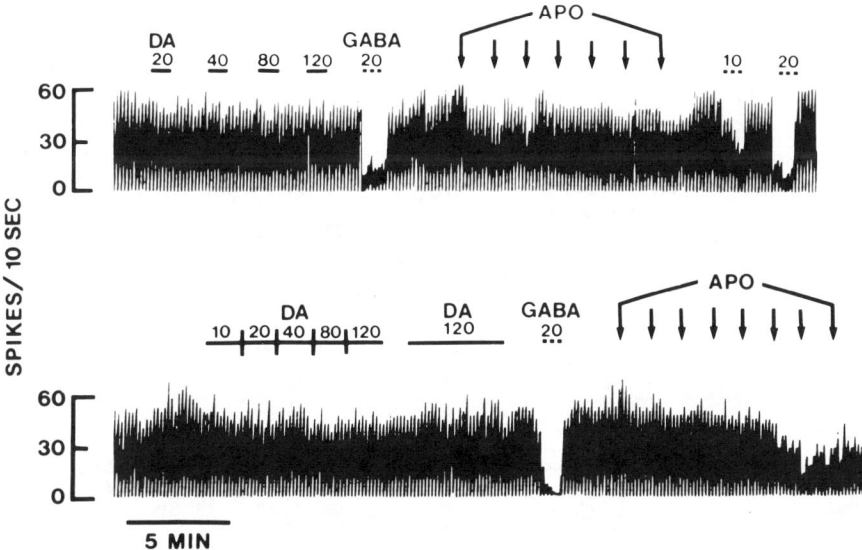

FIG. 7. Effects of microiontophoretically ejected DA and i.v. apomorphine (APO) on identified mesocortical A10 DA neurons. Top, rate histogram of a mesocortical DA cell demonstrating the lack of effect of iontophoretic DA and i.v. apomorphine (1, 2, 4, 8, 16, 32, 64 µg/kg injected at arrows) on cell firing rate. Bottom, rate histogram of another mesocortical A10 DA neuron showing lack of effect of even prolonged ejection of DA with high iontophoretic currents. High doses of apomorphine (1, 2, 4, 8, 16, 32, 64, 128 µg/kg at arrows) produced only weak inhibition of firing. Iontophoretic application of γ-aminobutyric acid (GABA, 0.01 M, pH 4.5) readily inhibited both cells. Horizontal bars and associated numbers indicate periods of iontophoretic ejection and the respective ejection currents (nA). (Taken from White and Wang, 1984a, with permission.)

In summary, there is a good correlation between the presence or absence of impulse-regulating autoreceptors and the DA turnover rate, baseline firing rate, degree of burst firing, and responsiveness to DA agonists (Roth, 1984). The validity of the finding is underscored by the report that an artificial increase in firing rate does not alter the responsiveness of A10 DA neurons to iontophoretic DA (White and Wang, 1984b). In contrast, a brief communication (Shepard and German, 1984) suggests that mesocortical DA neurons have neither elevated firing rates nor an altered response to a single bolus injection of apomorphine (5 µg/kg). The exact reasons for the differences between this study and the others described above are not clear, and the study is difficult to evaluate without a detailed presentation of the methodology employed (see below).

Whereas mesocortical DA neurons devoid of autoreceptors are necessarily unresponsive to low doses of apomorphine and microiontophoretically applied DA, they are readily inhibited by systemic administration of d-amphetamine (0.5–1.0 mg/kg), an effect that is reversed by haloperidol (Wang, 1981c; Chiodo et al., 1984; White and Wang, 1984b). Since both mechanical transection of the axons of A10 DA cells and neurochemical destruction of postsynaptic target sites do not alter the inhibitory action of d-amphetamine, the mode of action of the drug on these DA cells remains to be determined (Dalsass et al., 1979; Wang, 1981c).

In electrophysiological studies of the type discussed above, it is important that the technique of antidromic activation be used with great care so as to minimize "false" positives. In our opinion, studies that employ antidromic activation should incorporate the following details. First, small concentric bipolar stimulating electrodes should be used. Nonconcentric bipolar electrodes or monopolar electrodes produce a significantly greater current spread, which, in turn, increases the chance of stimulating axons some distance away from the electrode tip. Second, stimulating electrode placements should be shown in a composite histology figure. This is important in that it allows the reader to evaluate the possibility that adjacent structures were stimulated because of their proximity to the electrode tip. For example, when stimulating the prefrontal cortex (see Chiodo et al., 1984), if care is not taken and the stimulating electrodes are placed too deep within this region (against the forceps minor), the possibility of stimulating the far anterior pole of the nucleus accumbens is quite high. This possibility is only increased when nonconcentric bipolar electrodes are used. Third, the stimulating current employed should be kept as low as possible. Although small unmyelinated axons (such as those of monoaminergic neurons) are known to have a high chronaxie relative to myelinated fibers, stimulating currents greater than 3 mA are excessive and should be avoided for the sake of specificity. In general, the axons of dopaminergic neurons are readily stimulated to produce an antidromic spike with currents of 0.5–3 mA (Guyenet and Aghajanian, 1978; Grace and Bunney, 1980; Wang, 1981a; Chiodo and Bunney, 1983; Chiodo et al., 1984). Stimulating currents may be kept to a minimum by adjusting the dorsal–ventral position of the stimulating electrode while decreasing the current intensity until the lowest possible current level (which reliably produces an antidromic spike) is determined. Finally, in addition to the fixed latency of the antidromic spike and frequency following up to at least 50 Hz, collision of the antidromic spike with a spontaneously occurring action potential must be achieved for each cell tested.

The effects of both high and low doses of DA agonists on biochemical indices of A10 DA cell activity have also been studied. A number of years ago, it was reported that high doses of apomorphine (2–5 mg/kg) decreased the levels of the DA metabolites dihydroxyphenylacetic acid (DOPAC) and homovanillic acid (HVA), both in large frontal cortical dissections and in the striatum, as would be predicted if apomorphine inhibits DA cell firing (Westerink and Korf, 1976; Elchisak et al., 1976). More recently, Bacopoulos and Roth (1981) found that more moderate doses (0.1–0.2 mg/kg) of apomorphine significantly decreased striatal and olfactory tubercle DOPAC and HVA levels but had negligible effects on DA metabolite levels in a frontal cortical region. Similarly, low doses (30–50 μg/kg) of apomorphine (which selectively activate autoreceptors; Skirboll et al., 1979) lowered HVA levels in the striatum and olfactory tubercle, while HVA levels remained unchanged in a discrete prefrontal cortical region (Bannon et al., 1983a). The inability of autoreceptor-specific doses of apomorphine to decrease DA metabolite levels in the prefrontal cortex is consistent with the absence of impulse-regulating autoreceptors, as well as the absence of nerve terminal autoreceptors in mesoprefrontal DA neurons.

DA metabolite changes in terminal fields reflect not only the physiological activity of DA cells but also the influence of synthesis and/or release-modulating DA autoreceptors on DA terminals. In order to selectively study the effects of nerve terminal autoreceptors on DA synthesis *in vivo*, the influence of drug interactions at postsynaptic receptors (i.e., postsynaptic feedback loop mediated effects) must be removed. Impulse flow in nigrostriatal, mesolimbic, and mesocortical DA neurons can be interrupted pharmacologically by γ-butyrolactone (GBL) administration or by axotomy (Kehr et al., 1972; Walters et al., 1973; Walters and Roth, 1976; Bannon et al., 1982, 1983a). It is postulated that the subsequent decrease in DA release into the synaptic cleft decreases nerve terminal DA autoreceptor activation, which, in turn, leads to increased tyrosine hydroxylation and elevated intraneuronal DA levels (see Roth, 1979). In the striatum, limbic regions, and the piriform cortex, the increase in DA

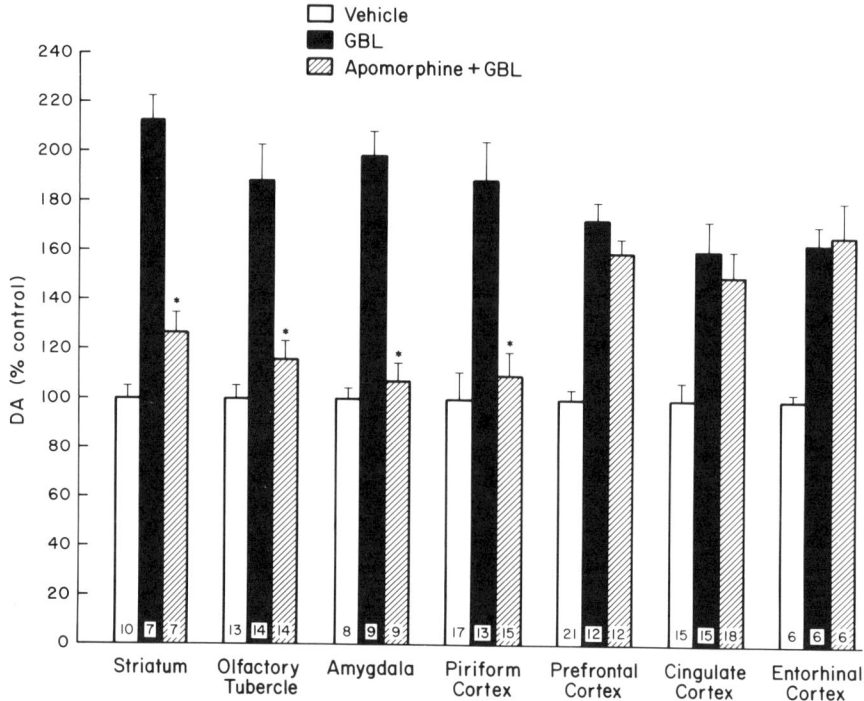

FIG. 8. Regional distribution of nerve terminal DA autoreceptors determined by the GBL model. Rats were decapitated 40 min after i.p. apomorphine (2 mg/kg) and 35 min after i.p. GBL (750 mg/kg). Vertical bars represent the mean (±SEM) percent of control DA levels, and the number below each bar equals the number of animals. $*p < .01$ versus GBL treatment, Student's t test. (From Roth, 1984.)

is prevented by apomorphine and other DA agonists through terminal autoreceptor activation (Fig. 8). The GBL- or axotomy-induced increase in prefrontal and cingulate DA is not the result of increased DA synthesis (Bannon et al., 1981) and is not prevented by DA agonists, which suggests that mesoprefrontal and mesocingulate DA cells lack nerve terminal synthesis-modulating autoreceptors (Bannon et al., 1981, 1982, 1983a; Chiodo et al., 1984). The use of very large cortical dissections, which would include a number of these distinct mesocortical DA nerve terminals (Andén et al., 1983a, 1983b), most likely obscures important differences with regard to mesocortical autoreceptors, DA turnover, and drug responsiveness (see Bannon and Roth, 1983). The absence of mesoprefrontal synthesis-modulating DA autoreceptors has been confirmed using the electrical stimulation model in which any effect of DA agonists on DA synthesis must be mediated at nerve terminal autoreceptors, since modulation of impulse flow is eliminated by driving DA neurons at a fixed frequency (Tam et al., 1983; Roth et al., 1984).

The accumulation of dihydroxyphenylalanine (DOPA) after inhibition of DOPA decarboxylase can also be used as an index of *in vivo* DA synthesis, but since DOPA serves as the precursor for norepinephrine (NE) as well as DA, it is difficult to know what portion of DOPA accumulation in NE-rich cortical regions actually represents tyrosine hydroxylation in DA neurons. Some recent work indicates that under pharmacological conditions in which DA formation is inhibited and DA levels in the nerve terminal are declining, DA agonists can modulate tyrosine hydroxylation in the prefrontal cortex. Fadda et al. (1984) have reported that autoreceptor-specific doses (25–50 µg/kg) of apomorphine inhibit DOPA accumulation in the prefrontal cortex of rats pretreated with a DOPA decarboxylase inhibitor. These results were interpreted by the authors as evidence for the presence of synthesis-modulating DA autoreceptors in the prefrontal cortex. More recent experiments (Galloway et al., 1986; Roth et al., 1984) have confirmed the inhibitory effects of DA agonists on DOPA accumulation in all DA systems studied, including the prefrontal cortex, but have suggested that DA agonists modulate synthesis indirectly by altering levels of DA within mesoprefrontal nerve terminals rather than acting directly through synthesis-modulating DA autoreceptors. These investigators propose that DA agonists act at release-modulating autoreceptors to inhibit ongoing DA release and thereby slow the very rapid decline in endogenous DA levels that occurs in prefrontal DA terminals after decarboxylase inhibition. This would elevate DA levels in the nerve terminal (relative to animals that received decarboxylase inhibitor but no DA agonist) and subsequently inhibit tyrosine hydroxylase through a feedback mechanism. This hypothesis is supported by the *in vitro* evidence that DA agonists inhibit K^+-stimulated release of [^{3}H]-DA from prefrontal cortical brain slices (Wolf and Roth, 1987).

In summary, the results obtained using the GBL, electrical stimulation, and DOPA accumulation models may best be reconciled by proposing that mesoprefrontal nerve terminals possess release-modulating, but not synthesis-modulating nerve terminal autoreceptors. This raises the interesting possibility that DA release and synthesis in other DA projections may be regulated by distinct presynaptic autoreceptors. One might speculate that in mesocortical DA nerve terminals, in which DA pools are small enough to be sensitive to agonist-induced changes in release, synthesis can be regulated indirectly by release-dependent changes in intraneuronal DA levels. In contrast, the high levels of striatal DA are normally unaltered by release, which suggests that striatal tyrosine hydroxylase would not be subject to release-dependent variations in feedback inhibition by intraneuronal DA pools. Under these conditions, a direct mechanism for autoregulation of tyrosine hydroxylase activity (e.g., synthesis-modulating autoreceptors) might be adaptive. However, it is important to keep in mind that the (release-modulating) effects of DA agonists on prefrontal cortical DA are apparent *in vivo* only under conditions of impaired DA synthesis and declining DA levels (e.g., after DOPA decarboxylase inhibition). Under normal physiological conditions, DA agonists have little or no effect on either the firing rate or the DA turnover of the mesoprefrontal DA neurons (Bannon *et al.*, 1983a; Chiodo *et al.*, 1984; White and Wang, 1984b; see above). Therefore, the physiological role of the hypothesized release-modulating autoreceptors is as yet unclear.

5.2. DA Receptor Antagonist Actions

In the following sections, we will examine the effects of both acute and chronic treatment with DA receptor blockers (antipsychotic drugs or neuroleptics), the treatment of choice for the major symptoms of psychosis (Klein *et al.*, 1980), on A10 DA neurons. In order to do this, it will be necessary also to review the actions of these drugs on the activity of A9 DA neurons.

In 1963, Carlsson and Lindqvist hypothesized that neuroleptics have a specific, selective action on central catecholamine systems and that these actions are mediated, in part, through long-loop feedback pathways from forebrain regions innervated by the catecholamine neurons. This initial observation was a major impetus behind the last two decades of research on the mode of action of neuroleptics.

5.2.1. Acute Administration

Numerous electrophysiological studies have demonstrated that the acute administration of neuroleptics increase the activity of A9 and A10 DA neurons (Bunney *et al.*, 1973a; see Bunney and Aghajanian, 1975b; Bunney, 1977, 1979; Chiodo and Bunney, 1984; and Bunney *et al.*, 1985 for reviews). Although these drugs are able to block DA autoreceptors, it appears that their rate-increasing effects on A9 DA neurons are primarily related to the blockade of postsynaptic DA receptors and a subsequent feedback activation, as proposed by Carlsson (see Bunney, 1979; Chiodo and Bunney, 1984). For A10 DA neurons, it is likely that both long-loop feedback pathways and autoreceptor effects of neuroleptics may be important (see Chiodo and Bunney, 1984). These early studies also noted that all neuroleptics tested were able to block or reverse the reduction in DA neuronal activity normally produced by DA agonists in both A9 and

A10. Only the nonantipsychotic phenothiazine analog mepazine was able to discriminate between these two regions. That is, mepazine reversed the d-amphetamine-induced inhibition of A9 but *not* A10 DA neuronal firing (Bunney and Aghajanian, 1975b).

By the late 1970s, it had been demonstrated that neuroleptics that were associated with a high incidence of extrapyramidal side effects (e.g., haloperidol and perphenazine) readily reversed agonist-induced suppression of A9 and A10 cell activity to levels above base line, whereas the antipsychotic compounds associated with a low incidence of side effects (e.g., clozapine and thioridazine) returned A9 cell activity only to a predrug base line (see Bunney, 1977, 1979; Chiodo and Bunney, 1984). Thus, this pattern of response of A9 and A10 DA neurons to acute neuroleptic administration appeared to provide a predictive model for screening antipsychotic drugs. Unfortunately, false positives were soon discovered. For example, the GABA receptor antagonist picrotoxin, which is not a neuroleptic, also reversed DA agonist-induced decreases in DA neuronal activity. Therefore, even though these electrophysiological studies confirmed the earlier hypothesis, based on biochemical data, that acute DA antagonists increase DA turnover (Carlsson and Lindqvist, 1963; Andén *et al.*, 1964; Nybäck *et al.*, 1968; Roth *et al.*, 1975), they were unable to establish a reliable model that would differentiate between clinical efficacy and side-effect potential.

In 1975, Scatton and colleagues reported a 10-fold higher dose of DA antagonist pretreatment was required to increase [^{3}H]-DA synthesis in cortical slices compared to striatal slices (Scatton *et al.*, 1975a). Since that report, the effects of acute administration of DA antagonists on the metabolism of DA in different brain regions have been studied: DA antagonist administration increases (250–400%) DA metabolite levels in the striatum, in limbic regions such as the olfactory tubercle and nucleus accumbens, and in the piriform cortex. In a carefully defined area of prefrontal or cingulate cortex, DOPAC and HVA generally increase only 30–95% in response to acute antipsychotic drugs (Fig. 9) (Westerink and Korf, 1976; Scatton, 1977; Wheeler and Roth, 1980; Bannon *et al.*, 1982, 1983a; see Bannon and Roth, 1983; Roth, 1984). Similarly, DOPA accumulation increases 200 to 400% in the striatum but only 30 to 90% in the prefrontal cortex (Bannon *et al.*, 1981; Fadda *et al.*, 1984). There is some evidence that although the neuroleptic-induced increase in DA cell firing does contribute to increased DA metabolite levels, the metabolite increase is primarily the result of nerve terminal autoreceptor blockade (Casu *et al.*, 1980; DiChiara *et al.*, 1977a,b; for a review, see Bannon and Roth, 1983). This could explain the diminished biochemical effects of neuroleptics in areas lacking nerve terminal synthesis-modulating autoreceptors, such as the prefrontal and cingulate cortices.

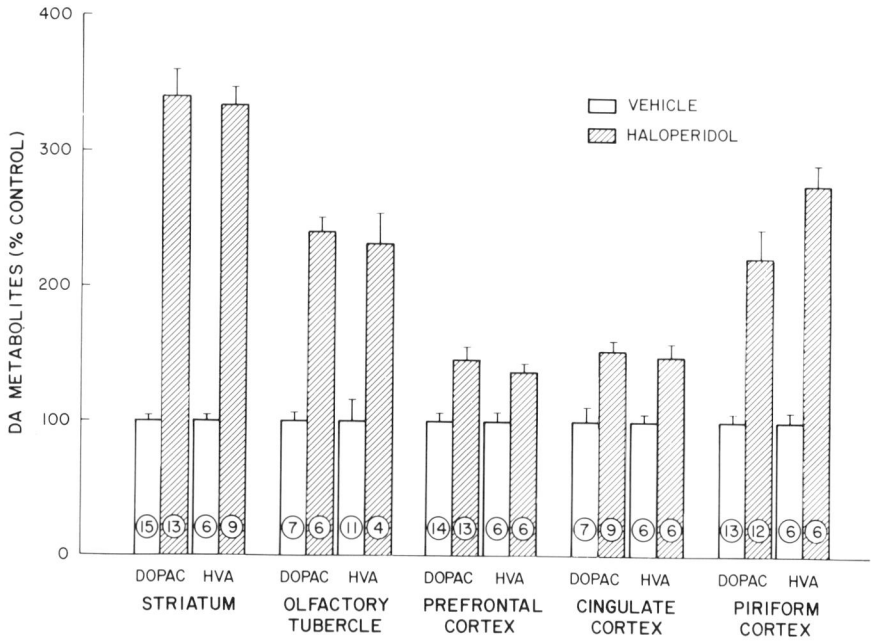

FIG. 9. The effects of haloperidol on dihydroxyphenylacetic acid (DOPAC) and homovanillic acid (HVA) levels. Haloperidol (1 mg/kg, i.p.) or vehicle was administered 60 min before decapitation. Numbers are expressed as a percentage (±SEM) of control DOPAC and HVA levels from either one experiment or two separate experiments. DOPAC: striatum 2430 ± 130 ng/g, 1342 ± 71 ng/g; olfactory tubercle 1160 ± 70 ng/g; prefrontal cortex 118 ± 13 ng/kg, 43 ± 3 ng/g; cingulate cortex 92 ± 11 ng/g; piriform cortex 146 ± 18 ng/g, 144 ± 13 ng/g. HVA: striatum 857 ± 48 ng/g, olfactory tubercle 440 ± 18 ng/g, prefrontal cortex 95 ± 6 ng/g, cingulate cortex 93 ± 6 ng/g, piriform cortex 99 ± 7 ng/g. (From Bannon et al., 1983a.)

5.2.2. Chronic Administration

After the acute effects of many neuroleptics were studied, the action of chronically administered neuroleptics on midbrain DA cell activity was examined. This is particularly important because the clinical efficacy of antipsychotic drugs usually takes days or even weeks to develop (Crane, 1973; Beckman et al., 1979). A technique was developed by which it was possible to sample populations of DA cells, recording the number of cells per electrode track while repeatedly lowering the electrode (at predetermined intervals) through a stereotaxically defined block of the midbrain known to contain DA neurons (Bunney and Grace, 1978; Nowycky et al., 1978). This methodological development was necessary, since current electrophysiological techniques do not allow us to record from the same neuron continuously during the entire period of chronic drug administration. However, by carefully employing the cells/track technique, it is possible to quantitatively measure the response of a given population of DA neurons to both acute and chronic drug treatment.

To date, several studies have used this new population sampling technique. The first of these studies sampled animals either 1 hr after a single subcutaneous injection of haloperidol (0.5 mg/kg) or on day 21 of repeated treatment (Bunney and Grace, 1978). Relative to controls, the acute treatment resulted in a significantly higher number of spontaneously active DA neurons in A9. The chronically treated animals, however, had significantly fewer cells/track than the control. Moreover, the DA neurons that were not firing in the chronically treated animals were inactive (or "silent") because of excessive depolarization (i.e., depolarization block). For example, the silent DA neurons of chronically treated animals could not be made to fire by the direct iontophoretic application of the excitatory amino acid glutamate, but they would begin to fire after the local application of the inhibitory substance γ-aminobutyric acid (GABA, Fig. 10) (Bunney and Grace, 1978; Chiodo and Bunney, 1982, 1983). *In vivo* intracellular recordings have confirmed that chronic administration of antipsychotic drugs reduces (10–15 mV) the resting membrane potential of DA cells (Grace and Bunney, 1986).

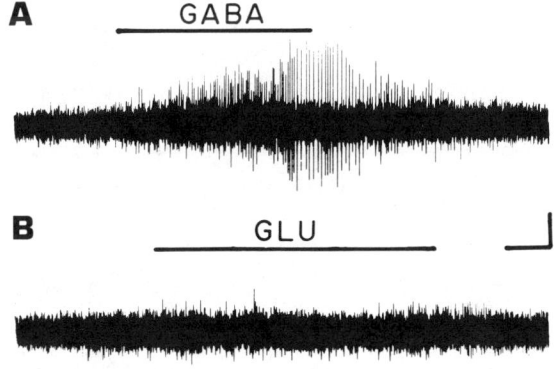

FIG. 10. Oscilloscope tracings show typical responses of a "silent" A10 DA neuron to glutamic acid (GLU) and γ-aminobutyric acid (GABA) in a rat chronically treated with chlorpromazine. (A) This cell was activated by the microiontophoretic application of GABA (3 nA). After a short delay, GABA caused the cell to appear out of the background noise. Continued GABA application resulted in a decrease in activity (action potential amplitude increases and duration decreases). When GABA was turned off, the firing rate markedly increased (amplitude decreases, duration increases), and the spikes merged with the background noise. (The changes in spike duration are not visible because of the paper speed employed.) (B) The excitatory amino acid GLU (ejected at 12 nA 1 min after the GABA ejection, shown in the upper trace, was unable to activate the silent DA neuron). Horizontal bars represent the duration of iontophoretic drug application. Calibration equals 400 μV and 2 sec. (From Chiodo and Bunney, 1983.)

We have recently extended these studies to include an investigation of the effects of chronic oral neuroleptic administration on the activity of *both* A9 and A10 DA neurons (Chiodo and Bunney, 1982, 1983). In these studies, animals were studied 1 hr after a single oral administration or on day 21 of continuous administration via the drinking water. All neuroleptics sampled to date that are associated with a high incidence of extrapyramidal side effects (e.g., haloperidol, chlorpromazine, *l*-sulpiride) increase the number of cells/track acutely but induce a state of depolarization inactivation (a decreased number of active DA neurons) in both A9 and A10 chronically. In contrast, those antipsychotic drugs associated with a low incidence of side effects (e.g., clozapine and mesoridazine), while increasing the cells/track in both areas acutely, inactivate A10, but *not* A9 DA neurons, when given chronically (Fig. 11). Qualitatively identical results have been reported by White and Wang (1983*a,b*).

The induction of depolarization inactivation appears to be specific to neuroleptics, since a nonneuroleptic phenothiazine (promethazine), the inactive isomer of sulpiride (*d*-sulpiride), an antidepressant (desmethylimipramine), and α-noradrenergic receptor blockers (prazosin and idazoxan) did not inactivate A9 or A10 DA neurons when chronically administered (Chiodo and Bunney, 1982, 1983, 1984; White and Wang, 1983*b*). By examining the population response of both A9 and A10 DA neurons to chronic treatment, it may be possible to predict whether a new compound will exert an antipsychotic action (because of the correlation between A10 DA cell inactivation and clinical efficacy) or induce extrapyramidal side effects (because of the correlation between inactivation of A9 DA cells and induction of clinical side effects) or produce both effects. In both regions, the presence of long-loop feedback pathways is necessary for the induction of depolarization inactivation by chronically administered neuroleptics (Bunney and Grace, 1978; White and Wang, 1983*a*). However, there may be a difference between the two areas in the importance of such feedback regulation in the maintenance of depolarization block once it has been induced (Chiodo and Bunney, 1983, 1984). That is, hemitransection of the forebrain (which destroys all long-loop feedback pathways from anterior structures) on day 21 of neuroleptic treatment abolishes the inactivation of A9, but not A10 DA neurons. Although most A10 DA neurons enter a state of depolarization inactivation during repeated treatment with neuroleptics, a small number of cells are found to remain active. The majority of these DA cells have been identified as mesocortical cells that project to the prefrontal cortex (Fig. 12) (Chiodo and Bunney, 1983). This finding is consistent with biochemical studies that show that the prefrontal lobe does not develop tolerance to the effects of DA antagonists (see below).

Scatton and co-workers conducted early studies on the effects of chronic administration of DA antagonists on [^{3}H]-DA synthesis in slices

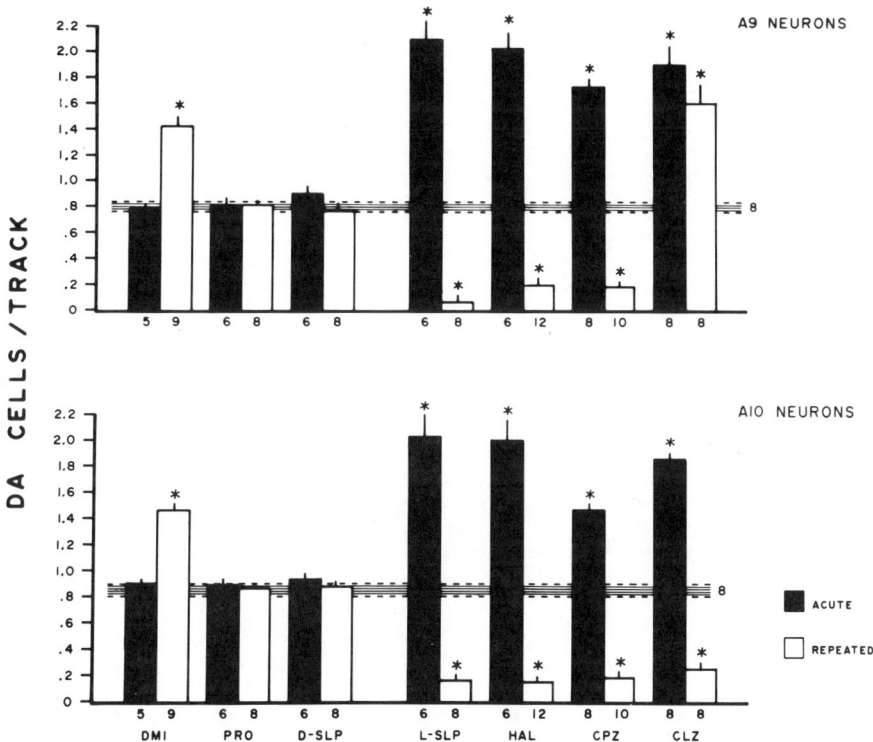

FIG. 11. The effects of both acute and repeated (21-day) oral neuroleptic administration on the mean (±SEM) number of spontaneously firing DA cells encountered per track in both A9 and A10. Shaded areas, control means (±SEM) obtained for untreated animals; DMI, desmethylimipramine; PRO, promethazine; D-SLP, d-sulpiride; L-SLP, l-sulpiride; HAL, haloperidol; CPZ, chlorpromazine; CLZ, clozapine. *$p < .01$ relative to untreated controls, two-tailed Dunnett test. The number below each bar indicates the number of animals studied. (From Chiodo and Bunney, 1983.)

and on DA metabolism in various brain areas. Tolerance developed to the neuroleptic-induced activation of [^{3}H]-DA synthesis in striatal slices following chronic neuroleptic pretreatment. However, no tolerance to this activation was observed in slices derived from limbic or cortical tissue (Scatton et al., 1975b, 1976). The time course of the development of tolerance to synthesis activation was determined following a single depot injection of the neuroleptic pipotiazine. In the striatum, an initial acceleration in DA synthesis was followed by a prolonged decrease in synthesis, which indicated the development of tolerance. In olfactory tubercle/nucleus accumbens slices, the initial increase was prolonged and was followed by an inhibitory phase of lesser duration and extent than in the striatum. No tolerance occurred in cortical slices, where only increased

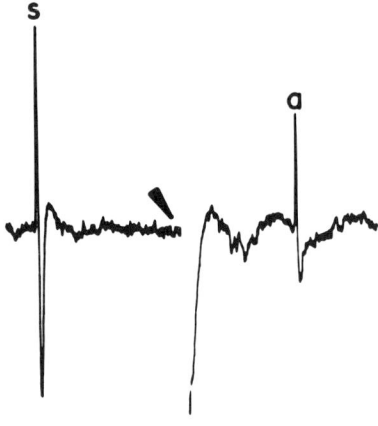

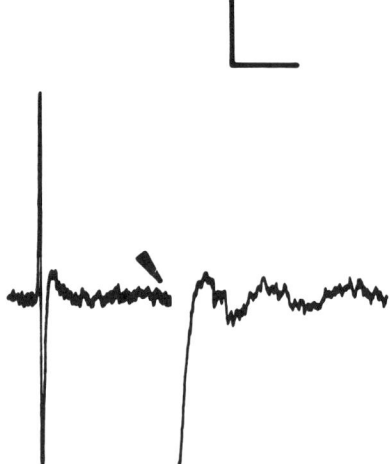

FIG. 12. A digital oscilloscope tracing showing the antidromic activation from the prefrontal cortex of a spontaneously active A10 DA neuron in an animal treated daily with haloperidol via the drinking water (0.56 ± 0.08 mg/kg per day) for 21 days. (Top) The spontaneously occurring action potential (s) triggers the electrical stimulation (1.9 mA, 500-μsec duration at arrows) after a delay of 24.0 msec. This produces an antidromic spike (a, 18.5 msec latency). The reduced amplitude of the antidromic spike compared to the spontaneous action potential is the result of the activation of only the initial segment component. (Bottom) Stimulation 21.5 msec after the spontaneous spike occurs fails to antidromically activate this cell, demonstrating that collision has occurred. Calibration equals 200 μV and 10 msec. (From Chiodo and Bunney, 1983.)

synthesis was observed (Scatton et al., 1977). A similar pattern of tolerance was observed to develop to the effects of repeated haloperidol treatment (0.2 mg/kg) on DOPAC levels. Tolerance to DOPAC elevation occurred within 11 days in the striatum and within 40 days in the olfactory tubercle/nucleus accumbens; the prefrontal cortex actually increased in responsiveness by 40 days (Scatton, 1977). Bannon et al. (1982) also reported that daily administration of haloperidol (0.5 mg/kg) induced a diminished responsiveness to acute haloperidol challenge in the striatum and olfactory tubercle but not in the prefrontal cortex by day 28 of treatment. It is interesting to note that tolerance can be induced in all brain areas in a relatively short time if the daily dose is increased to a level greater than that which produces maximal effects when given acutely

(Scatton, 1977; Wheeler and Roth, 1980; Bacopoulos, 1981a,b). Biochemical data in human and nonhuman primates also suggest the development of neuroleptic tolerance in the striatum and in limbic areas, without tolerance to moderate doses of DA antagonists in the prefrontal cortex (Bacopoulos *et al.*, 1978, 1979, 1980; Roth *et al.*, 1980).

It has been suggested (Bannon *et al.*, 1982) that the development of tolerance to neuroleptic-induced biochemical changes in DA systems is related to the induction of autoreceptor supersensitivity. This would enhance responsiveness of the DA neuron to the inhibitory effects of released DA. The electrophysiological and biochemical studies reveal that a population of DA neurons that lacks synthesis-modulating and somatodendritic autoreceptors (mesoprefrontal system) neither goes into depolarization inactivation nor exhibits an attenuated biochemical response following repeated treatment with DA antagonists. However, the relationship among the absence of autoreceptors, the resistance to depolarization inactivation and the induction of tolerance remains obscure at this time. The majority of other DA neurons are inactivated during chronic treatment and develop biochemical tolerance. However, even after tolerance occurs, DA metabolite levels are still elevated in chronically treated animals versus controls. Finally, as mentioned earlier, feedback mechanisms seem to be involved in neuroleptic-induced increases in DA cell firing and in the induction and perhaps maintenance of depolarization inactivation. In contrast, both the acute biochemical effects of neuroleptics and the development of tolerance to these effects occur in the absence of feedback mechanisms (Casu *et al.*, 1980; see Bannon and Roth, 1983).

6. EFFECTS OF NEUROTRANSMITTERS ON A10 DOPAMINE NEURON ACTIVITY

Several classes of neurotransmitters have been examined for their effects on A10 DA neurons. It is hoped that such studies will lead to an understanding of precisely how neuronal afferents are involved in the regulation of A10 DA systems.

6.1. The Influence of GABA on A10 DA Neurons

A number of electrophysiological and biochemical studies suggest that there are feedback pathways from various forebrain regions to the A10 area. Considerable effort has been devoted to the study of the role of GABA in the feedback control of these cells. Microiontophoretic application of GABA onto A10 DA neurons inhibits firing (Aghajanian and

Bunney, 1973). The firing of unidentified A10 neurons (presumed to be dopaminergic) is inhibited by electrical stimulation of the nucleus accumbens and by iontophoretically applied GABA (Wolf *et al.*, 1978; Yim and Mogenson, 1980*a,b*; Olpe *et al.*, 1977). All of the above effects are antagonized by the GABA antagonists bicuculline and picrotoxin. The stimulation-induced depression of neuronal firing is enhanced by the GABA uptake inhibitor nipecotic acid (Yim and Mogenson, 1980*b*). In the latter studies, rigorous identification of the cells sampled was not carried out, but the results are consistent with the possibility of GABAergic modulation of A10 DA neuronal activity.

Intravenous administration of GABA agonists results in dose-related increases in the firing rates of both A9 and A10 DA cells, which, however, are not blocked by the prior injection of picrotoxin (Walters and Lakoski, 1978; MacNeil *et al.*, 1978; Grace and Bunney, 1979; Waszczak *et al.*, 1980; Waszczak and Walters, 1980). Such an effect would be unexpected if GABAergic pathways exerted a direct inhibitory influence on these cells. The paradoxical excitatory effect of systemic GABA agonists on DA neurons in A9 is paralleled by a concomitant increase in caudate DA release and/or metabolite levels (see Grace and Bunney, 1979, for a review) and is apparently the result of inhibition of a nigral GABAergic neuron that provides tonic inhibitory control over DA cell firing (MacNeil *et al.*, 1978; Grace and Bunney, 1979). Iontophoretic experiments have revealed this neuron to be 20 times more sensitive than DA cells to the GABA agonist muscimol, so that the systemic administration of GABA results in disinhibition of nigral DA neurons (Grace and Bunney, 1979). It is possible that a similar influence on A10 DA neurons is provided by GABAergic neurons in that area. This possibility is supported by anatomical findings that show that GABAergic cells are found in proximity to DA neurons in the VTA (Oertel *et al.*, 1982; Nagai *et al.*, 1983). However, as outlined in Section 6.1.1, although GABA agonists increase A10 DA cell firing, they inhibit DA turnover in the nucleus accumbens and olfactory tubercle, areas that receive their dopaminergic innervation predominantly from the VTA. It is likely that actions of GABA at both A10 DA neuronal somatodendritic and terminal sites are responsible for their divergent effects on the electrophysiology and biochemistry of these cells.

6.1.1. Evidence for a GABA Pathway to A10

Similar inhibitory effects have been reported for GABA agonists, GABA transaminase inhibitors, and baclofen on the turnover of DA in limbic areas (Hökfelt *et al.*, 1975; Fuxe *et al.*, 1975, 1977, 1978; Kääriäinen, 1976; Pycock *et al.*, 1978; Palfreyman *et al.*, 1978; Scatton *et al.*, 1980*a*). GABA and its synthetic enzyme glutamic acid decarboxylase

(GAD) are present in A10 (Balcom et al., 1975; McGeer et al., 1976; Fonnum et al., 1977), and kainic acid lesions of the nucleus accumbens result in a diminution in the levels of GAD in A10 (Waddington and Cross, 1978). All these studies contribute to the notion that endogenous GABA may influence the activity of A10 DA neurons.

6.1.2. Evidence against a GABA Pathway to A10

Although the evidence cited for interactions of GABA with A10 DA systems is consistent with the possible existence of a GABAergic link participating in the modulation of A10 DA neuronal activity, little anatomical evidence for a descending GABAergic pathway to the VTA is provided. Therefore, although anatomical studies show that there are afferent inputs from limbic and cortical areas to the A10 region (Conrad and Pfaff, 1976; Nauta, 1978; Phillipson, 1979; Swanson, 1982), such inputs do not appear analogous to the rich GABAergic projection from the striatum to the substantia nigra (Precht and Yoshida, 1971; Kim et al., 1971; McNair et al., 1972; Hattori et al., 1975; Frigyesi and Szabo, 1975; Jessell et al., 1978). In fact, in contrast to the effects of kainic acid lesioning of the nucleus accumbens (Waddington and Cross, 1978), no changes in VTA GAD levels were found in rat brain following hemitransection (McGeer et al., 1976, 1977; Fonnum et al., 1977). In a later study, by Walaas and Fonnum (1980), electrocoagulation of the nucleus accumbens resulted in only a small decrease in GAD activity, which was localized to a region of the VTA that had few cells sending projections to the nucleus accumbens, a finding suggesting that A10 DA neurons are not influenced by GABA neurons originating in the nucleus accumbens.

Taken together, these studies illustrate that there is no clear consensus regarding the magnitude of the influence of GABA on A10 DA neuronal function. Although the existence of a GABAergic feedback system appears plausible on the basis of several of the biochemical and electrophysiological studies discussed, the data do not argue convincingly for a significant GABAergic projection originating in the forebrain and terminating on DA cell bodies/dendrites in the VTA. Nevertheless, drugs that interact with GABA receptors do influence the electrophysiological and biochemical activity of A10 DA neurons, though not in an easily interpretable manner.

One intriguing biochemical finding of the GABA–A10 cell interaction deserves mention here. Mild stressors selectively activate mesoprefrontal cortical, but not mesolimbic or nigrostriatal, DA neurons, as discussed in Section 6.4. This stress-induced activation is prevented by benzodiazepine agonists (Lavielle et al., 1978; Fadda et al., 1978; Reinhard et al., 1982) and mimicked by the administration of anxiogenic β-

carbolines (Tam and Roth, 1985). Thus, some benzodiazepine/GABA system (not localized to date) profoundly and selectively modulates mesoprefrontal DA cells.

6.2. The Effects of Serotonin on A10 DA Neurons

The A10 area receives serotonergic inputs from the raphe nuclei of the brain stem (Azmitia and Segal, 1978; Moore *et al.*, 1978; Phillipson, 1979; Simon *et al.*, 1979). The medial raphe innervates the midline VTA, and the dorsal raphe innervates most of the VTA. Although the dorsal raphe serotonergic projection has been shown to influence the electrical activity of A9 DA cells (see below), parallel experiments have not assessed the role of this nucleus on the firing of A10 DA cells (Chiodo, 1981; Bunney and DeRiemer, 1982; Chiodo and Bunney, unpublished data). Biochemical experiments indicate that serotonin (5-hydroxytryptamine, 5-HT) can also affect DA turnover. Intraperitoneal administration of the 5-HT agonist quipazine produces increases in the levels of HVA and DOPAC in limbic and striatal areas, whereas the 5-HT receptor antagonist metergoline causes decreased DA metabolism in those regions (Pycock *et al.*, 1978). Direct injection of 5-HT into the nucleus accumbens increased the concentrations of HVA and DOPAC in that area (Pycock *et al.*, 1978). Low doses of LSD produce more than a doubling in prefrontal cortical HVA levels, but striatal HVA remains unchanged (Bowers and Salomonssen, 1982). The accelerating effect of haloperidol on DA turnover in the frontal cortex, the striatum, and the nucleus accumbens/olfactory tubercle area (see Section 5) is potentiated by inhibitors of 5-HT reuptake, whereas the 5-HT antagonist mianserin blocks the haloperidol effect (Waldmeier, 1980). These results, however, are difficult to reconcile with the finding that electrolytic lesions of the dorsal raphe caused an increase in the DOPAC/DA ratio in the nucleus accumbens and, to a lesser degree, in the striatum but not in the frontal cortex (Herve *et al.*, 1979). Thus, in spite of biochemical studies that point to a stimulating effect of 5-HT receptor agonists on forebrain DA turnover, removal of the endogenous serotonergic influence on DA neurons also increases DA turnover. The possibility that there are differences between the effects of low versus high doses of 5-HT agonists and antagonists on DA biochemistry remains to be carefully determined.

Despite the identified serotonergic input and the demonstrated effects of 5-HT on DA biochemistry, there is no clear indication of what the effects of endogenous 5-HT on A10 DA cell electrophysiology may be. Intravenously administered LSD and lisuride interact with central 5-HT neurons in a manner that has been attributed to a 5-HT agonist action (Kehr, 1977; Pieri *et al.*, 1978; Silbergeld and Hruska, 1979; Walters *et* al., 1979; Rosenfeld and Makman, 1981). However, the divergent effects of the two drugs on the firing of A10 DA cells are apparently mediated by DA receptors and *not* by 5-HT receptors (White and Wang, 1983c). In addition, the 5-HT$_1$ receptor agonist 5-methoxy-N,N-dimethyltryptamine produces effects on A10 DA neuronal activity unrelated to interactions at DA receptors or at 5-HT$_1$ or 5-HT$_2$ receptors (White and Wang, 1983c). Evidence for the lack of a direct effect of 5-HT on A10 DA neurons is also demonstrated by the inability of 5-HT to alter the firing rate of these cells after iontophoretic application (Aghajanian and Bunney, 1974b). However, a modulatory role for 5-HT is suggested by the observation that iontophoretic 5-HT diminishes the excitatory effects of simultaneously applied glutamate (Aghajanian and Bunney, 1974b) or CCK (Grace and Bunney, 1986).

6.3. The Effects of Noradrenergic Agonists and Antagonists on A10 DA Neurons

Microiontophoretic application of the α-receptor agonist clonidine has no effect, and the β-receptor agonist isoproterenol has only a weak depressant action on A10 DA neuronal firing (Aghajanian and Bunney, 1977; White and Wang, 1984a). Although no other investigations of the effects of noradrenergic agents on A10 DA cell electrophysiology have been carried out, the results from studies on A9 DA cells can be summarized. The intravenous administration of certain noradrenergic drugs (e.g., clonidine, prazosin, WB4101) has been shown to reverse the inhibition of A9 DA neuronal firing produced by intravenous apomorphine or amphetamine but to have no effect when given alone (Bunney and DeRiemer, 1982). These effects of noradrenergic agents on A9 DA cell firing appear to be indirectly mediated via alterations in the influence of norepinephrine (NE)-containing neurons on the dorsal raphe serotonergic system. In this instance, reversal of DA agonist-induced suppression was apparently the result of either stimulation of α_2-NE autoreceptors or to a blockade of postsynaptic α_1 receptors. In either case, a diminished influence of NE cells on the 5-HT cells would result (Svensson et al., 1975; Cedarbaum and Aghajanian, 1976; Gallager and Aghajanian, 1976; Baraban and Aghajanian, 1980). This hypothesis is supported by the finding that dorsal raphe lesions abolish the ability of α_1-receptor blockers to reverse DA agonist-induced inhibition of DA neuronal firing (Bunney and DeRiemer, 1982).

A number of α_2-receptor antagonists (e.g., yohimbine, piperoxan, rauwolscine) increase striatal DA turnover after intravenous administration. However, these effects appear to be a result of the postsynaptic DA receptor blocking properties of the drugs (Scatton et al., 1980b, 1983).

6.4. The Effects of Substance P on A10 DA Neurons

The localization, neurochemistry, and possible functions of substance P (SP) in the nervous system have been reviewed in detail by Jessell (1983). A prominent SP system projects from the striatum to the globus pallidus, entopeduncular nucleus, and substantia nigra (both the zona compacta and the zona reticulata) (see Jessell, 1983). Following the intranigral administration of SP, DA turnover in A9 neurons is accelerated, and behaviors thought to be mediated through the nigrostriatal DA system are elicited (see Iversen, 1982; Jessell, 1983). Conversely, the intranigral infusion of antisera directed against SP decreases striatal DA turnover, suggesting that the striatonigral SP system exerts a tonic excitatory influence on A9 DA neurons (Cheramy et al., 1978; Michelot et al., 1979). The intranigral application of two putative SP antagonists also decreases GABA turnover in the deep layers of the colliculus, a terminal field of the GABAergic nigrotectal projection, suggesting that SP also exerts a tonic excitatory modulation of the GABA output neurons (Melis and Gale, 1984). However, questions about CNS toxicity and the efficacy of these SP antagonists (Hökfelt et al., 1981; Salt et al., 1982) raise some doubts about the specificity of these potentially useful antagonists.

Despite these data, the role of SP in the substantia nigra remains enigmatic. Microiontophoretically applied SP has only minimal direct effects on identified A9 DA neurons or cells of the zona reticulata (Pinnock and Dray, 1982; Pinnock et al., 1983). Given the high SP content of the substantia nigra, a very low number of SP binding sites are identified in this area by autoradiographic radioligand experiments (Quirion et al., 1983; Mantyh et al., 1984), although the limitations of this approach (especially in the presence of high concentrations of endogenous ligand) necessitate a cautious interpretation of these data. Further ultrastructural studies will be required to determine the specific substantia nigra cells directly innervated by SP inputs.

For many years, SP was thought to be the sole member of the tachykinin peptide family in mammalian tissue (Erspamer, 1981). Recently, however, a kassininlike peptide termed *substance K* (SK) was detected in spinal cord (Maggio et al., 1983) and soon after sequenced (Kimura et al., 1983). The use of cDNA clones derived from brain striatal mRNA has demonstrated that a number of distinct mRNAs derived from one preprotachykinin (PPT) gene by alternate splicing encode for both SP and SK (Nawa et al., 1983, 1984). Whether the presence of SK, which is localized with striatonigral SP (Lee et al., 1986), will help to explain the puzzling SP electrophysiological and binding data remains unclear. Just as SP apparently alters striatal DA turnover, the acute and chronic administration of DA agonists or antagonists alters the concentrations of SP in the striatum and/or substantia nigra in a complex manner (see Koshiya and Kato, 1983; Bannon and Goedert, 1984; and references therein), although the relationship between SP concentration and SP utilization remains obscure. Repeated administration of antipsychotic DA antagonist drugs consistently decreases the nigral concentration of SP (Hong et al., 1978; Hanson et al., 1981a,b; LeDouarin et al., 1983; Oblin et al., 1984; Bannon et al., 1986b) and SK (Bannon et al., 1986b). It has generally been accepted that the net decrease in SP after DA antagonists results from an imbalance between an increase in SP synthesis and an even greater acceleration of SP release (Hong et al., 1978). Contrary to this hypothesis, direct quantitation of striatonigral PPT (SP/SK-encoding) mRNA reveals that the DA antagonist-induced decrease in SP and SK is paralleled by a *decrease* in SP/SK mRNA, i.e., an apparent inhibition of tachykinin synthesis (Bannon et al., 1986b).

Another prominent target area for brain SP neurons is the VTA. Iversen and colleagues have found that infusion of SP or its stable analogs into the VTA increases exploratory behavior and locomotor activity and potentiates the induction of these behaviors by *d*-amphetamine. The behavioral effects of SP infusion can be prevented by destroying the mesolimbic DA neurons or by infusing DA antagonists into the nucleus accumbens locally (for a review, see Iversen, 1982). These studies suggest a role for SP in the regulation of A10 DA neuronal activity. Short periods of rather mild footshock also activate primarily mesocortical and secondarily mesolimbic (but not nigrostriatal) DA systems (see Bannon and Roth, 1983). Selective activation of the mesocortical DA system is also produced by reexposure to the environment previously paired with the footshock (Herman et al., 1982; Deutch et al., 1985b). During the period of footshock-induced mesoprefrontal DA cell activation, SP concentrations in the VTA rapidly decline (Lisoprawski et al., 1980; Bannon et al., 1986a), suggesting a role for SP in mediating the footshock-induced activation of A10 DA cells. In support of this hypothesis, footshock-induced activation of mesoprefrontal DA cells is mimicked by the local infusion of SP or SP analogs (Iversen et al., 1983; Elliott et al., 1986; Deutch et al., 1985a) and is prevented by immunoneutralization of released SP in the VTA (Bannon et al., 1983b). Surprisingly, during footshock, VTA SK levels remain unaltered (Bannon et al., 1986a). Similarly, SP levels rapidly rebound after footshock while SK levels remain constant. This apparent dissociation of cotransmitters may be the result of differential compartmentalization of the two tachykinins and the preferential release or processing of SP. Further molecular studies will be required to test this hypothesis. As in the case of SP in the substantia nigra, the precise identity of the VTA neurons innervated by SP afferents remains undetermined. The footshock studies and the effects of SP versus SK infusion on behavior and regional DOPAC changes suggest that SP primarily activates mesoprefrontal DA cells, whereas SK may primarily modulate mesoaccumbens DA neurons (Deutch *et al.*, 1985*a*). Nevertheless, many questions remain about the possible role of SK versus SP in regulating A10 DA cells. In short, even though DA cells and SP cells are two of the most intensively studied neurochemically identified neurons, our understanding of their interactions in the midbrain is still rudimentary.

7. SUMMARY

Over the last decade, there has been a progressive evolution of our understanding of the biochemistry and electrophysiology of midbrain DA neurons. Initially, it was believed that A9 and A10 DA cells formed two homogeneous populations. More recently, it has been shown that these cells are actually organized into distinct subgroups. Thus, they may be classified in terms of their (1) projection areas, (2) site of origin (e.g., A9 versus A10), (3) physiological profile (e.g., degree of bursting, turnover rates, presence of autoreceptors), and (4) pharmacological responsiveness. The recent recognition of these important differences makes it necessary for the basic researcher to carefully identify the specific DA subsystem being studied. This task is being accomplished by the utilization of such techniques as antidromic activation of DA neurons from their terminal regions in electrophysiological investigations, as well as more careful and discrete dissections in biochemical studies.

While differences among DA subsystems are being appreciated, it is becoming evident that complex interactions among these subsystems exist. For example, it is now known that A10 DA neurons project to the nucleus accumbens, which, in turn, projects to the substantia nigra (see Nauta, 1978). Further work on the extent of these interactions, as well as the importance of afferent inputs into these different DA systems, will be necessary over the next several years. In addition to the conceptual advances in the last decade, much of the promise of future research lies in technological advances. These range from techniques applicable to the freely moving animal, such as extracellular recording in conjunction with *in vivo* electrochemistry, to *in vitro* experiments, including intracellular studies on the basic ionic mechanisms underlying drug action on DA neurons and studies probing gene structure and regulation in these cells.

NOTE ADDED IN PROOF

This review appears essentially as submitted by the authors in June, 1984, with the exception that references to ongoing work by our research groups have been updated.

ACKNOWLEDGMENTS

We thank Drs. Marina Wolf and John Maggio for their most helpful comments on this manuscript, and Sue Mulready for manuscript preparation. This work was supported, in part, by NIH grants MH-08841, MH-08987, MH-28849, and MH-14092 and by the state of Connecticut.

8. REFERENCES

AGHAJANIAN, G. K., and BUNNEY, B. S., 1973, Central dopaminergic neurons: Neurophysiological identification and responses to drugs, in: *Frontiers in Catecholamine Research* (S. H. Snyder and E. Usdin, eds.), Pergamon Press, Elmsford, NY, pp. 643–648.

AGHAJANIAN, G. K., and BUNNEY, B. S., 1974a, Pre- and postsynaptic feedback mechanisms in central dopaminergic neurons, in: *Frontiers of Neurology and Neuroscience Research* (P. Seeman and G. M. Brown, eds.), University Toronto Press, Toronto, pp. 4–11.

AGHAJANIAN, G. K., and BUNNEY, B. S., 1974b, Dopaminergic and non-dopaminergic neurons of the substantia nigra: Differential responses to putative transmitters, in: *Proceedings 9th Congress of the Collegium Internationale Neuropsychopharmacologicum* (J. R. Boissier, H. Hippius, and P. Pichot, eds.), Excerpta Medica Foundation, Amsterdam, pp. 444–452.

AGHAJANIAN, G. K., and BUNNEY, B. S., 1977, Dopamine "autoreceptors": Pharmacological characterization by microiontophoretic single cell recording studies, *Naunyn-Schmiedeberg's Arch. Pharmacol.* **297**:1–7.

ANDÉN, N-E., ROOS, B. E., and WERDINIUS, B., 1964, Effects of chlorpromazine, haloperidol and reserpine on the levels of phenolic acids in rabbit corpus striatum, *Life Sci.* **3**:149–158.

ANDÉN, N-E., GRABOWSKA-ANDÉN, M., and LILJENBERG, B., 1983a, On the presence of autoreceptors on dopamine neurons in different brain regions, *J. Neural Trans.* **57**:129–137.

ANDÉN, N-E., GRABOWSKA-ANDÉN, M., and LILJENBERG, B., 1983b, Demonstration of autoreceptors on dopamine neurons in different brain regions of rats treated with gammabutyrolactone, *J. Neural Trans.* **57**:143–152.

AZMITIA, E. C., and SEGAL, M., 1978, Autoradiographic analysis of the differential ascending projections of the dorsal and median raphe nuclei in the rat, *J. Comp. Neurol.* **179**:641–668.

BACOPOULOS, N. G., 1981a, Biochemical mechanism of tolerance to neuroleptic drugs; regional differences in rat brain, *Eur. J. Pharmacol.* **70**:585–586.

BACOPOULOS, N. G., 1981b, Antipsychotic drug effects on dopamine and serotonin receptors: *In vitro* binding and *in vivo* turnover studies, *J. Pharmacol. Exp. Ther.* **219**:708–713.

BACOPOULOS, N. G., and ROTH, R. H., 1981, Apomorphine–haloperidol interactions: Different types of antagonism in cortical and subcortical brain regions, *Brain Res.* **205**:313–319.

BACOPOULOS, N. G., BUSTOS, G., REDMOND, D. E., BAULU, J., and ROTH, R. H., 1978, Regional sensitivity of primate brain dopaminergic neurons to haloperidol: Alterations following chronic treatment, *Brain Res.* **157**:396–401.

BACOPOULOS, N. G., SPOKES, E. G., BIRD, E. D., and ROTH, R. H., 1979, Antipsychotic drug action in schizophrenic patients: Effect on cortical dopamine metabolism after long-term treatment, *Science* **205**:1405–1407.

BACOPOULOS, N. G., REDMOND, D. E., BAULU, J., and ROTH, R. H., 1980, Chronic haloperidol or fluphenazine: Effects on dopamine metabolism in brain, cerebrospinal fluid and plasma of *Cercopithecus aethiops* (vervet monkey), *J. Pharmacol. Exp. Ther.* **212**:1–5.

BALCOM, G. J., LENOX, R. H., and MEYERHOFF, J. L., 1975, Regional γ-aminobutyric acid levels in rat brain determined after microwave fixation, *J. Neurochem.* **24**:609–613.

BANNON, M. J., and GOEDERT, M., 1984, Changes in substance P concentrations after protein synthesis inhibition provide an index of substance P utilization, *Brain Res.* **301**:184–186.

BANNON, M. P., and ROTH, R. H., 1983, Pharmacology of mesocortical dopamine neurons, *Pharmacol. Rev.* **35**:53–68.

BANNON, M. J., MICHAUD, R. L., and ROTH, R. H., 1981, Mesocortical dopamine neurons: Lack of autoreceptors modulating dopamine synthesis, *Mol. Pharmacol.* **19**:270–275.

BANNON, M. J., REINHARD, J. F., JR., BUNNEY, E. B., and ROTH, R. H., 1982, Unique response to antipsychotic drugs is due to the absence of terminal autoreceptors in mesocortical dopamine neurons, *Nature* **296**:444–446.

BANNON, M. P., WOLF, M. E., and ROTH, R. H., 1983a, Pharmacology of dopamine neurons innervating the prefrontal, cingulate and piriform cortices, *Eur. J. Pharmacol.* **91**:119–125.

BANNON, M. J., ELLIOTT, P. J., ALPERT, J. E., GOEDERT, M., IVERSEN, S. D., and IVERSEN, L. L., 1983b, Role of endogenous substance P in stress-induced activation of mesocortical dopamine neurones, *Nature* **306**:791–792.

BANNON, M. J., DEUTCH, A. Y., TAM, S.-Y., ZAMIR, N., LEE, J.-M., MAGGIO, J. E., ESKAY, R. L., and ROTH, R. H., 1986a, Mild footshock stress dissociates substance P from substance K and dynorphin from Met- and Leu-enkephalin, *Brain Res.* **381**:393–396.

BANNON, M. J., LEE, J.-M., GIRAUD, P., YOUNG, A. C., AFFOLTER, H.-U., and BONNER, T. I., 1986b, Dopamine antagonist haloperidol decreases substance P, substance K and preprotachykinin mRNAs in rat striatonigral neurons, *J. Biol. Chem.* **261**:6640–6642.

BARABAN, J. M., and AGHAJANIAN, G. K., 1980, Suppression of firing activity of 5-HT neurons in the dorsal raphe by alpha-adrenoceptor antagonists, *Neuropharmacology* **19**:355–363.

BEART, P. M., and MCDONALD, D., 1980, Neurochemical studies of the mesolimbic dopaminergic pathway: Somatodendritic mechanisms and GABAergic neurones in the rat ventral tegmental area, *J. Neurochem.* **34**:1622–1629.

BECKMAN, B., HIPPIUS, H., and RUTHER, E., 1979, Treatment of schizophrenia, *Prog. Neuro-Psychopharmacol.* **3**:47–52.

BENINGER, R. J., 1983, The role of dopamine in locomotor activity and learning, *Brain Res. Rev.* **6**:173–196.

BERGER, B., 1977, Histochemical identification and localization of dopaminergic axons in rat and human cerebral cortex, in: *Advances in Biochemical Psychopharmacology*, Vol. 16 (E. Costa and G. L. Gessa, eds.), Raven Press, New York, pp. 13–20.

BERGER, B., TASSIN, J. P., BLANC, G., MOYNE, M. A., and THIERRY, A. M., 1974, Histochemical confirmation for dopaminergic innervation of the rat cerebral cortex after destruction of the noradrenergic ascending pathway, *Brain Res.* **81**:332–337.

BERGER, B., THIERRY, A. M., TASSIN, J. P., and MOYNE, M. A., 1976, Dopaminergic innervation of the rat prefrontal cortex: A fluorescence histochemical study, *Brain Res.* **106**:133–145.

BJÖRKLUND, A., and LINDVALL, O., 1985, Dopamine-containing systems in the CNS, in: *Handbook of Chemical Neuronanatomy*, Vol. 2, P. 1 (A. BJÖRKLUND and T. HÖKFELT, eds.), Elsevier, Amsterdam, pp. 55–122.

BOWERS, M. B., JR., and SALOMONSSEN, L. A., 1982, LSD: Effect on monoamine metabolites in rat prefrontal cortex, *Biochem. Pharmacol.* **31**:4093–4096.

BROWDER, S., GERMAN, D. C., and SHORE, P. A., 1981, Midbrain dopamine neurons: Differential response to amphetamine isomers, *Brain Res.* **207**:333–342.

BROZOSKI, T. J., BROWN, R. M., ROSVOLD, H. E., and GOLDMAN, P. S., 1979, Cognitive deficit caused by regional depletion of dopamine in prefrontal cortex of rhesus monkey, *Science* **205**:929–931.

BUNNEY, B. S., 1977, Central dopaminergic systems: Two *in vivo* electrophysiological models for predicting therapeutic efficacy and neurological side effects of putative antipsychotic drugs, in: *Animal Models in Psychiatry and Neurology* (I. Hanin and E. Usdin, eds.), Pergamon Press, New York, pp. 91–105.

BUNNEY, B. S., 1979, The electrophysiological pharmacology of midbrain dopaminergic systems, in: *The Neurobiology of Dopamine* (A. S. Horn, J. Korf, and B. H. C. Westerink, eds.), Academic Press, New York, pp. 417–452.

BUNNEY, B. S., and AGHAJANIAN, G. K., 1975a, Evidence for drug actions on both pre- and postsynaptic catecholamine receptors in the CNS, in: *Pre- and Postsynaptic Receptors* (E. Usdin and W. E. Bunney, Jr., eds.), Dekker, New York, pp. 89–122.

BUNNEY, B. S., and AGHAJANIAN, G. K., 1975b, Antipsychotic drugs and central dopaminergic neurons: A model for predicting therapeutic efficacy and incidence of extrapyramidal side effects, in: *Predictability in Psychopharmacology: Preclinical and Clinical Correlations* (A. Sudilovsky, S. Gershon, and B. Beer, eds.), Raven Press, New York, pp. 225–245.

BUNNEY, B. S., and AGHAJANIAN, G. K., 1976, d-Amphetamine-induced inhibition of central dopaminergic neurons: Mediation by a striato-nigral feedback pathway, *Science* **192**:391–393.

BUNNEY, B. S., and AGHAJANIAN, G. K., 1978, d-Amphetamine-induced depression of central dopamine neurons: Evidence for mediation by both autoreceptors and a striatal-nigral feedback pathway, *Naunyn-Schmiedeberg's Arch. Pharmacol.* **304**:255–261.

BUNNEY, B. S., and DERIEMER, S., 1982, Effects of clonidine on dopaminergic neuron activity in the substantia nigra: Possible indirect mediation by noradrenergic regulation of the serotonergic raphe system, in: *Gilles de la Tourette Syndrome* (A. J. Friedhoff and T. N. Chase, eds.), Raven Press, New York, pp. 99–104.

BUNNEY, B. S., and GRACE, A. A., 1978, Acute and chronic haloperidol treatment: Comparison of effects on nigral dopaminergic cell activity, *Life Sci.* **23**:1715–1728.

BUNNEY, B. S., WALTERS, J. R., ROTH, R. H., and AGHAJANIAN, G. K., 1973a, Dopaminergic neurons: Effect of antipsychotic drugs and amphetamine on single cell activity, *J. Pharmacol. Exp. Ther.* **185**:560–571.

BUNNEY, B. S., AGHAJANIAN, G. K., and ROTH, R. H., 1973b, Comparison of effects of L-dopa, amphetamine and apomorphine on firing rate of rat dopaminergic neurons, *Nature New Biol.* **245**:123–125.

BUNNEY, B. S., CHIODO, L. A., GRACE, A. A., and SCHENK, J. O., 1985, In vivo effects of acute and chronic antipsychotic drug administration on midbrain dopaminergic neuron activity, in: *Behavioral Pharmacology: The Current Status* (L. S. Seiden and R. L. Balster, eds.), Liss, New York, pp. 205–220.

CARLSSON, A., 1975, Dopaminergic autoreceptors, in: *Chemical Tools in Catecholamine Research*, Vol. II (O. Almgren, A. Carlsson, and J. Engel, eds.), North Holland Publishing Co., Amsterdam, pp. 219–225.

CARLSSON, A., and LINDQVIST, M., 1963, Effects of chlorpromazine and haloperidol on formation of 3-methoxytyramine and normetanephrine in mouse brain, *Acta Pharmacol. Toxicol.* **20**:140–144.

CARTER, C. J., and PYCOCK, C. J., 1980, Behavioral and biochemical effects of dopamine and noradrenaline depletion within the medial prefrontal cortex of the rat, *Brain Res.* **192**:163–176.

CASU, M., KLIMEK, V., BIGGIO, G., and GESSA, G. L., 1980, Tolerance to haloperidol effect on dopamine (DA) synthesis is independent from postsynaptic DA receptors, *Pharmacol. Res. Commun.* **12**:393–396.

CEDARBAUM, J. M., and AGHAJANIAN, G. K., 1976, Noradrenergic neurons of the locus coeruleus: Inhibition by epinephrine and activation by the α-antagonist piperoxane, *Brain Res.* **112**:413–419.

CHERAMY, A., MICHELOT, R., LEVIEL, V., NIEOULLON, A., GLOWINSKI, J., and KERDELHUE, B., 1978, Effect of immunoneutralization of substance P in the cat substantia nigra on the release of dopamine from dendrites and terminals of dopaminergic neurons, *Brain Res.* **155**:404–408.

CHIODO, L. A., 1981, Studies on the regulation of the responsiveness of substantia nigra dopamine neurons to sensory stimuli. Doctoral dissertation, University of Pittsburgh.

CHIODO, L. A., and BUNNEY, B. S., 1982, Effects of chronic neuroleptic treatments on nigral dopamine cell activity, *Soc. Neurosci. Abstr.* **8**:482.

CHIODO, L. A., and BUNNEY, B. S., 1983, Typical and atypical neuroleptics: Differential effects of chronic administration on the activity of A9 and A10 midbrain dopaminergic neurons, *J. Neurosci.* **3**:1607–1619.

CHIODO, L. A., and BUNNEY, B. S., 1984, Effects of dopamine antagonists on midbrain dopamine cell activity, in: *Catecholamines* (E. Usdin, A. Carlsson, A. Dahlström, and J. Engel, eds.), Pergamon Press, Elmsford, NY, pp. 369–391.

CHIODO, L. A., BANNON, M. J., GRACE, A. A., ROTH, R. H., and BUNNEY, B. S., 1984, Evidence for the absence of impulse-regulating somatodendritic and synthesis-modulating nerve terminal autoreceptors on subpopulations of mesocortical dopamine neurons, *Neuroscience* **12**:1–16.

CONRAD, L. C. A., and PFAFF, D. W., 1976, Autoradiographic tracing of nucleus accumbens efferents in the rat, *Brain Res.* **113**:589–596.

COOPER, J. R., BLOOM, F. E., and ROTH, R. H., 1982, *The Biochemical Basis of Neuropharmacology*, 4th ed., Oxford University Press, New York.

CRANE, G. E., 1973, Persistent dyskinesia, *Br. J. Psychiatr.* **122**:395–405.

DAHLSTRÖM, A., and FUXE, K., 1964, Evidence for the existence of monoamine containing neurons in the central nervous system. I. Demonstration of monoamines in the cell bodies of brain stem neurons, *Acta Physiol. Scand.* **62**(Suppl. 232):1–55.

DALSASS, M., GERMAN, D. C., KISER, R. S., and SPECIALE, S., 1979, Effects of D-amphetamine on dopaminergic neurons in the ventral tegmental area of the rat, *Soc. Neurosci. Abstr.* **5**:553.

DENEAU, J. M., THIERRY, A. M., and FEGER, J., 1980, Electrophysiological identification of mesencephalic ventromedial tegmental (VTA) neurons projecting to the frontal cortex, septum and nucleus accumbens, *Brain Res.* **189**:315–326.

DEUTCH, A. Y., 1982, Behavioral organization of the A8 dopamine cell group, *Soc. Neurosci. Abstr.* **8**:391.

DEUTCH, A. Y., GOLDSTEIN, M., BUNNEY, B. S., and ROTH, R. H., 1984, The anatomical organization of the efferent projections of the A8 dopamine cell group, *Soc. Neurosci. Abstr.* **10**:9.

DEUTCH, A. Y., MAGGIO, J. E., BANNON, M. J., KALIVAS, P. W., TAM, S-Y., GOLDSTEIN, M., and ROTH, R. H., 1985a, Substance K and substance P differentially modulate mesolimbic and mesocortical systems, *Peptides* **6**(Suppl. 2):113–122.

DEUTCH, A. Y., TAM, S-Y., and ROTH, R. H., 1985b, Footshock and conditioned stress increase 3,4-dihydroxy-phenylacetic acid (DOPAC) in the ventral tegmental area but not substantia nigra, *Brain Res.* **333**:143–146.

DICHIARA, G., PORCEDDU, M. L., FRATTA, W., and GESSA, G. L., 1977a, Postsynaptic receptors are not essential for dopaminergic feedback regulation, *Nature* **267**:270–272.

DICHIARA, G., PORCEDDU, M. L., SPANO, P. F., and GESSA, G. L., 1977b, Haloperidol increases and apomorphine decreases striatal dopamine metabolism after destruction of striatal dopamine-sensitive adenylate cyclase by kainic acid, *Brain Res.* **130**:374–382.

ELCHISAK, M. A., MURRIN, L. C., and ROTH, R. H., 1976, Free and conjugated dihydroxyphenylacetic acid: Effect of alterations in impulse flow in rat neostriatum and frontal cortex, *Commun. Psychopharmacol.* **2**:411–420.

ELLIOTT, P. J., ALPERT, J. E., BANNON, M. J., and IVERSEN, S. D., 1986, Selective activation of mesolimbic and mesocortical dopamine metabolism by infusion of a stable substance P analogue into the ventral tegmental area in rat brain, *Brain Res.* **363**:145–147.

ERSPAMER, V., 1981, The tachykinin peptide family, *Trends Neurosci.* **4**:267–269.

FADDA, F., ARGOLAS, A., MELIS, M. R., TISSARI, A. H., ONALI, P. R., and GESSA, G. L., 1978, Stress-induced increase in 3,4-dihydroxyphenylacetic acid (DOPAC) levels in the cerebral cortex and in nucleus accumbens: Reversal by diazepam, *Life Sci.* **23**:2219–2224.

FADDA, F., GESSA, G. L., MARCOU, M., MOSCA, E., and ROSSETTI, Z., 1984, Evidence for autoreceptors in mesocortical dopamine neurons, *Brain Res.* **293**:67–72.

FALLON, J. H., 1981, Collateralization of monoamine neurons: Mesotelencephalic dopamine projections to caudate, septum and frontal cortex, *J. Neurosci.* **4**:1361–1368.

FONNUM, F., WALAAS, I., and IVERSEN, E., 1977, Localization of GABAergic, cholinergic and aminergic structures in the mesolimbic system, *J. Neurochem.* **29**:221–230.

FREEMAN, A. S., and BUNNEY, B. S., 1987, Activity of A9 and A10 dopaminergic neurons in unrestrained rats: Further characterization and effects of apomorphine and cholecystokinin, *Brain Res.* (in press).

FREEMAN, A. S., MELTZER, L. T., and BUNNEY, B. S., 1985, Firing properties of substantia nigra dopaminergic neurons in freely moving rats, *Life Sci.* **36**:1983–1994.

FRIGYESI, T. L., and SZABO, J., 1975, Caudate evoked synaptic activities in nigral neurons, *Exp. Neurol.* **49**:123–139.

FUXE, K., HÖKFELT, T., LJUNGDAHL, A., AGNATI, L., JOHANSSON, O., and PEREZ DE LA MORA, M., 1975, Evidence for an inhibitory GABAergic control of the meso-limbic dopamine neurons: Possibility of improving treatment of schizophrenia by combined treatment with neuroleptics and GABAergic drugs, *Med. Biol.* **53**:177–183.

FUXE, K., PEREZ DE LA MORA, M., HÖKFELT, T., AGNATI, L., LJUNGDAHL, A., and JOHANSSON, O., 1977, GABA-DA interactions and their possible relation to schizophrenia, in: *Psychopathology and Brain Dysfunction* (C. Shagass, S. Gershon, and A. J. Friedhoff, eds.), Raven Press, New York, pp. 97–111.

FUXE, K., ANDERSSON, K., OGREN, S. O., PEREZ DE LA MORA, M., SCHWARCZ, R., HÖKFELT, T., ENEROTH, P., GUSTAFSSON, J. A., and SKETT, P., 1978, GABA neurons and their interaction with monoamine neurons. An anatomical, pharmacological and functional analysis, in: *GABA-Neurotransmitters* (P. Krogsgaard-Larsen, J. Scheel-Krueger, and H. Kofod, eds.), Munksgaard, Copenhagen, pp. 74–94.

GALEY, D., SIMON, H., and LEMOAL, M., 1977, Behavioral effects of lesions in the A10 dopaminergic area of the rat, *Brain Res.* **124**:83–97.

GALLAGER, D. W., and AGHAJANIAN, G. K., 1976, Effect of antipsychotic drugs on the firing of dorsal raphe cells. I. Role of adrenergic system, *Eur. J. Pharmacol.* **39**:341–355.

GALLOWAY, M. P., WOLF, M. E., and ROTH, R. H., 1986, Regulation of dopamine synthesis in the medial prefrontal cortex is mediated by release modulating autoreceptors: Studies *in vivo*, *J. Pharmacol. Exp. Ther.* **236**:689–698.

GERMAN, D. C., DALSASS, M., and KISER, R. S., 1980, Electrophysiological examination of the ventral tegmental (A10) area in the rat, *Brain Res.* **181**:191–197.

GLOWINSKI, J., 1975, Effects of neuroleptics on the nigroneostriatal and mesocortical dopaminergic systems, in: *Biology of Major Psychosis* (D. X. Freedman, ed.), Raven Press, New York, pp. 233–246.

GRACE, A. A., and BUNNEY, B. S., 1979, Paradoxical GABA excitation of nigral dopaminergic cells: Indirect mediation through reticulata inhibitory neurons, *Eur. J. Pharmacol.* **59**:211–218.

GRACE, A. A., and BUNNEY, B. S., 1980, Nigral dopamine neurons: Intracellular recording and identification with L-dopa injection and histofluorescence, *Science* **210**:654–656.

GRACE, A. A., and BUNNEY, B. S., 1983, Intracellular and extracellular electrophysiology of nigral dopaminergic neurons. I. Identification and characterization, *Neuroscience* **10**:301–315.

GRACE, A. A., and BUNNEY, B. S., 1986, Induction of depolarization block in midbrain dopamine neurons by repeated administration of haloperidol: Analysis using *in vivo* intracellular recording, *J. Pharmacol. Exp. Ther.* **238**:1092–1100.

GROVES, P. M., WILSON, C. J., YOUNG, S. J., and REBEC, G. V., 1975, Self-inhibition by dopamine neurons, *Science* **190**:522–529.

GUYENET, P. G., and AGHAJANIAN, G. K., 1978, Antidromic identification of dopaminergic and other output neurons of the rat substantia nigra, *Brain Res.* **150**:69–84.

HANSON, G., ALPHS, L., PRADLAN, S., and LOVENBERG, W., 1981a, Response of striatonigral substance P systems to a dopamine receptor agonist and antagonist, *Neuropharmacology* **20**:541–548.

HANSON, G. R., ALPHS, L., WOLF, W., LEVINE, R., and LOVENBERG, W., 1981b, Haloperidol-induced reduction of nigral substance P-like immunoreactivity: A probe for the interactions between dopamine and substance P neuronal systems, *J. Pharmacol. Exp. Ther.* **218**:568–574.

HATTORI, T., FIBIGER, H. C., and MCGEER, P. L., 1975, Demonstration of a pallidonigral projection innervating dopaminergic neurons, *J. Comp. Neurol.* **162**:487–504.

HERMAN, J. P., GUILLONEAU, D., DANTZER, R., SCATTON, B., SEMERDJIAN-ROUQUIER, L., and LEMOAL, M., 1982, Differential effects of inescapable footshocks and of stimuli previously paired with inescapable footshocks on dopamine turnover in cortical and limbic areas of the rat, *Life Sci.* **30**:2207–2214.

HERVE, D., SIMON, H., BLANC, G., LISOPRAWSKI, A., LEMOAL, M., KIM, J., and TASSIN, J. P., 1979, Increased utilization of dopamine in the nucleus accumbens but not in the central cortex after dorsal raphe lesions in the rat, *Neurosci. Lett.* **15**:127–133.

HÖKFELT, T., FUXE, K., and GOLDSTEIN, M., 1973, Immunohistorical studies on monoamine containing cell systems, *Brain Res.* **62**:461–469.

HÖKFELT, T., FUXE, K., JOHANSSON, O., and LJUNGDAHL, A., 1974, Pharmaco-histochemical evidence of the existence of DA nerve terminals in the limbic cortex, *Eur. J. Pharmacol.* **25**:108–112.

HÖKFELT, T., AGNATI, L., FUXE, K., JOHANSSON, O., JONSSON, G., LJUNGDAHL, A., and LOFSTRÖM, A., 1975, Possible involvement of GABA synapses in the action of neuroleptic drugs on dopamine neurons, in: *Antipsychotic Drugs: Pharmacodynamics and Pharmacokinetics* (G. Sedvall, ed.), Pergamon Press, Oxford and New York, pp. 227–233.

HÖKFELT, T., VINCENT, S., HELLSTEN, L., ROSELL, S., FOLKERS, K., MARKEY, K., GOLDSTEIN, M., and CUELLU, C., 1981, Immunohistochemical evidence for a "neurotoxic" action of (D-Pro^2, D-Trp^{7,9})-substance P, an analogue with substance P antagonistic activity, *Acta Physiol. Scand.* **113**:571–573.

HONG, J. S., YANG, H.-Y. T., and COSTA, E., 1978, Substance P content of substantia nigra alter chronic treatment with antischizophrenic drugs, *Neuropharmacology* **17**:83–85.

IVERSEN, L. L., ELLIOTT, P. J., BANNON, M. J., ALPERT, J. E., and IVERSEN, S. D., 1983, Interaction of substance P with dopaminergic neurones in brain, in: *Substance P—Dublin 1983* (P. Skrabanek and D. Powell, eds.), Poole Press, Dublin, pp. 43–44.

IVERSEN, S. D., 1977a, Brain dopamine systems and behavior, in: *Handbook of Psychopharmacology*, Vol. 8 (L. L. Iversen, S. D. Iversen, and S. H. Snyder, eds.), Plenum Press, New York, pp. 333–384.

IVERSEN, S. D., 1977b, Striatal function and stereotyped behavior, in: *The Psychology of the Striatum* (A. R. Cools, A. H. M. Lohman, and J. H. L. van den Bercker, eds.), North Holland Publishing Co., Amsterdam, pp. 99–118.

IVERSEN, S. D., 1982, Behavioral effects of substance P through dopaminergic pathways in the brain, in: *Substance P in the Nervous System* (R. Porter and M. O'Conner, eds.), Pittman, London, pp. 307–324.

JESSELL, T. M., 1983, Substance P in the nervous system, in: *Handbook of Psychopharmacology*, Vol. 16 (L. L. Iversen, S. D. Iversen, and S. H. Snyder, eds.), Plenum Press, New York, pp. 1–105.

JESSELL, T. M., EMSON, P. C., PAXINOS, A., and CUELLO, A. C., 1978, Topographic projections of substance P and GABA pathways in the striato- and pallido-nigral system: A biochemical and immunohistochemical study, *Brain Res.* **152**:487–498.

KÄÄRIÄINEN, I., 1976, Effects of aminooxyacetic acid and baclofen on the catalepsy and on the increase of mesolimbic and striatal dopamine turnover induced by haloperidol in rats, *Acta Pharmacol. Toxicol.* **39**:393–400.

KEHR, W., 1977, Effects of lisuride and other ergot derivatives on monoaminergic mechanisms in the rat brain, *Eur. J. Pharmacol.* **41**:262–273.

KEHR, W., CARLSSON, A., LINDQVIST, M., MAGNUSSON, T., and ATACK, C. V., 1972, Evidence for a receptor-mediated feedback control of striatal tyrosine hydroxylase activity, *J. Pharm. Pharmacol.* **24**:744–746.

KIM, J-S., BAK, I. J., HASSLER, R., and OKADA, Y., 1971, Role of γ-aminobutyric acid in the extrapyramidal motor system. 2. Some evidence for the existence of a type of GABA-rich striato-nigral neurons, *Exp. Brain Res.* **14**:95–104.

KIMURA, S., OKADA, M., SUGITA, Y., KANAZAWA, I., and MUNEKATA, E., 1983, Novel neuropeptides, neurokinin α and β, isolated from porcine spinal cord, *Proc. Japan Acad.* **59**(Ser. B):101–104.

KLEIN, D. F., GITTELMAN, R., QUITKIN, F., and RITKIN, A., 1980, *Diagnosis and Drug Treatment of Psychiatric Disorders: Adults and Children*, Williams & Wilkins, Baltimore, MD.

KOSHIYA, K., and KATO, T., 1983, Acute changes in nigral substance P content induced by drugs acting on dopamine, muscarine and GABA receptors, *Naunyn-Schmiedeberg's Arch. Pharmacol.* **324**:223–227.

LAVIELLE, S., TASSIN, J. P., THIERRY, A. M., BLANC, G., HERVE, D., BATHELEMY, C., and GLOWINSKI, J., 1978, Blockade by benzodiazepines of the selective high increase in dopamine turnover induced by stress in mesocortical dopaminergic neurons of the rat, *Brain Res.* **168**:585–594.

LEDOUARIN, C., OBLIN, A., FAGE, D., and SCATTON, B., 1983, Influence of lithium on biochemical manifestations of striatal dopamine target cell supersensitivity induced by prolonged haloperidol treatment, *Eur. J. Pharmacol.* **93**:55–62.

LEE, J.-M., MCLEAN, S., MAGGIO, J. E., ZAMIR, N., ROTH, R. H., ESKAY, R. L., and BANNON, M. J., 1986, The localization and characterization of substance P and substance K in striatonigral neurons, *Brain Res.* **371**:152–154.

LEMOAL, M., CARDO, B., and STINUS, L., 1969, Influence of ventral mesencephalic lesions on various spontaneous and conditioned behaviors in the rat, *Physiol. Behav.* **4**:567–573.

LENARD, L., and NAUTA, W. J. H., 1979, Neostriatal and limbic projections of cell group A8, *Neurosci. Lett.* suppl. **3**:S70.

LINDVALL, O., 1979, Dopamine pathways in the rat brain, in: *The Neurobiology of Dopamine* (A. S. Horn, J. Korf, and B. H. C. Westerink, eds.), Academic Press, New York, pp. 319–342.

LINDVALL, O., and BJÖRKLUND, A., 1978a, Anatomy of the dopaminergic neuron systems in the rat brain, in: *Advances in Biochemical Psychopharmacology*, Vol. 19 (P. J. Roberts, G. N. Woodruff, and L. L. Iversen, eds.), Raven Press, New York, pp. 1–23.

LINDVALL, O., and BJÖRKLUND, 1978b, Organization of cataecholamine neurons in rat central nervous system, in: *Handbook of Psychopharmacology*, Vol. 9 (L. L. Iversen, S. D. Iversen, and S. H. Snyder, eds.), Plenum Press, New York, pp. 139–231.

LINDVALL, O., BJÖRKLUND, A., and DIVAC, I., 1977, Organization of mesencephalic dopamine neurons projecting to the neocortex and septum, in: *Advances in Biochemical Psychopharmacology*, Vol. 16 (E. Costa and G. L. Gessa, eds.), Raven Press, New York, pp. 39–46.

LINDVALL, O., BJÖRKLUND, A., and DIVAC, I., 1978, Organization of catecholamine neurons projecting to the frontal cortex in the rat, *Brain Res.* **142**:1–24.

LISOPRAWSKI, A., HERVE, D., BLANC, G., GLOWINSKI, J., and TASSIN, J. P., 1980, Selective activation of the mesocortical frontal dopaminergic neurons induced by lesion of the habenula in the rat, *Brain Res.* **183**:229–234.

LOUGHLIN, S. E., and FALLON, J. H., 1984, Substantia nigra and ventral tegmental area projections to cortex: Topography and collateralization, *Neuroscience* **11**:425–435.

MACNEIL, D., GOWER, M., and SZYMANSKA, I., 1978, Response of dopamine neurons in substantia nigra to muscimol, *Brain Res.* **154**:401–403.

MAGGIO, J. E., SANDBERG, B. E. B., BRADLEY, C. V., IVERSEN, L. L., SANTIKARU, S., WILLIAMS, D. H., HUNTER, J. C., and HANLEY, M. R., 1983, Substance K: A novel tachykinin in mammalian spinal cord, in: *Substance P—Dublin 1983* (P. Skrabenak and D. Powell, eds.), Poole Press, Dublin, pp. 20–21.

MANTYH, P. W., MAGGIO, J. E., and HUNT, S. P., 1984, The autoradiographic distribution of kassinin and substance K binding sites is different from the distribution of substance P binding sites in rat brain, *Eur. J. Pharmacol.* **102**:361–364.

MATTHYSSE, S., 1973, Antipsychotic drug actions: A clue to the neuropathology of schizophrenia? *Fed. Proc.* **32**:200–205.

MCGEER, E. G., PARKINSON, J., and MCGEER, P. L., 1976, Neonatal enzyme development in the interpeduncular nucleus and surrounding ventral tegmentum, *Exp. Neurol.* **53**:109–114.

MCGEER, P. L., MCGEER, E. G., and HATTORI, T., 1977, Dopamine-acetylcholine-GABA neuronal linkages in the extrapyramidal and limbic systems, in: *Advances in Biochemical Psychopharmacology*, Vol. 16 (E. Costa and G. L. Gessa, eds.), Raven Press, New York, pp. 397–402.

MCNAIR, J. L., SUTIN, J., and TSUBOKAWA, T., 1972, Suppression of cell firing in the substantia nigra by caudate nucleus stimulation, *Exp. Neurol.* **37**:395–411.

MELIS, M. R., and GALE, K., 1984, Evidence that nigral substance P controls the activity of the nigrotectal GABAergic pathway, *Brain Res.* **295**:389–393.

MELTZER, H. Y., 1980, Relevance of dopamine autoreceptors for psychiatry: Preclinical and clinical studies, *Schizophrenia Bull.* **6**:456–475.

MELTZER, H. Y., and STAHL, S. M., 1976, The dopamine hypothesis of schizophrenia: A review, *Schizophrenia Bull.* **2**:19–76.

MICHELOT, R., LEVIEL, V., GIORGIUEFF-CHESSELET, M. F., CHERAMY, A., and GLOWINSKI, J., 1979, Effects of the unilateral nigral modulation of substance P transmission on the activity of the two nigrostriatal dopaminergic pathways, *Life Sci.* **24**:715–724.

MILLER, J. D., FARBER, J., GOTZ, P., ROFFWARG, H., and GERMAN, D. C., 1983, Activity of mesencephalic dopamine and non-dopamine neurons across stages of sleep and waking in the rat, *Brain Res.* **273**:133–141.

MOORE, K. E., and KELLY, P. H., 1978, Biochemical pharmacology of mesolimbic and mesocortical dopaminergic neurons, in: *Psychopharmacology: A Generation of Progress* (M. A. Lipton, A. DiMascio, and K. F. Killam, eds.), Raven Press, New York, pp. 221–234.

MOORE, R. Y., HALARIS, A. E., and JONES, B., 1978, Serotonin neurons of the midbrain raphe: Ascending projections, *J. Comp. Neurol.* **180**:417–438.

NAGAI, T., MCGEER, P. L., and MCGEER, E. G., 1983, Distribution of GABA-T-intensive neurons in the rat forebrain and midbrain, *J. Comp. Neurol.* **218**:220–238.

NAUTA, W. J. H., 1978, Efferent connections and nigral afferents of the nucleus accumbens septi in the rat, *Neuroscience* **3**:385–401.

NAWA, H., HIROSE, T., TAKASHIMA, H., INAYAMA, S., and NAKANISHI, S., 1983, Nucleotide sequences of cloned cDNAs for two types of bovine brain substance P precursor, *Nature* **306**:32–36.

NAWA, H., KOTANI, H., and NOKANISHI, S., 1984, Tissue-specific generation of two preprotachykinin mRNAs from one gene by alternate RNA splicing, *Nature* **312**:729–734.

NOWYCKY, M. C., and ROTH, R. H., 1978, Dopaminergic neurons: Role of presynaptic receptors in the regulation of transmitter biosynthesis, *Prog. Neuro-Psychopharmacol.* **2**:139–158.

Nowycky, M. C., Walters, J. R., and Roth, R. H., 1978, Dopaminergic neurons: Effect of acute and chronic morphine administration on single cell activity and transmitter metabolism, *J. Neural Transmission* **42:**99–116.

Nyback, H., Borzecki, A., and Sedvall, G., 1968, Accumulation and disappearance of catecholamines formed from tyrosine-C^{14} in mouse brain: Effect of some psychiatric drugs, *Eur. J. Pharmacol.* **4:**395–403.

Oblin, A., Zivkovic, B., and Bartholini, G., 1984, Involvement of the D-2 receptor in the neuroleptic-induced decrease in nigral substance P, *Eur. J. Pharmacol.* **105:**175–177.

Oertel, W. H., Tappaz, M. L., Berod, A., and Mugnaini, E., 1982, Two-color immunohistochemistry for dopamine and GABA neurons in rat substantia nigra and zona incerta, *Brain Res. Bull.* **9:**463–474.

Olpe, H-R., Koella, W. P., Wolf, P., and Haas, H. L., 1977, The action of Baclofen on neurons of the substantia nigra and of the ventral tegmental area, *Brain Res.* **134:**577–580.

Palfreyman, M. G., Huot, S., Lippert, B., and Schechter, P. J., 1978, The effect of γ-acetylenic GABA, an enzyme-activated irreversible inhibitor of GABA-transaminase, on dopamine pathways of the extrapyramidal and limbic systems, *Eur. J. Pharmacol.* **50:**325–336.

Phillipson, O. T., 1979, Afferent projections to the ventral tegmental area of Tsai and interfascicular nucleus: A horseradish peroxidase study in the rat, *J. Comp. Neurol.* **187:**117–144.

Pieri, L., Keller, H. H., Burkard, W., and DaPrada, M., 1978, Effects of lisuride and LSD on cerebral monoamine systems and hallucinosis, *Nature* **252:**586–588.

Pinnock, R. D., and Dray, A., 1982, Differential sensitivity of presumed dopaminergic and non-dopaminergic neurones in rat substantia nigra to electrophoretically applied substance P, *Neurosci. Lett.* **29:**153–158.

Pinnock, R. D., Woodruff, G. N., and Turnbull, M. J., 1983, Actions of substance P, MIF, TRH and related peptides in the substantia nigra, caudate nucleus and nucleus accumbens, *Neuropharmacology* **22:**687–696.

Precht, W., and Yoshida, M., 1971, Blockade of caudate-evoked inhibition of neurons in the substantia nigra by picrotoxin, *Brain Res.* **32:**229–233.

Pycock, C. J., Horton, R. W., and Carter, C. J., 1978, Interactions of 5-hydroxytryptamine and γ-aminobutyric acid with dopamine, in: *Advances in Biochemical Psychopharmacology*, Vol. 19 (P. J. Roberts, G. N. Woodruff, and L. L. Iversen, eds.), Raven Press, New York, pp. 323–341.

Pycock, C. J., Kerwin, R. W., and Carter, C. J., 1980, Effect of lesion of cortical dopamine terminals on subcortical dopamine receptors in rats, *Nature* **286:**74–77.

Quirion, R., Shults, C. W., Moody, T. W., Pert, C. B., Chase, T. N., and O'Donohue, T. L., 1983, Autoradiographic distribution of substance P receptors in rat central nervous system, *Nature* **303:**714–716.

Rebec, G. V., and Groves, P. M., 1975, Apparent feedback from caudate nucleus to the substantia nigra following amphetamine administration, *Neuropharmacology* **14:**275–282.

Reinhard, J. F., Jr., Bannon, M. J., and Roth, R. H., 1982, Acceleration by stress of dopamine synthesis and metabolism in prefrontal cortex: Antagonism by diazepam, *Naunyn-Schmiedeberg's Arch. Pharmacol.* **318:**374–377.

Rosenfeld, M., and Makman, M. H., 1981, The interaction of lisuride, an ergot derivative, with serotonergic and dopaminergic receptors in rabbit brain, *J. Pharmacol. Exp. Ther.* **216:**526–531.

Roth, R. H., 1979, Dopamine autoreceptors: Pharmacology, function and comparison with postsynaptic dopamine receptors, *Commun. Psychopharmacol.* **3:**429–445.

Roth, R. H., 1984, Dopamine autoreceptors: Distribution, pharmacology and function, *Ann. NY Acad. Sci.* **689:**27–53.

ROTH, R. H., MORGENROTH, V. H., and MURRIN, L. C., 1975, The effects of antipsychotic drugs and impulse flow on the kinetics of striatal tyrosine hydroxylase, in: *Antipsychotic Drugs: Pharmacodynamics and Pharmacokinetics* (G. Sedvall, ed.), Pergamon Press, Elmsford, NY, pp. 133–145.

ROTH, R. H., BACOPOULOS, N. G., BUSTOS, G., and REDMOND, D. E., JR., 1980, Antipsychotic drugs: Differential effects on dopamine neurons in basal ganglia and mesocortex following chronic administration in human and nonhuman primates, in: *Advances in Biochemical Psychopharmacology*, Vol. 24 (F. Cattabeni, G. Racagni, P. F. Spano, and E. Costa, eds.), Raven Press, New York, pp. 513–520.

ROTH, R. H., GALLOWAY, M. P., TAM, S.-Y., ONO, N., and WOLF, M. E., 1986, Dopamine autoreceptors: Studies on their distribution and mode of action, in: *Dopaminergic Systems and Their Regulation* (G. N. Woodruff, J. A. Poat, and P. J. Roberts, eds.), Macmillan Press, London, pp. 45–61.

SALT, T. E., DEVRIES, G. J., RODRIGUEZ, R. E., CAHUSAC, P. M. B., MORRIS, R., and HILL, R. G., 1982, Evaluation of (D-Pro^2, D-Trp^{7,9})-substance P as an antagonist of substance P responses in the central nervous system, *Neurosci. Lett.* **30**:291–295.

SCATTON, B., 1977, Differential regional development of tolerance to increase in dopamine turnover upon repeated neuroleptic administration, *Eur. J. Pharmacol.* **46**:363–369.

SCATTON, B., THIERRY, A. M., GLOWINSKI, J., and JULOU, L., 1975a, Effects of thioproperazine and apomorphine on dopamine synthesis in the mesocortical dopaminergic systems, *Brain Res.* **88**:389–393.

SCATTON, B., GARRET, C., and JULOU, L., 1975b, Acute and subacute effects of neuroleptics on dopamine synthesis and release in the rat striatum, *Naunyn-Schmiedeberg's Arch. Pharmacol.* **289**:419–434.

SCATTON, B., GLOWINSKI, J., and JULOU, L., 1976, Dopamine metabolism in the mesolimbic and mesocortical dopaminergic systems after single or repeated administrations of neuroleptics, *Brain Res.* **109**:184–189.

SCATTON, B., BOIREAU, A., GARRET, C., GLOWINSKI, J., and JULOU, L., 1977, Action of the palmitic ester of pipotiazine on dopamine metabolism in the nigro-striatal, meso-limbic and meso-cortical systems, *Naunyn-Schmiedeberg's Arch. Pharmacol.* **296**:169–175.

SCATTON, B., ZIVKOVIC, B., and BARTHOLINI, G., 1980a, Differential influence of GABAergic agents on dopamine metabolism in extrapyramidal and limbic systems of the rat, *Brain Res. Bull.* **5**(suppl. 2):421–425.

SCATTON, B., ZIVKOVIC, B., and DEDEK, J., 1980b, Antidopaminergic properties of yohimbine, *J. Pharmacol. Exp. Ther.* **215**:494–499.

SCATTON, B., DEDEK, J., and ZIVKOVIC, B., 1983, Lack of involvement of α-adrenoceptors in the regulation of striatal dopaminergic transmission, *Eur. J. Pharmacol.* **86**:427–433.

SEDVALL, G., Receptor feedback and dopamine turnover in CNS, in: *Handbook of Psychopharmacology*, Vol. 6 (L. L. Iversen, S. D. Iversen, and S. H. Snyder, eds.), Plenum Press, New York, pp. 127–177.

SHEPARD, P., and GERMAN, D. C., 1984, A subpopulation of mesocortical dopamine neurons possesses autoreceptors, *Eur. J. Pharmacol.* **98**:455–456.

SILBERGELD, E. K., and HRUSKA, R. E., 1979, Lisuride and LSD: dopaminergic and serotonergic interactions in the "serotonergic syndrome," *Psychopharmacology* **65**:233–237.

SIMON, H., LEMOAL, M., and CALAS, A., 1979, Efferents and afferents of the ventral tegmental A10 region after local injection of ^{3}H-leucine and horseradish peroxidase, *Brain Res.* **178**:17–40.

SIMON, H., SCATTON, B., and LEMOAL, M., 1980, Dopaminergic A10 neurones are involved in cognitive functions, *Nature* **286**:150–151.

SKIRBOLL, L. R., GRACE, A. A., and BUNNEY, B. S., 1979, Dopamine auto- and postsynaptic receptors: Electrophysiological evidence for differential sensitivity to dopamine agonists, *Science* **206**:80–82.

SNYDER, S. H., 1972, Catecholamines in the brain as mediators of amphetamine psychosis, *Arch. Gen. Psychiatry* **27**:169–179.

SNYDER, S. H., BANNERJEE, S. P., YAMAMURA, H. I., and GREENBERG, D., 1974, Drugs, neurotransmitters and schizophrenia, *Science* **184**:1243–1253.

STEINFELS, G. F., HEYM, J., and JACOBS, B. L., 1981, Single unit activity of dopaminergic neurons in freely moving cats, *Life Sci.* **29**:1435–1442.

STEVENS, J. R., 1973, An anatomy of schizophrenia? *Arch. Gen. Psychiatr.* **29**:177–189.

SVENSSON, T., BUNNEY, B. S., and AGHAJANIAN, G. K., 1975, Inhibition of both noradrenergic and serotonergic neurons in brain by the α-adrenergic agonist clonidine, *Brain Res.* **92**:291–306.

SWANSON, L. W., 1982, The projections of the ventral tegmental area and adjacent regions: A combined fluorescent retrograde tracer and immunofluorescence study in the rat, *Brain Res. Bull.* **9**:321–353.

TAM, S.-Y., and ROTH, R. H., 1985, Selective increase in dopamine metabolism in the prefrontal cortex by the anxiogenic beta-carboline FG 7142, *Biochem. Pharmacol.* **34**:1595–1598.

TAM, S.-Y., BANNON, M. J., and ROTH, R. H., 1983, Apomorphine selectively reverses the impulse induced increase in dopamine synthesis in mesocortical dopamine neurons with autoreceptors, *Soc. Neurosci. Abstr.* **9**:1004.

TASSIN, J. P., STINUS, L., SIMON, H., BLANC, G., THIERRY, A. M., LEMOAL, M., CARDO, B., and GLOWINSKI, J., 1978, Relationship between the locomotor hyperactivity induced by A10 lesions and the destruction of the fronto-cortical dopaminergic innervation in the rat, *Brain Res.* **141**:267–281.

THIERRY, A. M., BLANC, G., SOBEL, A., STINUS, L., and GLOWINSKI, J., 1973a, Dopaminergic terminals in the rat cortex, *Science* **182**:499–501.

THIERRY, A. M., STINUS, L., BLANC, G., and GLOWINSKI, J., 1973b, Some evidence for the existence of dopaminergic neurons in the rat cortex, *Brain Res.* **50**:230–234.

THIERRY, A. M., TASSIN, J. P., BLANC, G., and GLOWINSKI, J., 1978, Studies on mesocortical dopamine systems, in: *Advances in Biochemical Psychopharmacology*, Vol. 19 (P. J. Roberts, G. N. Woodruff, and L. L. Iversen, eds.), Raven Press, New York, pp. 205–216.

TRULSON, M. E., and PREUSSLER, D. W., 1984, Dopamine-containing ventral tegmental area neurons in freely moving cats: Activity during the sleep-waking cycle and effects of stress, *Exp. Neurol.* **83**:367–377.

TRULSON, M. E., PREUSSLER, D. W., and HOWELL, G. A., 1981, Activity of substantia nigra units across the sleep-waking cycle in freely moving cats, *Neurosci. Lett.* **26**:183–188.

UNGERSTEDT, U., 1971, Stereotaxic mapping of the monoamine pathways in the rat brain, *Acta Physiol. Scand.* Suppl. **367**:1–48.

VON HUNGEN, K., and ROBERTS, S., 1973, Adenylate cyclase receptors for adrenergic neurotransmitters in rat cerebral cortex, *Eur. J. Biochem.* **36**:391–401.

WADDINGTON, J. L., and CROSS, A. J., 1978, Neurochemical changes following kainic acid lesions of the nucleus accumbens: Implications for a GABA-ergic accumbal-ventral tegmental pathway, *Life Sci.* **22**:1011–1014.

WALASS, I., and FONNUM, F., 1980, Biochemical evidence for γ-aminobutyrate containing fibres from the nucleus accumbens to the substantia nigra and ventral tegmental area in the rat, *Neuroscience* **5**:63–72.

WALDMEIER, P. C., 1980, Serotonergic modulation of mesolimbic and frontal cortical dopamine neurons, *Experentia* **36**:1092–1094.

WALTERS, J. R., and LAKOSKI, J. M., 1978, Effect of muscimol on single unit activity of substantia nigra dopamine neurons, *Eur. J. Pharmacol.* **47**:469–471.

WALTERS, J. R., and ROTH, R. H., 1976, Dopaminergic neurons: An *in vivo* system for measuring drug interactions with presynaptic receptors, *Naunyn-Schmiedeberg's Arch. Pharmacol.* **296**:5–14.

WALTERS, J. R., ROTH, R. H., and AGHAJANIAN, G. K., 1973, Dopaminergic neurons: Similar biochemical and histochemical effects of γ-hydroxybutyrate and acute lesions of the nigro-neostriatal pathway, *J. Pharmacol. Exp. Ther.* **186**:630–639.

WALTERS, J. R., BARING, M. D., and LAKOSKI, J. M., 1979, Effects of ergolines on dopaminergic and serotonergic single unit activity, in: *Dopaminergic Ergot Derivatives and Motor Function* (K. Fuxe and D. B. Calne, eds.), Pergamon Press, Elmsford, NY, pp. 207–221.

WANG, R. Y., 1981a, Dopaminergic neurons of the rat ventral tegmental area. I. Identification and characterization, *Brain Res. Rev.* **3:**123–140.

WANG, R. Y., 1981b, Dopaminergic neurons of the rat ventral tegmental area II. Evidence for autoregulation, *Brain Res. Rev.* **3:**141–151.

WANG, R. Y., 1981c, Dopaminergic neurons of the rat ventral tegmental area III. Effects of D- and L-amphetamine, *Brain Res. Rev.* **3:**153–165.

WANG, R. Y., WHITE, F. J., and VOIGT, M. M., 1984, Effects of dopamine agonists on midbrain dopamine cell activity, in: *Catecholamines* (E. Usdin, A. Carlsson, A. Dahlström, and J. Engel, eds.), Pergamon Press, Elmsford, NY, pp. 359–367.

WASZCZAK, E. L., and WALTERS, J. R., 1980, Intravenous GABA agonist administration stimulates firing of A10 dopaminergic neurons, *Eur. J. Pharmacol.* **66:**141–144.

WASZCZAK, B. L., ENG, N., and WALTERS, J. R., 1980, Effects of muscimol and picrotoxin on single unit activity of substantia nigra neurons, *Brain Res.* **188:**185–197.

WESTERINK, B. H. C., and KORF, J., 1976, Acidic dopamine metabolites in cortical areas of the rat brain: Localization and effects of drugs, *Brain Res.* **13:**429–434.

WHEELER, S. C., and ROTH, R. H., 1980, Tolerance to fluphenazine and supersensitivity to apomorphine in central dopaminergic systems after chronic fluphenazine treatment, *Naunyn-Schmiedeberg's Arch. Pharmacol.* **312:**151–159.

WHITE, F. J., and WANG, R. Y., 1983a, Comparison of the effects of chronic haloperidol treatment on A9 and A10 dopamine neurons in the rat, *Life Sci.* **32:**983–993.

WHITE, F. J., and WANG, R. Y., 1983b, Differential effects of classical and atypical antipsychotic drugs on A9 and A10 dopamine neurons, *Science* **221:**1054–1057.

WHITE, F. J., and WANG, R. Y., 1983c, Comparison of LSD and lisuride on A10 dopamine neurons in the rat, *Neuropharmacology* **22:**669–676.

WHITE, F. J., and WANG, R. Y., 1984a, Pharmacological characterization of dopamine autoreceptors in rat ventral tegmental area: Microiontophoretic studies, *J. Pharmacol. Exp. Ther.* **231:**275–280.

WHITE, F. J., and WANG, R. Y., 1984b, A10 dopamine neurons: role of autoreceptors in determining firing rate and sensitivity to dopamine agonists, *Life Sci.* **34:**1161–1170.

WOLF, M. E., and ROTH, R. H., 1987, Dopamine neurons projecting to the medial prefrontal cortex possess release-modulating autoreceptors, *Neuropharmacology* (in press).

WOLF, P., OLPE, H-R., AVRITH, D., and HAAS, H. L., 1978, GABAergic inhibition of neurons in the ventral tegmental area, *Experientia* **34:**73–74.

YIM, C. Y., and MOGENSON, G. J., 1980a, Electrophysiological studies of neurons in the ventral tegmental area of Tsai, *Brain Res.* **181:**301–313.

YIM, C. Y., and MOGENSON, G. J., 1980b, Effect of picrotoxin and nipecotic acid on inhibitory response of dopaminergic neurons in the ventral tegmental area to stimulation of the nucleus accumbens, *Brain Res.* **199:**466–472.

6

PSYCHOPHARMACOLOGY OF REPEATED SEIZURES: POSSIBLE RELEVANCE TO THE MECHANISM OF ACTION OF ELECTROCONVULSIVE THERAPY

A. Richard Green and David J. Nutt

1. INTRODUCTION

The last few years have seen a marked increase in the research on the biochemical and pharmacological consequences of repeated electroconvulsive shock (ECS), for several reasons. The first reason is that electroconvulsive therapy (ECT) is still acknowledged as the most successful treatment for severe depressive illness (see Brandon *et al.*, 1984: Royal College of Psychiatrists, 1977; Fink, 1979). The second reason is that greater insight has now been gained into the mechanism of action of antidepressant drugs, so it seems reasonable to determine whether the experimental effects of ECS are similar to those of the drugs. The third reason is that ECT remains a controversial treatment, and thus a greater understanding of its mechanism of action may eventually lead to the develop-

---

A. Richard Green • MRC Clinical Pharmacology Unit, Radcliffe Infirmary, Oxford OX2 6HE, England. Present address: Astra Neuroscience Research Unit, 1 Wakefield Street, London WC1N 1PJ, England.   *David J. Nutt* • Department of Psychiatry, Research Unit, Littlemore Hospital, Oxford OX4 4NX, England. Present address: National Institute for Alcohol Abuse and Alcoholism, Bethesda, Maryland 20205.

ment of a pharmacological agent with the efficacy of ECT but, it is to be hoped, fewer side effects and less public disquiet.

Although it is reasonable to try and compare and contrast the effects of ECS with those of antidepressant drugs in experimental animals, one should be aware of the potential pitfalls. Our own view is that the action of these drugs should be studied following chronic administration and while the drugs are still being administered, not, as is sometimes done, after withdrawal (see Goodwin *et al.*, 1984). However, the presence of the drug in the tissue can be a complicating factor. We say this because therapeutic effects normally occur while the patient is on medication. There is no such problem with ECS because there is no drug present. Furthermore, one should not assume that drugs and ECS should necessarily produce the same pharmacological effects. Although similarities may be important indicators of possible mechanisms of therapeutic action, differences may be equally important. After all, patients often respond to ECT when they have failed to improve on antidepressant drugs, and it may be that such differences will eventually lead to our understanding the mechanism of action of ECT.

Several years ago we adapted criteria suggested by Fink (1974) to be necessary to fulfill when searching for a possible therapeutic mechanism in experimental animals. These were published (Grahame-Smith *et al.*, 1978) and are reproduced below.

1. Generally a single treatment with ECT is insufficient to produce detectable clinical improvement. The effect of ECS should be to produce a change that evolves gradually, the ECS initiating the change that is sustained by repeated application.
2. The method of inducing the seizure is not important, rather the number and frequency of the seizures is.
3. Subconvulsive shocks should not induce the change. It is the seizure that is the essential component.
4. Neuromuscular blocking drugs do not alter the response.
5. Any hypothesis resulting from animal experiments should try to exclude nonspecific effects, such as hypoxia.

Although we feel that these criteria are still relevant, one caveat should be added. This is that important changes may be present after a single seizure. Presumably, some biochemical change must be occurring after even a single ECS, which initiates further changes and result in the long-term alterations responsible for the therapeutic effect of ECT. This therapeutic change is presumably consolidated by both further treatments and the passage of time, since both are necessary for the antidepressant activity of ECT (see Fink, 1979).

In this review we shall discuss predominantly the changes in CNS function and biochemistry that occur after repeated ECS but will, as necessary, outline changes that occur after a single ECS when we think they may be relevant to the longer-term effects. First, we shall deal with alterations of *in vivo* function as revealed by neurotransmitter-induced behavioral effects, and then we shall consider the biochemical pharmacological effects of ECS on *in vitro* preparations.

2. FUNCTIONAL CHANGES AFTER SEIZURES

2.1. 5-Hydroxytryptamine

In 1976, it was first reported that repeated ECS (one ECS daily for 10 days) administration to rats resulted in their displaying enhanced behavioral responses to administration of tranylcypromine/L-tryptophan 24 hr after the last shock (Evans *et al.*, 1976). Enhanced responses to the 5-hydroxytryptamine (5-HT) agonist 5-methoxy-*N,N*-dimethyltryptamine (5-MeODMT) were also seen, suggesting a postsynaptic change (Evans *et al.*, 1976). This work was extended to show that ECS enhanced the response to the agonist quipazine and that this enhancement lasted approximately 1 week after the last ECS (Green *et al.*, 1977). The enhancement does not require fully matured neuronal systems in the brain, since immature rats also display enhanced responses to 5-HT agonists after repeated ECS (Atterwill and Green, 1980).

Enhanced 5-HT-mediated behavioral changes could be elicited when ECS was given in a way closely mimicking the clinical administration of ECT; that is, enhancement was seen when five ECS were spread out over 10 days and the rats were given both an anesthetic and a muscle relaxant (Costain *et al.*, 1979). Furthermore, changing the features of the ECS administration that are not thought to be important in the clinical outcome (bilateral or unilateral electrode placement, fractional or sinusoidal current) did not in any way affect the appearance of the enhanced behavior. Conversely, when the ECS was given in ways that do not produce therapeutic improvement (several seizures in one day or a subconvulsant shock), enhanced 5-HT-mediated behaviors were not observed (Grahame-Smith *et al.*, 1978; Costain *et al.*, 1979). Increasing the duration of electric shock or the voltage used did not reduce the number of treatments necessary for the enhanced behavior to be observed (Cowen *et al.*, 1980*a*).

There is good evidence that it is the seizure that is necessary for clinical improvement, not the passage of electricity, and in this regard there are several clinical studies demonstrating that a course of seizures induced by the inhalant convulsant flurothyl has an antidepressant effect (see Fink, 1979). Repeated seizures in rats produced by flurothyl also led to enhanced 5-HT-mediated behavior (Green, 1978) as did a series of seizures produced by intravenous injection of the GABA antagonist drug bicuculline (Nutt et al., 1980a).

In 1981, Lebrecht and Nowak demonstrated that repeated ECS enhanced head-twitch behaviors in mice induced by 5-hydroxytryptophan (5-HTP) administration, and this was confirmed and extended by Green et al. (1983a), who showed that the behavior was enhanced by ECS over a wide range of doses of 5-HTP (Figure. 1).

Several procedures have been shown to interfere with the appearance of the enhanced 5-HT-mediated behavior seen in rats and mice after repeated ECS. A lesion of the locus ceruleus and ascending noradrenergic

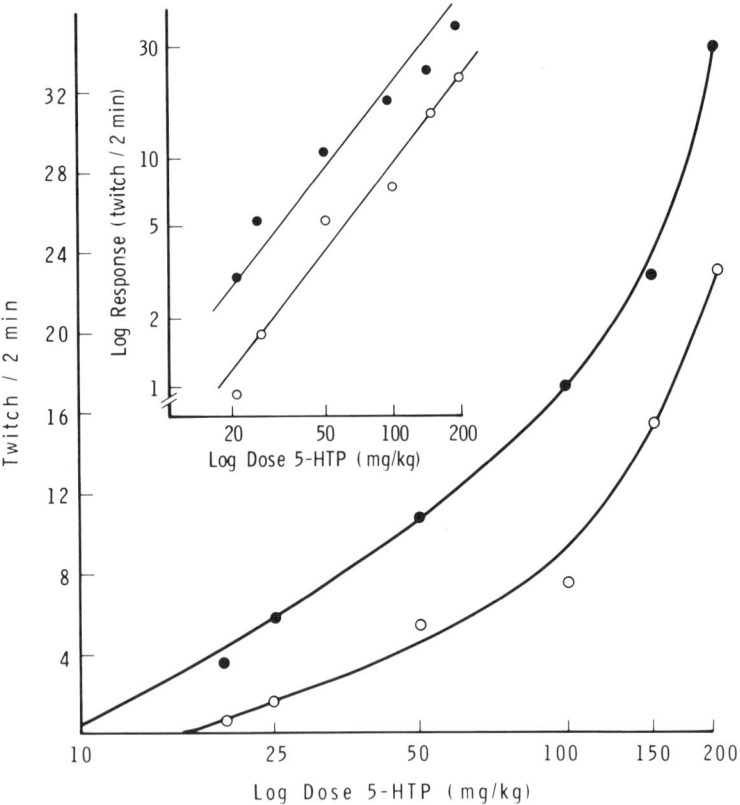

FIG. 1. Effect of repeated ECS on the behavioral response to carbidopa and 5-hydroxytryptophan (5-HTP). Mice were given either five ECS spread over 10 days (●) or five anesthetic exposures only (○). Twenty-four hours after the last treatment, both groups were given carbidopa (25 mg/kg) followed by various doses of 5-hydroxytryptophan. The main graph shows the log dose of 5-HTP versus the total number of head twitches in 2 min, 30 min after the 5-HTP. The small graph shows the log dose–log response curve. Experimental group significantly different from control group ($p < .05$ or better) at every dose. Eight animals used at each dose point.

bundles with 6-hydroxydopamine (6-OHDA), which markedly depleted brain noradrenaline (NA) concentration, did not, in itself, alter the behavioral response to the 5-HT agonist quipazine. It did, however, totally abolish the enhancement of this behavior by ECS (Green and Deakin, 1980; Green et al., 1980). This finding has recently been confirmed by Goodwin and Heal (1985), who used another agent, DSP-4 [N-(2-chloroeythyl-N-ethyl-bromobenzylamine)], to lesion NA pathways.

The administration of either p-chlorophenylalanine (PCPA) or the 5-HT antagonist methysergide during ECS administration also abolished the enhanced 5-HT-mediated behavior (Green et al., 1980). In addition, injection of subconvulsant doses of the GABA antagonist drugs bicuculline or pentylenetetrazol immediately before each ECS prevented the enhancement of the 5-HT-mediated behavior (Green et al., 1982), as did injection of diazepam (Bhavsar et al., 1981; Green and Mountford, 1985). The effect with diazepam did not appear to be merely an interference with the severity of the seizure, since it had the same effect when it was given postictally. This suggests that it is interfering with postconvulsion mechanisms, which are important in inducing changes in 5-HT function (Green and Mountford, 1985). This view is also supported by the work of Bhavsar et al. (1981), who found that administration of phenytoin, a potent antagonist of the tonic component of electrically induced seizures, did not block the ECS-induced enhancement of 5-HT-mediated behavior.

In contrast, hypophysectomy did not alter the ability of ECS to increase 5-HT-mediated behavior; this suggests that the pituitary hormone release seen following ECT administration (see Fink, 1979) is not responsible for the change in 5-HT-mediated behavior in rodents (Nutt et al., 1982).

Enhanced 5-HT-mediated responses have also been reported in a model not requiring locomotor activity. Vetulani et al. (1981) observed that repeated ECS enhanced the hyperpyrexia produced by 5-HT agonists in animals kept at a high ambient temperature. Repeated ECS also raises basal body temperature in rats (Horrell, 1981; Minchin and Nutt, 1984), perhaps because of increased tonic 5-HT function.

Very recently, this laboratory investigated the pharmacology of putative $5-HT_1$ agonists. 5-Methoxy-(1,2,3,6-tetrahydropyridin-4-yl)-1H-indole (RU 24969) produced marked locomotor activity (Green et al., 1984a) and this response was enhanced by repeated ECS. However, this might have been the result of an ECS alteration of dopamine function (see Section 2.2), since dopamine is involved in the RU 24969-induced locomotor response (Green et al., 1984a). Such proposals must remain fairly speculative, since the pharmacology of this compound is not well understood.

Another putative $5-HT_1$ agonist is 8-hydroxy-(di-N-propylamino)tetralin (8-OH-DPAT), and we have recently performed fairly extensive pharmacological investigations in the mouse on this compound

(Goodwin *et al.*, 1985*a*). Basically, in mice, it appears to be acting primarily as a presynaptic 5-HT$_1$ agonist, and it produces a marked hypothermic response. Antagonists of a variety of neurotransmitter receptors have no effect on this hypothermic response (Goodwin *et al.*, 1985*a*). Repeated ECS administration produced a marked and sustained attenuation of this hypothermic response, a change also seen after longer-term administration of several antidepressant drugs (Goodwin *et al.*, 1985*b*).

2.2. Dopamine

The first report of enhanced dopamine-mediated behavior following ECS was that of Modigh (1975), who reported that repeated ECS resulted in an enhanced response of mice to apomorphine. Recently, the ability of ECS to enhance this behavior over a wide range of apomorphine doses has been reported (Green *et al.*, 1983*a*). Evans *et al.* (1976) observed an enhancement of the behavioral responses of rats to tranylcypromine plus L-dopa, a finding confirmed by Deakin *et al.* (1981). Green *et al.* (1977) also found ECS-treated rats to be more responsive to the dopamine-releasing drug metamphetamine. Enhancement to dopamine agonists has also been reported by Wielosz (1981) and Bhavsar *et al.* (1981).

There are clear indications that the enhanced responses are not the result of a pharmacokinetic change in agonist distribution after ECS, since both Modigh and Jackson (1975) and Heal and Green (1978) observed that ECS-treated rats had greater locomotor responses to dopamine injected directly into the nucleus accumbens, a technique that bypasses the blood–brain barrier (Heal *et al.*, 1978).

It appears that intact presynaptic dopamine function is unnecessary for the enhanced responses to occur in rats after ECS, since unilateral nigrostriatal-lesioned rats showed increased circling responses not only to metamphetamine but also to apomorphine (Green *et al.*, 1977). The latter response is the result of apomorphine acting on the lesioned side, which implies that enhanced responses are being produced by changes "beyond" the dopamine synapse. This interpretation is supported by two studies. First, Heal and Green (1978) found that ECS-treated rats showed increased behavioral responses to dibutyryl cyclic AMP injected into the nucleus accumbens. This drug acts at the postsynaptic dopamine site but beyond the receptor; that is, it increases dopamine function even when haloperidol is present (Heal *et al.*, 1978). Second, it was observed that haloperidol administration shortly before each ECS did not prevent enhanced dopamine-mediated behaviors (Green *et al.*, 1980).

The studies cited all examined apomorphine- or amphetamine-induced locomotor responses. At higher doses, these drugs produced stereotyped behavior (stereotypy). In general, there is good agreement that ECS also enhances this behavior. Thus, enhanced stereotypy after ECS has been reported by Modigh (1979), Serra *et al.* (1981), Bhavsar *et al.* (1981), Globus *et al.* (1981), but not Wielosz (1981).

In an analogous manner to the effects of seizure on 5-HT-mediated behavior, it has been shown that repeated bicuculline-induced convulsions (Nutt *et al.*, 1980a) or flurothyl-induced convulsions (Green, 1978) both enhanced behavioral responses of rats to tranylcypromine/L-dopa or dopamine mimetic drugs. Indeed, the effects of flurothyl and ECS were additive over time, to produce the same final enhancement (Green, 1978); that is, ECS given for 4 days (which does not produce enhancement) plus flurothyl for 4 days produced an equivalent enhancement to that seen after 8 days of ECS.

Enhanced responses to tranylcypromine/L-dopa could be demonstrated after fewer bicuculline-induced seizures than were necessary to produce enhanced 5-HT-mediated behavior (Nutt *et al.*, 1980a; Cowen *et al.*, 1980a). Furthermore, fewer bicuculline-induced seizures were required to enhance dopamine-mediated behavior than ECS-induced seizures. However, there is evidence that this was the result of the anesthetic given with the ECS, which delayed the appearance of the enhanced behavior. Increased responses occurred more rapidly if ECS was given without anesthetic (Cowen *et al.*, 1980a). This effect did not appear to be due to the anesthetic modifying the seizure and making it less severe (which it does), because anesthetics given after an unmodified seizure had the same effect. It seems likely that the anesthetics were interfering with the postictal changes that are necessary to initiate the mechanisms responsible for enhanced behavior (Cowen *et al.*, 1980a; Nutt *et al.*, 1980a).

A 6-OHDA lesion of the noradrenergic system in the brain did not modify dopamine-mediated behavior but did abolish the ECS-induced enhancement of the behavior (Green and Deakin, 1980; Green *et al.*, 1980). Administration of pentylenetetrazol, bicuculline, or diazepam before each ECS (or after, in the case of diazepam) abolished the ECS-induced enhancement of dopamine-mediated responses (Green *et al.*, 1982; Green and Mountford, 1985). Hypophysectomy did not alter the ability of ECS to induce increased dopamine-mediated behavior (Nutt *et al.*, 1982).

All the above behavioral changes are almost certainly the result of postsynaptic dopamine receptor activation. Serra *et al.* (1981) have suggested that ECS may also alter presynaptic dopamine receptors. They found that repeated ECS attenuated the sedative response of a low dose of apomorphine. No change was seen after a single ECS, in contrast to the report of Chiodo and Antelman (1980), who observed long-term antagonism of sedation after a single ECS. Caution should be exercised, however, as to the site of the receptor in the light of the biochemical data of Serra *et al.* (1981) (see Section 3.2) and also the failure of Creese *et al.*

(1982) to observe evidence for dopamine autoreceptor subsensitivity after ECS.

In a model not relying on motor activity, White and Barnett (1981) have shown a greater sensitivity of rats to the discriminative stimulus properties of both amphetamine and apomorphine after ECS daily for 3 days. This would again suggest increased dopaminergic function.

2.3. Noradrenaline

2.3.1. α_2-Adrenoceptor Function

The administration of a low dose of clonidine to mice or rats produces a sedative response, which has been postulated to be the result of the activation of the presynaptic α_2-adrenoceptor (Drew *et al.*, 1979). We used this behavior to investigate the function of this receptor following ECS.

A single ECS had no effect on this behavioral response. However, repeated ECS partly attenuated the response (Fig. 2) in both rats and mice

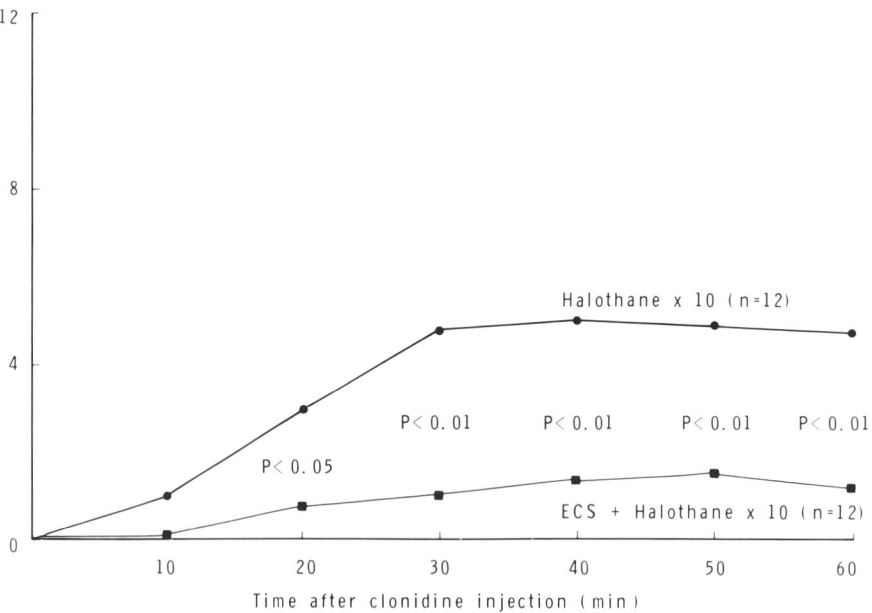

FIG. 2. Effect of repeated ECS on clonidine-induced hypoactivity in rats. Rats were given either a single ECS while under halothane anesthesia (■—■) or halothane anesthesia alone (●—●) once daily for 10 days. Both groups were injected with clonidine (0.1 mg/kg) 24 hr after the final treatment. Hypoactivity, shown as mean total score, was plotted against time after clonidine injection. Results were analyzed using the Wilcoxon's rank order test; where results are significantly different, significance levels are shown.

(Heal et al., 1981). This ECS-induced change is the same as that seen following the administration of several other antidepressant drugs (see Sugrue, 1982; Heal et al., 1983).

Pilc and Vetulani (1982) examined the hypothermic response to clonidine and found that repeated ECS attenuated this response as well.

There is also one indication that repeated ECS might alter postsynaptic α_2-adrenoceptors. Modigh (1975) demonstrated that, in reserpinized mice given apomorphine to restore dopamine function, the behavioral response to clonidine was enhanced after repeated ECS.

2.3.2. α_1-Adrenoceptor Function

Two models have been proposed as indicators of α_1-adrenoceptor function, and these yield conflicting data with regard to the effect of repeated ECS. Vetulani and Pilc (1982) proposed that quantification of postdecapitation convulsions in rats measures α_1-adrenoceptor function, since they are inhibited by α_1-adrenoceptor antagonists but not by either α_2- or β-adrenoceptor antagonists (see Vetulani, 1984). Vetulani (1984) reported that repeated ECS increases postdecapitation convulsion number, which suggests an increase in α_1-adrenoceptor function.

Heal (1984) used locomotor response in mice, following central injection of phenylephrine, as a measure of α_1-adrenoceptor function. This response is inhibited by α_1-adrenoceptor antagonists but not α_2-adrenoceptor antagonists, and the model has been quite extensively characterized pharmacologically (Heal, 1984). Using this model, Heal (1984) found no evidence for change in α_1-adrenoceptor function following repeated ECS.

2.4. GABA

Two main approaches have been used to determine whether GABA function is changed after repeated ECS. The first approach involved the effect of ECS on haloperidol-induced catalepsy. Low doses of haloperidol induce catalepsy in rats. This cataleptogenic effect of haloperidol is enhanced by increased GABA function (Keller et al., 1976; Worms and Lloyd, 1978; Davies and Williams, 1978) and decreased by GABA antagonists (Worms and Lloyd, 1978; Green et al., 1979). It was suggested, therefore, that one might be able to assess changes in GABA function by observing changes in the cataleptic response to haloperidol. A single ECS produced a modest and short-lasting attenuation of the cataleptic effect of haloperidol. Following longer-term (10 days) ECS administration, however, the attenuation was marked and lasted for several days after the last ECS (Fig. 3; Green et al., 1979).

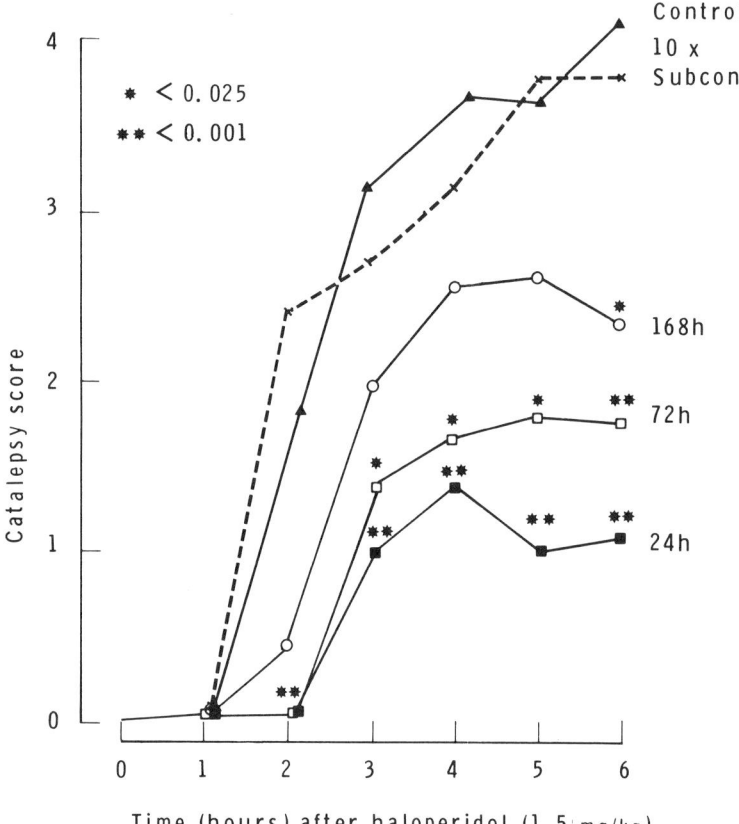

FIG. 3. Cataleptic response to haloperidol at various times following a single electroconvulsive shock given daily for 10 days (ECS × 10). Rats were given a single ECS daily for 10 days, and the cataleptic response during 6 hr following haloperidol (1.5 mg/kg) was measured 24 hr (■), 72 hr (□), and 168 hr (○) after the final shock. Anesthetic only (control) response (▲) and cataleptic response 24 hr after the final shock of 10 subconvulsive shocks (one daily for 10 days) (x) also shown. Significantly different from the control response *$p < .025$; **$p < .001$. Number of observations; control: 13; 24 hr: 16; 72 hr: 8; 168 hr: 7; subconvulsive: 6.

Nutt et al. (1981) used a very different approach. Seizure threshold can be determined by an infusion of convulsant drugs. It was felt, therefore, that changes in GABA receptor function might be reflected in changes in the seizure threshold measured by GABA antagonist drug infusion. A single ECS was found to produce a rise in seizure threshold of around 40%, which was maintained for 2–3 hr after the convulsion (Nutt et al., 1981; Fig. 4). This rise was also seen 30 min after the last of 10 once-daily ECS and seemed to be selective for convulsant drugs acting at the GABA–benzodiazepine receptor complex, since the threshold to strychnine and quipazine was unaltered. This finding of rise in seizure threshold after a single ECS has recently been confirmed by Tacke et al. (1984).

Investigations of GABA function using seizure threshold measurements have also been made 24 hr after the last of a course of 10 once-daily ECS (Nutt et al., 1980b). No change in threshold was detected to bicuculline or pentylenetetrazol. A reduced threshold to picrotoxin was observed, but this may have been artifactual, since later experiments with the potent picrotoxin-site ligand isopropylbicyclophosphate (IPTBO) showed no change (Cowen et al., 1980b).

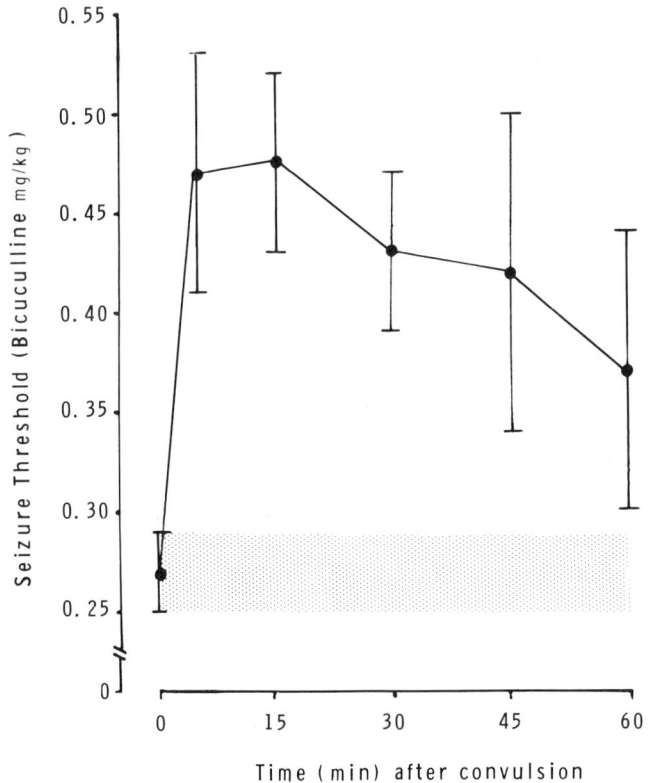

FIG. 4. The dose of bicuculline necessary to elicit a seizure at various times following an electroconvulsive shock. Rats were either handled or given an ECS. Results shown as mean dose; SD shown by vertical bars. Six or more determinations, each on a separate rat, were made for each value. Handled control values (mean ± SD) shown as stippled area. All values 5–45 min of experimental group different from controls $p < .001$, 60-min value different from control $p < .01$, and 60-min value lower than 15-min value $p < .05$. Ordinate seizure threshold (bicuculline mg/kg).

Using a somewhat different approach, Minchin and Nutt (1984) found that repeated ECS did not alter the anticonvulsant effect of THIP in rats, a GABA agonist, again suggesting that GABA receptor function in seizure control is unaltered by repeated ECS. However, the hypothermic effect of THIP was reduced, although the elevation of basal body temperature noted previously (Section 2.1) makes interpretation of this finding somewhat difficult.

The anticonvulsant effects of drugs acting at the other sites of the GABA/benzodiazepine receptor complex have also been studied following repeated ECS. Phenobarbitone and sodium valproate produced similar elevations in threshold in both ECS-treated rats, and controls. In contrast, the threshold elevation produced by diazepam was greater in ECS-treated animals (Cowen and Nutt, 1982). Subsequent work suggested that this latter effect was likely to have a pharmacokinetic basis, brain levels of diazepam were higher in the ECS group (Davies and Nutt, 1983).

2.5. Acetylcholine

The cholinomimetic arecoline also induces catalepsy (see Section 2.4), and it has been suggested that the locus of this action is the substantia nigra or globus pallidus (Costall and Olley, 1971). Repeated ECS also attenuates this cataleptic response (Green *et al.*, 1979), a finding supported by the observations of Stanley and Lerer (1985), who noted a similar effect with another cholinomimetic drug, pilocarpine. However, the mechanism involved in this change remains obscure.

2.6. Opioids

The effects of ECS on opiate receptor-induced changes have been studied by several groups. These studies were initiated by the observation that a single ECS produced a cataleptic response that was indistinguishable from morphine-or β-endorphin-induced catalepsy (Holaday and Belenky, 1980). Naloxone significantly attenuated the catalepsy without affecting seizure intensity or duration (Holaday *et al.*, 1978; Holaday and Belenky, 1980; Frenk *et al.*, 1979; Myslobodsky *et al.*, 1981). This is interpreted as indicating that ECS releases endorphins. In support of this, it was shown that ECS produced an increase in tail-flick and hotplate escape times, which was reversed by naloxone (Holaday and Belenky, 1980). The tail-flick test was subsequently difficult to replicate (see Belenky *et al.*, 1984).

Electroconvulsive shock was also observed to depress respiration (as do opiates), and this effect of ECS was also reversed by naloxone (Belenky and Holaday, 1979). A study of EEG following an ECS revealed that the seizure produced a period of postictal depression with high-voltage cortical synchrony similar to that seen after β-endorphin (Tortella et al., 1981).

This work was followed by studies on repeated ECS in rats. Twenty-four hours following the last ECS of a series given once daily for 9 days, rat sensitivity to morphine was determined. The rats showed a greater cataleptic response to morphine and increased tail-flick latencies. Repeated ECS had, therefore, clearly sensitized the rats to opiates (Belenky and Holaday, 1981). These authors also showed cross-sensitization, in that the postictal catalepic effect and tail-flick latency were increased in morphine-dependent rats (Belenky and Holaday, 1981). In both these situations, then, repeated ECS and morphine dependence, the animals showed greater sensitivity to morphine rather than less sensitivity or tolerance, as might have been expected. This apparent paradox has nevertheless been extended by the work of Myslobodsky and Mintz (1981), who showed that postictal rigidity and analgesia increased with repeated ECS.

2.7. Histamine

Impromidine, a potent histamine H_2-receptor agonist (Durant et al., 1978), produces hypothermia in rats (Pilc et al., 1980). This response was attenuated by repeated ECS (Vetulani, 1984).

3. BIOCHEMICAL CONSEQUENCES OF SEIZURES

3.1. 5-Hydroxytryptamine

There have been a variety of studies on the effect of single and repeated seizures on brain 5-HT concentrations and the synthesis rate of 5-HT.

There have been contradictory reports on changes in 5-HT concentration and synthesis in whole brain and brain regions, as well on the concentration of brain tryptophan (Essman, 1973; Shields, 1972; Gandolfi et al., 1978; Feighner et al., 1972; Evans et al., 1976; Lebrecht and Nowak, 1980b), after a single seizure. Although such changes may well be important to longer-term effects of ECS, contradictory data were obtained from different laboratories, so since the thrust of this chapter is on longer-term changes, a detailed review is not attempted here.

When repeated ECS therapy was given over a period of time, no marked differences in 5-HT concentration or synthesis rate, at least 24 hr following the last seizure (see, for example, Evans et al., 1976; Modigh,

1976), were observed. Although no alteration in 5-HT release was observed in brain slices obtained from rats given repeated ECS (Minchin et al., 1983), a change in uptake was observed. However, this change has proved elusive in subsequent studies in our laboratory (Minchin and Green, unpublished observations), and the original report should be treated with caution, particularly since Kellar (1984) has also failed to observe any change.

Initial binding studies suggested that the 5-HT receptor was also unchanged (Atterwill, 1980; Deakin et al., 1981). However, the identification of 5-HT receptor subtypes (Peroutka and Snyder, 1979) led to a reassessment of the effect of repeated ECS, which was prompted particularly by the observations of Peroutka and Snyder (1980) that repeated administration of various antidepressant drugs decreased the binding in the cortex of [^{3}H]spiperone, a ligand used for the 5-HT$_2$ receptor subtype. In 1981, two papers reported that repeated ECS increased the [^{3}H]spiperone receptor number (B_{max}) (Kellar et al., 1981a; Vetulani et al., 1981). It seemed reasonable to propose that this change in 5-HT$_2$ receptor number was responsible for the increase in 5-HT-mediated behaviors seen after repeated ECS (Section 2.1). This proposal was subsequently investigated. Vetulani et al. (1981) and Kellar et al. (1981a) investigated the effects of either a single ECS (no change in 5-HT$_2$ receptor number) or ECS given daily for 8–10 days without anesthetic (35–40% increase in 5-HT$_2$ receptor number). However, enhanced behavior is seen in rats following repeated ECS given with an anesthetic or indeed after five ECS given over 10 days (Costain et al., 1979). Green et al. (1983b) subsequently demonstrated that the 5-HT$_2$ receptor number also increased when ECS was given in these other treatment regimens (Table 1). In addition, there was a small change in K_D after ECS given five times in 10 days (Table 1); this may not be of much significance, however, since Kellar et al. (1981a) did not find any changes in K_D. Green et al. (1983b) also observed that the administration of pentylenetetrazol before each ECS abolished the increase in B_{max} of [^{3}H]spiperone binding (Table 1). Interestingly, this treatment also prevented the increase in 5-HT-mediated behavior (Section 2.1). Finally, using single-point binding studies, it was observed that administration of PCPA or α-methyl-p-tyrosine during the period of ECS also abolished the increase in binding (Table 2), and again these procedures prevented ECS from enhancing 5-HT-mediated behavior (Green et al., 1983b).

In a second study, the effect of repeated ECS was examined on 5-HTP-induced head-twitch behavior in mice (see Section 2.1) and [^{3}H]spiperone binding in mouse frontal cortex. This approach was chosen because head-twitch behavior is almost certainly 5-HT$_2$ receptor-mediated (see the review of Green and Heal, 1985; also Goodwin and Green, 1985), and it allowed a comparison with a study of the effects of antidepressant

TABLE 1
Effect of Various ECS Treatment Regimens on 5-HT$_2$ Receptor Binding Characteristics in Rat Frontal Cortex[a]

	5-HT$_2$ receptor binding characteristics	
	K_d (nM)	B_{max} (pmol mg^{-1} protein)
Control (handled)	1.23 ± 0.09 (3)	350 ± 15 (3)
ECS × 1	1.32 ± 0.17 (5)	379 ± 38 (5)
ECS × 10	1.63 ± 0.14 (6)	472 ± 32 (6)
Control (anesthetized × 5)	1.32 ± 0.01 (3)	356 ± 7 (3)
ECS × 5	1.65 ± 0.04 (4)*	494 ± 40 (4)**
Control (PTZ)	1.04 ± 0.07 (4)	275 ± 24 (4)
ECS × 5 + PTZ	1.02 ± 0.02 (4)	307 + 7 (4)

[a]All measurements were made 24 hr after the last treatment. ECS × 1 is a single ECS, ECS × 10 is ECS once daily for 10 days. ECS × 5 is 5 ECS spread over 10 days. Pentylenetetrazol (PTZ; 30 mg kg^{-1}) was given 3 min before the ECS. ECS × 5 treated rats were given halothane anesthesia. Results are expressed as mean ± SEM with the number of separate experiments in parentheses. Different from appropriate control: **$p < .05$; *$p < .01$. Correlation coefficient (r) 0.9 or better on every analysis.

drug administration. Repeated ECS increased both the behavior and 5-HT$_2$ receptor number in the mouse frontal cortex (Goodwin et al., 1984).

Studies of 5-HT$_1$ receptors (Bergström and Kellar, 1979) suggested that ECS did not produce any changes. However, since the discovery that there may be 5-HT$_1$ receptor subtypes (Pedigo et al., 1981), these data may require further evaluation.

Finally, the microiontophoretic study of de Montigny (1984) should be mentioned. He observed that repeated ECS, but not a single convulsion, markedly enhanced the effects of microiontophoretically applied 5-HT and 5-MeODMT, whereas the GABA and noradrenaline responses were unchanged.

TABLE 2
Effect of Monoamine Synthesis Inhibition on [^{3}H]Spiperone Binding of Rat Frontal Cortex after Repeated ECS[a]

	Specific bound [^{3}H]spiperone		Significance (p)
Injected	Control	ECS × 5	
Saline	236 ± 26 (6)	437 ± 28 (6)	<0.001
p-Chlorophenylalanine	296 ± 37 (6)	283 ± 58 (6)	NS
α-Methyl p-tyrosine	315 ± 12 (6)	272 ± 25 (6)	NS

[a]Results shown as mean ± SEM of the specifically bound [^{3}H]spiperone (fmol mg^{-1} protein) using a concentration of [^{2}H]spiperone of 1.66 nM (saline experiment). 1.69 nM (PCPA experiment) and 1.23 nM (AMPT experiment). NS = not significantly different from appropriate control.

3.2. Dopamine

The several clear demonstrations of altered dopamine-mediated behaviors following repeated ECS (Section 2.2) have initiated several studies on dopamine biochemistry in attempts to explain the behavioral changes. In general, however, there is little evidence of marked changes in dopamine biochemistry following repeated ECS.

Brain dopamine concentration did not change after repeated ECS (Evans *et al.*, 1976; Modigh, 1976), nor was there any change in the rate of synthesis of this transmitter (Modigh, 1976).

Studies on the dopamine receptor in the caudate using [^{3}H]spiperone as ligand did not detect any change after repeated ECS (Bergström and Kellar, 1979; Atterwill, 1980; Deakin *et al.*, 1981; Lerer *et al.*, 1982), nor was any change detected in the sensitivity of adenylate cyclase to dopamine (Green *et al.*, 1977).

Serra *et al.* (1981), as part of their study of the dopamine autoreceptor, studied the effect of a low dose of apomorphine on dopamine synthesis. Electroconvulsive shock did not affect the ability of apomorphine to inhibit dopamine synthesis. This raises questions as to the location of the receptor being studied in their experiments, since the sedation response to this dose of apomorphine was attenuated (see Section 2.2). It seems unlikely, therefore, that the two responses are mediated by the same autoreceptors.

3.3. Noradrenaline

The first reports on changes in noradrenaline-biochemistry following ECS were published nearly 20 years ago. Kety *et al.* (1967) reported that noradrenaline turnover increased after repeated ECS. This increase was also seen by Modigh (1976). The change seen by Modigh (1976) was, however, very small, and our own studies on noradrenaline turnover in whole brain failed to detect a significant change (Nimgaonkar *et al.*, 1986).

Modigh (1976) found a possible reduction in noradrenaline uptake into brain slices following repeated ECS. This finding did not, however, agree with the *in vitro* findings of Hendley (1976), who reported that following 14 ECS given over 7 days the V_{max} and the K_m of noradrenaline uptake increased. We reexamined this problem (Minchin *et al.*, 1983) giving ECS in a rather more "clinical" way, that is, five ECS spread over 10 days. There were no changes 30 min or 24 hr after a single ECS. However, 24 hr after the final ECS of a series, the K_m and the V_{max} for noradrenaline uptake were increased (Table 3), the degree of the changes being very similar to those seen by Hendley (1976). It is possible that these changes

TABLE 3
Effect of ECS on the Uptake of Noradrenaline in Rat Cortex Slices[a]

	Noradrenaline	
	K_m (nM)	V_{max} (nmol 6 min^{-1} g wet wt^{-1})
Naive	103 ± 25 (5)	0.82 ± 0.19 (5)
30 min after single ECS		
Control	226 ± 26 (5)	1.44 ± 0.21 (5)
ECS	217 ± 27 (4)	1.27 ± 0.13 (4)
24 hr after single ECS		
Control	190 ± 20 (5)	0.98 ± 0.10 (5)
ECS	237 ± 37 (5)	1.05 ± 0.13 (5)
24 hr after 5 ECS over 10 days		
Control	104 ± 18 (4)	0.83 ± 0.09 (4)
ECS	171 ± 6 (4)**	1.27 ± 0.15 (4)*

[a]The figures represent the mean ± SEM with the number of experiments in parentheses. *$p < .05$; **$p < .02$: statistics by the two-tailed t test.

would enhance reuptake into the nerve terminal and may be an adaptation to an increase in synaptic cleft concentration of the hormone.

Tyrosine hydroxylase activity was first reported to be elevated by repeated ECS by Musacchio et al. (1969) and confirmed by Modigh (1976) and by Masserano et al. (1981). The latter group found an increase in enzyme activity in selected brain regions, which lasted several days after the last ECS. They also found increased activity in the adrenal up to 24 hr after the last seizure.

The findings on the effect of repeated ECS on brain β-adrenoceptors are remarkably consistent. Vetulani and colleagues (1976) first reported that repeated administration of both antidepressant drugs and ECS led to a subsensitivity of the noradrenaline-sensitive adenylate cyclase system, a finding that was extended by Gillespie et al. (1979). This study was followed by a study by Bergström and Kellar (1979), who observed that repeated ECS also reduced the B_{max} of β-adrenoceptors in the rat frontal cortex. This change was confirmed by Pandey et al. (1979), Deakin et al. (1981), and Stanford and Nutt (1982). The receptor number reduction and the noradrenaline-sensitive adenylate cyclase decrease are also produced by a range of antidepressant drugs (see Sulser and Mobley, 1981). The β-adrenoceptor number decrease, however, following repeated ECS is not seen in all regions of rat brain. It occurs in both the cortex and hippocampus but not such regions as cerebellum, hypothalamus, and striatum (Kellar et al., 1981b; Stanford and Nutt, 1982). All these researchers studied β-adrenoceptors after daily ECS for several days whereas Belmaker et al. (1982) studied the cortical β-adrenoceptor number after intermittent ECS, to show that a decrease in receptor number also occurred with this treatment regimen, a finding confirmed by Nimgaonkar *et al.* (1985).

Electroconvulsive shock is also able to down-regulate β-adrenoceptors in reserpine-treated rats. Chronic reserpine administration increases both noradrenaline-stimulated cyclic AMP production and the density of β-adrenoceptors in the brain (Dismukes and Daly, 1974; U'Prichard and Snyder, 1978; Kellar *et al.*, 1981b). Vetulani and Sulser (1975) showed the ECS given concurrently with reserpine attenuated the increase in noradrenaline-stimulated cyclic AMP produced by the reserpine, and Kellar *et al.* (1981b) showed that ECS in rats treated chronically with reserpine accelerated the return of the receptor to normal.

The β-adrenoceptor changes produced by ECS seems to depend on 5-HT functions. Both Brunello *et al.* (1982) and Janowsky *et al.* (1982) reported that a lesion of serotonergic pathways to the cortex prevents tricyclic antidepressant drugs, such as imipramine, from down-regulating the β-adrenoceptor. This finding was confirmed (Green *et al.*, 1984b; Nimagaonkar *et al.*, 1985), but in addition, it was found by these workers that this lesion (produced by a central injection of 5,7-DHT) also prevented repeated ECS from down-regulating the β-adrenoceptor (Green *et al.*, 1984b; Nimgaonkar *et al.*, 1985). This finding reinforces the suggestion (Brunello *et al.*, 1982; Costa and Barbaccia, 1984) that 5-HT somehow permits the down-regulation of β-adrenoceptors produced not only by tricyclics but also by ECS.

Perumal and Barkai (1982) looked for a relationship between postictal EEG changes after repeated ECS and β-adrenoceptor density. Unfortunately, although their data did suggest a relationship, the fact that Scatchard analysis of the binding data was performed using only three points does preclude any serious evaluation of their data.

The effect of repeated ECS on α_2-adrenoceptors in rat brain is unfortunately nowhere near as clear as that of the β-adrenoceptor. Both Stanford and Nutt (1982) and Pilc and Vetulani (1982) reported a decrease in α_2-adrenoceptor number, which agrees with the decrease in the clonidine-induced sedation response (Section 2.3.1). However, Kellar *et al.* (1981b) and Deakin *et al.* (1981) found no change, and Garcia *et al.* (1982) reported an increase in receptor number. Similarly, conflicting data have been reported after the repeated administration of tricyclic antidepressant (Vetulani *et al.*, 1980; Smith *et al.*, 1981; Johnson *et al.*, 1980; Peroutka and Snyder, 1980; Stanford *et al.*, 1983). One problem with these binding studies is that they measure both pre- and postsynaptic binding sites (U'Prichard *et al.*, 1979). The attenuated clonidine sedation response (Section 2.3.1) suggests that presynaptic receptor function is reduced by ECS. It seems likely that clonidine sedation is mediated by way of presyn-

TABLE 4
Effect of Repeated ECS on Clonidine-Induced Changes in Rat Brain MOPEG-SO$_4$ Concentrations[a]

	MOPEG-SO$_4$ concentrations (pmol/g whole brain)	
	Saline-treated	Clonidine-treated
Untreated controls	443 ± 14 (8)	← $p < .001$ → 107 ± 22 (5)
Halothane × 10	416 ± 19 (4)	← $p < .001$ → 238 ± 21 (8)
	↑ NS ↓	↑ $p < .02$ ↓
ECS × 10	453 ± 76 (5)	NS 362 ± 35 (9)

[a]Rats were given a single ECS or halothane once daily for 10 days. 24 hr after the final treatment both of these groups plus a group of untreated controls were injected with clonidine (0.25 mg/kg) or saline. 60 min later brain MOPEG-SO$_4$ concentrations were determined. Results are shown as mean ± SE with the number of observations shown in parentheses. Data were analyzed using the Student's unpaired t test. NS = not significantly different.

aptic receptors, since brain 3-methoxy-4-dihydroxyphenylglycol-sulfate (MOPEG-SO$_4$) concentration is decreased by clonidine (Heal *et al.*, 1981). This decrease was attenuated after repeated ECS (Table 4). This observation was confirmed by Sugrue (1981, 1982), who also observed that chronic treatment with several antidepressant drugs produced a similar attenuation.

The reports on α_1-adrenoceptor binding are also contradictory. Vetulani *et al.* (1983) have reported an increase in [^{3}H]prazosin binding after repeated ECS and tentatively linked this with their observations of increased postdecapitation convulsions seen after this treatment (Section 2.3.2). However, most researchers found no change in α_1-adrenoceptor density (Bergström and Kellar, 1979; Deakin *et al.*, 1981), which is consistent with the failure of Heal (1984) to find a change in the behavioral response to phenylephrine after repeated ECS (Section 2.3.2).

3.4. GABA

Using a gas chromatographic–mass spectrometic technique (mass fragmentography) to measure GABA synthesis and turnover (Bertilsson and Costa, 1976), we first reported in 1978 that repeated ECS, but not a single ECS or a repeated subconvulsive shock, produced an increase in brain GABA concentrations. This increase was seen in the nucleus accumbens and nucleus caudatus but not in the substania nigra (Green *et al.*, 1978). Subsequently, Deakin *et al.* (1981) reported that they were unable to detect any change in GABA concentration when the rats were anesthetized. This led to a subsequent study using unanesthetized rats and rats given an anesthetic at the time of intermittent ECS administration (five ECS over 10 days). Although anesthetic administration alone raised GABA concentration in the striatum, ECS (administered either daily or intermittently) produced a further rise (Bowdler *et al.*, 1983). It is possible that Deakin *et al.* (1981) failed to see a change because they did not, as we did in both our studies, use microwave irradiation to kill the animals. It is therefore possible that the marked rise in brain GABA that occurs postmortem obscured the ECS-induced rise. Flurothyl-induced seizures also increased the GABA concentration in the striatum (Bowdler *et al.*, 1983).

GABA antagonist drugs given at the time of each ECS prevented the increase in 5-HT- and dopamine-mediated behavior (Green *et al.*, 1982). This procedure also prevented the increase in striatal GABA concentration normally produced by ECS (Green *et al.*, 1982). Although the striatal GABA concentration change is probably not associated with enhanced monoamine-mediated behavior, the finding that interfering with GABA function affects the ECS-induced alteration in GABA biochemistry, as well as the enhanced monoamine behaviors, suggests that the behavioral changes could be the result of altered GABA function. This is discussed further elsewhere (Section 5.4).

Another change seen after repeated ECS was a decrease in the synthesis rate of GABA. This decrease was observed in the nucleus accumbens and nucleus caudatus but not in the substantia nigra (Green *et al.*, 1978). This observation has recently been confirmed by the peripheral administration of a GABA transaminase inhibitor (amino oxyacetic acid, AOAA) and the subsequent measurement of the rate of rise in GABA concentration (Green *et al.*, 1985*b*). Repeated ECS therefore changes the biochemistry of GABA, and thus it seemed reasonable to examine the biochemical consequences of a single ECS.

Following a single ECS, the concentration of GABA rises in several brain regions (Bowdler and Green, 1982). We are currently investigating the possible causes of this rise. The rate of GABA synthesis in several brain regions has been measured by pretreating animals with AOAA and determining the rate of rise in GABA concentration. Five minutes following a single ECS, there is very little increase in GABA concentration, in contrast to the handled control rats (Fig. 5), which suggests that ECS almost totally inhibits synthesis. A flurothyl-induced seizure had the same inhibiting effect. No inhibition was seen 2 hr after ECS (Green *et al.*, 1985*b*).

We next studied the release of endogenous GABA from slices of rat brain prepared from animals given a single ECS. Release of GABA evoked

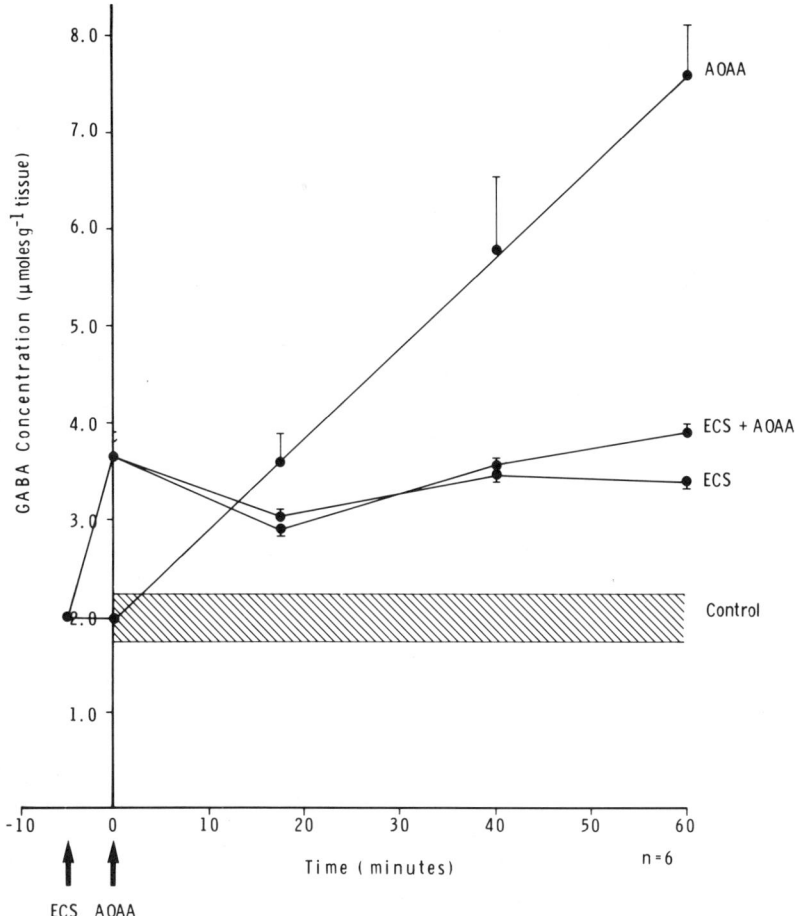

FIG. 5. The effect of a single ECS on the rate of accumulation of GABA in the hippocampus following injection of amino oxyacetic acid (AOAA). Rats were either handled (control) or handled and given AOAA. Another group was given a single ECS followed by either saline or AOAA. Note the almost total lack of increase in GABA concentration in the ECS animals given AOAA compared with control animals given the drug.

by K^+ (40 mM) was markedly inhibited in tissue taken from ECS-treated rats (Table 5). Interestingly, no such inhibition was seen in the release of [^{3}H]-GABA from slices preloaded with the transmitter (Table 6), which suggests that [^{3}H]-GABA was being released from a different pool than that of the endogenous GABA (Green et al., 1985c).

Overall, therefore, the work on GABA synthesis and GABA release, far from indicating that GABA function is increased by a seizure (as indi-

TABLE 5
Release of GABA in Slices of Rat Brain 30 Min Following a Single ECS[a]

	Endogenous GABA release (μmole g^{-1} hr^{-1})	
	Spontaneous	K^+ (40 nM)
Cortex		
Control	2.51 ± 0.36 (5)	7.72 ± 0.45 (5)
ECS	2.57 ± 0.61 (6)	5.43 ± 0.51 (6)*
Hippocampus		
Control	2.33 ± 0.39 (6)	7.01 ± 0.44 (6)
ECS	2.48 ± 0.17 (6)	4.86 ± 0.61 (6)*
Striatum		
Control	2.10 ± 0.57 (6)	6.48 ± 0.52 (6)
ECS	2.08 ± 0.43 (6)	3.21 ± 0.43 (6)*

[a]Values are mean ± SD with the number of experiments in parentheses. Different from control—K^+-induced release: *$p < .001$ two-tailed t test.

cated by the work on seizure threshold (Section 2.4), suggests that GABA function might be decreased by the seizure. The rise in seizure threshold might therefore reflect changes in other neurotransmitter systems as they compensate for the changes in GABA function. Alternatively, the switching off of GABA synthesis and release might be an attempt to compensate for the elevation of the threshold. Whether the immediate changes in GABA biochemistry initiate longer-term changes await further investigation.

Studies on glutamic acid decarboxylase activity following ECS have revealed no major change. Atterwill *et al.* (1981) observed a small, but statistically significant increase in activity following repeated ECS, but we have recently been unable to detect any change in the enzyme activity (in

TABLE 6
Release of [^{3}H]-GABA from Preloaded Slices of Rat Cortex 30 Min Following a Single ECS[a]

	[^{3}H]-GABA release fractional rate constant (min^{-1} × 10^{-3})	
	Spontaneous	K^+ (40 mM)
Control	5.5 ± 0.4 (7)	14.9 ± 2.2 (7)
ECS	5.6 ± 0.6 (7)	14.7 ± 2.8 (7)

[a]Values are mean ± SD with the number of experiments in parentheses.

both the absence and the presence of added pyridoxal phosphate cofactor) after either single or repeated ECS administration (Vincent and Green, unpublished observations).

GABA receptor binding has been studied following repeated ECS. Deakin et al. (1981) found no difference in [^{3}H]-GABA binding in rat cortex and Atterwill et al. (1981) found no difference in [^{3}H]muscimol binding in either cortex or striatum. The benzodiazepine binding site can modulate GABA function (see, for example, Costa, 1979). However, although the data are somewhat contradictory, overall they suggest few changes at this site after a single or repeated ECS. Paul and Skolnick (1978) did report a rise in [^{3}H]diazepam binding in vitro, using tissue from rats in which a single seizure was induced but this was not confirmed by Bowdler and Green (1982). McNamara et al. (1980) observed a rise in hippocampal benzodiazepine binding in vitro after 17 days of ECS treatment, but this was not seen after 10 ECS (Bowdler et al., 1983). Since the presence or absence of endogenous factors acting at the benzodiazepine binding site might account for these conflicting observations, Nutt and Minchin (1983) used the technique of in vivo diazepam binding (Minchin and Nutt, 1983) to investigate the effect of seizure on the benzodiazepine binding site. Neither a single ECS nor repeated treatment altered the binding of [^{3}H]diazepam or [^{3}H]ethyl-β-carboline carboxylate in vivo in the brain; this strongly suggests that the benzodiazepine binding site function is not changed by ECS (Nutt and Minchin, 1983).

Finally, there is now one preliminary and provocative finding by Lloyd et al. (1985), who reported that repeated ECS and repeated antidepressant drug administration increased the number of GABA$_B$ receptors. This is the GABA receptor for which baclofen is an agonist and which regulates the release of several monoamine neurotransmitters (Bowery et al., 1980).

3.5. Opioid Peptides

Repeated ECS but not a single seizure has been found to increase the concentration of Met^5-enkephalin in the caudate nucleus (Green et al., 1978). This finding was confirmed and extended by Hong et al. (1979), who showed that metenkephalin concentration also increased in several other brain regions and that the increase lasted for several days after the last convulsion. These authors also noted that the β-endorphin content of rat brain was not changed.

Current work by Yoshikawa et al. (1985) showed that the probable reason for the increase in metenkephalin following repeated ECS is an increase in the synthesis of this peptide. These authors observed a marked increase in preproenkephalin messenger RNA activity in both hypothalamus and striatum. They also observed that amygdaloid kindling altered opioid peptide concentration, with increases in hippocampal enkephalin-like immunoreactivity but decreases in dynorphinlike immunoreactivity (Hong et al., 1985).

Repeated ECS also changes opioid peptide receptor number. Belenky et al. (1984) observed that repeated seizures increased the B_{max} of [^{3}H]-D-ala2,D-leu-5-enkephalin ([^{3}H]-DADLE), a delta (γ)-opioid peptide receptor ligand. A single ECS had no effect, and interestingly, chronic morphine administration had the same effect. This result, therefore, may help explain the cross-sensitization noted between chronic morphine administration and repeated ECS (Section 2.6).

3.6. Acetylcholine

Atterwill (1984) recently reviewed the effects of seizures on brain cholinergic systems. In this section, we will discuss some of the more important or consistent changes that have been reported.

In general, there seems to be fairly transient changes in the acetylcholine (ACh) content of rodent brain during a seizure or shortly thereafter, and most reports suggest a reduction in content (see Atterwill, 1984). High-affinity uptake of choline (HAUC), which is postulated to be rate-limiting and regulatory in the control of ACh synthesis (Atweh et al., 1976), was unaltered in hippocampus or striatum preparations either 1 hr following a single ECS or 24 hr following the last ECS of repeated ECS (Atterwill, 1980).

The enzymes involved in ACh synthesis and degradation have been studied by several groups. In mice, choline acetyltransferase (ChAT) was reported to be transiently reduced after a single ECS (Essman, 1973); it was increased in rat cortex after a single ECS yet unchanged after repeated ECS (Longoni et al., 1976). Atterwill (1980, 1984) observed a small (10%) reduction in ChAT activity in rat striatum after repeated ECS but no changes in several other brain regions.

Acetylcholinesterase (AChE) activity has been reported to increase, again transiently, in whole rat brain after a single ECS or four ECS given over 96 hr (Adams et al., 1969). In a recent study of regional and temporal changes in AChE activity, Appleyard et al. (1984, 1986) examined specific AChE (both total and soluble) after a single ECS or a flurothyl-induced convulsion. There were transient changes (increased and decreased activity) in several brain regions after a single ECS. However, the most sustained change was decreased activity in the midbrain and hippocampal total AChE activity for up to 3 hr after a seizure. A flurothyl-induced seizure evoked the same change, but a subconvulsive shock had no effect. Preliminary data suggest that, in contrast, AChE activity in the CSF rises at this time (Appleyard et al., manuscript submitted). However, it is difficult to assess what functional consequences this change has on ACh metabolism, and this problem is compounded by the possible neuromodulatory role of the AChE protein in the substantia nigra (Greenfield, 1984). Preliminary data suggest that AChE activity is unchanged 30 min and 24 hr after the last of 10 ECS given once daily (Appleyard et al., unpublished observations).

Muscarinic cholinergic receptors have been studied after repeated ECS with the ligand [^{3}H]-quinuclidinylbenzylate ([^{3}H]-QNB). Deakin et al. (1981) and Kellar et al. (1981a) found no significant effect of ECS daily for 14 days on [^{3}H]-QNB binding in rat hippocampus or cortex. In contrast, Lerer et al. (1983) observed a small (15%), but statistically significant decrease after ECS daily for 7 days in both the hippocampus and cortex, and Dashieff et al. (1982) observed a 20% decrease in rats given ECS four times daily for 4 days. No change in nicotinic cholinergic receptors has been seen after repeated ECS (Kellar et al., 1981a).

3.7. Adenosine and Cyclic Nucleotides

In 1971, Sattin demonstrated that the adenosine 3'5'monophosphate (cyclic AMP, cAMP) concentration in the mouse forebrain was increased during seizures and that this increase was blocked by methylxanthines (theophylline or caffeine). He suggested that this change was caused by the liberation of free adenosine by hypoxia. It now seems that brain concentrations of both cAMP and cyclic guanosine monophosphate (cGMP) increase in most brain regions associated with the start of seizure activity (Chapman, 1981). However, the true course of these effects is different for the two nucleotides. The elevation of cGMP is seen just before the onset of convulsive activity, whereas cAMP increases as the seizure starts (Ferendelli and Kinscherf, 1977; Wasterlain and Csiszor, 1980). Seizures also markedly elevate adenosine levels in the cortex (Chapman, 1981; Lewin and Beck, 1981). Inosine and hypoxanthine levels are also elevated and seem to take longer to subside than do those of adenosine. Work on the effects of repeated ECS (Sattin, 1981) has shown that although noradrenaline-stimulated cAMP formation is reduced (see Section 3.3), the response to the adenosine analog N-ethyl-carboxamide adenosine (NECA) is enhanced (Sattin, 1981). Sattin suggested that the sensitivity of the adenosine A_2 receptor was enhanced after repeated ECS. However, in a study by Newman et al. (1984), his findings on cAMP-stimulated adenosine following ECS proved hard to replicate, and there were problems with regard to age and strain differences in the rats. Clearly, this work needs repeating to determine whether any changes in the A_2 adenosine receptor occur after repeated ECS.

3.8. Peptides

Although it has been known for many years that seizures significantly alter nucleic acid and protein synthesis (see Cupello *et al.*, 1981; Metafora *et al.*, 1977), relatively little work has been done on the effects of repeated ECS on brain peptides. Lighton *et al.* (1984) found that repeated ECS decreased the concentration of thyrotropin-releasing hormone (TRH) in the nucleus accumbens and lumbar spinal cord following repeated ECS in rats. The TRH content in several other brain regions was unchanged. A decrease in TRH release from slices prepared from the nucleus accumbens of animals treated with repeated ECS was seen but this decrease was not seen in slices prepared from the septal nuclei. In contrast, Lighton *et al.* (1985) found that repeated antidepressant drug administration increased the content of TRH in the nucleus accumbens and spinal cord. It is interesting that TRH and 5-HT coexist in these regions (Gilbert *et al.*, 1981) and that ECS increases 5-HT$_2$ receptor number, while antidepressant drugs decrease the number of these receptors (Section 3.1). However, whether this apparent inverse relationship between 5-HT$_2$ and TRH content is other than fortuitous will require further investigation.

Minchin and Emson (unpublished observations) found no change in substance P or neurotensin content after repeated ECS, although neuropeptide Y concentrations rose in the hippocampus and the cortex and somatostatin concentration in the hippocampus and the striatum.

Particularly interesting in the light of the "opposite" effects of ECS and antidepressant drugs on CNS TRH content is the recent work of Jones *et al.* (1985), who examined the responsiveness of cingulate cortex neurons to substance P after repeated ECS and antidepressant drug administration. The drugs (tranylcypromine, oxaprotiline, and carbamazepine) increased neuronal sensitivity, while ECS decreased it.

3.9. Calcium

Calcium concentrations in blood, urine, and CSF have been measured in patients undergoing ECT treatment. In all these fluids, it has been reported that the calcium concentration falls during the course of treatment (Flach *et al.*, 1960; Flach, 1964; Faragalla and Flach, 1970; Carman and Wyatt, 1977), and it has been suggested that the change in calcium disposition might be associated with the mood improvement (Carman et al., 1977). However, some data conflict with this straightforward story. First, not all patients show the decrease in serum calcium; also, the number of patients studied was small (e.g., Faragalla and Flach, 1970). Second, values tended to return toward normal after cessation of treatment (Carman et al., 1977); and third, Gour and Chaudhry (1957) observed only a transient hyperglycemia immediately following ECT.

In an attempt to reconcile the apparent differences, Bowdler et al. (1980) studied brain and serum calcium concentration in rats given ECS. Overall, few changes were observed in calcium content in either tissue following ECS. Anesthetic alone raised serum calcium concentration, whereas the intravenous injection of saline produced a decrease in serum calcium. No lasting effects were seen after repeated ECS. It seems possible, therefore, that anesthesia and premedication could have produced some of the changes seen in calcium content in the tissues of patients undergoing ECS.

4. NEUROENDOCRINE MARKERS OF NEUROTRANSMITTER CHANGES FOLLOWING ELECTROCONVULSIVE SHOCK

In humans, ECS produces a variety of neuroendocrine responses (see Fink, 1979). The purpose of this section is to review some of the work that has been performed using neuroendocrine responses to "challenge" tests. If selective pharmacological agents are used, then ECS-induced changes in the function of neurotransmitters may be revealed.

In studies with experimental animals and in clinical studies, attempts to demonstrate a decreased clonidine-induced neuroendocrine response analogous to the decreased behavioral response in rats and mice (Section 2.3) have produced conflicting data (see Steiner et al., 1982). For example, the growth hormone (GH) response to clonidine in baboons is enhanced (McWilliam et al., 1981, 1982), but there is no effect on GH secretion to clonidine in patients undergoing ECT (Slade and Checkley, 1980) or, indeed, in their sedation response to this drug (Checkley et al., 1981). However, it is generally thought that the α_2-adrenoceptor responsible for GH release is postsynaptic. If ECT selectively down-regulates presynaptic receptors, then this discrepancy may be explained.

The GH response to dopamine mimetics also produced conflicting data. In patients, ECT did not alter the euphoric, stimulant, or GH-releasing effects of methylamphetamine (Slade and Checkley, 1980). The GH response to apomorphine in patients who have received ECT was also shown to be unchanged in two studies (Christie et al., 1982; Balldin et al.,

1982) but enhanced in a third (Costain *et al.*, 1982). Equally controversial are the effects of ECS on the inhibition of prolactin release, produced in humans by apomorphine. Balldin *et al.* (1982) reported an enhancement; Christie *et al.* (1982) found no change.

In the one attempt to measure a 5-HT-mediated event, Steiner and Grahame-Smith (1980) observed an enhanced corticosteroid response to 5-HTP in rats undergoing repeated ECS.

This whole area has been reviewed in detail by Checkley *et al.* (1984), and Cowen (1985) has discussed the difficulties in interpretation of data obtained. Clearly, we require a better knowledge of the "wiring" of the neurotransmitters involved in neurohormone release. Stress and anesthetic administration can also markedly alter these responses (Steiner and Grahame-Smith, 1982). However, this approach still promises a means of investigating changes in neurotransmitter function in ECT patients.

5. ARE ANY BIOCHEMICAL AND FUNCTIONAL CHANGES ASSOCIATED?

To some extent there can be no definite answer to this question. However, one can point to strong possibilities of association.

5.1. 5-Hydroxytryptamine

It seems entirely reasonable that the enhancement of 5-HT-mediated behavior produced by administration of repeated ECS is the result of the increase in 5-HT_2 receptor number that also occurs. To date, the correlation between the appearance, or nonappearance, of increased behavioral responses and increase or no change in 5-HT_2 receptor number has been absolute. The mechanism that underlies the receptor change is uncertain but possibly reflects changes in GABA function. This is discussed in Section 5.4.

5.2. Dopamine

No clear-cut biochemical change has been observed in dopamine biochemistry following repeated ECS, which suggests that the action of other neurotransmitters modulating the effect of dopamine may have been altered. We examined the effect of decreasing GABA function and observed that acute picrotoxin administration at a subconvulsive dose did increase dopamine-mediated behavior (Green *et al.*, 1976). Following the daily injection of picrotoxin for 8 days, the rats did show enhanced dopamine-mediated behaviors (Cowen *et al.*, 1982). Repeated bicuculline administration, in contrast, had no effect (Cowen *et al.*, 1982), but this latter drug does have a short half-life.

5.3. Noradrenaline

Unfortunately, there are no good behavioral models for β-adrenoceptor function. With regard to α_2-adrenoceptor function, the decrease in the sedation response to clonidine and the attenuation of the clonidine-induced MOPEG-SO$_4$ decrease are consistent with the decrease in α_2-adrenoceptor number. However, as pointed out, not everyone finds a decrease in α_2-adrenoceptor number after ECS, and this discrepancy may reflect differences in methodologies and the fact that some α_2-adrenoceptors are postsynaptic. In this regard, the enhancement of the clonidine/apomorphine-induced behavior in reserpinized mice, the enhancement of the GH response in mice similarly treated, and the enhanced GH response to clonidine in baboons may all indicate changes in a postsynaptically located α_2-adrenoceptor.

As in the change in 5-HT-mediated behavior, there is just a hint that the altered clonidine-induced behavior is a consequence of changes in GABA function (see Section 5.4).

5.4. GABA

All the pharmacological indications suggest that the raised seizure threshold that occurs after an ECS (Section 2.4) is the result of an increase in function of the benzodiazepine/GABA system. However, the failure to find any change in benzodiazepine binding, either *in vitro* or *in vivo* after a convulsion, coupled with the evidence that both GABA synthesis and release are *decreased* after a single ECS (Section 3.4), cast some doubts on this. It is possible that GABA receptor binding is increased or that receptor efficacy is enhanced. Alternatively, neurotransmitter systems postsynaptic to the GABA/benzodiazepine receptor may be altered.

Nevertheless, on the basis of the seizure threshold data and the knowledge that GABA synthesis is changed after repeated ECS, we decided to see whether we could mimic any of the neuropharmacological effects of ECS by manipulating GABA function. We used the specific GABA mimetic drug progabide. This metabolizes to an acid, and both progabide and the acid are metabolized to GABA in the brain (Worms *et al.*, 1982). The acid has GABA-receptor agonist properties (Lloyd *et al.*, 1982). Peripheral progabide administration results in increased GABA

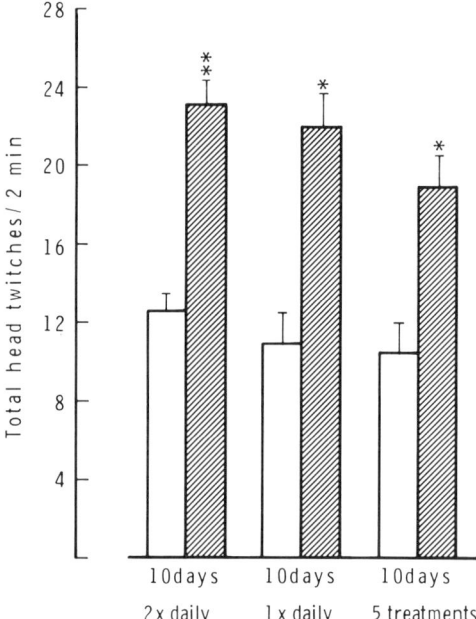

FIG. 6. Effect of progabide administration on 5-hydroxytryptophan-induced head-twitch. Mice were treated for 10 days with progabide (400 mg/kg, i.p.) either twice daily, once daily, or five times over the 10 days, and the head-twitch behavior was assessed 24 hr after the last dose. Results show median head twitch and bars the interquartile ranges in vehicle (open bars) and progabide (stippled bar)-treated groups of at least eight animals per group. Different from control: $*p < .05$; $**p < .01$.

concentration and function in the brain and hence raises seizure threshold (Worms et al., 1982). As shown earlier (Sections 2.4 and 3.4), both these changes occur after a single ECS.

Repeated injection of mice with progabide (400 mg/kg twice daily for 14 days) markedly increased 5-HTP-induced head-twitch behavior in mice, and this increase lasted for at least 8 days after the last progabide injection (Green et al., 1985a). Administration of progabide at this dose twice daily or once daily for 10 days also increased the head-twitch behavior, as did administration, in a manner analogous to ECS (that is, five injections spread over 10 days) (Fig. 6). Recently, we found that a similar enhancement occurred when progabide was given five times over 10 days at the much lower dose of 100 mg/kg (Gray et al., 1986). The probable reason for the behavioral enhancement is that progabide injection increased $5-HT_2$ receptor number in the brain (Table 7). Thus, repeated progabide produced the same changes in 5-HT biochemistry and function in the mouse as those seen after repeated ECS.

A further similarity to ECS was the finding (Green et al., 1985a) that repeated progabide injection resulted in the mice showing an attenuated sedation response to clonidine (Fig. 7). In contrast, however, repeated progabide injection did not down-regulate the β-adrenoceptor (Table 7) or enhance dopamine-mediated behavior (Green et al., 1985a). Repeated injection of sodium valproate, another drug that is anticonvulsant and that increases GABA function, produced similar results, whereas pheny-

TABLE 7
Characteristics of the 5-Hydroxytryptamine$_2$ (5-HT$_2$) Receptor in Frontal Cortex and β-Adrenoceptor in the Rest of the Cerebral Cortex Following Repeated Administration of Progabide to Mice[a]

	5-HT$_2$ receptor			β-Adrenoceptor		
	B_{max}	K_D		B_{max}	K_D	
Control	188 ± 8	2.40 ± 0.32	4	64.7 ± 1.0	0.78 ± 0.09	4
Progabide	253 ± 9**	1.47 ± 0.34	4	57.2 ± 6.0	0.97 ± 0.20	4

[a]β-Adrenoceptor characteristics were measured using [^{3}H]dihydroalprenolol binding and 5-HT$_2$ receptor characteristics using [^{3}H]spiperone. Mice were treated twice daily with progabide (400 mg/kg) or vehicle for 14 days. Twenty-four hours after the last dose, binding was performed on frontal cortex. Results are expressed as mean ± SEM with number of Scatchard analysis determinations shown (n). Different from control: **$p <$ .01. B_{max} expressed in fmol/mg protein and K_D in nM.

toin, which does not increase GABA function, had no effect. Since Schlicker *et al.* (1984) have shown that a GABA$_B$-receptor inhibits 5-HT release and that progabide was very active at that site, it is likely that progabide produces its 5-HT effects by an action at this site. A decrease in release would lead to a postsynaptic supersensitivity of 5-HT$_2$ receptors. This view is now perhaps strengthened by our recent finding that repeated administration of the GABA$_B$ agonist baclofen also increases the 5-HTP

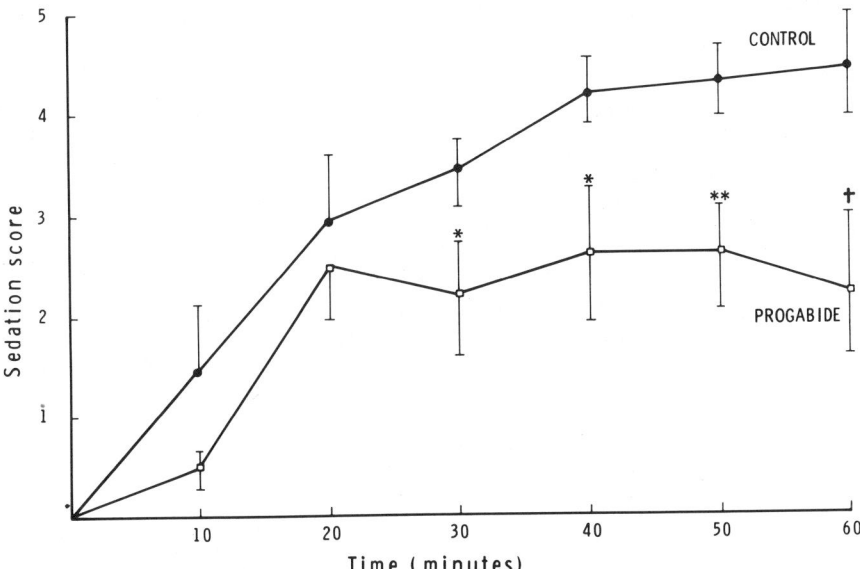

FIG. 7. Effect of valproate (400 mg/kg, i.p.) twice daily for 14 days (□) or saline (■) on the sedation response to clonidine (0.15 mg/kg, i.p.) in mice. The points show the median sedation response, the bars the interquartile ranges. Difference from the vehicle-treated mice at the same time point; *$p <$ .05; **$p <$ .001, with at least eight mice in each group.

head-twitch response in mice and the 5-HT$_2$ receptor number in the cortex (Metz *et al.*, 1985). Baclofen, however, did not attenuate clonidine-induced sedation (Gray *et al.*, 1986).

It seems possible, therefore, as proposed elsewhere (Green, 1986*a,b*), that at least some of the effects of repeated ECS on monoamine-mediated behavior are a consequence of the changes occurring in GABA function.

5.5. Acetylcholine

The fact that the mechanisms involved in the cataleptic response to cholinomimetics are obscure makes it difficult to associate this behavior with any biochemical change. Furthermore, it is difficult to assess what the changes in ACh biochemistry mean in terms of ACh function. It has been known for many years that ECS, and ECT, can cause memory impairment (see, for example, McGaugh, 1966; Weeks *et al.*, 1980; Frith *et al.*, 1983; Mellanby *et al.*, 1984; Lerer *et al.*, 1984). Anticholinergics also impair memory (Adams *et al.*, 1969). It is at least possible, therefore, that acetylcholine function is changed by ECS and that this change produces the memory impairment. The change in seizure threshold and the change in acetylcholinesterase activity seen after a convulsion are temporally similar, and alterations in acetylcholine function can induce seizures (Turski *et al.*, 1983; Olney *et al.*, 1983). The possibility exists, therefore, that these changes are in some way related, and this has been discussed more fully elsewhere (Appleyard *et al.*, 1985).

5.6. Opioid Peptides

The fact that ECS appears to increase enkephalin concentration and synthesis would certainly be compatible with the increased analgesia seen after a single ECS (Holaday and Belenky, 1980). A further point is that some opioid peptides and etophine are anticonvulsant in the rat (Tortella *et al.*, 1981), which raises the possibility that the changes in opioid peptide function are associated with the rise in seizure threshold. However, the complexity of this area was recently highlighted by the same group (Tortella *et al.*, 1984), who demonstrated that centrally administered opiates could both increase and decrease seizure threshold.

6. CAN BIOCHEMICAL OR BEHAVIORAL CHANGES BE ASSOCIATED WITH ANTIDEPRESSANT ACTION OF ELECTROCONVULSIVE SHOCK?

It is difficult to attempt to answer this question, since we are not sure what biochemical changes are important in antidepressant action. The fact that ECS increases 5-HT$_2$ receptor number, while most other antidepressant treatments decrease this parameter (Peroutka and Snyder, 1980; Kellar et al., 1981a; Goodwin et al., 1984) precludes any simple hypothesis linking changes in this receptor with antidepressant action. Because repeated diazepam administration also increases the 5-HT$_2$ receptor number (Green et al., 1985a), and ECT has been suggested to have a specific anxiolytic effect (Lambourn and Gill, 1978; Freeman et al., 1978), the effect of ECS in an animal model of anxiety was studied (File, 1980). However, although several changes in spontaneous behavior were noted, no specific anxiolytic effect was observed (File and Green, 1984).

It has been suggested that progabide, a drug that also increases the 5-HT$_2$ receptor number (Green et al., 1985a), had antidepressant properties (Lloyd et al., 1983), but then, as stated earlier, diazepam also increases the number of this receptor and this drug has never seriously been suggested as a good antidepressant drug.

The change we have recently seen in the sensitivity of mice to the drug 8-*OH*-DPAT, a putative 5-HT$_1$ agonist, is interesting, since a similar attenuation of this response was also noted after administration of various other antidepressant drugs (Goodwin et al., 1985b). However, it will take some time to determine whether this change is clinically important.

The change in β-adrenoceptor number seen after repeated ECS has, of course, been observed after most other antidepressant treatments, and indeed, it has been suggested to be a change necessary for antidepressant action (Sulser and Mobley, 1981), a hypothesis we have questioned elsewhere (Green and Nutt, 1983). Of interest is the fact that progabide administration does not produce either this change in number (Green et al., 1985a) or decrease the noradrenaline-sensitive adenylate cyclase (Zivkovic et al., 1982), although it may be antidepressant (Lloyd et al., 1983).

Attenuation of clonidine-induced sedation is seen after ECS and several antidepressant drugs (Heal et al., 1981, 1983; Sugrue, 1981, 1982), but again it is not a change seen with all treatments (see Green and Nutt, 1983, 1985). The clinical evaluation of selective drugs such as idazoxan, an α_2-adrenoceptor antagonist, may give further insight into the importance of changes in this receptor in antidepressant action.

The changes in GABA function may have therapeutic importance either because of the other changes induced in neurotransmitter systems, as argued elsewhere (Green, 1986a,b) and in this chapter, or because of the change in the seizure threshold (Sackheim et al., 1983; Green, 1986b).

In contrast, it is difficult to argue for the changes in acetylcholine biochemistry as having an antidepressant effect, but they may be responsible for some of the cognitive deficits induced by ECT (Lerer, 1985).

Changes in enkephalinergic biochemistry may be important, as has been argued (Hong et al., 1979; Belenky et al., 1984), but this is tentative, with rather little supporting evidence at present (Emrich and Höllt, 1984). It is difficult to evaluate the other peptide changes seen, even though a whole hypothesis has been advanced for the importance of ECT-induced peptide changes in the therapeutic process (Fink and Ottosson, 1980; Fink, 1984).

Changes in dopamine function are a major feature of repeated ECS, but few clear hypotheses link these changes with antidepressant activity. However, an increase in dopamine function may increase "'drive," an amphetaminelike action important in the overall effect of ECT. It is particularly likely to explain the effects that ECT has on the biological symptoms of depression. Chronically, it is well recognized that appetite reduction and motor retardation often respond faster to ECT than does depressed mood. The former symptoms may well reflect a relative deficiency of dopamine function, and it is interesting that in animal experiments, ECS changes dopamine function before 5-HT or α_2-adrenoceptor function (Section 2.2).

In conclusion, therefore, we do not advance any single hypothesis for the mechanism of the therapeutic effect of ECT; we think that, at this stage, it would be naive to do so. Nevertheless, the changes reported in this chapter do perhaps provide important pointers to a therapeutic mechanism. The development of drugs with more selective actions may provide a start toward producing a treatment with the therapeutic action of ECT but fewer side effects. However, it is possible that ECT has its marked efficacy because of the many effects it produces on neurotransmitter systems in the brain.

Acknowledgment

This chapter reviews much of our work performed in the MRC Clinical Pharmacology Unit, Oxford, over the last 10 years. This would have been impossible without the collaboration of our colleagues, Drs. Atterwill, Bowdler, Costain, Cowen, Goodwin, Heal, Minchin, Nimgaonkar, Steiner, and Vincent and the enthusiastic interest and support of Professor David Grahame-Smith. We thank them all for their collaboration and friendship.

7. REFERENCES

ADAMS, H. E., HOBLIT, P. R., and SULKER, P. D., 1969, Electroconvulsive shock, brain acetylcholinesterase activity and memory, *Physiol. Behav.* **4:**113–116.

APPLEYARD, M. E., GREEN, A. R., and SMITH, A. D., 1984, Regional acetylcholinesterase activity in rat brain following a convulsion, *Br. J. Pharmacol.* **82:**248P.

APPLEYARD, M. E., GREEN, A. R., and SMITH, A. D., 1985, Acetylcholinesterase activity in regions of the rat brain following a convulsion, *J. Neurochem.* **46:**1789–1793.

ATTERWILL, C. K., 1980, Lack of effect of repeated electroconvulsive shock on [^{3}H]-5-hydroxytryptamine binding and cholinergic parameters in rat brain, *J. Neurochem.* **35:**729–734.

ATTERWILL, C. K., 1984, The effects of ECS on central cholinergic and interrelated neurotransmitter systems, in: *ECT: Basic Mechanisms* (B. Lerer, R. D. Weiner, and R. H. Belmaker, eds.), John Libbey & Co., London, pp. 79–88.

ATTERWILL, C. K., and GREEN, A. R., 1980, Responses of developing rats to L-tryptophan plus an MAOI. II: Effects of repeated electroconvulsive shock, *Neuropharmacology* **19:**337–341.

ATTERWILL, C. K., BATTS, C., and BLOOMFIELD, M. R., 1981, Effect of single and repeated convulsions on glutamate decarboyxlase (GAD) activity and [^{3}H]-muscimol binding in the rat brain, *J. Pharm. Pharmacol.* **33:**329–331.

ATWEH, S., SIMON, J. R., and KUHAR, J. J., 1976 Utilisation of sodium-dependent high affinity choline uptake *in vitro* as a measure of the activity of cholinergic neurons *in vivo, Life Sci.* **17:**1535–1544.

BALLDIN, J., GRANERUS, A. K., LINDSTEDT, G., MODIGH, K., and WALINDER, J., 1982, Neuroendocrine evidence for increased responsiveness of dopamine receptors in humans following electroconvulsive therapy, *Psychopharmacology* **76:**371–376.

BELENKY, G. L., and HOLADAY, J. W., 1979, The opiate antagonist naloxone modifies the effect of electroconvulsive shock (ECS) on respiration, blood pressure and heart rate, *Brain Res.* **117:**414–417.

BELENKY, G. L., and HOLADAY, J. W., 1981, Repeated electroconvulsive shock (ECS) and morphine tolerance: Demonstration of cross-sensitivity in the rat, *Life Sci.* **29:**553–563.

BELENKY, G. L., TORTELLA, F. C., HITZEMANN, R. J., and HOLADAY, J. W., 1984, The role of endorphine systems in the effects of ECS, in: *ECT: Basic Mechanisms* (B. Lerer, R. D. Weiner, and R. H. Belmaker, eds.), John Libbey & Co., London, pp. 89–97.

BELMAKER, R. H., LERER, B., BANNET, J., and BIRMAHER, B., 1982, The effect of electroconvulsive shock at a clinically equivalent schedule on rat cortical β-adrenoceptors, *J. Pharm. Pharmacol.* **34:**275.

BERGSTRÖM, D. A., and KELLAR, K. J., 1979, Effect of electroconvulsive shock on monoaminergic receptor binding sites in rat brain, *Nature* **278:**464–466.

BERTILSSON, L., and COSTA, E., 1976, Mass-fragmentographic quantification of glutamic acid and γ-aminobutyric acid in cerebellar nuclei and sympathetic ganglia of rats, *J. Chromatogr.* **118:**395–402.

BHAVSAR, V. H., DHUMAL, V. R., and KELKAR, V. V., 1981, The effect of some anti-epilepsy drugs on enhancement of the monoamine-mediated behavioural responses following the administration of electroconvulsive shocks to rats, *Eur. J. Pharmacol.* **74:**243–247.

BOWDLER, J. M., and GREEN, A. R., 1982, Regional rat brain benzodiazepine receptor number and γ-aminobutyric acid concentration following a convulsion, *Br. J. Pharmacol.* **76:**291–298.

BOWDLER, J. M., GREEN, A. R., and RAWLE, F. C., 1980, Brain and serum calcium concentrations following electroconvulsive shock or bicuculline-induced convulsions in rats, *Br. J. Pharmacol.* **71:**321–325.

BOWDLER, J. M., GREEN, A. R., MINCHIN, M. C. W., and NUTT, D. J., 1983, Regional GABA concentrations and [^{3}H]-diazepam binding in rat brain following repeated electroconvulsive shock, *J. Neural Transm.* **56:**3–12.

BOWERY, N. G., HILL, D. R., HUDSON, A. L., DOBLE, A., MIDDLEMISS, D. N., SHAW, J., and TURNBULL, M., 1980, (−)-Baclofen decreases neurotransmitter release in the mammalian CNS by an action at a novel GABA receptor, *Nature* **283:**92–94.

BRANDON, S., COWLEY, P., MCDONALD, C., NEVILLE, P., PALMER, R., and WELLSTOOD-EASON, S., 1984, Electroconvulsive therapy: Results in depressive illness from the Leicestershire trial, *Br. Med. J.* **188:**22–25.

BRUNELLO, N., BARBACCIA, M. L., CHUANG, D. M., and COSTA, E., 1982, Down-regulation of β-adrenergic receptors following repeated injections of desmethylimipramine: Permissive role of serotonergic axons, *Neuropharmacology* **21:**1145–1149.

CARMAN, J. S., and WYATT, R. J., 1977, Alterations in cerebrospinal fluid and serum total calcium with changes in psychiatric state, in: *Neuroregulators and Psychiatric Disorders* (E.

Usdin, D. Hamburg, and J. Barchas, eds.), Oxford University Press, New York, pp. 488–494.
CARMAN, J. S., POST, R. M., GOODWIN, F. K., and BUNNEY, W. E., 1977, Calcium and electroconvulsive therapy of severe depressive illness, *Biol. Psychiatry* **12:**5–17.
CHAPMAN, A. G., 1981, Free fatty acid release and metabolism of adenosine and cyclic nucleotides during prolonged seizures, in: *Neurotransmitters, Seizures and Epilepsy* (P. L. Morselli, P. G. Lloyd, W. Löscher, B. Meldrum, and E. H. Reynolds, eds.) Raven Press, New York, pp. 165–173.
CHECKLEY, S. A., SLADE, A. P., and SHUR, E., 1981, Growth hormone and other response to clonidine in patients with endogenous depression, *Br. J. Psychiatry* **138:**51–55.
CHECKLEY, S. A., MELDRUM, B. S., and McWILLIAM. J. R., 1984. Mechanisms of action of ECT: Neuroendocrine studies, in: *ECT: Basic Mechanisms* (B. Lerer, R. D. Weiner, and R. H. Belmaker, eds.), John Libbey & Co., London, pp. 101–106.
CHIODO, L. A., and ANTELMAN, S. M., 1980, Electroconvulsive shock: progressive dopamine autoreceptor subsensitivity independent of repeated treatment, *Science* **210:** 799–801.
CHRISTIE, J. E., WHALLEY, L. J., Brown, N. S., *et al.*, 1982, Effect of ECT on the neuroendocrine response to apomorphine in severely depressed patients, *Br. J. Psychiatry* **140:**268–273.
COSTA, E., 1979, The role of gamma-amino butyric acid in the action of 1,4-benzodiazepines, *Trends Pharm. Sci.* **1:**41–45.
COSTA, E., and BARBACCIA, M. L., 1984, Regulation of 5-hydroxy-tryptamine (5-HT) uptake: Endocoid modulators and the action of imipramine, in: *Proceedings of the 9th International Congress of Pharmacology*, Vol. 3 (W.D.M. Paton, J. F. Mitchell, and P. Turner, eds.), Macmillan Press, Basingstoke, England, pp. 109–116.
COSTAIN, D. W., Green, A. R., and Grahame-Smith, D. G., 1979, Enhanced 5-hydroxytryptamine-mediated behavioural responses in rats following repeated electroconvulsive shock: Relevance to the mechanism of the antidepressive effect of electroconvulsive therapy, *Psychopharmacology* **61:**167–170.
COSTAIN, D. W., COWEN, P. J., GELDER, M. G., and GRAHAME-SMITH, D. G., 1982, Electroconvulsive therapy and the brain: Evidence for increased dopamine-mediated responses, *Lancet* **2:**360–362.
COSTALL, B., and OLLEY, J. E., 1971, Cholinergic and neuroleptic-induced catalepsy: Modification by lesions in the caudate putamen, *Neuropharmacology* **10:**297–306.
COWEN, P. J., 1985, Neuroendocrine responses as a probe into the mechanisms of action of ECT, *Ann. NY Acad. Sci.* **462:**163–171.
COWEN, P. J., and NUTT, D. J., 1982, Repeated electroconvulsive shock enhances the anticonvulsant effect of benzodiazepines, *Br. J. Pharmacol.* **75:**44P.
COWEN, P. J., NUTT, D. J., and GREEN, A. R., 1980a, Enhanced 5-hydroxytryptamine- and dopamine-mediated behavioural responses following convulsion. II: The effects of anaesthesia and current conditions on the appearance of the enhanced responses following electroconvulsive shock, *Neuropharmacology* **19:**901–906.
COWEN, P. J., NUTT, D. J., and GREEN, A. R., 1980b, Repeated electroconvulsive shock does not increase the susceptibility of rats to a cage convulsant (isopropylbicyclophosphate), *Neuropharmacology* **19:**1025–1026.
COWEN, P. J., NUTT, D. J., BATTS, C. C., GREEN, A. R., and HEAL, D. J., 1982, Repeated administration of subconvulsant doses of GABA antagonist drugs. II: Effect on monoamine-mediated behaviour, *Psychopharmacology* **76:**88–91.
CREESE, I., KUCZENSKI, R., and SEGAL, D., 1982, Lack of behavioural evidence for dopamine autoreceptor subsensitivity after acute electroconvulsive shock, *Pharmacol. Biochem. Behav.* **17:**375–376.
CUPELLO, A., FERMILLO, F., and ROZADINI, G., 1981, Long lasting effects of electroconvulsive shock on the pattern of poly(A)-RNA synthesis in rabbit cerebral cortex, *Neurochem. Res.* **6:**175–182.

DASHIEFF, R. M., SAVAGE, D. D., and McNAMARA, J. O., 1982, Seizures down-regulate muscarinic cholinergic receptors in hippocampal formation, *Brain Res.* **235**:327–334.

DAVIES, C. L., and NUTT, D. J., 1983, Repeated electroconvulsive shock alters diazepam pharmacokinetics in rats, *Br. J. Pharmacol.* **78**:114P.

DAVIES, J. A., and WILLIAMS, J., 1978, The effect of baclofen on α-flupenthixol-induced catalepsy in the rat, *Br. J. Pharmacol.* **62**:303–305.

DEAKIN, J. F. W., OWEN, F., CROSS, A. J., and DASHWOOD, M. J., 1981, Studies on possible mechanisms of action of electroconvulsive therapy: Effects of repeated electrically-induced seizures on rat brain receptors for monoamines and other neurotransmitters, *Psychopharmacology* **73**:345–349.

de MONTIGNY, C., 1984, Electroconvulsive shock treatments enhance responsiveness of forebrain neurons to serotonin, *J. Pharmacol. Exp. Ther.* **228**:230–236.

DISMUKES, R. K., and DALY, J. W., 1974, Norepinephrine-sensitive systems generating adenosine 3'5'-monophosphate: Increased responses in cerebral cortical slices from reserpine-treated rats, *Mol. Pharmacol.* **10**:933–940.

DREW, G. M., GOWER, A. J., and MARRIOTT, A. S., 1979, α_2-Adrenoceptors mediate clonidine-induced sedation in the rat, *Br. J. Pharmacol.* **67**:133–141.

DURANT, C. J., DUNCAN, N. A. M., GANNELIN, C. R., PARSONS, M. E., BLAKEMORE, R., and RASMUSSEN, A., 1978, Impromidine (SK&F-92676) is a very potent and specific agonist for histamine H_2 receptors, *Nature* **276**:403–405.

EMRICH, H. M., and HÖLLT, V., 1984, Effect of ECT on endorphinergic systems: Clinical aspects, in: *ECT: Basic Mechanisms* (B. Lerer, R. D. Weiner, and R. H. Belmaker, eds.), John Libbey & Co., London, pp. 98–100.

ESSMAN, W. B., 1974, *Neurochemistry of Cerebral Electroshock*, John Wiley, New York.

EVANS, J. P. M., GRAHAME-SMITH, D. G., GREEN, A. R., and TORDOFF, A. F. C., 1976, Electroconvulsive shock increases the behavioural response of rats to brain 5-hydroxytryptamine accumulation and central nervous system stimulant drugs, *Br. J. Pharmacol.* **56**:193–199.

FARAGALLA, F. F., and FLACH, F., 1970, Studies of mineral metabolism in mental depression. I. The effects of imipramine and electric convulsive therapy on calcium balance and kinetics, *J. Nerv. Ment. Dis.* **151**:120–129.

FEIGHNER, J. P., LOW, L., KING, L. J., and ROSS, W. J., 1972, Brain serotonin and norepinephrine after convulsions and reserpine, *J. Neurochem.* **19**:905–907.

FERENDELLI, J. A., and KINSCHERF, D. A., 1977, Cyclic nucleotides in epileptic brain: Effects of pentylenetetrazol on regional cyclic AMP and cyclic GMP *in vivo*, *Epilepsia* **18**:525–531.

FILE, S. E., 1980, The use of social interaction as a method of detecting anxiolytic activity of chlordiazepoxide-like drugs, *J. Neurosci. Methods* **2**:219–238.

FILE, S. E., and GREEN, A. R., 1984, Repeated electroconvulsive shock has no specific anxiolytic effect but reduces social interaction and exploration in rats, *Neuropharmacology* **23**:95–99.

FINK, M., 1974, Induced seizures and human behaviour, in: *Psychobiology of Convulsive Therapy* (M. Fink, S. Kety, J. McGaugh, and T. A. Williams, eds.), V. H. Winston & Sons, Washington, DC, pp. 1–17.

FINK, M., 1979, *Convulsive Therapy: Theory and Practice*, Raven Press, New York.

FINK, M., 1984, Theories of convulsive therapy: a neuroendocrine hypothesis, in: *ECT Basic Mechanisms* (B. Lerer, R. D. Weiner, and R. H. Belmaker, eds.), John Libbey & Co., London, pp. 115–123.

FINK, M., and OTTOSSON, J.-O., 1980, A theory of convulsive therapy in endogenous depression: Significance of hypothalamic functions, *Psychiatr. Res.* **2**:49–61.

FLACH, F. F., 1964, Calcium metabolism in states of depression, *Br. J. Psychiatry* **110**:588–593.

FLACH, F. F., LIANG, E., and STOKES, P. E., 1960, Effects of electric convulsive treatments on nitrogen, calcium and phosphorous metabolism in psychiatric patients, *J. Ment. Sci.* **106**:638–647.

FREEMAN, C. P. L., BASSON, J. V., and CRICHTON, A., 1978, Double-blind controlled trial of electroconvulsive therapy (ECT) and simulated ECT in depressive illness, *Lancet* **1**:738–740.

FRENK, H. J., ENGEL, J., ACKERMAN, R. F., SHAVIT, Y., and LIEBESKIND, J. C., 1979, Endogenous opiates may mediate post-ictal behavioural depression in amygdaloid-kindled rats, *Brain Res.* **167**:435–440.

FRITH, C. D., STEVENS, M., JOHNSTONE, E. C., DEAKIN, J. F. W., LAWLER, P., and CROW, T. J., 1983, Effects of ECT and depression on varous aspects of memory, *Br. J. Psychiatry* **142**:610–617.

GANDOLFI, O., DALL'OLIO, R., and MONTANARO, N., 1978, Early changes in rat brain 5-HT synthesis after a single electro-convulsive shock, *Pharmacol. Res. Commun.* **10**:75–79.

GARCIA, A., WANG, C. H., SALAMA, A. I., and U'PRICHARD, D.C., 1982, Regulation of rat cerebral cortex α_2-receptor affinity states after electroconvulsive shock and antidepressant treatment, *Soc. Neurosci. Abstr.* **8**:525.

GILBERT, R. F. T., EMSON, P. C., HUNT, S., BENNETT, G. W., MARSDEN, C. A., SANDBERG, B. E. B., and STEINBUSCH, H. W., 1981, The effect of monoamine neurotoxins on peptides in the rat spinal cord, *Neuroscience* **7**:69–87.

GILLESPIE, D. D., MANIER, D. H., and SULSER, F., 1979, ECT: Rapid subsensitivity of NA adenylate cyclase system in brain linked to down regulation of beta-receptors, *Commun. Psychopharmacology* **3**:191–195.

GLOBUS, M., LERER, B., HAMBURGER, R., and BELMAKER, R., 1981, Chronic electroconvulsive shock and chronic haloperidol are not additive in effects on dopamine receptors, *Neuropharmacology* **20**:1125–1128.

GOODWIN, G. M., and GREEN, A. R., 1985, A behavioural and biochemical study in mice and rats of putative agonists and antagonists for 5-HT$_1$ and 5-HT$_2$ receptors, *Br. J. Pharamacol.* **84**:743–753.

GOODWIN, G. M., and HEAL, D. J., 1985, DSP-4 lesioning abolishes the enhanced monoamine-mediated behaviour following repeated electroconvulsive shock, *Br. J. Pharmacol.* **84**:538.

GOODWIN, G. M., GREEN, A. R., and JOHNSON, P., 1984, 5-HT$_2$ receptor characteristics in frontal cortex and 5-HT$_2$ receptor-mediated head-twitch behaviour following antidepressant treatment to mice, *Br. J. Pharmacol.* **83**:235–242.

GOODWIN, G. M., De SOUZA, R. J., and GREEN, A. R., 1985a, The pharmacology of the hypothermic response in mice to 8-hydroxy-(di-*N*-propylamino)tetralin (8-OH-DPAT): A model of presynaptic 5-HT$_1$ function, *Neuropharmacology* **24**:1187–1194.

GOODWIN, G. M., De SOUZA, R. J., and GREEN, A. R., 1985b, Presynaptic serotonin receptor-mediated response in mice attenuated by antidepressant drugs and electroconvulsive shock, *Nature* **317**:531–533.

GOUR, K. N., and CHAUDHRY, H. M., 1957, Study of calcium metabolism in electric convulsive therapy (ECT) in certain mental diseases, *J. Ment. Sci.* **103**:275–285.

GRAHAME-SMITH, D. G., GREEN, A. R., and COSTAIN, D. W., 1978, Mechanism of the antidepressant action of electroconvulsive therapy, *Lancet* **1**:254–256.

GRAY, J. A., METZ, A., GOODWIN, G. M., and GREEN, A. R., 1986, The effects of the GABA-mimetic drugs Progabide and Baclefen on the biochemistry and function of 5-hydroxytryptamine and noradrenaline, *Neuropharmacology* **25**:711–716.

GREEN, A. R., 1978, Repeated exposure of rats to the convulsant agent flurothyl enhanced 5-hydroxytryptamine- and dopamine-mediated behavioural responses, *Br. J. Pharmacol.* **62**:325–331.

GREEN, A. R., 1986a, Changes in GABA biochemistry and seizure threshold, *Ann. NY Acad. Sci.* **462**:105–119.

GREEN, A. R., 1986b, Electroconvulsive therapy: A GABAergic mechanism? in: *GABA and Mood Disorders: Animal and Clinical Studies* (K. G. Lloyd, G. Bartholini, and P. L. Morselli, eds.), Raven Press, New York, pp. 51–60.

GREEN, A. R., and DEAKIN, J. F. W., 1980, Brain noradrenaline depletion prevents ECS-induced enhancement of serotonin- and dopamine-mediated behaviour, *Nature* **285**:232–233.

GREEN, A. R., and HEAL, D. J., 1985, The effects of drugs on serotonin-mediated behavioural models, in: *Neuropharmacology of Serotonin* (A. R. Green, ed.), Oxford University Press, Oxford, pp. 326–365.

GREEN, A. R., and MOUNTFORD, J. A., 1985, Diazepam administration to mice prevents some of the changes in monoamine-mediated behaviour produced by repeated electroconvulsive shock treatment, *Psychopharmacology* **86**:190–193.

GREEN, A. R., and NUTT, D. J., 1983, Antidepressants, in: *Psychopharmacology,* Vol. I (D. G. Grahame-Smith and P. J. Cowen, eds.), Elsevier/Excerpta Medica, Amsterdam, pp. 1–37.

GREEN, A. R., and NUTT, D. J., 1985, Antidepressants, in: *Psychopharmacology,* Vol. II (D. G. Grahame-Smith and P. J. Cowen, eds.), Elsevier/Excerpta Medica, Amsterdam, pp. 1–33.

GREEN, A. R., TORDOFF, A. F. C., and BLOOMFIELD, M. R., 1976, Elevation of brain GABA concentrations with amino-oxyacetic acid: Effect on the hyperactivity syndrome produced by increased 5-hydroxytryptamine synthesis in rats, *J. Neural Transm.* **39**:103–112.

GREEN, A. R., HEAL, D. J., and GRAHAME-Smith, D. C., 1977, Further observations on the effect of repeated electroconvulsive shock on the behavioural responses of rats produced by increases in the functional activity of brain 5-hydroxytryptamine and dopamine, *Psychopharmacology* **52**:195–200.

GREEN, A. R., PERALTA, E., HONG, J. S., MAO, C. D., ATTERWILL, C. K., and COSTA, E., 1978, Alterations in GABA metabolism and met-enkephalin content in rat brain following repeated electroconvulsive shocks, *J. Neurochem.* **31**:607–611.

GREEN, A. R., BLOOMFIELD, M. R., ATTERWILL, C. K., and COSTAIN, D. W., 1979, Electroconvulsive shock recuces the cataleptogenic effects of both haloperidol and arecoline in rats, *Neuropharmacology* **18**:447–451.

GREEN, A. R., COSTAIN, D. W., and DEAKIN, J. F. W., 1980, Enhanced 5-hydroxytryptamine- and dopamine-mediated behavioural response following convulsions. III: The effects of monoamine antagonists and synthesis inhibitors on the ability of electroconvulsive shock to enhance responses, *Neuropharmacology* **19**:907–914.

GREEN, A. R., SANT, K., BOWDLER, J. M., and COWEN, P. J., 1982, Further evidence for a relationship between changes in GABA concentrations in rat brain and enhanced monoamine-mediated behaviours following repeated electroconvulsive shock, *Neuropharmacology* **21**:981–984.

GREEN, A. R., HEAL, D. J., JOHNSON, P., LAURENCE, B. E., and NIMGAONKAR, V. L., 1983a, Antidepressant treatments: effects in rodents on dose-response curves of 5-hydroxytryptamine- and dopamine-mediated behaviours and 5-HT$_2$ receptor number in frontal cortex, *Br. J. Pharmacol.* **80**:377–385.

GREEN, A. R., JOHSON, P., and NIMGAONKAR, V. L., 1983b, Increased 5-HT receptor number in brain as a probable explanation for the enhanced 5-hydroxytryptamine-mediated behaviour following repeated electroconvulsive shock administration to rats, *Br. J. Pharmacol.* **80**:173–177.

GREEN, A. R., GUY, A. P., and GARDNER, C. R., 1984a, The behavioural effects of RU 24969, a suggested 5-HT$_1$ agonist in rodents and the effect on the behaviour of treatment with antidepressants, *Neuropharmacology* **23**:655–661.

GREEN, A. R., NIMGAONKAR, V. L., and GOODWIN, G. M., 1984b, β-Adrenoceptor agonists,

ECT and other antidepressants: Effects on serotonin biochemistry and function, in: *Proceedings of the 9th International Congress of Pharmacology*, Vol. 3 (W. D. M. Paton, J. F. Mitchell, and R. Turner, eds.), Macmillan Press, Basingstoke, England, pp. 117–124.

GREEN, A. R., JOHNSON, P., MOUNTFORD, J. A., and NIMGAONKAR, V. L., 1985a, Some anticonvulsant drugs alter monoamine-mediated behaviour in mice in ways similar to electroconvulsive shock: Implications for antidepressant therapy, *Br. J. Pharmacol.* **82**:337–346.

GREEN, A. R., HAYES, C., METZ, A., MINCHIN, M. C. W., WILLIAMS, H., and VINCENT, N. D., 1985b, Decreased GABA synthesis in regions of rat brain following a convulsion, *Br. J. Pharmacol.* **84**:88P.

GREEN, A. R., MINCHIN, M. C. W., and VINCENT, N. D., 1985c, GABA release in rat brain following a seizure, *Br. J. Pharmacol.* **84**:89P.

GREENFIELD, S. A., 1984, Acetylcholinesterase may have novel functions in the brain, *Trends Neurosci.* **7**:364–368.

HEAL, D. J., 1984, Phenylephrine-induced activity in mice as a model of central α_1-adrenoceptor function. Effects of acute and repeated administration of antidepressant drugs and electroconvulsive shock, *Neuropharmacology* **23**:1241–1251.

HEAL, D. J., and GREEN, A. R., 1978, Repeated electroconvulsive shock increases the behavioural responses of rats to injection of both dopamine and dibutyryl cyclic AMP into the nucleus accumbens, *Neuropharmacology* **17**:1085–1087.

HEAL, D. J., PHILLIPS, A. G., and GREEN, A. R., 1978, Studies on the locomotor activity produced by injection of dibutyryl cyclic 3'5'-AMP into the nucleus accumbens of rats, *Neuropharmacology* **17**:265–270.

HEAL, D. J., AKAGI, H., BOWDLER, J. M., and GREEN, A. R., 1981, Repeated electroconvulsive shock attenuates clonidine-induced hypoactivity in rodents, *Eur. J. Pharmacol.* **75**:231–237.

HEAL, D. J., LISTER, S., SMITH, S. L., DAVIES, C. L., MOLYNEUX, S. G., and GREEN, A. R., 1983, The effects of acute and repeated administration of various antidepressants on clonidine hypoactivity in mice and rats, *Neuropharmacology* **22**:983–992.

HENDLEY, E. D., 1976, Electroconvulsive shock and norepinephrine uptake kinetics in rat brain, *Psychopharmacol. Commun.* **2**:17–25.

HOLADAY, J. W., and BELENKY, G. L., 1980, Opiate-like effects of electroconvulsive shock in rats: A differential effect of naloxone on nociceptive measures, *Life Sci.* **27**:1929–1938.

HOLADAY, J. W., BELENKY, G. L., LOH, H. H., and MEYERHOFF, J. L., 1978, Evidence for endorphin release during electroconvulsive shock, *Soc. Neurosci. Abstr.* **4**:409.

HONG, J. S., GILLIN, J. C., YANG, H-Y. T., and COSTA, E., 1979, Repeated electroconvulsive shocks and the brain content of endorphins, *Brain Res.* **177**:273–278.

HONG, J. S., KANAMATSU, T., MCGINTY, J. F., OBIE, J., DYER, R. S., and MITCHELL, C. L., 1985, Amygdaloid kindling increases enkephalin-like immunoreactivity but decreases dynorphin A-like immunoreactivity in rat hippocampus, *Fed. Proc.* **9**:2535–2539.

HORRELL, R. I., 1981, Specific antidepressant-like behavioural consequences of ECS in experimental animals, in: *Electroconvulsive Therapy, an Appraisal* (R. L. Palmer, ed.), Oxford University Press, Oxford, pp. 125–136.

JANOWSKY, A., OKADA, F., MANIER, D. H., APPLEGATE, C. D., SULSER, F., and STERANKA, L. R., 1982, Role of serotonergic input in the regulation of the β-adrenergic receptor-coupled adenylate cyclase system, *Science (Washington)* **218**:900–901.

JOHNSON, R. W., REISINE, T., SPOTNITZ, S., WEICH, N., URSILLO, R., and YAMAMURA, H. I., 1980, Effects of desipramine and yohimbine on alpha$_2$- and beta-adrenoceptor sensitivity, *Eur. J. Pharmacol.* **67**:123–127.

JONES, R. S. G., MONDADORI, C., and OLPE, H-R., 1985, Neuronal sensitivity to substance P is increased after repeated treatment with tranylcypromine, carbamazepine or oxaprotaline but decreased after repeated electroconvulsive shock, *Neuropharmacology* **24:**627–633.

KELLAR, K. J., 1984, ECS: effects on serotonergic and β-adrenergic receptor binding sites in brain, in: *ECT: Basic Mechanisms* (B. Lerer, R. D. Weiner, and R. H. Belmaker, eds.), John Libbey & Co., London, pp. 46–56.

KELLAR, K. J., CASCIO, C. S., BUTLER, J. A., and KURTZKE, R. W., 1981a, Differential effects of electroconvulsive shock and antidepressant drugs on serotonin-2-receptors in rat brain, *Eur. J. Pharmacol.* **69:**515–518.

KELLAR, K. J., CASCIO, C. S., BERGSTROM, D. A., BUTLER, J. A., and IADAROLA, P., 1981b, Electroconvulsive shock and reserpine: Effects on β-adrenergic receptors in rat brain, *J. Neurochem.* **37:**830–836.

KELLER, H. H., SCHAFFNER, R., and HAEFELY, W., 1976, Interactions of benzodiazepines with neuroleptics at central dopamine neurones, *Naunyn-Schmiedeberg's Arch. Pharmac.* **294:**1–7.

KETY, S. S., JAVOY, F., THIERRY, A. M., JULOU, Z., and GLOWINSKI, J., 1967, A sustained effect of electroconvulsive shock on the turnover of norepinephrine in the central nervous system of the rat, *Proc. Natl. Acad. Sci. USA* **58:**1249–1254.

LAMBOURN, J., and GILL, D., 1978, A controlled comparison of simulated and real ECT, *Br. J. Psychiatry* **133:**514–519.

LEBRECHT, U., and NOWAK, J. Z., 1980a, Effect of single and repeated electroconvulsive shock on serotonergic system in rat brain. II: Behavioural studies, *Neuropharmacology* **19:**1049–1053.

LEBRECHT, U., and NOWAK, J. Z., 1980b, Effect of single and repeated electroconvulsive shock on serotonergic system in rat brain. II: Behavioural studies, *Neuropharmacology* **19:**1055–1061.

LERER, B., 1985, Studies on the role of brain cholinergic systems in the therapeutic mechanisms and adverse effects of ECT and lithium, *Biol. Psychiatry* **20:**20–40.

LERER, B., JABOTINSKY-RUBIN, K., BANNET, J., EBSTEIN, R. P., and BELMAKER, R. H., 1982, Electroconvulsive shock prevents dopamine receptor supersensitivity, *Eur. J. Pharmacol.* **80:**131–134.

LERER, B., STANLEY, M., DEMETRIOU, S., and GEERSHON, S., 1983, Effect of electroconvulsive shock on [³H]-QNB binding in rat cerebral cortex and hippocampus, *J. Neurochem.* **41:**1680–1683.

LERER, B., STANLEY, M., MCINTYRE, I., and ALTMAN, A., 1984, Electroconvulsive shock and brain muscarinic receptors: Relationship to anterograde amnesia, *Life Sci.* **35:**2659–2664.

LEWIN, E., and BLECK, V., 1981, Electroshock seizures in mice: Effect on brain adenosine and its metabolites, *Epilepsia* **22:**577–581.

LIGHTON, K. G., MARSDEN, C. A., BENNETT, G. W., MINCHIN, M. C. W., and GREEN, A. R., 1984, Decrease in levels of thyrotropin-releasing hormone (TRH) in the n. accumbens and lumbar spinal cord following repeated electroconvulsive shock, *Neuropharmacology* **23:**963–966.

LIGHTON, C., BENNETT, G. W., and MARSDEN, C. A., 1985, Increase in levels and *ex vivo* release of thyrotrophin-releasing hormone (TRH) in specific regions of the CNS of the rat by chronic treatment with antidepressants, *Neuropharmacology* **24:**401–406.

LLOYD, K. G., and PILC, A., 1984, Chronic antidepressants and GABA-B receptors, Poster; 9th International Congress on Pharmacology, London.

LLOYD, K. G., ARBILLA, S., BEAUMONT, K., BRILEY, M., DEMONTIS, G., SCATTON, B., LANGER, S. Z., and BARTHOLINI, G., 1982, γ-Aminobutyric acid (GABA) receptor stimulation. II: Specificity of progabide (SL 76002) and SL 75102 for the GABA receptor, *J. Pharmacol. Exp. Ther.* **220:**672–677.

LLOYD, K. G., MORSELLI, P. L., DEPOORTERE, H., FOURNIER, V., ZIVCOVIC, B., SCATTON, B.,

BROEKKAMP, C., WORMS, P., and BARTHOLINI, G., 1983, The potential use of GABA agonists in psychiatric disorders, evidence from studies with progabide on animal models and clinical trials, *Pharmacol. Biochem. Behav.* **18**:957–966.

LLOYD, K. G., THURET, F., and PILC, A., 1985, Upregulation of gamma-aminobutyric acid (GABA)$_B$ binding sites in rat frontal cortex: A common action of repeated administration of different classes of antidepressants and electroshock, *J. Pharmacol. Exp. Therap.* **235**:191–199.

LONGONI, R., MULAS, A., ODERFELD, B., PEPEU, I. M., and PEPEU, G., 1976, Effect of single and repeated electroshock applications on brain acetylcholine levels and choline acetyltransferase activity in the rat, *Neuropharmacology* **15**:283–286.

MASSERANO, J. M., TAKIMOTO, G. S., and WEINER, N., 1981, Electroconvulsive shock increases tyrosine hydroxylase activity in the brain and adrenal gland of the rat, *Science (Washington)* **214**:662–665.

McGAUGH, J. L., 1966, Time-dependent processes in memory storage, *Science (Washington)* **153**:1351–1358.

McNAMARA, J. O., PEPER, A. M., and PATRONE, V., 1980, Repeated seizures induce long-term increase in hippocampal benzodiazepine receptors, *Proc. Natl. Acad. Sci. USA* **77**:3029–3032.

McWILLIAM, J. R., MELDRUM, B. S., and CHECKLEY, S. A., 1981, Enhanced growth hormone response to clonidine after repeated electroconvulsive shock in a primate species, *Psychoneuroendocrinology* **6**:77–79.

McWILLIAM, J. R., MELDRUM, B. S., and CHECKLEY, S. A., 1982, Changes in noradrenergic neuroendocrine responses following repeated seizures and the mechanisms of action of ECT, *Psychopharmacology* **77**:53–57.

MELLANBY, J., GREEN, A. R., IMPEY, L., OATES, C., and TRAYNOR, L., 1984, The effect of electroconvulsive shock on learning and memory in rats, *Acta Neurol. Scand.* **69**(99):115–118.

METAFORA, S., PERSICO, M., FELSANI, A., FERRAIUOLO, R., and GUIDITTA, A., 1977, On the mechanism of the electroshock-induced inhibition of protein synthesis in rabbit cerebral cortex, *J. Neurochem.* **28**:1335–1346.

METZ, A., GOODWIN, G. M., and GREEN, A. R., 1985, The administration of baclofen to mice increases 5-HT$_2$-mediated head-twitch behaviour and 5-HT$_2$ receptor number in frontal cortex, *Neuropharmacology* **24**:257–260.

MINCHIN, M. C. W., and NUTT, D. J., 1983, Studies on [^{3}H]-diazepam and [^{3}H]-ethyl-β-carboline carboxylate binding to rat brain *in vivo*. I: Regional variations in displacement, *J. Neurochem.* **41**:1507–1512.

MINCHIN, M. C. W., and NUTT, D. J., 1984, The effect of repeated electroconvulsive shock on the function of THIP, a GABA agonist, *Pharmacol. Biochem. Behav.* **21**:491–493.

MINCHIN, M. C. W., WILLIAMS, J., BOWDLER, J. M., and GREEN, A. R., 1983, The effect of electroconvulsive shock on the uptake and release of noradrenaline and 5-hydroxytryptamine in rat brain slices, *J. Neurochem,* **40**:765–768.

MODIGH, K., 1975, Electroconvulsive shock and postsynaptic catecholamine effects: Increased psychomotor stimulant action of apomorphine and clonidine in reserpine pretreated mice by repeated ECS, *J. Neural Transm.* **36**:19–32.

MODIGH, K., 1976, Long-term effects of electroconvulsive shock therapy on synthesis, turnover, and uptake of brain monoamines, *Psychopharmacology* **49**:179–185.

MODIGH, K., 1979, Long lasting effects of ECT on monoaminergic mechanisms, in: *Neuropsychopharmacology* (B. Saletu, P. Berner, and L. Hollister, eds.), Pergamon Press, Oxford.

MODIGH, K., and JACKSON, P. M., 1975, Evidence for a sustained effect of ECS on neuronal structures connected to brain catecholamine neurones, *6th International Congress on Pharmacology, Helsinki*, Abstract, p. 172.

MUSACCHIO, J. M., JULOU, I., KETY, S. S., and GLOWINSKI, J., 1969, Increase in rat brain tyrosine hydroxylase activity produced by electroconvulsive shock, *Proc. Natl. Acad. Sci. USA* **63:**1117–1119.

MYSLOBODSY, M. S., and MINTZ, M., 1981, Postictal behavioral arrest in the rat: "Catalepsy" or "catatonia"? *Life Sci.* **28:**2287–2293.

MYSLOBODSKY, M., KOFMAN, O., and MINTZ, M., 1981, Convulsant-specific architecture of the postictal behaviour syndrome in the rat, *Epilepsia* **22:**559–568.

NEWMAN, M., ZOHAR, J., KALIAN, M., and BELMAKER, R. H., 1984, Effects of ECS on adenosine receptor systems in the brain, in: *ECT: Basic Mechanisms* (B. Lerer, R. D. Weiner, and R. H. Belmaker, eds.), John Libbey & Co., London, pp. 57–61.

NIMGAONKAR, V. L., GOODWIN, G. M., DAVIES, C. L., and GREEN, A. R., 1985, Down-regulation of β-adrenoceptors in rat cortex by repeated administration of desipramine, electroconvulsive shock and clenbuterol requires 5-HT neurones but not 5-HT, *Neuropharmacology* **24:**279–283.

NIMGAONKAR, V. L., HEAL, D. J., DAVIES, C. L., and GREEN, A. R., 1986, Studies on rat brain catecholamine synthesis and B-adrenoceptor number following administration of electroconvulsive shock, desipramine and clenbuterol, *J. Neurol. Transm.* **65:**245–259.

NUTT, D. J., and MINCHIN, M. C. W., 1983, Studies of [^{3}H]-diazepam and [^{3}H]-ethyl-β-carboline carboxylate binding to rate brain *in vivo*. II: Effects of electroconvulsive shock, *J. Neurochem.* **41:**1514–1517.

NUTT, D. J., GREEN, A. R., and GRAHAME-SMITH, D. G., 1980*a*, Enhanced 5-hydroxytryptamine- and dopamine-mediated behavioural responses following convulsions. 1: The effects of single and repeated bicuculline-induced seizures, *Neuropharmacology* **19:**897–900.

NUTT, D. J., COWEN, P. J., and GREEN, A. R., 1980*b*, On the measurement of rats of the convulsant effect of drugs and the changes which follow electroconvulsive shock, *Neuropharmacology* **19:**1018–1023.

NUTT, D. J., COWEN, P. J., and GREEN, A. R., 1981, Studies on the post-ictal rise in seizure threshold, *Eur. J. Pharmacol.* **71:**287–295.

NUTT, D. J., SMITH, S. L., and HEAL, D. J., 1982, Hypophysectomy does not prevent the enhanced monoamine-mediated behavioural responses following repeated electroconvulsive shocks, *Neuropharmacology* **21:**881–884.

OLNEY, J. W., DE GUBANEFF, T., and LABRUYERE, J., 1983, Seizure-related brain damage induced by cholinergic agents, *Nature* **310:**520–522.

PANDEY, G. N., HEINZE, W. J., BROWN, B. D., and DAVIS, J. M., 1979, Electroconvulsive shock treatment decreases beta-adrenergic receptor sensitivity in rat brain, *Nature* **280:**234–235.

PAUL, S. M., and SKOLNICK, P., 1978, Rapid changes in brain benzodiazepine receptors after experimental seizures, *Science* **202:**892–894.

PEDIGO, N. W., YAMAMURA, H. I., and NELSON, D. L., 1981, Discrimination of multiple [^{3}H]-5-hydroxytryptamine binding sites by the neuroleptic spiperone in rat brain, *J. Neurochem.* **36:**220–226.

PEROUTKA, S. J., and SNYDER, S. H., 1979, Multiple serotonin receptors: Differential binding of [^{3}H]-hydroxytryptamine, [^{3}H]-lysergic acid diethylamide and [^{3}H]-spiroperidol, *Mol. Pharmacol.* **16:**687–699.

PEROUTKA, S. J., and SNYDER, S. H., 1980, Long term antidepressant treatment decreases spiroperidol-labelled serotonin receptor binding, *Science* **210:**88.

PERUMAL, A. S., and BARKAI, A. I., 1982, β-Adrenergic receptor binding in different regions of rat brain after various intensities of electroshock: Relationship to postictal EEG, *J. Neurosci. Res.* **7:**289–296.

PILC, A., and VETULANI, J., 1982, Depression by chronic electroconvulsive treatment of clonidine hypothermia and [^{3}H]-clonidine binding to rat cortical membranes, *Eur. J. Pharmacol.* **80:**109–113.

PILC, A., ROGÓZ, Z., and BYRSKA, B., 1980, Some central effects of impromidine, a potent agonist of histamine H_2 receptor, *Neuropharmacology* **19**:947–950.

ROYAL COLLEGE OF PSYCHIATRISTS, 1977, The Royal College of Psychiatrists memorandum on the use of electroconvulsive therapy, *Br. J. Psychiatry* **131**:261–272.

SACKHEIM, H. A., DECINA, P., PROHOVNIK, I., MALITZ, S., and RESOR, S. K., 1983, Anticonvulsant and antidepressant properties of electroconvulsive therapy: A proposed mechanism of action, *Biol. Psychiatry* **18**:1301–1310.

SATTIN, A., 1971, Increase in the content of adenosine 3',5'-monophosphate in mouse forebrain during seizures and prevention of the increase by methylxanthines, *J. Neurochem.* **18**:1087–1096.

SATTIN, A., 1981, Adenosine as a mediator of antidepressant treatment, in: *Chemisms of the Brain* (R. Rodnight, H. S. Bachelard, and W. L. Stahl, eds.), Churchill-Livingstone, Edinburgh, pp. 265–275.

SCHLICKER, E., CLASSEN, K., and GOTHERT, M., 1984, GABA receptor-mediated inhibition of serotonin release in the rat brain, *Naunyn-Schiedeberg's Arch. Pharmac.* **326**:99–105.

SERRA, G., ARGIOLAS, A., FADDA, F., MELIS, M. R., and GESSA, G. L., 1981, Repeated electroconvulsive shock prevents the sedative effect of small doses of apomorphine, *Psychopharmacology* **73**:194–196.

SHIELDS, P. J., 1972, Effects of electroconvulsive shock on the metabolism of 5-HT in the rat brain, *J. Pharm. Pharmacol.* **23**:919–920.

SLADE, A. P., and CHECKLEY, S. A., 1980, A neuroendocrine study of the mechanism of action of ECT, *Br. J. Psychiatry* **137**:217–221.

SMITH, C. G., GARCIA-SEVILLA, J. A., and HOLLINGSWORTH, P. J., 1981, α_2-Adrenoceptors in rat brain are decreased after long-term tricyclic antidepressant drug treatment, *Brain Res.* **210**:413–418.

STANFORD, S. C., and NUTT, D. J., 1982, Comparison of the effects of repeated electroconvulsive shock on α_2-adrenoceptors in different regions of rat brain, *Neuroscience* **7**:1753–1757.

STANFORD, C., NUTT, D. J., and COWEN, P. J., 1983, Comparison of the effects of chronic desmethylimipramine administration on α_2- and β-adrenoceptors in different regions of rat brain, *Neuroscience* **8**:161–164.

STANLEY, M., and LERER, B., 1985, Electroconvulsive shock and cholinergic function: Role of striatal muscarinic receptors, *Convulsive Ther.* **1**:158–166.

STEINER, J. A., and GRAHAME-SMITH, D. G., 1980, The effect of repeated electroconvulsive shock on corticosterone responses to centrally acting pharmacological stimuli in the male rate, *Psychopharmacology* **71**:205–212.

STEINER, J. A., EVANS, G., and GRAHAME-SMITH, D. G., 1982, The effect of repeated electroconvulsive shocks on growth hormone secretion and growth hormone responses to clonidine in the intact rat, *Psychopharmacology* **76**:98–100.

SUGRUE, M. F., 1981, Effects of acutely and chronically administered antidepressants on the clonidine-induced decrease in rat brain 3-methoxy-4-hydroxyphenylethyleneglycol sulphate content, *Life Sci.* **28**:377–384.

SUGRUE, M. F., 1982, A study of the sensitivity of rat brain α_2-adrenoceptors during chronic antidepressant treatments, *Naunyn-Schmiedeberg's Arch. Pharmacol.* **320**:90–96.

SULSER, F., and MOBLEY, P. L., 1981, Regulation of central noradrenergic receptor functions: New vistas on the mode of action of antidepressant treatments, in: *Neuroregulators: Basic and Clinical Aspects* (E. Usdin, J. M. Davis, and W. E. Bunney, eds.), John Wiley & Sons, Chichester, pp. 55–83.

TACKE, U., PAANANEN, A., and TUOMISTO, J., 1984, Seizure thresholds and their postictal changes in audiogenic seizure (AGS)-susceptible rats, *Eur. J. Pharmacol.* **104**:85–92.

TORTELLA, F. C., COWAN, A., BELENKY, G. L., and HOLADAY, J. W., 1981, Opiate-like electroencephalographic and behavioural effects of electroconvulsive shock in rats, *Eur. J. Pharmacol.* **76**:121–128.

TORTELLA, F. C., COWAN, A., and ADLER, M. W., 1984, Studies on the excitatory and inhibitory influence of intracerebroventricularly injected opioids on seizure thresholds in rats, *Neuropharmacology* **23**:749–754.

TURSKI, W. A., CZUCZWAR, S. J., KLEINVOK, Z., and TURSKI, L., 1983, Cholinomimetics produce seizures and brain damage in rats, *Experientia* **39**:1408.

U'PRICHARD, D. C., and SNYDER, S. H., 1978, [^{3}H]-Catecholamine binding to α-receptors in rat brain: Enhancement by reserpine, *Eur. J. Pharmacol.* **51**:145–155.

U'PRICHARD, D., BECHTEL, W., ROUST, B., and SNYDER, S. H., 1979, Multiple apparent alpha noradrenergic receptor binding sites in rat brain: Effect of 6-hydroxydopamine, *Mol. Pharmacol.* **16**:47–60.

VETULANI, J., 1984, Changes in responsiveness of central aminergic structures after chronic ECS, in: *ECT: Basic Mechanisms* (B. Lerer, R. D. Weiner, and R. H. Belmaker, eds.), John Libbey & Co., London, pp. 33–45.

VETULANI, J., and PILC, A., 1982, Postdecapitation convulsions in the rat measured with an Anime motility meter: Relation to central α-adrenoceptors, *Eur. J. Pharmacol.* **85**:269–275.

VETULANI, J., and SULSER, F., 1975, Action of various antidepressant treatments reduced reactivity of noradrenergic cyclic AMP generating system in limbic forebrain, *Nature* **257**:495–496.

VETULANI, J., STAWARZ, R. J., DINGELL, J. V., and SULSER, F., 1976, A possible common mechanism of action of antidepressant treatments. Reduction in the sensitivity of noradrenergic cyclic AMP generating system in the rat limbic forebrain, *Naunyn-Schmiedeberg's Arch. Pharmacol.* **293**:109–144.

VETULANI, J., ANTKIEWICZ-MICHALUK, L., GOLEMBIOWSKA-NIKITIN, K., MICHALUK, J., PILC, A., and ROKOSZ, A., 1980, The effect of multiple imipramine administration on monoaminergic systems of the rat brain, *Pol. J. Pharmacol.* **32**:523–530.

VETULANI, J., LEBRECHT, U., and PILC, A., 1981, Enhancement of responsiveness of the central serotonergic system and serotonin-2-receptor density in rat frontal cortex by electroconvulsive treatments, *Eur. J. Pharmacol.* **76**:81–85.

VETULANI, J., ANTKIEWICZ-MICHALUK, L., ROKOSZ-PELC, A., and PILC, A., 1983, Chronic electroconvulsive treatment enhances density of [^{3}H]-prazosin binding sites in the central nervous system of the rat, *Brain Res.* **275**:392–395.

WASTERLAIN, C. G., and CSISZOR, E., 1980, Cyclic nucleotide metabolism in mouse brain during seizures induced by bicuculline or dibutyryl cyclic guanosine monophosphate, *Exp. Neurol.* **70**:260–268.

WEEKS, D., FREEMAN, C. P. L., and KENDELL, R. E., 1980, ECT III: Enduring cognitive defects, *Br. J. Psychiatry* **137**:26–37.

WEILOSZ, M., 1981, Increased sensitivity to dopaminergic agonists after repeated electroconvulsive shock in rats, *Neuropharmacology* **20**:941–945.

WHITE, D. K., and BARRETT, R. J., 1981, The effects of electroconvulsive shock on the discriminative stimulus properties of *d*-amphetamine and apomorphine: Evidence for dopamine receptor alteration subsequent to ECS, *Psychopharmacology* **73**:211–214.

WORMS, P., and LLOYD, K. G., 1978, Influence of GABA-agonists and antagonists on neuroleptic-induced catalepsy in rats, *Life Sci.* **23**:475–478.

WORMS, P. H., DEPOORTERE, A., DURAND, P. L., MORSELLI, M. G., LLOYD, K. G., and BARTHOLINI, G., 1982, γ-Aminobutyric acid (GABA) receptor stimulation. I: Neuropharmacological profiles of progabide (SL 76002) and SL 75102 with emphasis on their anticonvulsant spectra, *J. Pharmacol. Exp. Ther.* **220**:660–671.

YOSHIKAWA, K., HONG, J. S., and SABOL, S. L. 1985, Electroconvulsive shock increases preproenkephalin messenger RNA abundance in rat hypothalamus, *Proc. Natl. Acad. Sci. U.S.A.* **82**:589–593.

ZIVKOVIC, B., SCATTON, B., DEDEK, J., and BARTHOLINI, G., 1982, GABA influence on noradrenergic and serotonergic transmissions: Implications in mood regulation, in: *New Vistas in Depression, Advances in Bioscience*, Vol. 40, Pergamon Press, Oxford, pp. 195–201.

7

PSYCHOPHARMACOLOGY OF NICOTINE: STIMULUS EFFECTS AND RECEPTOR MECHANISMS

I. P. Stolerman

1. INTRODUCTION

1.1. Historical Background

The paradoxical status of the pharmacology of nicotinic mechanisms as a research problem has both stimulated and frustrated psychopharmacologists. The paradox is the dissonance between the practical importance of understanding a significant aspect of brain function and the actual amount of interest shown in the problem. People smoke tobacco mainly to obtain the effects of nicotine; a more effective, rational way of dealing with the pharmacological component of tobacco addiction can only come from advances in understanding both the behavioral mechanisms involved and the mode of action of nicotine in the CNS. There is also growing interest in the relation that central nicotinic mechanisms may have to certain pathological states, notably Alzheimer's disease (in which disturbances in cholinergic systems have been investigated mainly with regard to muscarinic systems) and parkinsonism (which is negatively correlated with cigarette smoking). Why has nicotine research been so much

---

I. P. Stolerman • Departments of Pharmacology and Psychiatry, Institute of Psychiatry, London SE5 8AF, England.

neglected until recent years? This chapter begins with a brief consideration of the reasons for this state of affairs; it then details recent advances made in understanding ways in which nicotine helps to maintain tobacco smoking and in knowledge of relevant CNS mechanisms.

The most obvious reason for the relative neglect of nicotinic mechanisms is historical. First, nicotine was discovered so long ago, its therapeutic value was so limited, and the peripheral cholinergic mechanisms seemed so well understood that there was little incentive, on purely scientific grounds, for extensive studies. Second, it was commonly thought that there were relatively few nicotinic–cholinergic receptors in the CNS, as compared with the relatively easily identified muscarinic–cholinergic sites. Third, the role of nicotine as the main addictive agent in tobacco use was widely misunderstood. One substantial group of researchers believed that this role was so well established, and that brain nicotinic sites and mechanisms were so well defined, that there was little more to be learned. Another, perhaps larger, number of scientists believed that tobacco use was primarily based on nonpharmacological sources of reinforcement, including the taste and smell of smoke and social factors, and that nicotine was so obviously nonaddictive that further work on its effects would be irrelevant. Thus, for one reason or another, research on central effects of nicotine was unpopular and attracted limited amounts of funding.

The change in the situation began in the late 1960s when Jarvik started to examine nicotine as a primary reinforcer of smoking, in the face of determined opposition from influential supporters of the then-prevailing view that pharmacological reinforcement was unimportant in tobacco use (Jarvik, 1968). Armitage *et al.* (1968) also argued cogently that the effects of nicotine were at the root of the smoking habit. One of the problems with the hypothesis of pharmacological reinforcement was the difficulty that many workers had in obtaining nicotine self-administration behavior in animals, which contrasted with findings for indisputably addictive agents. The scientific stimulation and controversy provoked by studies of the binding of nicotinic ligands to brain tissue and, in the last 5 years, the greater priority assigned to smoking research by funding agencies have encouraged more interest in nicotinic mechanisms.

This chapter reviews the recent work that was aimed at two main questions. What can behavioral studies contribute to knowledge of the addictiveness of nicotine and, if it is addictive, how do its behavioral effects contribute to the maintenance and regulation of tobacco use? What are the underlying neuropharmacological mechanisms? It will be argued that recent behavioral studies show that under suitable conditions, nicotine can be a very effective reinforcer and that there is justification for qualified optimism with regard to identification of relevant receptors.

1.2. Behavioral Background

It has been known for about 15 years that under suitable conditions, laboratory animals will self-administer doses of most drugs abused by humans. Included in this work were opioids, amphetamines, cocaine, barbiturates, and alcohol (Schuster and Thompson, 1969; Griffiths *et al.*, 1980). The most frequently used methods have involved implanting a venous catheter and then training the subject (often a small primate) to emit a typical operant response, such as pressing a bar, to obtain an intravenous injection of drug. Experiments of this type have been carried out with nicotine, and for a long time, they met with very little success. Response rates for nicotine either did not differ much from those for saline, or they were very low and variable in comparison with those maintained by other drugs. It was, therefore, difficult to argue that such work provided much evidence for the addictiveness of nicotine. Largely because of the work carried out by Goldberg, Spealman, and their colleagues, this situation has changed considerably in recent years (Henningfield and Goldberg, 1984); the progress made is outlined in Section 2.

Drugs may, of course, function as internal stimuli in several ways and not only as positive reinforcers. Several agents have aversive effects, as shown in punishment, negative reinforcement, or conditioned taste aversion paradigms. Included in this category are many addictive drugs, which, under different conditions, may serve as positive reinforcers (Stolerman and D'Mello, 1981). Nicotine is one such drug, since it is active in all three behavioral paradigms used to test for aversive effects. It has been suggested that such aversive effects of nicotine contribute to regulating the extent of exposure to tobacco smoke, perhaps by setting an upper limit to the amounts of nicotine sought (Kumar and Stolerman, 1977; Russell, 1979). The progress made in this area will be reviewed in Section 3.

Another behavioral technique, focusing on the discriminative stimulus effects of drugs, has also been extensively applied to nicotine. Drug discrimination experiments involve training animals to make different behavioral responses depending on whether they have been injected with a particular drug. Correct discriminations are reinforced by presenting either food or another of the conventional stimuli much used in behavioral research. The observation that nicotine is well discriminated from the nondrug condition does not itself indicate whether it is "addictive" or reinforcing. However, the nicotine discriminative stimulus or cue has been very useful as a behavioral assay in studies primarily concerned with nicotine's neuropharmacological mode of action, and this work is surveyed in Section 4. There is another reason why these studies may be of interest: With many classes of drug, there is a remarkable correlation between discriminative effects in animals and subjective effects in humans. The proper interpretation of this relationship remains controversial, but a reasonable case can be made that discriminative effects of drugs represent the closest known analog in animals of subjective effects and mood changes in humans.

From the earliest days of research on drugs as reinforcers, the possibility of parallels with the reinforcing effects of intracranial electrical stimulation was considered. The main hypothesis has been that both drugs and electrical stimuli may bring about their reinforcing effects by activating similar brain mechanisms, which may or may not be the same as those activated by conventional reinforcing events. Work with intracranial electrical stimulation in both self-stimulation and other paradigms may, therefore, be of some value in elucidating mechanisms of drug-produced reinforcement. These studies, and others that may bear on the same question, are discussed in Section 5.

1.3. Neurochemical Background

The two main questions concerning the neuropharmacology of nicotine have been, first, does nicotine act primarily through cholinergic mechanisms in the CNS and, second, how and where in the brain does nicotine act to bring about the effects sought by tobacco users? In the peripheral nervous system, it seems that all the major pharmacological effects of nicotine are achieved by mimicking the effects of acetylcholine at nicotinic–cholinergic receptors. Both stimulatory and blocking effects at cholinergic receptors are well documented, but only the former is thought to occur with concentrations of nicotine obtained from tobacco smoke. The main sites of action are in the autonomic ganglia, the adrenal medulla, and on sensory receptors such as those in the carotid body. It would be unwise to extrapolate from this knowledge to the CNS. In recent years, attempts have been made to identify and characterize putative nicotinic receptors in the CNS by means of ligand-binding studies. This strategy, which was so successfully used with other classes of drugs, was only slowly applied to nicotine.

During the late 1970s, a lengthy series of papers on the binding of α-bungarotoxin (ABTX) was published (reviewed by Brown, 1979; Schmidt et al., 1980; Morley, 1981). This ligand was selected because it had been extremely valuable in work on nicotinic–cholinergic receptors at the neuromuscular junction. ABTX binding in mammalian brain was specifically displaced by nicotine and other cholinergic agonists, and detailed descriptions of its distribution across different brain regions are available (e.g., Hunt and Schmidt, 1978). Volpe et al. (1979) reported on the regional distribution of ABTX binding sites in human brain and on possible changes in patients suffering from Parkinson's disease or senile dementia. However, this approach has several serious limitations. It is difficult to be certain that ABTX specifically labels all CNS nicotinic receptors. If the aim is to determine whether nicotine acts through noncholinergic mechanisms, using another cholinergic ligand instead of nicotine itself could give very misleading results.

Almost all the central effects of nicotine, be they electrophysiological, biochemical, or behavioral, are prevented by drugs that block the effects of nicotine at autonomic ganglia (e.g., mecamylamine). This suggests that central nicotinic receptors, if they are cholinergic, may resemble the receptors at ganglia rather than those at the neuromuscular junction. ABTX blocks transmission at the neuromuscular junction but not in autonomic ganglia. Only one study suggests that ABTX can block transmission in rat ganglia (Toldi *et al.*, 1983). Furthermore, the binding of ABTX in mammalian brain is potently inhibited by neuromuscular blocking drugs, whereas ganglionic blockers are inactive. ABTX has also been repeatedly found to be ineffective in blocking drug effects mediated through nicotinic–cholinergic receptors in mammalian CNS and in inhibiting nicotine binding in brain; these findings also suggest that it probably does not block most of the receptors through which nicotine acts. The neuroanatomical distributions of ABTX and nicotine binding sites are quite different (Marks and Collins, 1982; Clark *et al.*, 1985). In view of the problems mentioned, it is clear that ABTX is an inadequate marker for central nicotinic sites.

Two toxins that do seem to block neuronal effects of nicotinic agonists are κ-bungarotoxin and neosurugatoxin (Dryer and Chiappinelli, 1983; Hayashi *et al.*, 1984; Rapier *et al.*, 1985); these are potentially valuable agents about which only limited information is presently available. Neosurugatoxin was also found to inhibit nicotine binding in rat brain (Hayashi *et al.*, 1984; Rapier *et al.*, 1985). There is also a possibility that some samples of ABTX may have contained κ-bungarotoxin, since both are derived from venom of the same snake.

It follows that when the aim is to find out how and where nicotine acts in the CNS, it is necessary to use nicotine itself as the ligand. The earliest attempts to do so were hampered by several problems, not least the low specific activity of [^{3}H]nicotine available at the time (Schleifer and Eldefrawi, 1974; Yoshida and Imura, 1979). Not until 1980 was a binding site for nicotine identified with characteristics resembling those expected for a receptor, i.e., saturable binding displaceable by unlabeled nicotine and with some evidence for stereospecificity (Romano and Goldstein, 1980). The ligand used in this work was [^{3}H]-($\pm$)-nicotine, whereas the product in tobacco is (−)-nicotine. Most subsequent studies have also used labeled racemic nicotine as the ligand, and the qualitative aspects of the binding found by Romano and Goldstein have been confirmed by many workers (e.g., Marks and Collins, 1982). The binding is displaced by other nicotinic–cholinergic agonists (e.g., anabasine, carbachol, cytisine, dimethyl-phenylpiperazinium, and lobeline). (−)-Nicotine is at least 10 times more potent than (+)-nicotine in displacing [^{3}H]-(±)-nicotine. Drugs acting at other neurotransmitter receptors (including muscarinic–cholinergic compounds) were all ineffective except at very large concentrations.

Surprisingly, all the well-established nicotinic blocking drugs (mecamylamine, pempidine, hexamethonium, chlorisondamine, tubocurarine, and ABTX) also failed to inhibit nicotine binding. Similar findings have been obtained in several laboratories, including some in which autoradiographic techniques were used to compile a very detailed atlas of nicotine binding sites in rat brain (Clarke *et al.*, 1984, 1985). Binding sites were spread widely through many areas of the brain, with particularly high densities in the thalamus, interpeduncular nucleus, superior colliculus, medial habenula, cerebral cortex, substantia nigra, and dentate gyrus of the hippocampus (Fig. 1). Some structures were almost devoid of binding sites (e.g., globus pallidus).

The ability of nicotinic–cholinergic agonists to displace the binding of nicotine suggests that if the binding site is a receptor and not merely an acceptor site with no functional significance, then the endogenous ligand may well be acetylcholine. High-affinity binding sites for acetylcholine have been identified in the presence of atropine (which inhibits binding to muscarinic sites). This remaining acetylcholine binding is inhibited by nicotine, and the characteristics of the site, including its regional distribution, are almost identical to those of sites for nicotine itself (Schwartz *et al.*, 1982; Rainbow *et al.*, 1984; Clark *et al.*, 1985). The failure of such blocking drugs as mecamylamine to displace nicotine has been explained either as an artifact of the *in vitro* procedures or as an indication that in the presence of nicotine, the sites are placed in an "agonist-selective" state. There is no evidence directly supporting either of these explanations. Some reports that nicotinic–cholinergic agonists fail to displace nicotine have been interpreted as supporting the view that nicotine acts through nonnicotinic mechanisms (Sershen *et al.*, 1981; Abood *et al.*, 1978, 1981). These reports are in the minority, and their explanation was discussed by Marks and Collins (1982).

Another problem with the nicotine binding studies has been disagreement between laboratories on quantitative aspects of the binding. Table 1 shows the wide variations in K_d and B_{max} values reported to date. To some extent, these reflect differences in procedures and conditions used, and as more information becomes available, one might expect some of the discrepancies to be more easily understood. There is also disagreement as to whether the binding studies suggest the presence of multiple types of nicotinic receptors. Scatchard plots have sometimes suggested that both

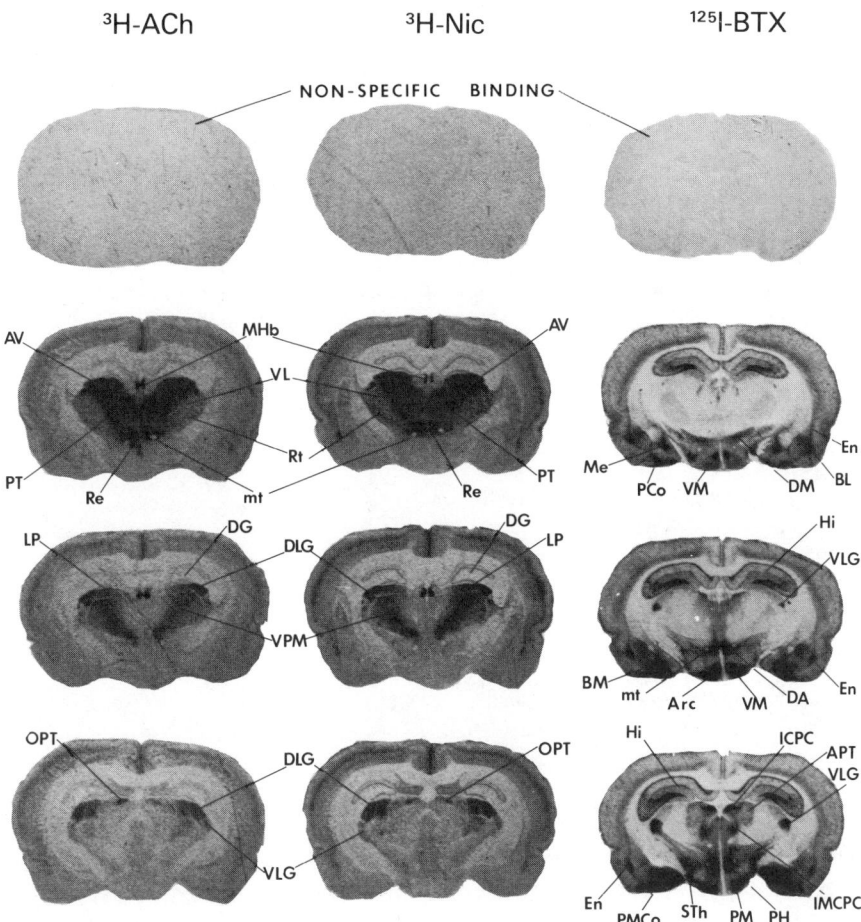

FIG. 1. Distribution of sites labeled by [³H]acetylcholine, [³H]-(±)-nicotine, and [¹²⁵I]-α-bungarotoxin as determined by autoradiography. Unfixed, nearly adjacent rat brain sections were prepared and incubated with radioligand. The patterns of binding produced by acetylcholine and nicotine were very similar and quite distinct from that produced by the toxin (from Clarke et al., 1985). Nonspecific binding was assessed in the presence of excess (−)-nicotine or carbachol. APT, anterior pretectal area; Arc, arcuate hypothalamic nucleus; AV, anteroventral thalamic nucleus; BL, basolateral amygdaloid nucleus; BM, basomedial amygdaloid nucleus; DA, dorsal hypothalamic area; DG, dentate gyrus; DLG, dorsal lateral geniculate nucleus; DM, dorsomedial hypothalamic nucleus; En, endopiriform nucleus; Hi, hippocampus; ICPC, intracommissural nucleus of posterior commissure; IMCPC, interstitial magnocellular nucleus of posterior commissure; LP, lateral posterior thalamic nucleus (pulvinar); MHb, medial habenular nucleus; mt, mammillothalamic tract; PCo, posterior cortical amygdaloid nucleus; PH, posterior hypothalamic nucleus; PM, paramedian lobule; PMCo, posteromedial cortical amygdaloid nucleus; PT, paratenial thalamic nucleus; Re, reuniens thalamic nucleus; Rt, reticular thalamic nucleus; STh, subthalamic nucleus; VL, ventrolateral thalamic nucleus; VLG, ventrolateral geniculate nucleus; VM, ventromedial thalamic nucleus; VPM, ventroposterior thalamic nucleus, medial part.

TABLE 1
Characteristics of High-Affinity Nicotine Binding to Brain

Reference	Ligand[a]	K_d^b	B_{max}^c	Specific binding[d]	Stereospecificity[e]
Abood et al., 1978	(±)	20	—	45	1.8
Abood et al., 1979	(±)	19	—	—	—
Abood et al., 1980	(±)	5.6	20	10	8
Romano and Goldstein, 1980	(±)	43	4.4	65–80	63
Martin and Aceto, 1981	(−)	60	—	68	1
Vincek et al., 1980	(+)	260	—	—	1
Sershen et al., 1981	(±)	40	170	50	1.3
Marks and Collins, 1982	(±)	59	88	60	—
Abood et al., 1983a	(−)	0.2	5.1	—	3
	(−)	1.7	29	—	3
Balfour and Benwell, 1983	(±)	3.6	15	—	—
Costa and Murphy, 1983	(±)	24	76	60	63
Marks et al., 1983	(±)	14	45	—	—
Marks and Collins, 1982	(±)	18	32	—	—
Sloan et al., 1984	(±)	5.2	—	55	100
Clarke et al., 1984	(±)	3.5	7	90	17
Jenner et al., 1986	(±)	12	90	65	—
	(−)	6.3	74	80	15

[a]Indicates use of [^{3}H]-(−)-nicotine or [^{3}H]-(±)-nicotine.
[b]Dissociation constant determined from Scatchard plot (nmol).
[c]Specific binding (fmoles/mg protein).
[d]Proportion of total binding displaceable by unlabeled (−)-nicotine.
[e]Ratio of concentrations of (+) to (−)-nicotine that inhibited binding of [^{3}H]nicotine by 50%.

low- and high-affinity receptors may be found, and usually studies have concentrated on the higher-affinity sites. One group of workers has reported as many as five different sites, but the pharmacological significance of several of the sites was not determined, and some of the evidence was rather indirect (Sloan et al., 1984). The matter remains open for clarification in further work. It will probably be necessary to use [^{3}H]-(−)-nicotine as the ligand, instead of racemic nicotine, to exclude erroneous conclusions associated with binding sites for (+)-nicotine or their interaction with (−)-nicotine sites. Few studies have used [^{3}H]-(−)-nicotine as the ligand (e.g., Abood et al., 1983a; Jenner et al., 1986).

Some recent studies have used classic nicotinic–cholinergic antagonists as ligands. This is a fresh approach, which will undoubtedly be pursued further. The drugs used were d-[^{3}H]tubocurarine and [^{3}H]dihydro-β-erythroidine (Nordberg and Larsson, 1980; Williams and Robinson, 1984). The characteristics of the binding are not yet fully established. In the peripheral nervous system, tubocurarine acts mainly at the neuromuscular junction rather than at autonomic ganglia. Dihydro-β-erythroidine may not be selective for either type of receptor. This will influence the relevance of the binding to central effects of nicotine itself. Specific binding with compounds selective for the ganglionic type of receptor seems not to have been reported.

2. NICOTINE AS A POSITIVE REINFORCER

2.1. Introduction

If people smoke tobacco mainly to obtain the effects of nicotine, then it should be possible to show that nicotine can serve as a primary positive reinforcer in self-administration experiments. The use of pure nicotine solutions in such work eliminates the main problem with all studies utilizing preparations of tobacco itself, namely, that the effects of other pharmacological or nonpharmacological reinforcers may be confounded with those of nicotine. The published work using this approach will be examined in terms of three objective criteria: (1) the absolute rates of responding maintained by nicotine expressed in responses per second; (2) the rate of responding for nicotine expressed as a percentage of the rate for saline, which is taken as 100%; and (3) the absolute hourly amount of nicotine self-administered in mg/kg. The use of these three criteria for assessing studies greatly facilitates comparisons between different experiments and emphasizes certain aspects of the data that were not previously apparent. An excellent review of nicotine self-administration studies has appeared recently (Henningfield and Goldberg, 1984), and the general discussion given there will not be repeated.

2.2. Studies in Animals

Data from 18 studies in rats, rhesus and squirrel monkeys, baboons and dogs have been analyzed. Only studies in which nicotine was administered by intravenous injection have been considered. The results are presented in Table 2. Both conventional reinforcers, such as food, and injections of known addictive drugs, such as cocaine, can maintain overall response rates of one response a second (rs/sec) or more, when presented under suitable schedules.

First, Table 2 shows that in all studies carried out before 1981, nicotine injections maintained very low rates of responding. In this period, the greatest absolute response rate recorded was no more than 0.015 rs/sec, and even this was only twice as fast as the rate of responding for saline injections (Griffiths *et al.*, 1979). In other studies, response rates were 2.5–25 times greater than those for saline, but absolute response rates

TABLE 2
Summarized Results of Nicotine Self-Administration Studies

Species	Schedule[a]	Response rate[b] rs/sec	%	Dose[c] mg/kg per hr	Reference
Monkey	FR 1	0.0006	—	0.05	Deneau and Inoki, 1967
Monkey	FR 1	0.006	680	0.4	Yanagita, 1977
Rat	FR 1[d]	0.0025	490	1.2	Lang et al., 1977
Rat	FR 1[d]	0.003	260	1.2	Singer et al., 1978
Rat	FR 1	0.003	2500	0.25	Hanson et al., 1979
Monkey	FR 160	0.015	200	0.3	Griffiths et al., 1979
Rat	FR 1[d]	0.006	300	2.1	Lattif et al., 1980
Rat	FR 1[d]	0.008	520	7.1	Smith and Lang, 1980
Rat	FR 1	0.0005	—	0.2	Dougherty et al., 1981
Monkey	FR(FI)	0.2	1000	4.3	Dougherty et al., 1981
Monkey	FI 5 min	0.15	600	3.3	Goldberg et al., 1981
Rat	FR 1[d]	0.007	—	2.5	Singer et al., 1982
Monkey	FR(FI)	1	400	—	Spealman and Goldberg, 1982
Monkey	FR 2	0.01	200	0.6	Ator and Griffiths, 1983
Human	FR 10	0.014	—	0.1	Henningfield et al., 1983a
Human	FR 10	0.01	200	0.2	Henningfield and Goldberg, 1983
Dog	FR 15	0.3	1500	—	Risner and Goldberg, 1983
Rat	FR 1	0.0012	500	0.1	Cox et al., 1984

[a]Schedule of nicotine infusion. FR = fixed ratio; FI = fixed interval; FR(FI) = second-order schedule of nicotine infusions available on fixed-interval basis, with responding in intervening periods maintained by brief presentations of light on an FR schedule.
[b]Highest rate of responding maintained by nicotine in responses per second (rs/sec) and, where possible, as percentage of responding maintained by saline (the latter defined as 100%).
[c]Nicotine dose self-administered in mg/kg per hr.
[d]Supplementary inducing schedule of food presentation also used.

were always extremely low (0.0005–0.008 rs/sec). However, despite the rather unimpressive nature of these data, nicotine did seem to maintain responding at levels consistently above those of saline. The absolute amounts of nicotine taken varied from 0.05 to 7.1 mg/kg per hr. In several studies, food deprivation and an inducing schedule of food presentation were used (cf. Cherek and Brauchi, 1981); these factors increased response rates for nicotine, although they were not necessary for self-administration to occur (references in Table 2). Few studies controlled for the possibility that nicotine would have increased rates of responding if given according to a predetermined program, in a manner not contingent upon responding.

Changes in experimental technique subsequently yielded much clearer evidence that nicotine could have a powerful reinforcing effect. Goldberg et al. (1981) and Spealman and Goldberg (1982), working with squirrel monkeys, were able to maintain response rates of 0.15–1 rs/sec; these rates of responding were four to six times greater than response rates for saline in the same animals. Figure 2 shows that the characteristics of responding under the second-order schedule were similar regardless of whether the reinforcer was nicotine or cocaine. The self-administered doses of nicotine were sufficient to produce vomiting in some monkeys, but this did not seem to influence the amounts of the drug self-administered subsequently. Risner and Goldberg (1983) obtained response rates of 0.3 rs/sec in dogs, 15 times above response rates for saline. Dougherty et al. (1981) also obtained 0.2 rs/sec, 10 times above baseline, in a monkey, although these data were of a very preliminary nature. Absolute amounts of nicotine obtained in this group of studies were 3.3–4.3 mg/kg per hr.

The reasons for the increases in response rates have not been fully analyzed. These improvements in nicotine self-administration behavior did not require the use of food deprivation or an inducing schedule. Perhaps the most important factor was the schedule of nicotine presentation.

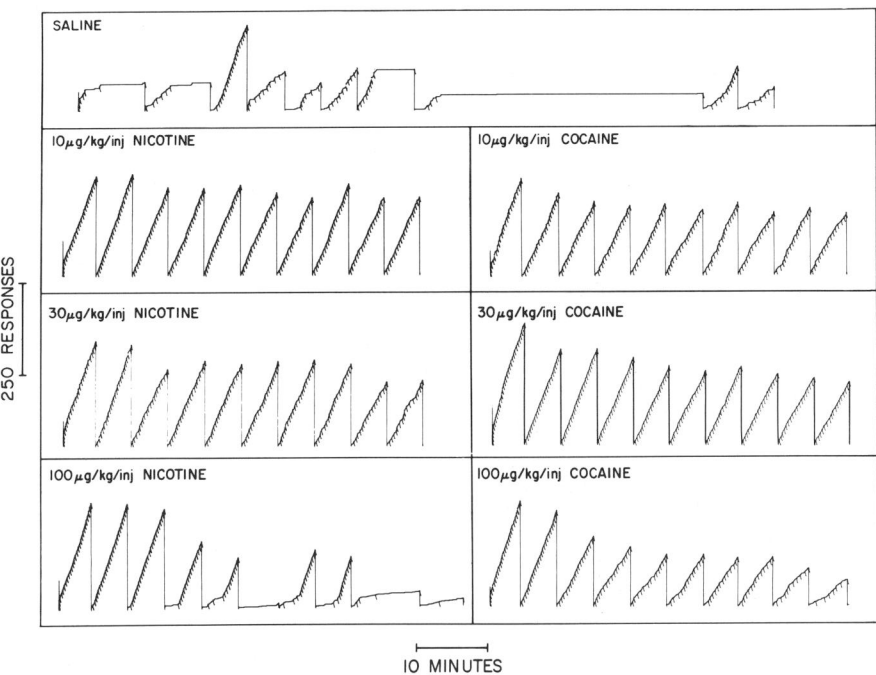

FIG. 2. Representative performance maintained by i.v. injections of nicotine or cocaine under a second-order fixed-interval (fixed-ratio) schedule in a squirrel monkey. Abscissae, time; ordinates, cumulative responses. Diagonal marks, presentations of the 1-sec visual stimulus. The recorder was reset after each injection. Each panel shows a complete record at the doses specified or when saline was substituted for the drug (from Spealman and Goldberg, 1982). These data establish similarities between the self-administration of nicotine and a standard addictive drug.

All studies with low response rates used fixed ratio schedules with a simple proportional relationship between response rate and number of injections. The cumulative dose of nicotine may well have had a response-rate decreasing effect upon such behavior, as it does on responding maintained by conventional reinforcers. Many of these studies utilized a fixed ratio 1 (i.e., continuous) reinforcement schedule, which again tends to minimize response rates. Most studies maintaining higher rates of responding utilized either fixed-interval or second-order schedules. In the fixed-interval schedule, nicotine was injected only after the first response following a 5-min period during which responding had no consequences. This manipulation limits the maximum rate of injections without directly limiting response rates. In the second-order schedule, nicotine was injected only after the tenth response following an interval of 5 min. During the interval itself, every tenth response produced a brief (3-sec) flash of light. This schedule maintained response rates averaging 1 rs/sec, which were very similar to response rates maintained by conventional reinforcers or cocaine. Omitting injections of nicotine or the brief light presentations considerably reduced response rates. These considerations can also explain why Risner and Goldberg (1983) obtained good responding with a FR 10 schedule of nicotine presentation in dogs, since in this study nicotine was not available during a lengthy time-out after each infusion.

2.3. Studies in Human Subjects

Recent experiments have used human subjects given the opportunity to self-administer nicotine solutions under conditions similar to those in studies with animal subjects. The subjects all have histories of tobacco use, and some of them had had extensive exposure to addictive drugs. Response rates of 0.01 rs/sec were maintained by nicotine solutions, about double those maintained by saline. The results were quite variable, and in some subjects, rates of responding for saline were equal to or higher than those for nicotine. The actual doses of nicotine obtained were small (0.1–0.2 mg/kg per hr). Despite these severe limitations, these experiments established for the first time that pure nicotine could serve as a reinforcer in human subjects. Subjective reports emphasized euphoria and likened the effects of nicotine to those of cocaine. Presumably, cigarette smokers who had not used cocaine would have described the effects of nicotine differently. The modest rates of responding maintained to date by nicotine in human subjects probably reflect the very considerable ethical and practical problems that need to be overcome for such work to be at all possible. Among these were the limitation of 16 experimental sessions in any one subject, as compared with the hundreds of sessions used in animal experiments. It appears that further work would greatly benefit if a device could be developed for delivering controlled amounts of nicotine by inhalation, thus mimicking tobacco smoking more closely and avoiding the problems associated with repeated venous cannulations in humans. In both the human and the animal experiments, remarkably little attention has been given to the actual amounts of nicotine obtained; for example, it is not known whether the plasma concentrations of nicotine match those in cigarette smokers.

2.4. Conclusions

The work on nicotine self-administration serves two purposes in addition to providing evidence that nicotine may be the reinforcer maintaining tobacco use. First, knowledge of the conditions under which nicotine functions as a reinforcer may aid understanding of tobacco use. Although it has been argued strongly that nicotine is an effective positive reinforcer, it cannot be denied that considerable difficulties have attended the demonstration of such effects. In contrast to other addictive drugs, nicotine maintains responding well only under a rather narrow range of conditions, principally under fixed-interval or second-order schedules (Henningfield and Goldberg, 1984). Under these conditions, however, nicotine appears equivalent to standard addicting drugs. This may be considered surprising in view of the apparently wide range of conditions under which humans use tobacco. It is also not clear whether these particular schedules model any specific human situation. Cigarette smokers normally have nicotine available for every puff; why does the best self-administration of nicotine by animal subjects take place under second-order schedules in which drug delivery is relatively infrequent? Perhaps the brief stimuli presented in these schedules serve a discriminative or secondary reinforcing function that may be analogous to functions of the sight, taste, or smell of cigarette-related stimuli, but this needs to be tested formally.

Second, studies of nicotine self-administration are potentially able to clarify CNS mechanisms and receptors through which nicotine acts to maintain smoking behavior. Very limited research efforts have been made in this direction. It is known that the reinforcing effects of nicotine in both animal and human subjects are blocked by mecamylamine, which blocks transmission through autonomic ganglia and which penetrates to the CNS. Ganglion-blocking drugs that do not penetrate well to the CNS fail to block the reinforcing effect of nicotine in animal subjects (e.g., Goldberg *et al.*, 1981; Spealman and Goldberg, 1982). Mecamylamine also blocks some central effects of nicotine in humans, whereas compounds that act only peripherally do not (Stolerman *et al.*, 1973; Henningfield *et al.*, 1983*b*). These results provide a very strong indication that nicotine's reinforcing effect is primarily central. They do not show unequivocally that nicotinic–cholinergic receptors are involved because of the doubts about how mecamylamine blocks nicotine, as discussed in detail elsewhere in this chapter.

3. NICOTINE AS AN AVERSIVE STIMULUS

3.1. Introduction

Drugs, like conventional exteroceptive events, can have multiple stimulus effects, and work with nicotine exemplifies this principle to a greater extent than work with any other compound. Kumar and Stolerman (1977) and Russell (1979) suggested that, in addition to its positive reinforcing effects, nicotine may be able to serve as an aversive stimulus. The implication was that aversive effects of nicotine might set an upper limit to smoke exposure in tobacco users, with the overall dose of nicotine being determined by the balance between its positive reinforcing and aversive effects in any given situation. Both pharmacological and behavioral variables may be expected to alter this balance. Animal studies provide three pieces of evidence from different behavioral paradigms, each of which supports the view that nicotine may have aversive effects. The paradigms are (1) punishment, (2) negative reinforcement, and (3) conditioned taste aversion.

3.2. Nicotine as a Punisher

A stimulus may be defined as punishing when behavior that leads to its presentation is suppressed. Squirrel monkeys responded to obtain food under a two-component fixed-ratio schedule. In the nonpunishment component, a green light was present and food was delivered after every thirtieth bar-pressing response. In the punishment component, a red light was present, and the first response in each fixed ratio produced an injection of nicotine through a chronic venous cannula (Goldberg and Spealman, 1982, 1983). When nicotine was injected at doses of 10–30 µg/injection, rates of responding were markedly suppressed in the punishment component but not in the alternating nonpunishment component. When saline was injected instead of nicotine, rates of responding in the two components were similar. The effect of nicotine was not nonspecific suppression, since responding was under stimulus control and recovered as soon as the green light signaled the end of the punishment component. Thus, nicotine acted as a punisher to produce behavioral suppression similar to that produced by electric shock. The effect of nicotine was attenuated either by the ganglion-blocking drug mecamylamine or by chlordiazepoxide, which attenuates the punishing effects of shock.

3.3. Nicotine as a Negative Reinforcer

Postponement of scheduled injections of nicotine can also maintain behavior. This negatively reinforcing effect of nicotine can also be used to assess its aversive action. Such work provides especially convincing evidence, since the observed effect is an increase in behavioral output rather than suppression of responding, which could sometimes be attributable to nonspecific effects. Spealman (1983) carried out such work in squirrel monkeys. In the absence of any bar-pressing responses, the monkeys received injections of nicotine (30 µg/kg) every 20 sec through a venous cannula. Each bar-pressing response postponed the next injection for 60 sec. After behavior stabilized, different doses of nicotine were tested. Nicotine in doses of 10–56 µg/kg maintained rates and patterns of bar pressing that were similar to those maintained under similar schedules of electric shock postponement. Larger doses of nicotine produced vomiting and disrupted responding. Pretreatment with mecamylamine markedly shifted the nicotine dose–response curve to the right, whereas hexamethonium had only a very limited blocking action, suggesting that the negatively reinforcing effect of nicotine was of primarily central origin (Spealman, 1983). Further work with a wider range of blocking drugs might help to clarify these results.

3.4. Conditioned Taste Aversions

Nicotine can also produce conditioned taste aversions. This type of effect provides another possible method for studying aversive actions of drugs, although it is not certain that the effects detected are equivalent to those that motivate conventional punished or negatively reinforced behavior (Stolerman and D'Mello, 1981). In rats, nicotine produced powerful taste aversions that were directly related to dose and to the number of conditioning sessions (Kumar *et al.*, 1983). Rats were allowed to drink distinctively flavored solutions (salt or saccharin) for 15 min; immediately afterward either nicotine or saline was injected subcutaneously. For any one rat, one of the flavors was repeatedly "paired" with nicotine in this way, whereas the other flavor was repeatedly paired with saline. Flavor-injection pairings were counterbalanced in each group of rats. Figure 3 shows the development of conditioned taste aversions in three groups of rats conditioned with different doses of nicotine. The mean intake of fla-

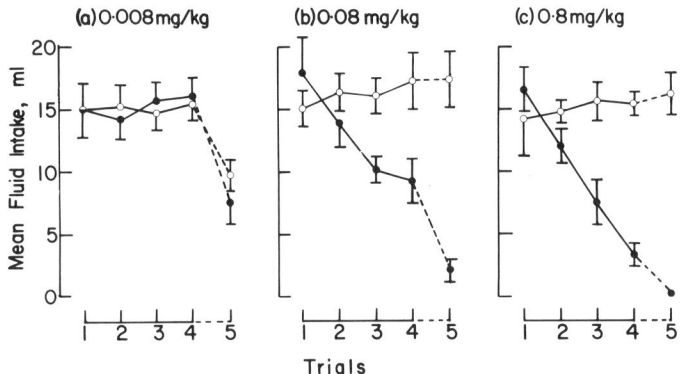

FIG. 3. Conditioned taste aversions to nicotine-paired flavored solutions in three groups of rats (●, $n = 8$), in which intakes of saline-paired flavored solutions were not suppressed (○). Trials 1–4, conditioning sessions; trial 5, simultaneous presentation of both flavored solutions, hence the fall apparent in the consumption of each solution in (a). Vertical bars, ±SEM; overlapping bars and those shorter than the diameters of the symbols are not shown (from Kumar et al., 1983). These data show the potency of nicotine in a procedure widely used to test for aversive drug effects.

vored solutions paired with nicotine (0.08 mg/kg) fell steadily over the sessions, whereas the intake of saline-paired flavors by the same rats remained relatively constant (Fig. 3b). Nicotine did not produce a detectable degree of taste aversion at a dose of 0.008 mg/kg; a dose of 0.8 mg/kg, however, had a more marked effect.

These observations support those obtained in punishment and negative reinforcement procedures in suggesting that nicotine may have aversive effects over a wide range of conditions. The taste aversions produced by nicotine were specifically blocked by mecamylamine but not by hexamethonium, suggesting central mediation. Since hexamethonium blocks vomiting produced by nicotine in other species, it appears that emetic mechanisms are not involved in the taste aversion effect of nicotine (Kumar et al., 1983). Iwamoto and Williamson (1984) obtained similar results; they have also demonstrated that previous exposure to nicotine attenuates its taste aversion effect. Etscorn (1980) has reported briefly on taste aversions conditioned in mice at the fairly large dose of 2 mg/kg.

3.5. Conclusions

Animal studies using three different experimental paradigms have consistently suggested that nicotine can have aversive effects as defined operationally in terms of behavioral changes. More preliminary data from human subjects also seem consistent with this idea (Henningfield and

Goldberg, 1984), and, of course, humans have often reported subjectively noxious effects or vomiting produced by sufficiently large doses of nicotine. The aversive behavioral effects in animals have been reported at small dose levels. The punishing and negatively reinforcing effects of nicotine were obtained with doses per injection that in other experiments had positive reinforcing effects. The doses of nicotine that produced taste aversions in rats resulted in plasma nicotine concentrations close to those found in cigarette smokers who inhale. Careful consideration will have to be given to the possible role of aversive effects in the regulation of nicotine intake by cigarette smokers.

4. DISCRIMINATIVE STIMULUS EFFECTS OF NICOTINE

4.1. Introduction

Nicotine, like many psychoactive drugs, has powerful discriminative stimulus (cue) effects, which have been extensively studied in animal experiments. The main aim of much of this work has been to clarify the CNS mechanisms upon which nicotine acts. Discriminative effects of drugs are particularly suitable for use as "behavioral assays" because they can be assessed in an objective, quantitative manner, they may be very specific in a pharmacological sense, and they may be extremely robust and reproducible.

Remarkably, the first major publication on the nicotine cue was also one of the first papers to introduce the two-bar drug discrimination task. Refined versions of this task subsequently became standard for the majority of experiments on the discriminative effects of drugs. Morrison and Stephenson (1969) trained rats to discriminate the effects of nicotine (0.4 mg/kg s.c.) from saline. This was done in the now conventional manner: Presses on one of two bars were reinforced with food in sessions after nicotine injections, whereas presses on the other bar were reinforced in sessions after saline injections. Presses on the incorrect bar had no consequences. Generalization tests and pretreatment experiments with a range of drugs were then carried out to determine the characteristics of the nicotine cue. Overton (1969) also obtained discriminative control with nicotine in a T-maze shock-escape task, although the dose used was very large. These and all subsequent experiments have used the naturally occurring (−)-nicotine isomer for training.

Rosecrans and his co-workers carried out a lengthy series of studies using both maze and two-bar operant techniques. This work established the nicotine cue as an exceptionally reliable and valid method for assessing the sensitivity of subjects to central effects of nicotine. One major

4.2. Generalization Tests: Nicotinic Agonists

Figure 4 shows typical dose–response functions for rats trained to discriminate nicotine in a two-bar task with food reinforcement. An intermittent schedule of food reinforcement was used (tandem variable interval 1, fixed ratio 10), although the schedule is not thought to greatly influence the outcome of such work. It can be seen from Fig. 4a that the numbers of responses on the bar appropriate for nicotine were strongly related to dose, reaching a maximum of 88% after the 0.4 mg/kg dose of nicotine used for training, as compared with 3% after saline. Doses of nicotine up to 0.4 mg/kg had little effect on the total numbers of responses on both bars (Fig. 4b), showing the superior sensitivity of the discriminative index of response. The mean plasma nicotine concentrations asso-

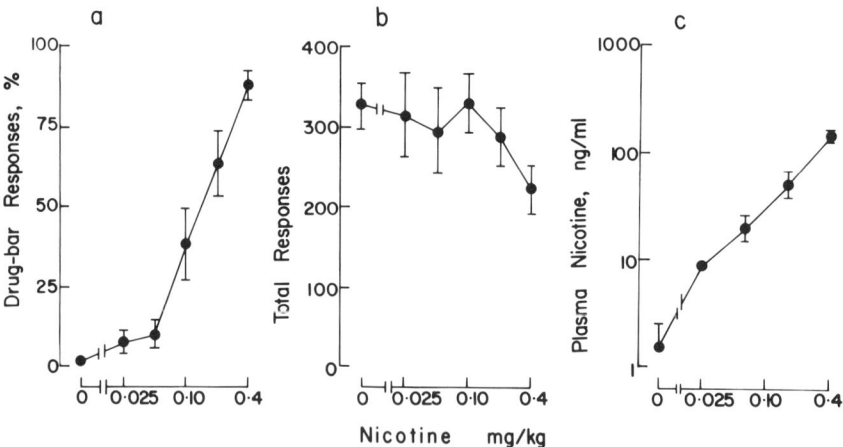

FIG. 4. Nicotine dose–response determinations in rats trained to discriminate 0.4 mg/kg nicotine from saline ($n = 8$). The discriminative stimulus (cue) effect of nicotine is shown in (a) by dose-related increases in percentages of responding on the drug-appropriate bar. The weak reduction in overall response rate is shown in (b) by total numbers of responses on both bars. Corresponding mean plasma nicotine concentrations determined in groups of six to seven untrained rats are shown in (c). All injections (s.c.) 15 min before sampling behavior or plasma (from Pratt et al., 1983). Vertical bars, ± SEM. These data show the powerful discriminative effect of nicotine, much used as a behavioral assay in studies of its mode of action.

ciated with nicotine administration were determined in other rats of the same sex, strain, and age. Figure 4c shows that, at the 0.4 mg/kg training dose, the peak plasma nicotine concentration was 146 ng/ml. In other experiments, nicotine-appropriate responding increased as early as 2.5 min after s.c. injections; it became maximal between 2.5–20 min and disappeared at 80–160 min; these results also correlated well with the time course for nicotine in plasma (Pratt et al., 1983). Doses as low as 0.1 mg/kg of nicotine have been used successfully for training (Chance et al., 1977; Stolerman et al., 1984).

Drugs that produce nicotinelike responding in trained rats are said to be generalized with nicotine, and they may help to elucidate the ways in which nicotine acts in the brain. Chance et al. (1978) tested several nicotine analogs in an investigation of structure–activity relationships, thus introducing an important experimental strategy into work on the nicotine cue. Only one compound, (3)-pyridyl-methylpyrollodine, was generalized with nicotine. Using rats trained in a T-maze shock-escape task, Romano et al. (1981) presented preliminary evidence of generalization with the nicotine analog anabasine; this was an important observation because anabasine inhibited the binding of nicotine to a recently discovered site in rat brain. The analog cytisine was behaviorally inactive, possibly because of its poor penetration into the CNS. Subsequently, a clear dose-related generalization to both anabasine and cytisine was obtained in a conventional two-bar procedure. Figure 5 illustrates these findings, which were clearest in rats trained with a small (0.1 mg/kg) dose of nicotine (Pratt et al., 1983; Stolerman et al., 1984). It can be seen that virtually complete generalization was obtained with both quantitative (Fig. 5a) and quantal (Fig. 5c) response indices, at doses of the analogs that had minimal effects on overall numbers of responses. Another compound that has been reported to generalize with nicotine is its stereoisomer, (+)-nicotine, which was about nine times less potent than (−)-nicotine (Table 3A). The stereoisomers of nornicotine are also generalized fully, and are approximately equipotent.

These findings with (+)-nicotine, anabasine, and cytisine provide a very strong indication that the site at which these compounds inhibit the binding of (±)-nicotine is a functional receptor mediating at least the discriminative effect of nicotine. The relative potencies of the two isomers of nicotine and nornicotine, and of cytisine, in the behavioral and biochemical procedures correlate reasonably well when allowances are made for pharmacokinetic factors (Romano et al., 1981; Martin et al., 1983; Jenner et al., 1986). The possibility of a similar correlation for anabasine cannot be tested because pharmacokinetic data are not available. The clearest generalization to anabasine and cytisine was obtained in rats trained with a small (0.1 mg/kg) dose of nicotine, which produced a peak plasma nicotine concentration of 35 ng/ml; this is similar to plasma nicotine concentration found in cigarette smokers who inhale (range = 4–72 ng/ml; Rus-

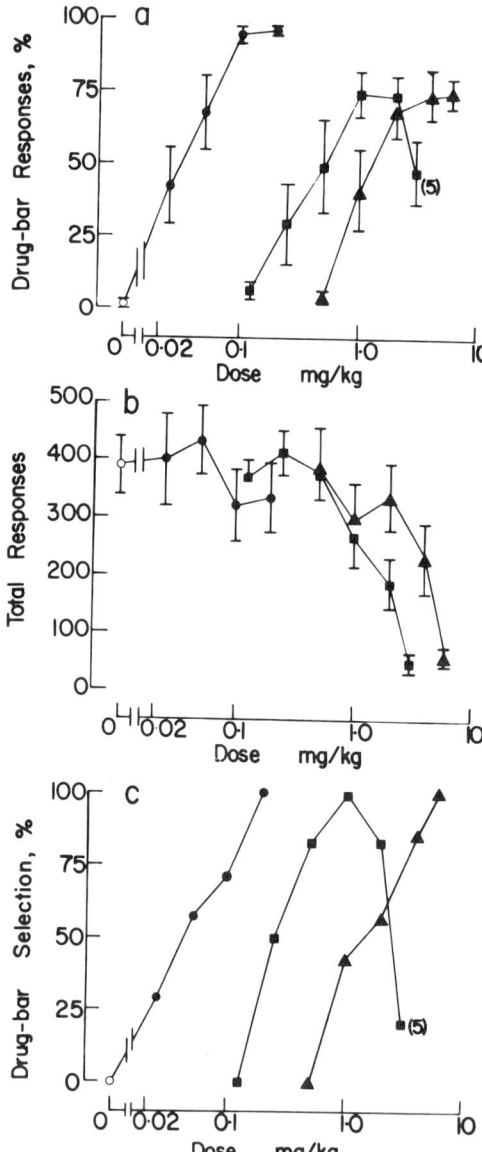

FIG. 5. Dose–response generalization tests with nicotine (●) and the nicotine analog cytisine (■) and anabasine (▲), in rats trained to discriminate 0.1 mg/kg of nicotine from saline ($n = 6$–8). Generalization to anabasine and cytisine is shown by a quantitative index, percentage of responses on the nicotine-appropriate bar (top), and by a quantal index, percentage of rats selecting the nicotine-appropriate bar (bottom). Generalization occurred with doses of the analogs producing only minimal reductions in overall rates of responding (middle). All injections (s.c.) 15 min before tests (from Stolerman et al., 1984). Vertical bars ± SEM. These data indicate that the analogs produce a specific, nicotine-like behavioral effect.

sell et al., 1980). Thus, only nicotinic–cholinergic agonists can both inhibit nicotine binding and generalize with nicotine. It follows that there is an important cholinergic link in the central mediation of nicotine's effects, in the dose range relevant to the human use of tobacco.

Some generalization experiments have failed to support the cholinergic hypothesis. Lobeline inhibits nicotine binding but is not generalized

TABLE 3
Characteristics of the Nicotine Discriminative Stimulus: Generalization Tests

Reference	Test drugs
A. Drugs that can fully generalize with the (−)-nicotine discriminative stimulus	
Chance et al., 1978	(3)-Pyridyl-methylpyrrollodine
Meltzer et al., 1980	(+)-Nicotine
Romano et al., 1981	Anabasine, (+)-nicotine
Stolerman et al., 1984	Anabasine, cytisine
Garcha et al., 1986	(−)- and (+)-nornicotine, (+)-nicotine
B. Drugs that increase nicotine-appropriate responding to at least 50% but do not fully generalize with the nicotine discriminative stimulus	
Chance et al., 1977	(+)-Amphetamine
Rosecrans and Chance, 1977	Cotinine (intraventricular)
Stolerman et al., 1984	(+)-Amphetamine
C. Drugs that do not generalize with the discriminative stimulus effect of nicotine	
Morrison and Stephenson, 1969	Adrenaline, (+)-amphetamine, apomorphine, caffeine, chlorisondamine, chlordiazepoxide, gallamine, mecamylamine, pentobarbitone, physostigmine
Schechter and Rosecrans, 1971a	Arecoline, atropine
Schechter and Rosecrans, 1971b	Hexamethonium, mecamylamine
Schechter and Rosecrans, 1972b	(+)-Amphetamine, arecoline, lobeline, nicotine methiodide
Hirschhorn and Rosecrans, 1974	Mecamylamine
Chance et al., 1978	Pyridine derivatives of nicotine
Overton, 1978	Dimenhydrinate, diphenhydramine, pyrilamine
Rosecrans and Chance, 1978	Caffeine, haloperidol
Rosecrans et al., 1978	(−)-Amphetamine, cotinine, lobeline
Meltzer et al., 1980	Atropine, hexamethonium, mecamylamine
Romano et al., 1981	Cytisine, lobeline, morphine, 2-nicotine, 4-nicotine, piperidine
Rosecrans and Meltzer, 1981	Physostigmine-atropine-hexamethonium mixture
Pratt et al., 1983	(+)-Amphetamine, apomorphine, atropine, cocaine, fenfluramine, midazolam, oxotremorine, physostigmine, quipazine
Stolerman et al., 1983	Metergoline
Stolerman et al., 1984	Apomorphine, chlordiazepoxide, cocaine hexamethonium, mecamylamine, oxotremorine, picrotoxin, quipazine
Stolerman et al., unpublished observations	Physostigmine–atropine mixture, clenbuterol, phencyclidine, pimozide

(Table 3C); however, there is no evidence that lobeline penetrates to the CNS, nor has it been tested in rats trained to discriminate small (0.1 mg/kg) doses of nicotine. Mixtures of physostigmine, atropine, and hexamethonium or of physostigmine and atropine also failed to generalize, although they would be expected to selectively increase cholinergic stimulation at central nicotinic–cholinergic sites (Table 3). The results of such complex manipulations have led Rosecrans and Meltzer (1981) to speculate that the nicotine cue is mediated through noncholinergic mechanisms.

4.3. Generalization Tests: Nonnicotinic Drugs

Tests of generalization to nicotine analogs would be practically uninterpretable in terms of receptor mechanisms if the nicotine cue were pharmacologically nonspecific. Figure 6a shows results of some generalization tests carried out over a range of doses with two nonnicotinic drugs. It can be seen that neither the convulsant picrotoxin nor the benzodiazepine chlordiazepoxide increased nicotine-appropriate responding. The

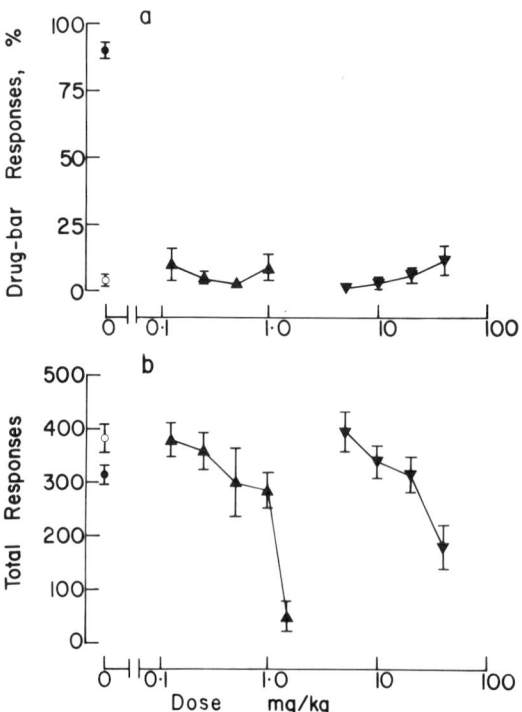

FIG. 6. Generalization tests with two nonnicotinic drugs in rats trained to discriminate 0.4 mg/kg of nicotine from saline ($n = 8$). Neither picrotoxin nor chlordiazepoxide (a) produced an increase in nicotine-appropriate responding at any of the doses tested (Pratt and Stolerman, unpublished data). Both drugs reduced overall rates of responding, as shown in (b). Injections (s.c.) were either 15 min (picrotoxin, ▲) or 30 min before tests (chlordiazepoxide, ▼). Vertical bars ±SEM. These data illustrate the type of evidence used to establish the specificity of the nicotine cue.

doses of picrotoxin and chlordiazepoxide included some that may themselves be discriminable when used to train animals, and their behavioral activity in the experiments shown was confirmed by reductions in overall numbers of responses (Fig. 6b). Such experiments not only establish that the nicotine cue has some specificity but also help to characterize the nature of the cue. If some form of subconvulsant "aura" formed the basis of the cue, one would expect generalization to subconvulsant doses of other convulsant agents. Similarly, if the putative tranquilizing effect of nicotine was being discriminated, then one would expect generalization to other antianxiety agents. Neither type of generalization occurred; hence, it is unlikely that the discriminative effect of nicotine is based primarily on either its convulsant or its tranquilizing effects.

Many other studies have shown that rats trained to discriminate nicotine do not identify nonnicotinic drugs as nicotinelike. Table 3C summarizes experiments, from 16 publications, that establish the remarkable specificity of the nicotine cue. Drugs from many different pharmacological classes either failed to increase nicotine-appropriate responding or produced small increases that were easily distinguishable from those produced by nicotine itself. Among the drugs tested were compounds acting at receptors for catecholamines, opioids, 5-hydroxytryptamine, benzodiazepines, and muscarinic–cholinergic agonists. Similar negative results were obtained with nicotinic antagonists and certain nicotine analogs (cotinine and lobeline). In some cases, the negative findings would have been more convincing if a wider range of doses had been tested. There was no evidence for an overall loss of specificity when very small doses of nicotine were used for training (Stolerman et al., 1984).

A very small number of drugs have yielded equivocal results: Intraventricular administration of cotinine produced partially nicotinelike effects. Systemic amphetamine also increased nicotine-appropriate responding, apparently to a greater extent in rats trained with small (0.1 mg/kg doses) of nicotine (Table 3B). Both nicotine and amphetamine can increase arousal, but it is not known whether this is relevant. Such an effect of amphetamine also occurs in rats trained to discriminate small doses of some nonnicotinic drugs, and its interpretation remains unclear.

Another, less direct, way of testing the specificity of nicotine's discriminative effects involves generalization tests with nicotine carried out in rats trained to discriminate nonnicotinic drugs. Such tests have been carried out in subjects trained to discriminate each of 10 different drugs, and the results have been almost uniformly negative (Table 4). Even in rats trained to discriminate the muscarinic–cholinergic agonist arecoline, nicotine failed to generalize, indicating that muscarinic and nicotinic receptors are distinguishable behaviorally. In a small proportion of subjects trained with cocaine, nicotine has been found to generalize. This

TABLE 4
Drugs That Do Not Generalize to Nicotine When the Latter Is Given in a Cross-Test

Training drug	Species	Reference
(+)-Amphetamine	Rat	Schechter and Rosecrans, 1973
(+)-Amphetamine	Rat	Ho and Huang, 1975
Fentanyl	Rat	Colpaert et al., 1975
Cocaine	Monkey[a]	Ando and Yanagita, 1978
Pentylenetetrazol	Rat	Shearman and Lal, 1979
Arecoline	Rat	Meltzer and Rosecrans, 1981
Caffeine	Rat	Modrow et al., 1981
Morphine	Rat	Romano et al., 1981
Phencyclidine	Rat	Browne, 1982
Fentanyl	Rat	Koek and Slangen, 1982
Fentanyl or cocaine	Rat	Colpaert and Janssen, 1982
Cocaine	Monkey[a]	de la Garza and Johanson, 1983
Naltrexone	Bird	Valentino et al., 1983
Midazolam	Rat	Rose and Stolerman, 1984
Cocaine	Bird[a]	de la Garza and Johanson, 1985

[a]Generalization in one of two subjects used.

work strengthens the evidence that the discriminative effects of nicotine differ from those of drugs in any other pharmacological class.

4.4. Pretreatment Experiments

Pretreatment studies with drugs thought to act specifically on particular neurotransmitter receptors are equally important as generalization tests in characterizing a drug-produced cue. The only drugs that to date have been found to block the nicotine cue are compounds that block nicotinic–cholinergic receptors in autonomic ganglia. This extremely reliable effect has been obtained consistently in several laboratories; only a few of the many references are cited in Table 5. The active drugs are those ganglion blockers that penetrate well into the CNS, i.e., mecamylamine and pempidine. Mecamylamine also blocks the generalization response to cytisine (Stolerman et al., 1983, 1984). Such studies provide evidence that the receptor mediating the discriminative effect of nicotine may resemble the nicotinic–cholinergic receptor in autonomic ganglia. A variety of drugs that act on a wide range of other neurotransmitter systems have failed to attenuate the nicotine cue (Table 5).

These observations are all the more interesting because of the failure of mecamylamine and pempidine to inhibit binding of nicotine to rat brain membranes (Section 1). This suggests that the drugs may act through noncompetitive mechanisms. One would expect the block of nicotine's effects to be reversed by increasing the dose of nicotine if mecamylamine acted competitively. Figure 7a shows that the block of the nicotine cue by mecamylamine could not be fully reversed by increasing nicotine doses. The block of the response rate-reducing effect of nicotine was reversible (Fig. 7b), but response rate decreases do not indicate specific nicotinelike effects. Effects of nicotine that cannot reflect nonspecific behavioral depression (e.g., self-administration and increases in response rates generally) seem irreversible, whereas response rate decreases seem reversible (Spealman and Goldberg, 1982; Spealman et al., 1981; Stolerman et al., 1983). These studies are, therefore, consistent with the possibility that mecamylamine acts through noncompetitive mechanisms and generally fit in with the results of the ligand-binding work.

Quaternary ganglion-blocking drugs such as hexamethonium and chlorisondamine do not penetrate well into the CNS, and when injected systemically, they do not block the nicotine cue except at very large doses. This suggests that the nicotine cue is primarily of central origin, thus con-

TABLE 5
Characteristics of the Nicotine Discriminative Stimulus: Pretreatment Studies

Reference	Test drugs
A. Drugs that can fully block the nicotine discriminative stimulus	
Morrison and Stephenson, 1969	Mecamylamine
Overton, 1969	Mecamylamine
Schechter and Rosecrans, 1971*b*	Mecamylamine
Schechter and Rosecrans, 1972*c*	Mecamylamine
Romano et al., 1981	Pempidine, mecamylamine
Garcha et al., 1985	Chlorisondamine (i.v.t.)
B. Drugs that do not block the nicotine discriminative stimulus	
Morrison and Stephenson, 1969	Chlorisondamine
Schechter and Rosecrans, 1971*a*	Atropine
Schechter and Rosecrans, 1971*b*	Hexamethonium
Hirschhorn and Rosecrans, 1974	Atropine, dibenamine, propanolol
Rosecrans and Chance, 1977	Alpha-methyl-*p*-tyrosine, *p*-chlorophenylalanine, 6-hydroxydopamine
Chance et al., 1978	Pyridine analogs of nicotine
Hazell et al., 1978	Hexamethonium (i.v.t.)
Rosecrans et al., 1978	Haloperidol
Meltzer et al., 1980	Atropine
Romano et al., 1981	Lobeline, naloxone, nicotine analogs
Overton, 1983	Haloperidol, naltrexone, pimozide, pyrilamine, reserpine, scopolamine
Stolerman et al., 1983	Metergoline, hexamethonium (i.v.t.)

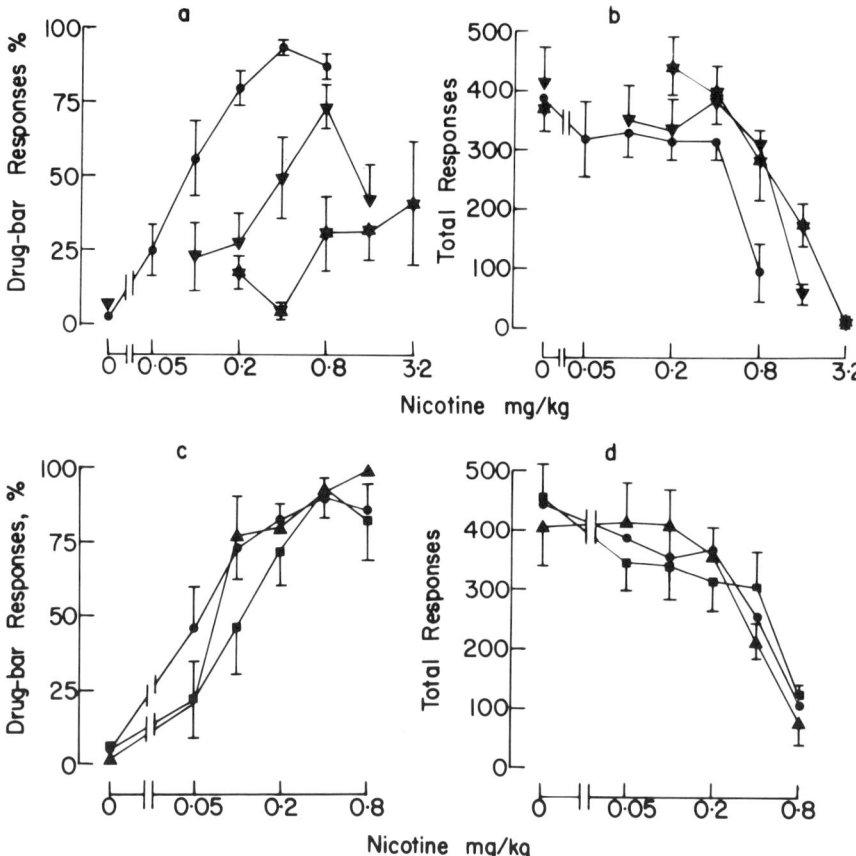

FIG. 7. Dose–response curves for the discriminative and response-rate reducing effects of nicotine in rats trained to discriminate 0.4 mg/kg of nicotine from saline ($n = 7-8$). Mecamylamine blocked both effects, but only the block of response-rate decreases could be reversed by increasing the dose of nicotine. (a) Discriminative effect of nicotine after pretreatment with saline (●) or mecamylamine in doses of 0.25 (▼) or 0.75 mg/kg (★); (b) total numbers of responses in the same rats. Hexamethonium did not affect either response to nicotine. (c) Discriminative effects after pretreatment with saline (●) or hexamethonium in doses of 2.5 (▲) or 7.5 mg/kg (■); (d) total numbers of responses (from Stolerman et al., 1983). Vertical bars ±SEM.

firming the conclusion also reached from generalization tests with nicotine methiodide, which also acts mainly in the periphery. However, intraventricular (i.v.t.) injection of small (2–5 µg) doses of chlorisondamine can block the nicotine cue for a period of several weeks (Garcha et al., 1985). Similar injections of chlorisondamine can also block both the facilitatory and inhibitory effects of nicotine on locomotor activity in rats, again for long periods of time (Clarke and Kumar, 1983a; Clarke, 1984). Surprisingly, hexamethonium has not been found to block the nicotine cue when injected i.v.t. (Table 5), and this work should be repeated using procedures like those used to show the effects of chlorisondamine.

Further studies of how antagonists such as mecamylamine and chlorisondamine block the discriminative effects of nicotine may make useful contributions to understanding of central nicotinic mechanisms. The value of such work will be largely dependent on the specificity of the blocking effects. Evidence to date indicates that the ability of mecamylamine to block the nicotine cue is highly specific: Mecamylamine had no antagonistic action in rats trained to discriminate arecoline, methysergide, morphine, pentobarbitone, phencyclidine, quipazine, or scopolamine (Schechter and Rosecrans, 1972c; Poling et al., 1979; Meltzer and Rosecrans, 1981; Overton, 1983; Stolerman et al., 1983). Much less information is available about chlorisondamine, although it appears not to block amphetamine, apomorphine, or midazolam when injected i.v.t. in doses that block nicotine (Clarke, 1984; Garcha et al., 1985). To date, there is no evidence that any of the ganglion-blocking drugs which block the nicotine cue have nonspecific central effects in the doses normally used.

4.5. Conclusions

The work outlined here shows that the discriminative effect of nicotine is centrally mediated and highly specific. Evidence from generalization tests with nicotinic agonists and from pretreatment studies with ganglion-blocking drugs supports the view that it is mediated through binding sites for nicotine that seem, therefore, to be functional receptors and not merely acceptor sites. Since nicotinic–cholinergic agonists are active biochemically and produce nicotinelike behavioral effects, it appears that the nicotine cue is mediated primarily through cholinergic mechanisms. However, certain enigmas remain, notably the lack of generalization to lobeline and to mixtures of physostigmine with atropine. It is also unclear why the training dose of nicotine should critically determine whether generalization to anabasine and cytisine occurs. It may be noted that, in the case of opioid drugs, some compounds thought to act upon different subclasses of receptors have discriminative effects that can be distinguished only if careful attention is given to the choice of training dose (Holtzman, 1982). Future work on the discriminative effects of nicotinic compounds should further examine the possibility that the nicotine cue may not be mediated solely through a single population of receptors.

The studies of the nicotine discriminative stimulus have generally been directed to neuropharmacological questions, but they may have wider significance. Rosecrans et al. (1978b) have suggested that state-dependent learning produced by nicotine may contribute to its ability to produce dependence. If behavior initially acquired under the influence of nicotine was not available to smokers in its absence, then the improved performance associated with smoking could contribute to nicotine's positive reinforcing effect. However, little work explicitly attempted to produce state-dependent phenomena with nicotine. Peters and McGee (1982) reported on state-dependent effects associated with the human use of tobacco but did not establish that nicotine was responsible. Many workers believe that drug discrimination and state-dependency effects are closely related phenomena, but it is not even clear that nicotine can function as a discriminative stimulus in formal drug discrimination experiments in human subjects. The only work related to this question was an experiment in which smokers were required to distinguish between cigarettes thought to deliver different amounts of nicotine (Kallman *et al.*, 1982). Although the discrimination was acquired, there was no evidence to confirm that nicotine was responsible. Another study referring to the discriminability of nicotine for human subjects simply confirms that the perceived strength of cigarettes may be related to the amounts of nicotine thought to be delivered (Rose, 1984).

5. NICOTINE AND BRAIN MECHANISMS OF REWARD

5.1. Introduction

It has often been suggested that drugs produce their positive reinforcing effects by acting directly on brain reinforcement mechanisms (as mapped by studies of electrical self-stimulation behavior). Most of the relevant studies have dealt with opioid or with psychomotor stimulant drugs. Very limited information is available about nicotine in this context, and much of it is only indirectly relevant. Some of these studies will be surveyed briefly because a full understanding of nicotine dependence will come from the study not only of specific nicotinic mechanisms but also of such commonalities as may exist with other abused substances. The indirect evidence from studies of self-stimulation, intake of palatable substances, place conditioning, and neuropharmacological observations is considered first.

5.2. Studies of Intracranial Self-Stimulation

Nicotine may either increase or decrease rates of responding when intracranial self-stimulation (ICSS) is the reinforcer (Pradhan and Bowling, 1971). Pharmacological and behavioral factors can both influence the direction and magnitude of effect. Such changes in response rates tell us little about nicotine's effects on reinforcement mechanisms. Changes in rate cannot be interpreted in terms of specific effects of nicotine on ICSS behavior, since the drug has similar, powerful effects on behavior maintained by conventional reinforcers. Only from direct comparisons of similar patterns of responding maintained by different events can inferences possibly be made about event-specificity and motivational mechanisms. Changes in response rate also do not index the positive reinforcing or aversive stimulus effects of nicotine. Both increases and decreases in ICSS response rates have sometimes been cited as evidence for drugs having positive reinforcing effects. In the former case, the drug effects have been said to enhance the reinforcing value of the electrical stimuli; in the latter, the drug effects were said to substitute for or mimic the effects of the electrical stimuli. A paradigm in which two diametrically opposite outcomes yield similar conclusions cannot advance knowledge significantly. The reinforcing effects of drugs can only be assessed in procedures in which exposure to a drug (or, possibly, to a stimulus previously associated with the drug) is contingent upon some behavioral response.

Some techniques for assessing the reinforcing value of brain stimulation in a manner independent of simple response rate changes have been developed (e.g., Atrens, 1970). Two such methods were developed by Clarke and Kumar, utilizing quite different experimental paradigms. In each case, responding was maintained by electrical stimuli delivered through electrodes inplanted in the medial forebrain bundle. In the first experiment, ICSS behavior involved discriminative responses to different arms of a Y-shaped runway. Measures of time spent in particular parts of the runway served as the dependent variables. In this case, there was no evidence that small doses of nicotine decreased thresholds for ICSS behavior, although the doses used produced marked changes in indices of locomotor activity (Clarke and Kumar, 1983b). In the second experiment, rats were required to move between two sections of a shuttle box to maintain ICSS, and the relative amounts of time spent in each section were measured. Nicotine apparently enhanced the reinforcing effects of ICSS in this experiment (Clarke and Kumar, 1984b).

There was no clear explanation for the different outcomes in these two experiments, and it seemed unlikely that nicotine had robust, selective effects on the form of ICSS studied. An analysis of this work from the viewpoint of operant conditioning would emphasize the totally different and extremely complex schedules of reinforcement used in the two situations. Schedule-associated variables are known to influence the effects of nicotine on behavior maintained by conventional reinforcers, and the same may apply to ICSS. It appears that studies on ICSS need considerably more development before they can tell us much about how nicotine may act upon brain reinforcement mechanisms.

5.3. Intake of Palatable Substances

Another method has been proposed recently as a means for assessing drug effects on hedonic mechanisms, which may possibly be linked with reinforcement processes and with dependence. This involves assessing a subject's intake of a highly palatable liquid, for example, a sucrose or saccharin solution. Changes in intake of the flavored solutions are interpreted as changes in their hedonic value. The practical simplicity of this approach is appealing, but ruling out alternative interpretations of the data is not simple.

Nicotine has not been formally tested in these procedures, although closely related work has been done. Small doses of nicotine can decrease the intake of ordinary food or water in laboratory rats (Munster and Battig, 1975; McNair and Bryson, 1983; Clarke and Kumar, 1984a). However, in both rats and humans, these same doses had a much greater depressant effect on intake of highly palatable, sweetened foods (Grunberg, 1982; Grunberg et al., 1984). This result is interesting in relation to the increases in appetite and weight gain associated with cessation of cigarette smoking. Reductions in weight possibly produced by nicotine may be a contributory factor maintaining dependence on it. However, it is difficult to see how a drug such as nicotine, hypothesized to act by facilitating CNS reinforcement mechanisms, should selectively decrease a proposed index of such effects.

5.4. Conditioned Place Preferences

Place conditioning may offer an alternative approach that is quicker and technically easier than self-administration. Only one such study with nicotine has been reported to date. Rats were injected with the drug or saline and then placed in distinctive environments: There was a dose-related increase in the time spent in the environment previously associated with nicotine (Fudala et al., 1985). The place preference produced by nicotine was blocked by mecamylamine but not by hexamethonium. Such procedures assess the reinforcing effects of drugs indirectly, through responses to drug-paired stimuli, and there is no contingent relationship between a behavioral response and drug administration. Nevertheless, they may usefully supplement self-administration studies, especially those studies involving direct manipulation of brain regions.

5.5. Neuropharmacological Observations

Many workers believe that the neurotransmitter dopamine plays a very significant role in CNS reinforcement mechanisms, and others have attached great significance to enkephalins. Although it will probably take many more years of research for these matters to be sorted out, it is intriguing to note that nicotine can be linked to both dopamine and opioid mechanisms.

Nicotine can release dopamine from mammalian brain tissue both *in vitro* and *in vivo* (de Belleroche and Bradford, 1978; Giorguieff-Chesselet *et al.*, 1980; Andersson *et al.*, 1981; Westfall *et al.*, 1983). Much of the evidence points to the existence of presynaptic nicotinic–cholinergic receptors in the striatum. There is also electrophysiological evidence consistent with actions of nicotine on dopamine systems (Misgeld *et al.*, 1980; Lichtensteiger *et al.*, 1982). Nicotine has also been reported to modestly increase rotational behavior in rats with unilateral lesions of the substantia nigra, a well-established test for actions on dopaminergic mechanisms (Kaakkola, 1981). The incidence of Parkinson's disease is also lower in smokers or ex-smokers than in people who have never smoked (Godwin-Austen *et al.*, 1982).

None of these effects is yet sufficiently compelling or clearly enough linked to any powerful behavioral effect of nicotine for any definite conclusions to be reached. For example, drugs impairing the synthesis of or blocking receptors for dopamine have not been found to block the discriminative or conditioned taste aversion effects of nicotine (Table 5) (Pratt and Stolerman, 1984). If the effects of nicotine on dopaminergic mechanisms play a role in, for example, mediation of the nicotine discriminative effect or conditioned taste aversion, it must be subtle or indirect. Nevertheless, the negative correlation between cigarette smoking and parkinsonism, the locomotor activity increases produced by nicotine, and the evidence specifically linking nicotine to striatal dopamine suggest that further work in this area is needed.

Evidence for a connection between nicotinic and opioid mechanisms has recently been obtained. Enkephalinlike opioid peptides are stored in bovine splanchnic nerves and may act as a cotransmitter, modulating the effects of acetylcholine released from the same nerves (Costa *et al.*, 1983). The acetylcholine acts upon nicotinic sites to release catecholamines, and opioid receptor agonists counteract this effect. The action of the opioids is stereoselective and is blocked by naloxone. This entirely peripheral type of interaction may or may not provide a useful guide to what happens in the CNS. Kammerling *et al.* (1982) studied certain possible nicotine–opioid interactions in dogs. The opioid antagonist naltrexone potentiated increases in respiratory rate produced by nicotine, but attenuated miosis and tachycardia. These observations again suggest that there may be functional nicotine–opioid interactions, although the extent of CNS involvement is unclear. Naloxone has also been reported to reduce cigarette smoking, but whether this effect is reproducible or involves nicotine remains to be determined. At present, there does not seem to be any evidence directly linking behavioral effects of nicotine to opioid mechanisms.

Balfour (1982b) has provided a general review of the effects of nicotine on neurotransmitters in the brain.

5.6. Evidence from Nicotine Self-Administration

Almost without exception, all the work reviewed up to this point bears only indirectly on the question of nicotine's effects on CNS reinforcement mechanisms. The most direct approach to the question seems to involve studies of the CNS mechanisms mediating the positive reinforcing effect of nicotine, as shown in self-administration experiments. The virtual lack of such studies is hardly surprising. Only in the last few years have techniques for developing reliable nicotine self-administration behavior been described. Combining this fairly complex, time-consuming behavioral procedure with manipulations involving brain structures, lesions, or microinjections is a formidable task. Even in the case of drugs for which self-administration behavior was established much longer ago, comparatively few such studies have appeared.

In one recent study, the effects of lesions in the nucleus accumbens on nicotine self-administration in rats were investigated (Singer et al., 1982). The neurotoxin 6-hydroxydopamine was injected bilaterally in doses shown to substantially deplete dopamine in the nucleus accumbens. Self-injection of nicotine in food-deprived rats was examined in the presence of an inducing schedule of food presentation. Response rates for nicotine were much lower in lesioned than in sham-lesioned rats. Since similar results for other schedule-induced behaviors have been obtained, interpretation of the study in any terms specific to drug self-administration is not possible. Nevertheless, one might expect to see, in the next few years, further studies along similar lines with more elaborate analyses of the behavioral effects. There is preliminary evidence that the locomotor activity response to nicotine is enhanced in rats with lesions of the ventral pallidum, a proposed model of Alzheimer's disease (Ksir and Benson, 1983). Nicotine self-injected into the lateral hypothalamus may also serve as a positive reinforcer (Iwamoto and Williamson, 1983).

6. GENERAL CONCLUSIONS

6.1. Integration of Different Approaches

Work on various aspects of the stimulus effects of nicotine was outlined in earlier sections. Each type of stimulus effect provides information relating to a different aspect of the psychopharmacology of nicotine.

Each, in its own way, helps to provide a more complete picture of the brain and behavioral mechanisms involved in maintaining tobacco use.

At the heart of the matter is the ability of nicotine to act as a positive reinforcer. Controlled laboratory experiments on the self-administration of pure nicotine solutions have shown that nicotine can indeed serve as a positive reinforcer; most of the evidence has come from animal experiments, although the main findings have been replicated in a weaker form in humans. Such work complements studies of tobacco use in which the role of nicotine has been difficult to isolate. The nature of nicotine's reinforcing effect needs further attention. Some workers have emphasized changes in arousal and improvements in the performance of tasks requiring high degrees of vigilance (Wesnes and Warburton, 1983). Balfour (1982a) has developed a model that depends heavily on a proposed ability of nicotine to attenuate the effects of stress.

Other experiments employing all known behavioral paradigms for testing putative aversive effects of drugs have clearly shown that nicotine can serve as an aversive stimulus. These effects are clear and unequivocal, they can be produced by small doses of nicotine, and they have been shown to occur in rat, mouse, monkey, and human subjects. It follows that a strong case can be made that aversive actions of nicotine may set an upper limit to the doses of nicotine that are self-administered by tobacco users. No experiments in which pure nicotine solutions are self-administered have yet been attempted to evaluate this proposition. It is also not known whether nicotine actually has two different effects, one reinforcing and the other aversive, or whether precisely the same effects can be reinforcing in one context and aversive in another. Interestingly, the ability of a particular dose of nicotine to produce vomiting did not indicate whether it would serve as a reinforcing or aversive stimulus. If aversive control is a significant factor in the regulation of smoke exposure, it will be necessary to look beyond nausea to identify the nature of the reinforcers involved.

The situation of a drug having multiple stimulus effects is not unique to nicotine, although the evidence may be stronger than with any other compound. There is evidence that many self-administered drugs have aversive effects under certain conditions (Stolerman and D'Mello, 1981). This is no more surprising than the fact that a given drug can either increase or decrease response rates depending on pharmacological and behavioral factors and the previous history of the organism. Henningfield and Goldberg (1984) have summarized this situation very clearly:

> The studies of nicotine's positively and negatively reinforcing properties also reveal more similarities than differences when nicotine is compared to other drugs of abuse, and when results obtained from studies involving animal subjects are compared to those obtained from studies involving human volunteers. . . . If there is a difference it is that nicotine appears to be an even more malleable stimulus than other drugs of abuse.

The discriminative stimulus, or cueing effect, of nicotine does not relate in such a direct way to the regulation of human use of tobacco. Only indirectly, by virtue of the link to the related, but distinct state-dependent effects, has it been suggested that the cue function of nicotine contributes to the reinforcing effectiveness of tobacco. Instead, studies of the nicotine cue have been providing much information about CNS mechanisms, as discussed in Section 4. The nicotine cue has proved particularly suitable for such work because of its remarkable pharmacological specificity, both in generalization tests and as a procedure for testing putative specific antagonists. At this point, it is appropriate to ask whether the nicotine cue can be related to either the reinforcing or the aversive effect of the drug. No clear answer can be given, since the pharmacological mechanisms mediating these different effects cannot themselves be dissociated at the present time. The evidence from studies of the nicotine cue generally supports the view that the main behavioral effects of nicotine are mediated through cholinergic receptors. It was originally reported that cholinergic antagonists (e.g., mecamylamine) did not block the "prostration syndrome" produced by the intraventricular injection of small doses of nicotine (Abood *et al.*, 1978; 1979), but Schwab and Kritzer (1982) were able to demonstrate block.

6.2. Models of the CNS Nicotinic Receptor

Evidence presented here suggested that the receptor site upon which nicotine acts to produce its main behavioral and psychological effects (as assayed by the nicotine cue) is cholinoceptive. Biochemical (ligand-binding) studies and behavioral observation are in reasonably good agreement on this point. Whether only a single population of nicotine receptor sites exists is unclear, and upon this possibility rests many of the hopes for producing agonists with actions more selective than those of nicotine itself. Presently, chewing gum delivering nicotine is a useful aid to smoking cessation (Jarvis *et al.*, 1982); nicotinic agonists that produce only desirable effects, such as positive reinforcement or relief of withdrawal symptoms, would presumably be advantageous, involving, as they would, fewer peripheral or unwanted central effects.

The overall structure of the receptor may resemble those in autonomic ganglia because most of the central effects of nicotine can be prevented by ganglion-blocking drugs. This argument would be strengthened if drugs blocking nicotinic receptors at the neuromuscular junction could be shown not to block behavioral effects of nicotine. Such information is not available, although the convulsant effect of nicotine is prevented by ganglion, but not neuromuscular blockers (Caulfield and Higgins, 1983).

In contrast, Wonnacott *et al.* (1982) have reported a 5% immunological cross-reactivity between a partly purified ABTX-binding component of rat brain and antibodies for rat muscle. Immunological studies with monoclonal antibodies to nicotinic receptors from chick muscle also suggest some similarity of CNS nicotinic receptors to those at the neuromuscular junction (Mehraban *et al.*, 1984). The immunological studies reopen the question of whether central nicotinic receptors resemble more closely the ganglionic or the neuromuscular receptors; comparative studies of immunological cross-reactivity with ganglionic receptors will be needed before a definite answer can be given. The possibility that both types of receptor have their analogs in brain cannot be discounted.

Several pieces of evidence suggest that the central effects of nicotine involve more than simply a recognition site for nicotine. Such highly effective nicotine antagonists as mecamylamine, pempidine, and chlorisondamine appear to act through noncompetitive mechanisms and do not inhibit nicotine binding. Nicotine binding in brain tissue is not displaceable by ABTX, yet binding of the toxin itself is specific and displaceable by nicotine; this suggests the possible existence in brain of material resembling the peripheral nicotinic receptors to which ABTX binds. There is strong evidence that peripheral nicotinic receptors are linked to ion channels that play a crucial role in the chain of events leading from a drug effect at the nicotine recognition site to an observed pharmacological effect. The possibility that nicotine acts centrally not simply through a single site but rather through a receptor complex must be considered. The different elements in the complex may be in close physical proximity to each other and pharmacological responses would be influenced by events at any one of them.

The idea of a central nicotinic receptor complex parallels work on the central actions of benzodiazepines. Many of the effects of benzodiazepines are now thought to involve not only a benzodiazepine recognition site but also a closely linked GABA receptor, which, in turn, controls an ion channel (Paul *et al.*, 1981). At least some of the compounds that resemble benzodiazepines behaviorally (e.g., depressant barbiturates) may act at the ion channel, as may certain compounds (e.g., picrotoxin) that block effects of GABA and benzodiazepines. The complex nature of currently available information on central nicotinic mechanisms suggests the possible existence of an analogous central nicotinic receptor complex. It is very difficult at present to make specific suggestions as to the form of the complex. Only some speculations can be presented in the form of a model that may have heuristic value.

The most elaborate form of the model is shown schematically in Fig. 8. As explained earlier, the primary site in the proposed receptor complex is that at which nicotine and other cholinergic agonists bind. The widely used nicotine antagonists probably act elsewhere because they do not

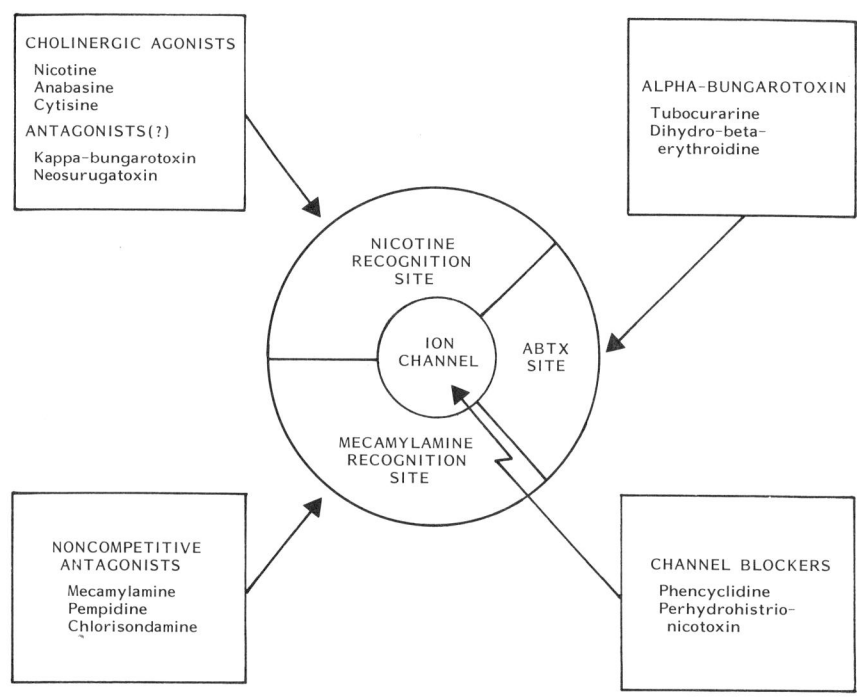

FIG. 8. Speculative model of a CNS nicotinic receptor complex, indicating the maximum number of sites suggested by present evidence, arranged schematically around an ion channel. Drugs proposed to act at each site are also shown.

inhibit nicotine binding and because the antagonism exhibits noncompetitive characteristics. Only some recently identified toxins may possibly act as antagonists at this site, although even this is in doubt (Yamada *et al.*, 1985). Presumably, therefore, there is a second site through which antagonists such as mecamylamine act (Marks and Collins, 1982). Ligand-binding studies with such drugs have not been published. Identification of such a site could introduce a substantial new element into knowledge of central nicotinic mechanisms. Presumably, any endogenous agonist for such a site would not be acetylcholine; hence the idea may help to resolve the controversy about mediation of nicotine effects by showing the involvement of both cholinergic and noncholinergic mechanisms. Third, there is the matter of possible linkage to an ion channel. This idea is firmly established in studies of nicotinic mechanisms at the neuromuscular junction, and various channel blockers, including phencyclidine and perhydro-histrionicotoxin, have been identified (Albuquerque *et al.*, 1980). The relevance of the idea to the CNS can only be assessed if more information becomes available.

Fourth, there is a need to resolve the question of ABTX binding. Insofar as ABTX binding is displaceable by nicotine, and blocks a limited range of nicotinic effects, the possibility that there is an ABTX binding component in some central nicotinic receptors must be taken seriously. The ABTX site cannot be identical to either the nicotine or the antagonist recognition sites; ABTX does not itself inhibit nicotine binding, nor do antagonists such as mecamylamine or chlorisondamine inhibit ABTX binding. However, in view of the very limited overlap in the neuroanatomical distributions of nicotine and ABTX binding sites, it seems hardly credible that all central nicotinic receptor complexes could contain an ABTX site. Thus, the elaborate model comprises four sites; the nicotine recognition site, the antagonist site, an ion channel, and the ABTX site.

The simplest feasible model comprises only two sites: the nicotine recognition site and the antagonist site. In this case, it is assumed either that no ion channel is involved in the central nicotinic receptor complex or that the antagonist site is the ion channel. The latter assumption gains credibility from studies in peripheral tissues that suggest that some nicotinic antagonists, including mecamylamine and chlorisondamine, act as channel blockers (Ascher et al., 1979; Lingle, 1983). However, it cannot be assumed that this situation applies to the CNS, especially because the other proposed nicotinic ion-channel blockers (e.g., phencyclidine, a dissociative anesthetic with hallucinogenic effects) do not seem to show much pharmacological resemblance to the nicotine antagonists. Finally, no separate site is allocated for ABTX on the assumption that, in brain, it binds mainly to an acceptor site that is functionally insignificant. Alternative models assume two populations of nicotinic sites, in which case the failure of ABTX to displace nicotine binding would have to be explained (Marks and Collins, 1982; Clarke et al., 1985). If distinct nicotinic sites are labeled by ABTX and resemble the receptor at the neuromuscular junction, then these are probably not the sites that mediate the main behavioral effects of nicotine, all of which are sensitive to ganglion blockers.

Finally, it may be noted that the acceptance of the idea of the nicotine receptor complex may be independent of the issue concerning single or multiple nicotinic receptors. The primary nicotine recognition sites in a complex could be either homogenous or heterogeneous without damaging the model. Answers to all these questions will only come from studies of central nicotinic mechanisms, which range from *in vitro* experiments to tests of functional significance in intact, behaving subjects. It is reported that a nicotine-binding site from rat brain has been partly purified, with a resultant 800-fold increase in binding capacity as compared with crude synaptosomal preparations (Abood et al., 1983b). The complete amino-acid sequences in all subunits of the receptor at the neuromuscular junction are known, and the time when similar knowledge of central sites becomes available cannot be far away.

ACKNOWLEDGMENTS

I thank my colleagues, Dr. R. Kumar, Dr. C. Reavill, and Dr. R. M. Marchbanks, for their thoughtful comments on an earlier draft of the manuscript, and the Medical Research Council for financial support. The literature surveyed for this article includes publications up to December 1984, with limited coverage of subsequent work.

7. REFERENCES

ABOOD, L. G., LOWY, K., TOMETSKO, A., and BOOTH, H., 1978, Electrophysiological, behavioral, and chemical evidence for a noncholinergic, stereospecific site for nicotine in rat brain, *J. Neurosci. Res.* **3**:327–333.

ABOOD, L. G., LOWY, K., TOMETSKO, A., and MACNEIL, M., 1979, Evidence for a noncholinergic site for nicotine's action in brain: Psychopharmacological, electrophysiological and receptor binding studies, *Arch. Int. Pharmacodyn.* **237**:213–229.

ABOOD, L. G., REYNOLDS, D. T., and BIDLACK, J. M., 1980, Stereospecific [^{3}H]-nicotine binding to intact and solubilized rat brain membranes and evidence for its noncholinergic nature, *Life Sci.* **27**:1307–1314.

ABOOD, L. G., REYNOLDS, D. T., BOOTH, H., and BIDLACK, J. M., 1981, Sites and mechanisms for nicotine's action in the brain, *Neurosci. Biobehav. Rev.* **5**:479–486.

ABOOD, L. G., GRASSI, S., and COSTANZA, M., 1983a, Binding of optically pure (−)-[^{3}H]nicotine to rat brain membranes, *FEBS Lett.* **157**:147–149.

ABOOD, L. G., LATHAM, W., and GRASSI, S., 1983b, Isolation of a nicotine binding site from rat brain by affinity chromatography, *Proc. Natl. Acad. Sci. U.S.A.* **80**:3536–3539.

ALBUQUERQUE, E. X., TSAI, M-C., ARONSTAM, R. S., WITKOP, B., ELDEFRAWI, A. T., and ELDEFRAWI, M. E., 1980, Phencyclidine interactions with the ionic channel of the acetylcholine receptor and electrogenic membrane, *Proc. Natl. Acad. Sci. USA* **77**:1224–1228.

ANDERSON, K., FUXE, K., and AGNATI, L. F., 1981, Effects of single injections of nicotine on the ascending dopamine pathways in the rat, *Acta Physiol. Scand.* **112**:345–347.

ANDO, K., and YANAGITA, T., 1978, The discriminative stimulus properties of intravenously administered cocaine in rhesus monkeys, in: *Stimulus Properties of Drugs: Ten Years of Progress* (F. C. Colpaert and J. A. Rosecrans, eds.), Elsevier, Amsterdam, pp. 125–136.

ARMITAGE, A. K., HALL, G. H., and MORRISON, C. F., 1968, Pharmacological basis for the tobacco smoking habit, *Nature* **217**:331–334.

ASCHER, P., LARGE, W. A., and RANG, H. P., 1979, Studies on the mechanism of action of acetylcholine antagonists on rat parasympathetic ganglion cells, *J. Physiol.* **295**:139–170.

ATOR, N. A., and GRIFFITHS, R. R., 1983, Nicotine self-administration in baboons, *Pharmacol. Biochem. Behav.* **19**:993–1003.

ATRENS, D. M., 1970, Reinforcing and emotional consequences of intracranial self-stimulation of subcortical limbic-forebrain, *Physiol. Behav.* **5**:1461–1471.

BALFOUR, D. J. K., 1982a, The pharmacology of nicotine dependence: A working hypothesis, *Pharmacol. Ther.* **15**:239–250.

BALFOUR, D. J. K., 1982b, The effects of nicotine on brain neurotransmitter systems, *Pharmacol. Ther.* **16**:269–282.

BALFOUR, D. J. K., and BENWELL, M. E. M., 1983, Localization and properties of nicotine binding sites in selected regions of rat brain, *Br. J. Pharmacol.* **78**:117P.

BROWN, D. A., 1979, Neurotoxins and the ganglionic (C6) type of nicotinic receptor, in:

Advances in Cytopharmacology, Vol. 3 (B. Ceccarelli and F. Clementi, eds.), Raven Press, New York, pp. 225–230.

BROWNE, R. G., 1982, Discriminative stimulus properties of phencyclidine, in: *Drug Discrimination: Applications in CNS Pharmacology* (F. C. Colpaert and J. L. Slangen, eds.), Elsevier, Amsterdam, pp. 109–122.

CAULFIELD, M. P., and HIGGINS, G. A., 1983, Mediation of nicotine-induced convulsions by central nicotinic receptors of the "C_6" type, *Neuropharmacology* **22:**347–351.

CHANCE, W. T., MURFIN, D., KRYNOCK, G. M., and ROSECRANS, J. A., 1977, A description of the nicotine stimulus and tests of its generalization to amphetamine, *Psychopharmacology* **55:**19–26.

CHANCE, W. T., KALLMAN, M. D., ROSECRANS, J. A., and SPENCER, R. M., 1978, A comparison of nicotine and structurally related compounds as discriminative stimuli, *Br. J. Pharmacol.* **63:**609–616.

CHEREK, D. R., and BRAUCHI, J. T., 1981, Schedule-induced cigarette smoking behavior during fixed-interval monetary reinforced responding, in: *Quantification of Steady-State Operant Behaviour* (C. M. Bradshaw, E. Szabadi, and C. F. Lowe, eds.), Elsevier, Amsterdam, pp. 389–392.

CLARKE, P. B. S., 1984, Chronic central nicotinic blockade after a single administration of the bisquaternary ganglion-blocking drug chlorisondamine, *Br. J. Pharmacol.* **83:**527–535.

CLARKE, P. B. S., and KUMAR, R., 1983a, Characterization of the locomotor stimulant action of nicotine in tolerant rats, *Br. J. Pharmacol.* **80:**587–594.

CLARKE, P. B. S., and KUMAR, R., 1983b, Nicotine does not improve discrimination of brain stimulation reward by rats, *Psychopharmacology* **79:**271–277.

CLARKE, P. B. S., and KUMAR, R., 1984a, Some effects of nicotine on food and water intake in undeprived rats, *Br. J. Pharmacol.* **82:**233–239.

CLARKE, P. B. S., and KUMAR, R., 1984b, Effects of nicotine and d-amphetamine on intracranial self-stimulation in a shuttle box test in rats, *Psychopharmacology* **84:**109–114.

CLARKE, P. B. S., PERT, C. B., and PERT, A., 1984, Autoradiographic distribution of nicotine receptors in rat brain, *Brain Res.* **323:**390–395.

CLARKE, P. B. S., SCHWARTZ, R. D., PAUL, S. M., PERT, C. B., and PERT, A., 1985, Nicotinic binding in rat brain: Autoradiographic comparison of ^{3}H-acetylcholine, ^{3}H-nicotine and ^{125}I-alpha-bungarotoxin, *J. Neurosci.* **5:**1307–1315.

COLPAERT, F. C., and JANSSEN, P. A. J., 1982, OR discrimination: A new drug discrimination method, *Eur. J. Pharmacol.* **78:**141–144.

COLPAERT, F. C., NIEMEGEERS, C. J. E., and JANSSEN, P. A. J., 1975, The narcotic cue: Evidence for the specificity of the stimulus properties of narcotic drugs, *Arch. Int. Pharmacodyn.* **218:**268–276.

COSTA, E., GUIDOTTI, A., HANBAUER, I., and SAIANI, L., 1983, Modulation of nicotinic receptor function by opiate recognition sites highly selective for Met^5-enkephalin[Arg^{6}Phe^7], *Fed. Proc.* **42:**2946–2952.

COSTA, L. G., and MURPHY, S. D., 1983, [^{3}H]Nicotine binding in rat brain: Alteration after chronic acetylcholinesterase inhibition, *J. Pharmacol. Exp. Ther.* **226:**392–397.

COX, B. M., GOLDSTEIN, A., and NELSON, W. T., 1984, Nicotine self-administration in rats, *Br. J. Pharmacol.* **83:**49–55.

DE BELLEROCHE, J., and BRADFORD, H. F., 1978, Biochemical evidence for the presence of presynaptic receptors on dopaminergic nerve terminals, *Brain Res.* **142:**53–68.

DE LA GARZA, R., and JOHANSON, C. E., 1983, The discriminative stimulus properties of cocaine in the rhesus monkey, *Pharmacol. Biochem. Behav.* **19:**145–148.

DE LA GARZA, R., and JOHANSON, C. E., 1985, Discriminative stimulus properties of cocaine in pigeons, *Psychopharmacology* **85:**23–30.

DENEAU, G. A., and INOKI, R., 1967, Nicotine self-administration in monkeys, *Ann. NY Acad. Sci.* **142:**277–279.

DOUGHERTY, J., MILLER, D., TODD, G., and KOSTENBAUDER, H. B., 1981, Reinforcing and other behavioral effects of nicotine, *Neurosci. Biobehav. Rev.* **5**:487–495.
DRYER, S. E., and CHIAPPINELLI, V. A., 1983, Kappa-bungarotoxin: An intracellular study demonstrating blockade of neuronal nicotinic receptors by a snake neurotoxin, *Brain Res.* **289**:317–321.
ETSCORN, F., 1980, Sucrose aversions in mice as a result of injected nicotine or passive tobacco smoke inhalation, *Bull. Psychon. Soc.* **15**:54–56.
FUDALA, P. J., TEOH, K. W., and IWAMOTO, E. T., 1985, Pharmacologic characterization of nicotine-induced conditioned place preference, *Pharmacol. Biochem. Behav.* **22**:237–241.
GARCHA, H. S., KUMAR, R., NORRIS, E. A., REAVILL, C., and STOLERMAN, I. P., 1985, Long-term blockade of nicotine cue by chlorisondamine in rats, *Br. J. Pharmacol.* **85**:245P.
GARCHA, H. S., GOLDBERG, S. R., REAVILL, C., and STOLERMAN, I. P., 1986, Behavioral effects of the optical isomers of nicotine and nornicotine, and of cotinine, in rats, *Br. J. Pharmacol.* **88**:298P.
GIORGUIEFF-CHESSELET, M. F., CHERAMY, A., and GLOWINSKI, J., 1980, *In vivo* and *in vitro* studies on the presynaptic control of dopamine release from nerve terminals of the nigrostriatal dopaminergic neuron, in: *Neurotransmitters and Their Receptors* (U. Z. Littauer, Y. Dudai, I. Silman, V. I. Teichberg, and Z. Vogel, eds.), Wiley, New York, pp. 33–47.
GODWIN-AUSTEN, R. B., LEE, P. N., MARMOT, M. G., and STERN, G. M., 1982, Smoking and Parkinson's disease, *J. Neurol. Neurosurg. Psych.* **45**:577–581.
GOLDBERG, S. R., and SPEALMAN, R. D., 1982, Maintenance and suppression of behavior by intravenous nicotine injections in squirrel monkeys, *Fed. Proc.* **41**:216–220.
GOLDBERG, S. R., and SPEALMAN, R. D., 1983, Suppression of behavior by intravenous injections of nicotine or by electric shocks in squirrel monkeys: Effects of chlordiazepoxide and mecamylamine, *J. Pharmacol. Exp. Ther.* **224**:334–340.
GOLDBERG, S. R., SPEALMAN, R. D., and GOLDBERG, D. M., 1981, Persistent behavior at high rates maintained by intravenous self-administration of nicotine, *Science* **214**:573–575.
GRIFFITHS, R. R., BRADY, J. V., and BRADFORD, L. D., 1979, Predicting the abuse liability of drugs with animal drug self-administration procedures: Psychomotor stimulants and hallucinogens, in: *Advances in Behavioral Pharmacology*, Vol. 2 (T. Thompson and P. B. Dews, eds.), Academic Press, New York, pp. 163–208.
GRIFFITHS, R. R., BIGELOW, G. E., and HENNINGFIELD, J. E., 1980, Similarities in animal and human drug-taking behavior, in: *Advances in Substance Abuse: Behavioral and Biological Research* (N. K. Mello, ed.), JAI Press, Greenwich, CT, pp. 1–90.
GRUNBERG, N. E., 1982, The effects of nicotine and cigarette smoking on food consumption and taste preferences, *Addict. Behav.* **7**:317–331.
GRUNBERG, N. E., BOWEN, D. J., and MORSE, D. E., 1984, Effects of nicotine on body weight and food consumption in rats, *Psychopharmacology* **83**:93–98.
HANSON, H. M., IVESTER, C. A., and MORTON, B. R., 1979, Nicotine self-administration in rats, in: *Cigarette Smoking as a Dependence Process* (N. A. Krasnegor, ed.), NIDA Monograph 23, pp. 70–90, U.S. Department of Health, Education and Welfare, Rockville, MD.
HAYASHI, E., ISOGAI, M., KAGAWA, Y., TAKAYANAGI, N., and YAMADA, S., 1984, Neosurugatoxin, a specific antagonist of nicotinic acetylcholine receptors, *J. Neurochem.* **42**:1491–1494.
HAZELL, P., PETERSON, D. W., and LAVERTY, R., 1978, Inability of hexamethonium to block the discriminative stimulus (S^D) property of nicotine, *Pharmacol. Biochem. Behav.* **9**:137–140.
HENNINGFIELD, J. E., and GOLDBERG, S. R., 1983, Nicotine as a reinforcer in human subjects and laboratory animals, *Pharmacol. Biochem. Behav.* **19**:989–992.
HENNINGFIELD, J. E., and GOLDBERG, S. R., 1985, Stimulus properties of nicotine in animals

and human volunteers: A review, in: *Behavioral Pharmacology: The Current Status* (L. S. Seiden and R. L. Balster, eds.), Liss, New York, pp. 433-449.

HENNINGFIELD, J. E., MIYASOTO, K., and JASINSKI, D. R., 1983a, Cigarette smokers self-administer intravenous nicotine, *Pharmacol. Biochem. Behav.* **19**:887-890.

HENNINGFIELD, J. E., MIYASOTO, K., JOHNSON, R. E., and JASINSKI, D. R., 1983b, Rapid physiologic effects of nicotine in humans and selective blockade of behavioral effects by mecamylamine, in: *Problems of Drug Dependence* (L. S. Harris, ed.), NIDA monograph 43, pp. 259-265, U.S. Department of Health, Education and Welfare, Rockville, MD.

HIRSCHHORN, I. D., and ROSECRANS, J. A., 1974, Studies on the time course and the effect of cholinergic and adrenergic receptor blockers on the stimulus effect of nicotine, *Psychopharmacologia*, **40**:109-120.

HO, B. T., and HUANG, J.-T., 1975, Role of dopamine in d-amphetamine induced discriminative responding, *Pharmacol. Biochem. Behav.* **3**:1085-1092.

HOLTZMAN, S. G., 1982, Discriminative stimulus properties of opioids in the rat and squirrel monkey, in: *Drug Discrimination: Applications in CNS Pharmacology* (F. C. Colpaert and J. L. Slangen, eds.), Elsevier, Amsterdam, pp. 17-36.

HUNT, S., and SCHMIDT, J., 1978, Some observations on the binding patterns of α-bungarotoxin in the central nervous system of the rat, *Brain Res.* **157**:213-232.

IWAMOTO, E. T., and WILLIAMSON, E. C., 1983, Self-administration of nicotine by microinfusion into the lateral hypothalamus of rats, *Fed. Proc.* **42**:769.

IWAMOTO, E. T., and WILLIAMSON, E. C., 1984, Nicotine-induced taste aversion: Characterization and preexposure effects in rats, *Pharmacol. Biochem. Behav.* **21**:527-532.

JARVIK, M. E., 1968, The role of nicotine in the smoking habit, in: *Learning Mechanisms in Smoking* (W. A. Hunt, ed.), Aldine, Chicago, pp. 155-190.

JARVIS, M. J., RAW, M., RUSSELL, M. A. H., and FEYERABEND, C., 1982, Randomised controlled trial of nicotine chewing-gum, *Br. Med. J.* **285**:537-540.

JENNER, P. G., KUMAR, R., MARSDEN, C. D., REAVILL, C., and STOLERMAN, I. P., 1986, Characteristics of [^{3}H]-(−)-nicotine binding to rat brain, *Br. J. Pharmacol.* **88**:297P.

KAAKKOLA, S., 1981, Effect of nicotinic and muscarinic drugs on amphetamine- and apomorphine-induced circling behaviour in rats, *Acta Pharmacol. Toxicol.* **48**:162-167.

KALLMAN, W. M., KALLMAN, M. J., HARRY, G. J., WOODSON, P. P., and ROSECRANS, J. A., 1982, Nicotine as a discriminative stimulus in human subjects, in: *Drug Discrimination: Applications in CNS Pharmacology* (F. C. Colpaert and J. L. Slangen, eds.), Elsevier, Amsterdam, pp. 211-218.

KAMMERLING, S. G., WETTSTEIN, J. G., SLOAN, J. W., SU, T.-P., and MARTIN, W. R., 1982, Interaction between nicotine and endogenous opioid mechanisms in the unanesthetized dog, *Pharmacol. Biochem. Behav.* **17**:733-740.

KOEK, W., and SLANGEN, J. L., 1982, Effects of reinforcement differences between drug and saline sessions on discriminative stimulus properties of fentanyl, in: *Drug Discrimination: Applications in CNS Pharmacology* (F. C. Colpaert and J. L. Slangen, eds.), Elsevier, Amsterdam, pp. 343-354.

KSIR, C., and BENSON, D. M., 1983, Enhanced behavioral response to nicotine in an animal model of Alzheimer's disease, *Psychopharmacology* **81**:272-273.

KUMAR, R., and STOLERMAN, I. P., 1977, Experimental and clinical aspects of drug dependence, in: *Handbook of Psychopharmacology*, Vol. 7 (L. L. Iversen, S. D. Iversen, and S. H. Snyder, eds.), Plenum Press, New York, pp. 321-367.

KUMAR, R., PRATT, J. A., and STOLERMAN, I. P., 1983, Characteristics of conditioned taste aversion produced by nicotine in rats, *Br. J. Pharmacol.* **79**:245-253.

LANG, W. J., LATIFF, A. A., MCQUEEN, A., and SINGER, G., 1977, Self-administration of nicotine with and without a food delivery schedule, *Pharmacol. Biochem. Behav.* **7**:65-70.

LATTIF, A. A., SMITH, L. A., and LANG, W. J., 1980, Effects of changing dosage and urinary pH in rats self-administering nicotine on a food delivery schedule, *Pharmacol. Biochem. Behav.* **13**:209-213.

LICHTENSTEIGER, W., HEFTI, F., FELIX, D., HUWYLER, T., MELAMED, E., and SCHLUMPF, M., 1982, Stimulation of nigrostriatal dopamine neurones by nicotine, *Neuropharmacology* **21**:963–968.

LINGLE, C., 1983, Blockade of cholinergic channels by chlorisondamine on a crustacean muscle, *J. Physiol.* **339**:395–417.

MARKS, M. J., and COLLINS, A. C., 1982, Characterization of nicotine binding in mouse brain and comparison with the binding of α-bungarotoxin and quinuclidinyl benzilate, *Mol. Pharmacol.* **22**:554–564.

MARKS, M. J., BURCH, J. B., and COLLINS, A. C., 1983, Effects of chronic nicotine infusion on tolerance development and nicotinic receptors, *J. Pharmacol. Exp. Ther.* **226**:817–825.

MARTIN, B. R., and ACETO, M. D., 1981, Nicotine binding sites and their localization in the central nervous system, *Neurosci. Biobehav. Rev.* **5**:473–478.

MARTIN, B. R., TRIPATHI, H. L., ACETO, M. D., and MAY, E. L., 1983, Relationship of the biodisposition of the stereoisomers of nicotine in the central nervous system to their pharmacological actions, *J. Pharmacol. Exp. Ther.* **226**:157–163.

MCNAIR, E., and BRYSON, R., 1983, Effects of nicotine on weight change and food consumption in rats, *Pharmacol. Biochem. Behav.* **18**:341–344.

MEHRABAN, F., KEMSHEAD, J. T., and DOLLY, J. O., 1984, Properties of monoclonal antibodies to nicotinic acetylcholine receptor from chick muscle, *Eur. J. Biochem.* **138**:53–61.

MELTZER, L. T., and ROSECRANS, J. A., 1981, Discriminative stimulus properties of arecoline: A new approach for studying central muscarinic receptors, *Psychopharmacology* **75**:383–387.

MELTZER, L. T., ROSECRANS, J. A., ACETO, M. D., and HARRIS, L. S., 1980, Discriminative stimulus properties of the optical isomers of nicotine, *Psychopharmacology* **68**:283–286.

MISGELD, U., WEILER, M. H., and BAK, I. J., 1980, Intrinsic cholinergic excitation in the rat neostriatum: Nicotinic and muscarinic receptors, *Exp. Brain Res.* **39**:401–409.

MODROW, H. E., HOLLOWAY, H. E., and CARNEY, J. M., 1981, Caffeine discrimination in the rat, *Pharmacol. Biochem. Behav.* **14**:683–688.

MORLEY, B. J., 1981, The properties of brain nicotine receptors, *Pharmacol. Ther.* **15**:111–122.

MORRISON, C. F., and STEPHENSON, J. A., 1969, Nicotine injections as the conditioned stimulus in discrimination learning, *Psychopharmacologia* **15**:351–360.

MUNSTER, G., and BÄTTIG, K., 1975, Nicotine-induced hypophagia and hypodipsia in deprived and hypothalamically stimulated rats, *Psychopharmacologia* **41**:211–217.

NORDBERG, A., and LARSSON, C., 1980, Studies on muscarinic and nicotinic binding sites in brain, *Acta Physiol. Scand.* (Suppl.) **479**:19–23.

OVERTON, D. A., 1969, Control of T-maze choice by nicotinic, antinicotinic, and antimuscarinic drugs, *Proceedings, 77th Annual Convention, American Psychological Association*, pp. 869–870.

OVERTON, D. A., 1978, Discriminable effects of antihistamine drugs, *Arch. Int. Pharmacodyn.* **232**:221–226.

OVERTON, D. A., 1983, Test for a neurochemically specific mechanism mediating drug discriminations and for stimulus masking, *Psychopharmacology* **81**:340–344.

PAUL, S. M., MARANGOS, P. J., and SKOLNICK, P., 1981, The benzodiazepine–GABA–chloride ionophore receptor complex: Common site of minor tranquilizer action, *Biol. Psychiatry* **16**:213–229.

PETERS, R., and MCGEE, R., 1982, Cigarette smoking and state-dependent memory, *Psychopharmacology* **76**:232–235.

POLING, A. D., WHITE, F. J., and APPEL, J. B., 1979, Discriminative stimulus properties of phencyclidine, *Neuropharmacology* **18**:459–463.

PRADHAN, S. N., and BOWLING, C., 1971, Effects of nicotine on self-stimulation in rats, *J. Pharmacol. Exp. Ther.* **176:**229–243.

PRATT, J. A., and STOLERMAN, I. P., 1984, Pharmacologically specific pretreatment effects on apomorphine-mediated conditioned taste aversions in rats, *Pharmacol. Biochem. Behav.* **20:**507–511.

PRATT, J. A., STOLERMAN, I. P., GARCHA, H. S., GIARDINI, V., and FEYERABEND, C., 1983, Discriminative stimulus properties of nicotine: Further evidence for mediation at a cholinergic receptor, *Psychopharmacology* **81:**54–60.

RAINBOW, T. C., SCHWARTZ, R. D., PARSONS, B., and KELLAR, K. J., 1984, Quantitative autoradiography of nicotinic [^{3}H]acetylcholine binding sites in rat brain, *Neurosci. Lett.* **50:**193–196.

RAPIER, C., HARRISON, R., LUNT, G. G., and WONNACOTT, S., 1985, Neosuragatoxin blocks nicotinic acetylcholine receptors in the brain, *Neurochem. Int.* **7:**389–396.

RISNER, M. E., and GOLDBERG, S. R., 1983, A comparison of nicotine and cocaine self-administration in the dog: Fixed-ratio and progressive-ratio schedules of intravenous drug infusion, *J. Pharmacol. Exp. Ther.* **224:**319–326.

ROMANO, C., and GOLDSTEIN, A., 1980, Stereospecific nicotine receptors on rat brain membranes, 1980, *Science* **210:**647–650.

ROMANO, C., GOLDSTEIN, A., and JEWELL, N. P., 1981, Characterization of the receptor mediating the nicotine discriminative stimulus, *Psychopharmacology* **74:**310–315.

ROSE, I. C., and STOLERMAN, I. P., 1984, Discriminative stimulus effects of midazolam in rats, *Br. J. Pharmacol.* **82:**239P.

ROSE, J. E., 1984, Discriminability of nicotine in tobacco smoke: Implications for titration, *Addict. Behav.* **9:**189–193.

ROSECRANS, J. A., and CHANCE, W. T., 1977, Cholinergic and non-cholinergic aspects of the discriminative stimulus properties of nicotine, in: *Discriminative Stimulus Properties of Drugs* (H. Lal, ed.), Plenum Press, New York, pp. 155–185.

ROSECRANS, J. A., and CHANCE, W. T., 1978, The discriminative stimulus properties of N- and M-cholinergic receptor stimulants, in: *Drug Discrimination and State Dependent Learning* (B. T. Ho, D. W. Richards, and D. L. Chute, eds.), Academic Press, New York, pp. 119–130.

ROSECRANS, J. A., and MELTZER, L. T., 1981, Central sites and mechanisms of action of nicotine, *Neurosci. Biobehav. Rev.* **5:**497–501.

ROSECRANS, J. A., KALLMAN, M. J., and GLENON, R., 1978, The nicotine cue: An overview, in: *Stimulus Properties of Drugs: Ten Years of Progress* (F. C. Colpaert and J. A. Rosecrans, eds.), Elsevier, Amsterdam, pp. 69–81.

RUSSELL, M. A. H., 1979, Tobacco dependence: Is nicotine rewarding or aversive? in: *Cigarette Smoking as a Dependence Process* (N. A. Krasnegor, ed.), NIDA Monograph 23, pp. 100–122, U.S. Department of Health, Education and Welfare, Rockville, MD.

RUSSELL, M. A. H., JARVIS, M., IYER, R., and FEYERABEND, C., 1980, Relation of nicotine yield of cigarettes to blood nicotine concentrations in smokers, *Br. Med. J.* **280:**972–976.

SCHECHTER, M. D., and ROSECRANS, J. A., 1971a, CNS effect of nicotine as the discriminative stimulus for the rat in a T-maze, *Life Sci.* **10:**821–832.

SCHECHTER, M. D., and ROSECRANS, J. A., 1971b, Behavioral evidence for two types of cholinergic receptors in the CNS, *Eur. J. Pharmacol.* **15:**375–378.

SCHECHTER, M. D., and ROSECRANS, J. A., 1972a, Nicotine as a discriminative stimulus in rats depleted of norepinephrine or 5-hydroxytryptamine, *Psychopharmacologia* **24:**417–429.

SCHECHTER, M. D., and ROSECRANS, J. A., 1972b, Nicotine as a discriminative cue in rats: inability of related drugs to produce a nicotine-like cueing effect, *Psychopharmacologia* **27:**379–387.

SCHECHTER, M. D., and ROSECRANS, J. A., 1972c, Effect of mecamylamine on discrimination between nicotine- and arecoline-produced cues, *Eur. J. Pharmacol.* **17:**179–182.
SCHECHTER, M. D., and ROSECRANS, J. A., 1973, d-Amphetamine as a discriminative cue: Drugs with similar stimulus properties, *Eur. J. Pharmacol.* **21:**212–216.
SCHLEIFER, L. S., and ELDEFRAWI, M. E., 1974, Identification of the nicotinic and muscarinic acetylcholine receptors in subcellular fractions of mouse brain, *Neuropharmacology* **13:**53–63.
SCHMIDT, J., HUNT, S., and POLZ-TEJERA, G., 1980, Nicotinic receptors of the central and autonomic nervous system, in: *Neurotransmitters, Receptors and Drug Action* (W. B. Essman, ed.), Spectrum, New York, pp. 1–45.
SCHUSTER, C. R., and THOMPSON, T., 1969, Self-administration of and behavioral dependence on drugs, *Annu. Rev. Pharmacol.* **9:**483–502.
SCHWAB, L. S., and KRITZER, M. F., 1982, The effect of cholinergic antagonists on a central response to nicotine, *Experientia* **38:**119–120.
SCHWARTZ, R. D., MCGEE, R., and KELLAR, K. J., 1982, Nicotinic cholinergic receptors labelled by [^{3}H]acetylcholine in rat brain, *Mol. Pharmacol.* **22:**56–62.
SERSHEN, H., REITH, M. E. A., LAJTHA, A., and GENNARO, J., 1981, Noncholinergic, saturable binding of ($\pm$)-[^{3}H]nicotine to mouse brain, *J. Receptor Res.* **2:**1–15.
SHEARMAN, G. T., and LAL, H., 1979, Discriminative stimulus properties of pentylenetetrazol and bemegride: Some generalization and antagonism tests, *Psychopharmacology* **64:**315–319.
SINGER, G., SIMPSON, F., and LANG, W. J., 1978, Schedule induced self-injections of nicotine with recovered body weight, *Pharmacol. Biochem. Behav.* **9:**387–389.
SINGER, G., WALLACE, M., and HALL, R., 1982, Effects of dopaminergic nucleus accumbens lesions on the acquisition of schedule induced self-injection of nicotine in the rat, *Pharmacol. Biochem. Behav.* **17:**579–581.
SLOAN, J. W., TODD, G. D., and MARTIN, W. R., 1984, Nature of nicotine binding to rat brain P$_2$ fraction, *Pharmacol. Biochem. Behav.* **20:**899–909.
SMITH, L. A., and LANG, W. J., 1980, Changes occurring in self-administration of nicotine by rats over a 28-day period, *Pharmacol. Biochem. Behav.* **13:**215–220.
SPEALMAN, R. D., 1983, Maintenance of behavior by postponement of scheduled injections of nicotine in squirrel monkeys, *J. Pharmacol. Exp. Ther.* **227:**154–159.
SPEALMAN, R. D., and GOLDBERG, S. R., 1982, Maintenance of schedule-controlled behavior by intravenous injections of nicotine in squirrel monkeys, *J. Pharmacol. Exp. Ther.* **223:**402–408.
SPEALMAN, R. D., GOLDBERG, S. R., and GARDNER, M. L., 1981, Behavioral effects of nicotine: schedule-controlled responding by squirrel monkeys, *J. Pharmacol. Exp. Ther.* **216:**484–491.
STOLERMAN, I. P., and D'MELLO, G. D., 1981, Oral self-administration and the relevance of conditioned taste aversions, in: *Advances in Behavioral Pharmacology*, Volume 3 (T. Thompson, P. B. Dews, and W. A. McKim, eds.), Academic Press, New York, pp. 169–214.
STOLERMAN, I. P., GOLDFARB, T., FINK, R., and JARVIK, M. E., 1973, Influencing cigarette smoking with nicotine antagonists, *Psychopharmacologia* **28:**247–259.
STOLERMAN, I. P., PRATT, J. A., GARCHA, H. S., GIARDINI, V., and KUMAR, R., 1983, Nicotine cue in rats analysed with drugs acting on cholinergic and 5-hydroxytryptamine mechanisms, *Neuropharmacology* **22:**1029–1037.
STOLERMAN, I. P., GARCHA, H. S., PRATT, J. A., and KUMAR, R., 1984, Role of training dose in discrimination of nicotine and related compounds by rats, *Psychopharmacology* **84:**413–419.
TOLDI, J., JOO, F., ADAM, G., FEHER, O., and WOLFF, J. R., 1983, Inhibition of synaptic transmission in the rat superior cervical ganglion by intracarotid infusion of bungarotoxin, *Brain Res.* **262:**323–327.

VALENTINO, R. J., HERLING, S., and WOODS, J. H., 1983, Discriminative stimulus effects of naltrexone in narcotic-naive and morphine-treated pigeons, *J. Pharmacol. Exp. Ther.* **224**:307–313.

VINCEK, W. C., MARTIN, B. R., ACETO, M., and BOWMAN, E. R., 1980, Synthesis and preliminary binding studies of 4,4-ditritio-(−)-nicotine of high specific activity, *J. Med. Chem.* **23**:960–962.

VOLPE, B. T., FRANCIS, A., GAZZANIGA, M. S., and SCHECHTER, N., 1979, Regional concentration of putative nicotinic-cholinergic receptor sites in human brain, *Exp. Neurol.* **66**:737–744.

WESNES, K., and WARBURTON, D. M., 1983, Smoking, nicotine and human performance, *Pharmacol. Ther.* **21**:189–208.

WESTFALL, T. C., GRANT, H., and PERRY, H., 1983, Release of dopamine and 5-hydroxytryptamine from rat striatal slices following activation of nicotinic cholinergic receptors, *Gen. Pharmacol.* **14**:321–325.

WILLIAMS, M., and ROBINSON, J. L., 1984, Binding of the nicotinic cholinergic antagonist, dihydro-β-erythroidine, to rat brain tissue, *J. Neurosci.* **4**:2906–2911.

WONNACOTT, S., HARRISON, R., and LUNT, G. C., 1982, Immunological cross-reactivity between the α-bungarotoxin binding component from rat brain and nicotinic acetylcholine receptor, *J. Neuroimmunology* **3**:1–13.

YAMADA, S., ISOGAI, M., KAGAWA, Y., TAKAYANAGI, N., HAYASHI, E., TSUJI, K., and KOSUGE, T., 1985, Brain nicotinic acetylcholine receptors: Biochemical characterization by neosurugatoxin, *Mol. Pharmacol.* **28**:120–127.

YANAGITA, T., 1977, Brief review on the use of self-administration techniques for predicting drug dependence potential, in: *Predicting Dependence Liability of Stimulant and Depressant Drugs* (T. Thompson and K. R. Unna, eds.), University Park Press, Baltimore, pp. 231–242.

YOSHIDA, K., and IMURA, H., 1979, Nicotinic cholinergic receptors in brain synaptosomes, *Brain Res.* **172**:453–459.

8

THE BEHAVIORAL EFFECTS OF OPIATES

David J. Mayer

1. INTRODUCTION

This chapter will examine the effects of opiates on behavior, which immediately raises the questions of what are "opiates" and what constitutes "behavior." Although both these terms can encompass widely varying domains, for the purpose of this chapter, they will not be very rigidly defined. *Opiate* will be used to denote chemicals with opium or morphine-like effects regardless of whether they are derived from plant or animal sources or whether they are synthetic. The term *opioid* will be used in a more restrictive sense, being reserved for substances endogenous to the mammalian central nervous system and synthetic analogs of them that have opiatelike properties. *Behavior* will be used in a broad sense of the word, including any response of striated, smooth, or cardiac muscle, as well as secretion of glands. This approach will allow the examination of topics that are relatively simple and about which an instructive amount is known and may provide useful models for the examination of the role of opiates in more complex behaviors.

1.1. Historical Perspective

The earliest definitive references to opium come from the Greek and Latin literatures, although there is more controversial reference to it in

---

David J. Mayer • Department of Physiology and Biophysics, Medical College of Virginia, Virginia Commonwealth University, Richmond, Virginia 23298.

the Bible and Talmud (Macht, 1915). The compound spread from its origins in the Middle East by way of Arab traders to India and China possibly as early as the tenth century (Macht, 1915). Opium was used primarily as a treatment for dysentery and for its general calming effect until the nineteenth century. Two developments at this time extended and transformed the usage of opiates (Musto, 1973). First, the isolation of the active ingredients in opium, primarily morphine, made more potent compounds available. Second, the invention of the hypodermic needle allowed a method of administration that dramatized some of the psychoactive effects of opiates. These developments led to two of the major uses of opiates today, as analgesics and for the production of euphoria.

A number of critical discoveries about the neurobiology of opiate action have been made in the past few years: (1) the demonstration of stereospecific and saturable binding sites for opiates in the central nervous system (Hiller *et al.*, 1973; Pert and Snyder, 1973; Terenius, 1973); (2) the associated demonstration of multiple binding sites for opiates (see Martin, 1983, for an excellent review of this topic); (3) the discovery of endogenous ligands for opiate receptors (Hughes, 1975); and (4) the concept of using opiate antagonists to antagonize endogenous behavioral repetoires (Akil *et al.*, 1972). These findings, along with the extensive utilization of the intracerebral microinjection technique to localize the site of action of neurochemicals within the central nervous system (Tsou and Jang, 1964), have, in turn, had an important impact on theoretical and methodological research strategies utilized for the study of the effects of opiates on behavior.

1.2. Methodological Considerations

Before these discoveries, the field of the behavioral pharmacology of opiates was primarily phenomenological; the behavioral effects of opiates were catalogued and seen in the light of designing drugs with more therapeutically desirable and fewer therapeutically undesirable effects for clinical application. Although clinical utility certainly remains an important concern of opiate research, the discoveries just described have resulted in research that is conceptually broader. The current overall view is that opiates often act on endogenous biological substrates for behaviors. Hence, the behavioral pharmacology of opiates now addresses the organization of the neurobiological substrates of behavior. Much of the research in this area now proceeds in the following pattern: (1) Can a behavior elicited by opiates be elicited by exogenous environmental manipulations? For example, can analgesia be induced by transcutaneous nerve stimulation? (2) If so, can the behavior, when initiated by nonpharmacological means, be shown to utilize endogenous opiates? This question is generally approached by determining whether the behavior can be antagonized by opiate antagonists and reduced by the induction of tolerance to opiates (that is, does cross-tolerance occur?). Additional support for a role of endogenous opiates is provided by the demonstration of a correlation between the release of endogenous opiates and the occurrence of the behavior under study. (3) If the behavior is shown to involve endogenous opiates, the precise neuroanatomical foci underlying the behavior are investigated, utilizing the microinjection of opiate agonists and antagonists into restricted central nervous system loci. (4) The opiate receptor type involved in the behavior is determined by administering opiate agonists and antagonists at least partially selective for particular receptor subtypes (e.g., mu, kappa, delta). (5) Ideally, steps 3 and 4 are combined to determine the anatomical locus of specific receptor types involved in the behavior being studied. (6) An attempt is made to determine the precise endogenous ligand (e.g., β-endorphin, metenkephalin, dynorphin) involved in a particular behavior. Again, an attempt is made to find the anatomical locus of action of the particular ligand.

This is, of course, an idealized outline of the path followed to investigate opiate involvement in a behavior. More often than not, the actual course of research is less direct than this, and the final conclusions are not usually simple. Nevertheless, keeping the general approach described in mind will aid the reader to see the overall progression of the field.

The remainder of this chapter will first examine in some but not comprehensive detail three diverse effects elicited by exogenous opiates and environmental situations that elicit these behaviors by calling into play endogenous opioids: analgesia, reward, and cardiovascular effects. It is hoped that the diverse nature of these behaviors will exemplify the approaches, successes, and failures of the behavioral pharmacology of opiates, as well as behavioral pharmacology, in general. A final section of the chapter will catalogue in less detail the broad range of behavioral effects of opiates.

2. THE EFFECTS OF OPIATES ON PAIN

As discussed in Section 1, one of the most important uses of opiates has been for the alleviation of pain. Pain is a biomedical problem that may well be viewed as a hidden epidemic. Bonica (1980) has estimated that over 80,000,000 persons in the United States suffer from some painful syndrome at any given time. Of these, approximately 60,000,000 suffer at least a partial disability. This is approximately 25% of the population. The cost to the economy in the United States is estimated to be over 60 billion dollars. Reliable estimates of the magnitude of the problem in other countries are not available, but there is good reason to believe that the problem may be even worse in less developed countries because overall health care is generally not as advanced as in the United States.

As the epidemiology of pain was studied, the biomedical importance of pain research became apparent. Thus, pain research, in general, and research on the involvement of opiates in pain, in particular, has undergone an impressive expansion in the past decade. A complete review of the literature in this field will not be attempted here (for more detailed reviews see Kruger and Liebeskind, 1984). In this section, the neurobiology of afferent pain transmission from the periphery central to and including the dorsal horn will be briefly reviewed to provide the reader with the background necessary to understand the mechanisms of opiate modulation of pain transmission. Then the extensive literature on the mechanisms of pain modulation by opiates and the involvement of endogenous opioids in analgesia will be reviewed in considerable detail. Because pain modulation is probably the most studied of opiate effects on behavior, this section will provide a very detailed discussion of opiate effects on pain and a model for the discussion of the effects of opiates on other behaviors.

2.1. The Neurobiology of Afferent Pain Transmission

In this section, a concise review of portions of the afferent pathways involved in pain transmission for readers unfamiliar with this topic is provided. Readers familiar with this topic may find they will skim or skip this section.

Pain is generally analyzed as a sensory system, and this approach will be followed here, although there are good reasons for alternative analytical approaches (see Mayer and Price, 1982, and Melzack and Wall, 1965, for more detailed discussion of this point). An analysis of a sensory system will involve a discussion of the receptors, primary afferents, and central nervous system synapses involved in the processing of information about stimuli in the environment that produce or threaten to produce tissue damage.

2.1.1. Receptors and Primary Afferents for Pain

Receptors that signal impending tissue damage fall into several categories, depending of their responses to mechanical, thermal, and chemical stimulation and on the conduction velocities of the axons that supply them (Price and Dubner, 1977). Although nociceptive afferents have been shown to innervate several types of tissue, those innervating the skin have been most extensively studied and are strongly implicated in pain mechanisms. Their essential characteristics are summarized below.

A-delta high-threshold mechanoreceptive (A-delta HTM) afferents that respond only to intense mechanical stimuli and have conduction rates between 4 and 40 m/sec have been described in the skin of the cat and in the extremities of the monkey. Many respond only to stimulus intensities that produce overt tissue damage; others give threshold responses to nondamaging pressure applied to the skin. Most important, all such HTM primary afferents respond to noxious or potentially damaging skin stimuli with the highest impulse frequency. They are particularly sensitive to excitation by sharp objects but relatively insensitive to heat. Therefore, they seem well adapted for transmitting information that is related to the localized pricking pain produced by mechanical stimuli.

A-delta heat-nociceptive afferents that conduct between 3 and 20 m/sec have been identified in the limb and facial skin of monkeys (Price *et al.*, 1977). Like A-delta HTM afferents, these afferents respond to intense mechanical stimulation. However, unlike A-delta HTM afferents, A-delta heat-nociceptive afferents respond monotonically to increases in receptive-field skin temperature. Threshold temperatures for these afferents are usually below noxious or painful levels (40–44°C), but highly noxious skin temperatures (>50°C) evoke maximum responses. The role of these neurons in signaling pain is clearly established. They are the only myelinated primary afferents innervating the skin of the extremities that can be reliably activated by noxious heat. Thus, heat-induced first pain, the latency of which corresponds to the activity in the small myelinated A-delta fibers, must be initiated by impulses in the A-delta heat afferents. Neither this first pain, nor the responses of the A-delta heat afferents, outlasts the duration of the heat stimulus. Both the intensity of the first pain in humans and the response of the A-delta heat afferents in monkeys are progressively reduced during brief repeated application of heat stimuli to the same spot on the hand. Thus, the characteristics of heat-induced first pain can be largely accounted for by the response characteristics of A-delta heat-nociceptive afferents. It has been shown that these afferents excite neurons of origin of the spinothalamic tract of monkeys (Price *et al.*, 1978). Therefore, A-delta heat-nociceptive afferents have central connections consistent with a role in pain.

C-fiber polymodal nociceptive afferents are an extremely important group of peripheral fibers, since they constitute 80–90% or more of the C-fiber population of primates. They innervate the skin of the monkey (Beitel and Dubner, 1976) and humans (Torebjork, 1974) and are characterized by their responses to noxious mechanical, noxious heat, and chemical irritant stimuli. Some also respond to intense cold (<10°C). These polymodal nociceptive afferents have several important properties, such as sensitization after repeated applications of low-intensity noxious stimuli and response suppression by high-intensity noxious stimuli. They respond with their highest frequency to two or more forms of intense cutaneous stimuli but also respond weakly to mechanical (1–10 g) and thermal (38–

43°C) stimuli that clearly do not appear painful to human observers. They may, therefore, provide some information about nonpainful sensations.

There is little doubt that C-fiber polymodal nociceptive afferents signal tissue damage and contribute directly to pain sensations in man. Brief heat pulses evoke distinct first and second pain (Price *et al.*, 1977). Except for the very small population of C warm afferents that respond to noxious heat, polymodal nociceptive afferents are the predominant C afferent group activated by this stimulus in primates and are the peripheral population that is most likely to account for heat-induced second pain. C-fiber polymodal nociceptive afferents excite many of the same spinothalamic tract neurons that are activated by A-delta heat-nociceptive afferents (Price *et al.*, 1978). Therefore, their central synaptic connections are adapted to play a role in pain mechanisms.

There is little doubt that all the major classes of primary nociceptive afferents activate all dimensions of pain. The different types of pain evoked by selective stimulation of each class result in sensations with sensory–discriminative characteristics, arousal, feelings of unpleasantness,

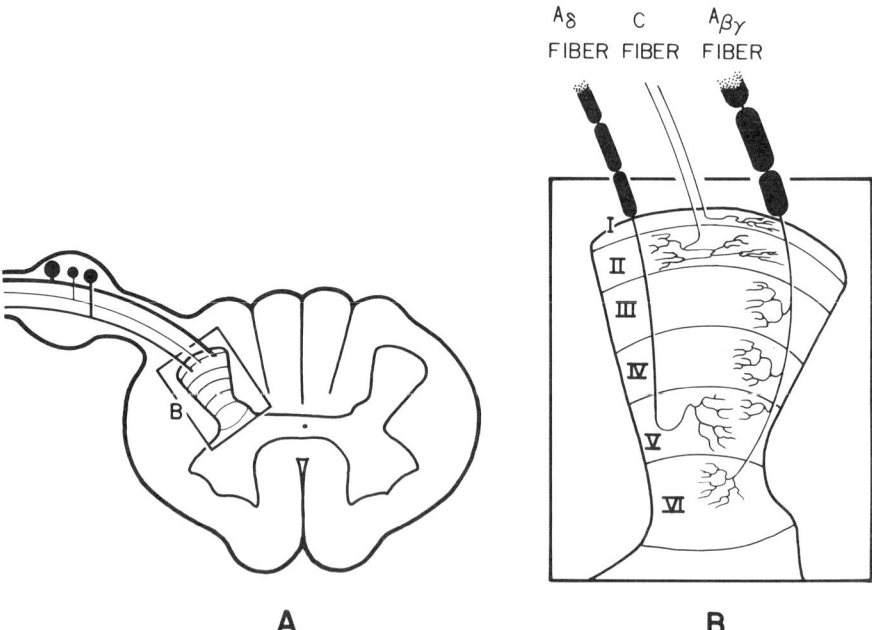

FIG. 1. Course and termination of primary afferent fibers involved in the transmission of pain. (A) Course through the dorsal root and entry into the dorsal horn of primary afferent fibers involved in pain; (B) termination of large (A-beta, gamma) and small (A-delta and C) primary afferents in the dorsal horn; Roman numerals left of Panel B, Rexed's laminae I–VI.

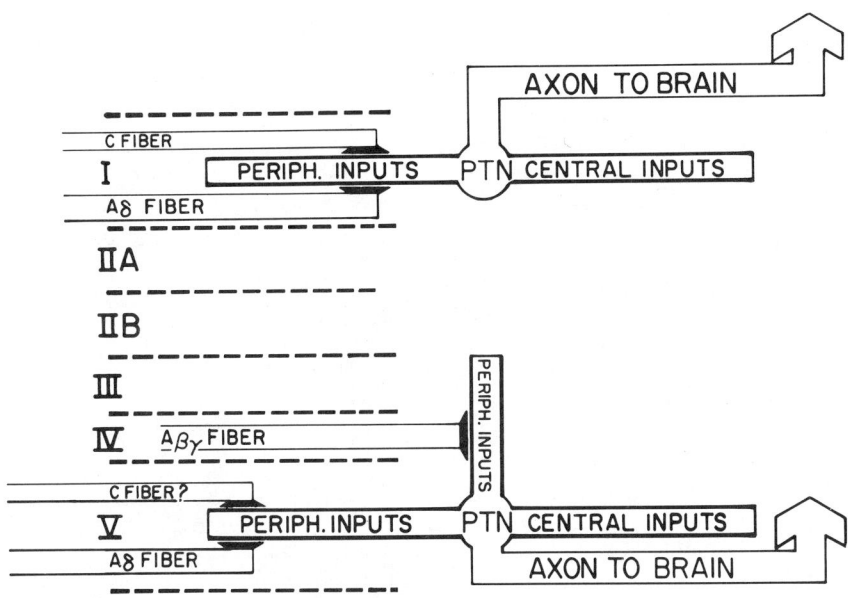

FIG. 2. Schematic diagram of the termination of primary afferent fibers in the dorsal horn. Roman numerals left of figure, Rexed's laminae I–V; filled terminals, excitatory connections. Note that the C fiber entering lamina V is followed by a "?". This indicates that the evidence for C-fiber input to lamina V is indirect. PTN, pain transmission neuron.

and motoric responses. It would be inappropriate to compare the extent to which each pain component is activated by the different types of primary afferents, since different types of pain depend on the parameters of stimulation. For example, if one brief heat stimulus is given, the initial pricking pain is more unpleasant than the second pain. If several heat stimuli are given, second pain may summate to a point where it is definitely more unpleasant than first pain. The peripheral path of these different primary afferent fibers is illustrated in Fig. 1A, and their termination in the spinal cord is illustrated in Figs. 1B and 2.

2.1.2. Classes of Spinothalamic Nociceptive Neurons

It has become increasingly apparent that radical transformations take place between input from primary nociceptive afferents and outputs of second-order sensory neurons (Price and Dubner, 1977; Price et al., 1978). This effect is probably accounted for by the complex anatomical arrangements in the dorsal horn (see Fig. 3). These transformations account for the lack of simple relationships between impulse frequencies

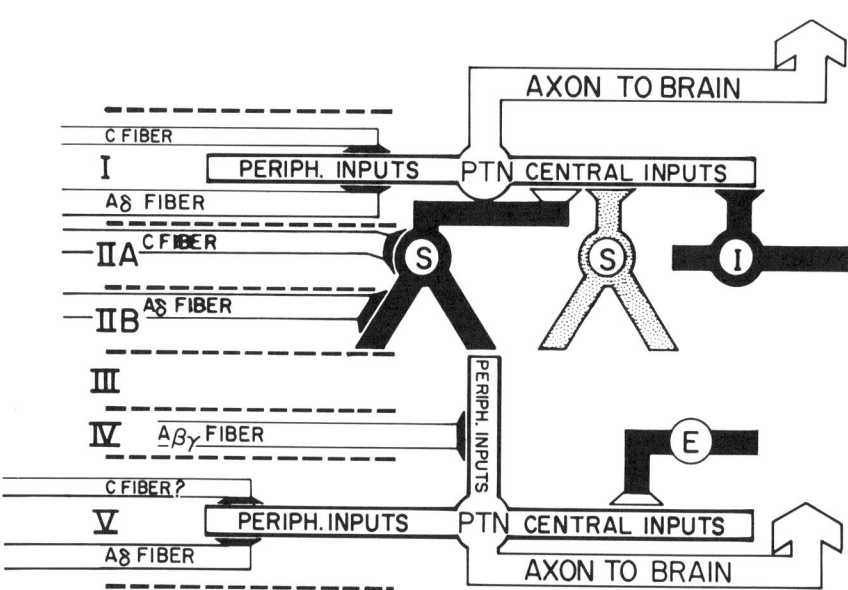

FIG. 3. Schematic diagram of the organization of the dorsal horn, including peripheral inputs, interneurons, and inputs originating from the central nervous system. Roman numerals left of figure, Rexed's laminae I–V; filled terminals, excitatory connections; unfilled terminals, inhibitory connections. The filled cells indicate cells containing endogenous opioids. E, endorphin; I, islet cell; S, stalked cell; PTN, pain transmission neuron.

in primary nociceptive afferents and pain perception (e.g., the evident lack of a simple one-to-one relationship between C-fiber polymodal nociceptive responses and second pain). The objective of this section is to explain some aspects of pain experience that are not accounted for by the responses of primary afferent neurons. This explanation focuses on the functional characteristics of spinothalamic and trigeminothalamic tract neurons that could be involved in pain.

There are two major types of these neurons found in primates that could convey information about tissue injury (Price and Dubner, 1977). The first type, wide-dynamic-range (WDR) neurons, respond with progressively higher-impulse frequencies as stimulus intensities progress from weak and innocuous (i.e., <100 mg force) to definitely noxious. Thus, maximum frequencies are evoked in these neurons by either penetration of the skin or noxious skin temperatures above 44°C. They receive excitatory synaptic inputs from large myelinated (A-beta) low-threshold mechanoreceptive afferents, A-delta high-threshold mechanoreceptive (HTM) afferents, and C-fiber polymodal nociceptive afferents (Fig. 3). As a result of this extensive convergence, these cells respond with increasingly higher frequencies of impulse discharge to touch, firm pressure, and noxious pinching. The responses of many of these cells are monotonic functions of increases in skin temperature within the noxious range (44–52°C), similar to the perceived magnitude of pain intensity over this same temperature range.

The receptive fields of WDR neurons often have extensive gradients of sensitivity. These receptive fields usually have a central zone wherein the neuron responds differentially to gentle touch, firmer pressure, and noxious stimulation. Surrounding this relatively small zone is an area in which the neuron responds differentially to firm pressure (greater than or equal to 1 g von Frey force) and pinching. This area, in turn, is surrounded by another region in which only definitely noxious stimuli, such as a pinch or 49–51°C skin temperatures, will cause impulse discharge. The total receptive field area of these neurons is sometimes quite large, extending across more than one trigeminal division in the case of nucleus caudalis trigeminothalamic neurons and across several spinal dermatomes in the case of spinothalamic tract neurons.

A second type of dorsal horn spinothalamic neuron, termed *nociceptive specific* (NS), is relatively specific for responses to intense mechanical and/or thermal stimuli and is located primarily in superficial (laminae I–II) and, to some degree, in deeper layers (V–VI) of the dorsal horn. This type of neuron typically receives excitatory synaptic effects exclusively from one or more types of primary nociceptive afferents. One subcategory of nociceptive-specific neurons receives excitatory input from A-delta HTM, A-delta heat-nociceptive afferents, and C-fiber polymodal nociceptive afferents. As a result of these inputs, this type of neuron responds to firm pressure and pinching with an increasingly higher frequency of impulse discharge. These neurons also respond to noxious skin temperatures. The receptive fields of these neurons are generally smaller than those of WDR neurons but have a similar gradient of sensitivity. Thus, their receptive fields can sometimes be divided into a central zone, in which firm pressure and pinching result in progressively higher frequency of impulse discharge, and other zones, in which only pinch will cause a discharge. Another subcategory of nociceptive-specific spinothalamic tract neuron is unequivocally specific for responses to noxious skin stimuli. It appears to receive input only from A-delta HTM, since it responds only to noxious mechanical stimulation of the skin or to electrical stimulation of A-delta afferents. Its responses do not outlast the stimulus nor do they summate with repeated application. Therefore, like the A-delta HTM, this type of neuron is probably related to mechanically induced pain, such as that evoked by needle prick. Its receptive field does not appear to have a gradient of sensitivity.

The nociceptive stimulus-response functions and other physiological characteristics of WRD and NS neurons make it appear that these neurons are important for pain. However, a critical question concerning these categories of neurons is whether their activation is necessary and/ or sufficient to give rise to the conscious perception of pain. This question has been examined in a series of experiments in which spinothalamic tract axons within the cervical spinal cord were electrically stimulated in awake humans, and the parameters of stimulation were adjusted so as to stimulate only the axons of WDR neurons (Mayer *et al.*, 1975). This stimulus condition was inferred by comparing electrical threshold and refractory period of monkey spinothalamic tract axons with similar parameters required to evoke pain in awake humans (Price and Mayer, 1975). The refractory periods and electrical thresholds of WDR neurons (but not of NS neurons) matched the refractory period and electrical thresholds of anterolateral-quadrant-evoked pain. Since the electrical thresholds of NS axons were higher than current levels required to evoke pain in humans, it appears that activation of WDR neurons is sufficient to evoke pain.

In the context of determining which types of spinal cord neurons projecting to the brain are sufficient to evoke pain, several observations were made that have direct bearing on pain mechanisms in man. First, it is of considerable significance that pain evoked by stimulation of projection neurons was similar to that evoked by naturally occurring stimuli. Most of the reports were of burning pain, but dull, aching pain, cramping, and sharp pain were also described. These types of pain were evoked by 50-Hz trains of regularly spaced pulses, a pattern that is not likely to be generated by natural stimuli. Therefore, it is unlikely that pain is subserved by some special temporal pattern that depends on the exact intervals of impulses in spinal cord nociceptive neurons. However, the intensity of pain was found to depend on the overall frequency in projection neurons over a range of 5–100 Hz. A linear relationship was found between stimulation frequency and percentage of subjects reporting pain. At 25 Hz, 100% of subjects reported pain, whereas none reported pain at 5 Hz. Similarly, monkey WDR neurons responded to graded noxious heat with a frequency of 5–25 Hz over skin temperature range of 44–46.5°C (Price *et al.*, 1978), the range over which most human heat pain threshold values are distributed (Hardy *et al.*, 1952). In contrast, the frequency of nociceptive-specific responses extends from 5 to 25 Hz over a skin temperature range of 46–48°C. These temperature values evoke suprathreshold pain in most human subjects. Thus, pain appears to depend critically on the overall frequency of impulse in WDR neurons.

These studies also support the concept that central spatial summation is especially critical for pain. When the frequency was held constant (50 Hz), it was found that the perception of projection-neuron-evoked pain invariably required larger stimulus intensities and, presumably, the activation of a larger number of axons than required for the perception of tingle, warmth, or cooling. The amount of spatial summation was critical, since stimulus intensities just sufficient to evoke tingle would do so even when stimulus frequencies extended up to 500 Hz. In contrast, when stimulus intensities were increased to activate a critical number of axons, much lower frequencies (5–25 Hz) evoked pain. These results fit well with other lines of evidence indicating that pain requires central spatial summation.

Another finding in this same study was that projection-neuron-evoked pain was clearly aversive although certainly tolerable. Behavioral responses and reports indicating that the pain was unpleasant (i.e., "bad," "hurts") were given without provocation or suggestion. Since the currents and frequencies were adjusted so as to activate mainly the axons of WDR neurons, these reports of aversion are significant. They support the inference that WDR neurons activate central mechanisms related to the affective–motivational dimension of pain as well as central mechanisms related to sensory discrimination.

Given these sensory and affective effects of stimulation of the spinothalamic pathway, one may begin to question whether all dimensions of pain are uniformly represented in this pathway or whether there is some functional separation within the spinothalamic tract. The idea of functional separation is strongly indicated by the popular assertion that the paleospinothalamic pathway is more important for affective–motivational aspects of pain and the neospinothalamic pathway carries mainly sensory–discriminative information (Melzack and Casey, 1968; Melzack, 1973). This idea is based mainly on anatomical grounds (Melzack, 1973); it suggests that the spinothalamic pathway has two components ascending in the brain stem. The medial component of this pathway (paleospinothalamic tract) gives off numerous collaterals to brain stem structures thought to be involved in arousal (e.g., reticular formation structures) or affect (central gray, tectal area). The lateral component (neospinothalamic tract) is thought to have fewer collaterals to medial brain stem structures and to project to areas that are mostly involved in sensory–discriminative functions.

Several lines of evidence support a more uniform representation of function within the spinothalamic pathway. First, as we saw earlier, stimulation of spinothalamic tract axons within the cervical spinal cord gives rise to pain with both sensory–discriminative and affective components. Second, numerous lesions within the human cervical spinal cord only partially interrupt the spinothalamic tract (Nathan and Smith, 1979). Such lesions produce a restricted zone of analgesia in which all the components of pain are interrupted at once (Nathan and Smith, 1979). Thus, there is no selective loss of aversive components of pain as compared to sensory components. Third, spinothalamic tract axons, the terminals of which end within the sensory thalamic nucleus, ventroposteriolateralis, are now known to have collaterals to such medial brain stem structures as the central gray (Price *et al.*, 1978). Individual spinothalamic neurons, then, appear to have multiple functions. These neurons, which include WDR and NS types, have physiological characteristics similar to those neurons that do not appear to have collaterals to the medial brain stem and to those neurons that only project as far as the mesencephalon. Spinal cord afferent neurons with similar physiological characteristics project to varying levels of the brain stem. All these observations indicate that classic functional subdivisions of the spinothalamic pathways are oversimplified and misleading (Noordenbos, 1959; Melzack, 1973). The spinothalamic pathway appears to contain many neurons that participate in different components of pain and some neurons with more restricted outputs. There does not appear to be sharp functional subdivision of the different components of pain within the spinothalamic pathway.

2.2. The Effects of Opiates on Pain Transmission

Until the early 1970s, in spite of evidence to the contrary (Dewey *et al.*, 1969; Irwin *et al.*, 1951; Tsou and Jang, 1964), the generally accepted theory of opiate analgesic action (Lim, 1966) was that opiates produced analgesia by a central nervous system mechanism analogous to the action of local anesthetics on a peripheral nerve (see Fig. 4). Since then, a major advance in our conception of the neural processing of pain has occurred.

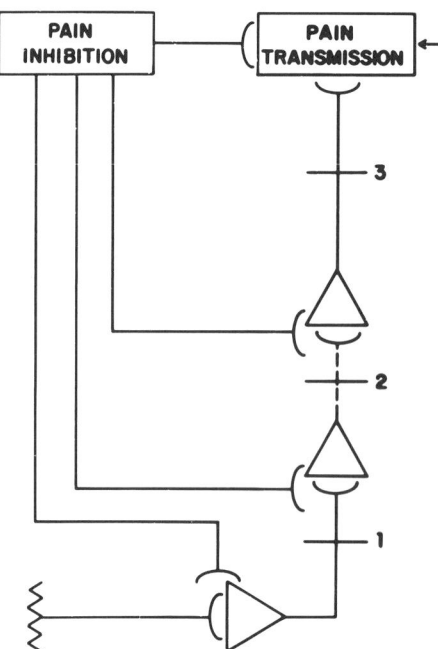

FIG. 4. Schematic diagram of potential mechanisms of action of centrally acting analgesic manipulations. An analgesic manipulation acts either by incapacitating a component in a pain transmission system (points 1–4) or by activating a pain inhibitory system. Lim (1966) proposed the former mechanism. (Reprinted from Mayer and Price, 1976.)

It has become clear that information about tissue damage is not passively received by the nervous system. Rather, it is filtered, even at the first synapse, by complex modulatory systems. The discovery of these systems has fostered, and has, in turn, been fostered by, the notion that the central nervous system contains endogenous substances, endorphins, that possess analgesic properties virtually identical to opiates of plant and synthetic origin. In this section, the development of these concepts is examined. Then the existence of opiate and nonopiate central nervous system pain modulatory mechanisms activated by environmental stimuli will be discussed.

2.2.1. Historical Perspective

It has long been recognized that a simple invariant relationship between stimulus intensity and the magnitude of pain perception is often not present. Two general classes of observations support the complexity of this relationship. The first is the clinical observation that pain is often present without any apparent precipitating pathology. This situation represents the clinical problem of pain treatment. More important for the topic of this section is the common observation that pain may not be experienced in the presence of factors that should produce it; that is, under a variety of circumstances, total or partial analgesia is seen. These observations were explicitly recognized in earlier models of pain perception in spite of the lack of direct evidence supporting the theoretical models (e.g., Noordenbos, 1959; Melzack and Wall, 1965). Thus, the concept that the nervous system possesses intrinsic pain inhibitory mechanisms was recognized when only indirect evidence was available.

The earliest work indicating that opiates produce analgesia, at least in part, by activation of endogenous pain inhibitory systems was done by Irwin *et al.* (1951). They demonstrated that morphine was not effective in inhibiting the spinally mediated tail-flick response in spinalized rats. They reasoned, based on this result, that morphine must activate supraspinal neural circuitry that has an output to the spinal cord and that modulates the processing of nociceptive information at spinal level (see Fig. 4). This work was largely ignored until the early 1970s, even though it was replicated in the mouse (Dewey *et al.*, 1969).

The first impetus for the detailed study of pain-modulatory circuitry was the observation that electrical stimulation of the brain could powerfully suppress the perception of pain (Reynolds, 1969; Mayer *et al.*, 1971). Further investigation of stimulation-produced analgesia provided considerable detail about the neural circuitry involved (see Mayer and Watkins, 1984, for a detailed review of this topic).

Significantly, at that time, several similarities were recognized between these observations and data from a concomitant resurgence of interest in the mechanisms of opiate analgesia (Mayer *et al.*, 1971). The most important parallel facts revealed by these studies were the following: (1) Effective loci for both opiate microinjection analgesia (Tsou and Jang, 1964) and stimulation-produced analgesia (Mayer *et al.*, 1971) lie within the periaqueductal and periventricular gray matter of the brain stem. (2) Opiate analgesia and stimulation-produced analgesia are both mediated, in part, by the activation of a centrifugal control system that exits from the brain and modulates pain transmission at the level of the spinal cord (Irwin *et al.*, 1951; Dewey *et al.*, 1969). (3) The ultimate inhibition of the transmission of nociceptive information occurs, at least in part, at the initial processing stages in the spinal cord dorsal horn and homologous trigeminal nucleus caudalis by selective inhibition of nociceptive neurons (Satoh and Takagi, 1971).

In addition to these correlative observations, studies of stimulation-produced analgesia provided direct evidence indicating that mechanisms extant in the central nervous system depended upon endogenous opiates: (1) Subanalgesic doses of morphine were shown to synergize with subanalgesic levels of brain stimulation to produce behavioral analgesia (Saminin and Valzelli, 1971). (2) Tolerance, a phenomenon invariably associated with repeated administration of opiates, was observed to the analgesic effects of brain stimulation (Mayer and Hayes, 1975). (3) Cross-tolerance between the analgesic effects of brain stimulation and opiates was demonstrated (Mayer and Hayes, 1975). (4) Stimulation-produced analgesia (SPA) could be antagonized by naloxone, a specific narcotic antagonist (Akil *et al.*, 1972, 1976*b*). This last observation, in particular, could be most parsimoniously explained if electrical stimulation resulted in the release of an endogenous opiatelike factor. Indeed, naloxone antagonism of SPA was critical to the eventual discovery of such a factor (Hughes, 1975).

Coincidental with the work of SPA, another discovery of critical importance for our current concepts of endogenous analgesia systems was made. Several laboratories, almost simultaneously, reported the existence of stereospecific binding sites for opiates in the central nervous system (Hiller *et al.*, 1973; Pert and Snyder, 1973; Terenius, 1973). These "receptor" sites were subsequently shown to be localized to neuronal synaptic regions (Pert *et al.*, 1974) and to overlap anatomically with loci involved in the neural processing of pain (Pert *et al.*, 1975). The existence of an opiate receptor again suggested the likelihood of an endogenous compound with opiate properties to occupy it.

In 1974, Hughes and Kosterlitz (Hughes, 1975) reported the isolation from neural tissue of a factor (enkephalin) with such properties. An immense amount of subsequent work has characterized this and other neural and extraneural compounds as having opiate properties. As with the opiate receptor, the anatomical distribution of endogenous opiate ligands overlaps with sites involved in pain processing (see Akil *et al.*, 1984, for a recent review of these studies).

To summarize these important historical developments, the existence of an endogenous opiate analgesia system is suggested by several lines of evidence. Electrical stimulation of the brain produces analgesia. The anatomical structures and neural mechanisms involved in stimulation-produced analgesia parallel those involved in opiate analgesia. The central nervous system contains opiate binding sites and endogenous ligands capable of interacting with those sites. These binding sites and ligands are found at anatomical loci consistent with sites at which stimulation-produced analgesia and opiate microinjection analgesia are elicited.

2.2.2. Neural Circuitry Involved in Analgesia Resulting from the Administration of Exogenous Opiates

In this section, data on the sites and mechanisms involved in the modulation of pain by the administration of exogenous opiates are reviewed. Primarily, two lines of experimentation will be examined: (1) the locations in the CNS at which administration of opiates results in analgesia and the administration of opiate antagonists blocks analgesia; (2) the locations in the CNS at which lesions block the action of exogenous opiates.

Following the work of Tsou and Jang (1964), it was not until the early 1970s, with one exception (Lotti *et al.*, 1965), that opiate microinjection mapping studies began. Initially, these studies concentrated on the periaqueductal–periventricular regions of the mesencephalon and diencephalon (Jacquet and Lajtha, 1973; Pert and Yaksh, 1974; Yaksh *et al.*, 1976). This resurgence of interest in these particular sites of opiate action probably was the result of work showing that analgesia resulted from electrical stimulation of the periaqueductal gray matter (Mayer *et al.*, 1971), as well as the lead provided by the results of Tsou and Jang (1964). Overall, these and other studies confirmed the importance of the periaqueductal–periventricular region in opiate analgesia and provided an impetus for the examination of other brain areas.

A second brain area shown to be of considerable importance for opiate action is the anatomically complex region of the ventromedial medulla. In Fig. 5, this region is seen to consist of at least three distinct nuclei: the medially located nucleus raphe magnus (NRM), the more laterally situated nucleus reticularis paragigantocellularis (NRP), and the dorsolaterally located nucleus reticularis gigantocellularis (NRG). Based on retrograde labeling criteria, Watkins *et al.* (1980) have proposed the term *nucleus raphe alatus* for the combined cell groups in NRM and NRP. Takagi *et al.* (1976) were the first group to map this region for analgesia by morphine microinjection. Overall (Takagi, 1980), this group found the NRP to be approximately 20 times more sensitive to morphine that the

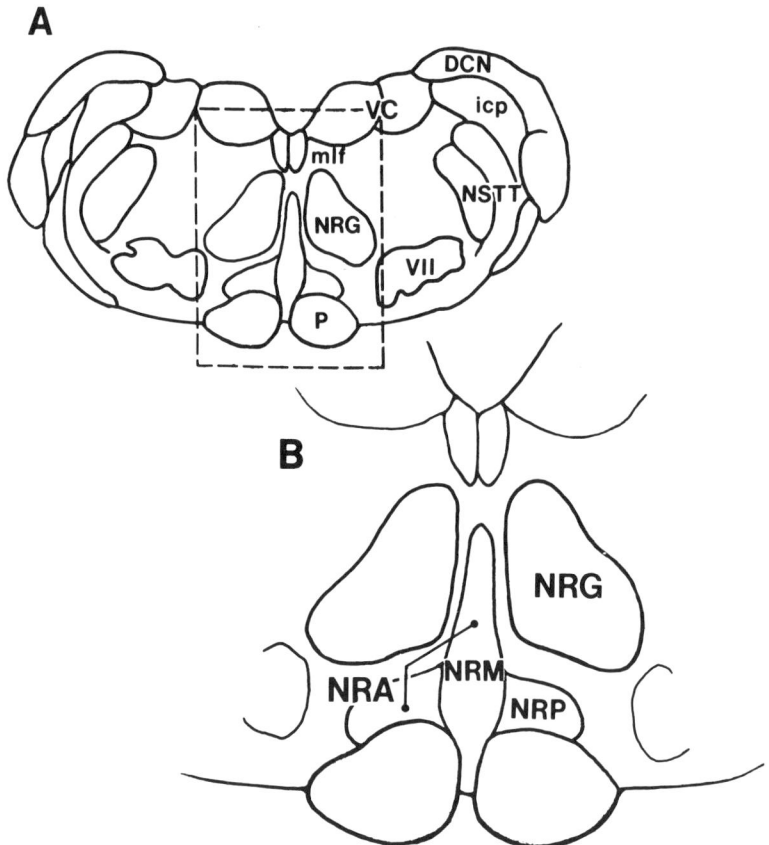

FIG. 5. Detailed anatomy of the rat ventromedial medulla. (A) Frontal section through the rostral medulla of the rat; (B) enlargement of the box enclosed by the dashed line in A. The nucleus raphe alatus, NRA, is the combined cell groups of the nucleus raphe magnus NRM, and the nucleus reticularis paragigantocellularis, NRP. mlf, Medial longitudinal faciculus; NRG, nucleus reticularis gigantocellularis; VII, nucleus of the facial nerve.

NRG. They found that microinjection of morphine into the NRM did not produce analgesia. This point is controversial, since other groups (Azami et al., 1982; Zorman et al., 1982) have reported analgesia from microinjection into NRM. Azami et al. (1982) did find, however, that the NRM was less sensitive than the NRP.

A number of other brain areas, including the amygdala (Rodgers, 1977, 1978), the medial lemniscus (Van Ree, 1977), the nucleus medialis dorsalis of the thalamus (Van Ree, 1977), the mesencephalic reticular formation (Haigler and Spring, 1978; Pert and Yaksh, 1974), and the nucleus of the solitary tract (Oley et al., 1982), have been shown to produce analgesia upon injection with opiates. However, little work has been done on these areas compared with those discussed earlier, and the relative potency of injections into these areas has not been explored.

A final, but crucial point concerns the analgesic effects of microinjections of opiates directly into the intrathecal space of the spinal cord. Although Tsou and Jang (1964) reported no analgesia from direct spinal application of morphine, subsequent work has consistently demonstrated relatively potent effects of intrathecal morphine microinjection (Yaksh and Rudy, 1976, 1977). This observation has had important clinical applications, since direct intrathecal application of opiates has been shown to have analgesic effects without the concomitant psychoactive effects observed with systemic administration.

From this line of evidence it appears, then, that at least three general areas of the CNS are involved in opiate analgesia: the periaqueductal–periventricular gray matter, the ventromedial medulla, and the spinal cord. This observation indicates that the analgesic effects of a systemically administered opiate may produce analgesia by acting at any, all, or some combination of these distinct regions. Studies in which the microinjection of narcotic antagonists are utilized have provided at least a partial answer to this question.

In a number of early studies, it was concluded that supraspinal sites of opiate action are the effective ones, since analgesia induced by systemically administered opiates was antagonized by either intracranioventricular or intracerebral narcotic antagonists (Albus *et al.*, 1970; Jacquet and Lajtha, 1974; Tsou, 1963; Vigouret *et al.*, 1973). Later work, however, demonstrated that intrathecal naloxone could antagonize the analgesia resulting from even relatively high doses of systemically administered opiates (Yaksh and Rudy, 1977). Thus, these studies lead to the paradoxical conclusion that both supraspinal sites and spinal sites of opiate action are involved in analgesia.

This seeming paradox was resolved in a series of complex, but unusually important studies by Yeung and Rudy (1980*a,b*). They demonstrated that, by simultaneously injecting various doses of morphine intrathecally (spinal cord) and intraventricularly (brain), a multiplicative dose–response function was observed. That is, simultaneous spinal and supraspinal morphine resulted in greater analgesia than the same total dose at either location alone. The effect is quite large, with the multiplicative factor being as high as 45 under certain circumstances (Yeung and Rudy, 1980*b*). This type of multiplicative interaction, as will be seen below, may turn out to be a confounding factor in many pharmacological and physiological analyses of the involvement of opiates in various behaviors. Thus, the reader should keep in mind, when evaluating the literature on this and other topics, the potential for complex interactions between the same or various neurotransmitters and/or neuromodulators.

Although the experiments just described elucidate the contribution of spinal versus supraspinal sites of opiate analgesia, the relative contribution of the various supraspinal sites at which opiates act to produce analgesia is less clear. The only work to examine this issue utilizing microinjection of narcotic antagonists was done by Azami et al. (1982). They found, as did Takagi's group, that the NRP was more sensitive to morphine than the NRM for elicitation of analgesia. Surprisingly, however, they found that when analgesia was produced by systemically administered morphine, naloxone injected into the NRM antagonized analgesia more effectively than when it was injected into more lateral medullary regions including the NRP. They concluded that NRP does not contribute significantly to the analgesia resulting from systemic administration of morphine. The relative contribution of medullary versus more rostral mesencephalic sites has not been studied.

An approach similar to the one just described for disecting the neural circuitry for opiate analgesia utilized the selective destruction of nuclei and pathways. Opiates, injected systemically or at discrete sites in the nervous system, and the effect of particular lesions were studied. Table 1 lists these experiments. An overview of this work supports the conclusion reached in the work utilizing injection of antagonists. It appears that several brain areas, including the periaqueductal gray matter, NRM, and NRP, must be intact for the full expression of opiate analgesia.

TABLE 1
The Effect of Various CNS Lesions on Opiate Analgesia Resulting from Various Routes of Administration[a]

Lesion site	Systemic injection	PAG microinjection	NRM microinjection	NRP microinjection
DLF	< Hayes et al., 1978b	< Murfin et al., 1976		
	< Barton et al., 1980			
NRM	< Azami et al., 1982	< Young et al., 1984		< Azami et al., 1982
	< Young et al., 1984			
	< Proudfit and Anderson, 1975			
NRP	= Azami et al., 1982			
	< Kishioka et al., 1983			
	< Lai and Chan, 1982			
NRA	%< Young et al., 1984			
PAG	%< Yeung et al., 1975			
	< Dostrovsky and Deakin, 1977			
LC	< Hammond and Proudfit, 1980			
POF	< Pottoff et al., 1979			

[a] <, attenuates analgesia; %<, partially attenuates analgesia; =, no effect on analgesia. Citations are listed alphabetically in the references. DLF, dorsolateral funiculus; LClocus coeruleus; NRA, nucleus raphe alatus; NRM, nucleus raphe magnus; NRP, nucleus raphe paragigantocellularis; PAG, mesencephalic periaqueductal gray matter; POF, preoptic forebrain.

2.3. Environmental Activation of Endogenous Analgesia Systems

The demonstration that opiates activate well-defined neural systems capable of blocking pain transmission suggests, but by no means proves, that this system functions to dynamically modulate the perceived intensity of noxious stimuli. If this system has such a physiological role, then one might expect that the level of activity within the system would be influenced by environmental stimuli. If environmental situations that produce analgesia could be identified, it would give credibility to the idea that invasive procedures, such as brain stimulation or narcotic drugs administration, inhibit pain by mimicking the natural activity of these pathways.

A systematic search for environmental stimuli that activate pain inhibitory systems was begun by Hayes *et al.* (1976, 1978a,b). They observed that potent analgesia could be produced by such diverse stimuli as brief footshock, centrifugal rotation, and intraperitoneal saline injection. These effects appeared to be specific to pain perception insofar as normal motor behavior, righting and corneal reflexes, vocalization, startle responses, and response to touch were unimpaired (Hayes *et al.*, 1978a). Two other important concepts emerged from this work. First, exposure to "stress" was not sufficient to produce analgesia. Although almost all analgesia-inducing environmental stimuli studied to date are stressors (Table 2), the failure of classical stressors, such as ether vapors and horizontal oscillation, to produce pain inhibition indicated that stress was not the critical variable responsible. Second, it was found rather unexpectedly that the opiate antagonist naloxone did not block environmentally induced analgesia (Hayes *et al.*, 1978a). Therefore, it appeared that nonopiate systems, in addition to the system activated by opiates described earlier, must exist.

Although the stimuli studied by Hayes *et al.* (1978a,b) did not appear to activate an opiate system, subsequent investigations found clues that endogenous opioids might be involved in at least some types of environmentally induced analgesia. Akil *et al.* (1976b) studied the analgesic effects of prolonged footshock. In contrast to the results of Hayes *et al.* (1978a, b), naloxone did partially antagonize the analgesia. This initial indication of opiate involvement led Akil and co-workers to look for biochemical evidence that footshock effected the released brain opiates. The changes in brain opiate levels did indeed parallel the development of footshock-induced analgesia (Akil *et al.*, 1976a). When tolerance developed to the analgesic effects of footshock, brain opiate levels returned to control values.

The controversy over the involvement of opiates in footshock-induced analgesia was resolved, in part, by Lewis *et al.* (1980). They noted

TABLE 2
Summary of Currently Available Data on Endogenous Analgesia Systems[a]

	Opiate								Hormone		Circuitry					Neurochemistry					
	Sys. Nal.	IT Nal.	Mu Antag.	Delta Ant.	Kappa Ant.	Dyn. Antis.	Enk. Antis.	Bend. Antis.	X Tolerance	Plas. Level	CNS Level	Adrenal X	Adr. Demed.	Hypox	Spinalize	DLF Les.	NRA Les.	PAG Les.	Decereb.	5 HT CNS	Spin. 5 HT	CNS NE	Spinal NE	Dopamine	CNS ACH	CCK 8	Histamine	GABA
Neural/opiate																												
Brief FPFS	V	V					V					∧	×	○	V	V	V	○	○	V	V	V	V		○	V		
CCA	V	V	V	○			V					∧	×	○	×	V	V	V	○	V	V	V	○		V			
Systemic morph	V	○	○	○			V	?	?			∧	○	∧	V	V	?	○	○									
IC morph (PAG)	V	V	○	○			V					○	×	○	×	V	V	×	×		○							
IT morph	V	○	○	V			V	×	×			×	×	×	×	×	×	×	×	○	○							
ECS	V	V				V						○	○	○	×	V	V	×	×	×								
Conditioned fear												○	×	○			?			?								
Defeat												○	○	○	V	V	V	○	○	○		○						
Neural/nonopiate																												
Brief HPFS	○	○	○	○			○	○		∧		○	×	∧	V	V	V	○	○	○	○	○	○	V	V	V	V	V
≤OR=3 min 4-PFS	○	×	○	○				V				○	○	○		V	V	○	V	V		V	V		○	○		
2DG	?																	?				V						
Horm/opiate																												
Acupunc (lo freq)	V	V	V				V	V		∧	∧	V	V	V		V	○	∧	∧	○	?	○	V	V	V	V	V	V
30 min 4-PFS	V	V	○	○			V	V		○		V	V	V	V		○	V	V	V		V	V	V	V	V	V	V

486   DAVID J. MAYER

BEHAVIORAL EFFECTS OF OPIATES

Immobilization	
15 min cold (4 C)	
Exercise	
Pregnancy	
Cond helpless	
CCA	
Food dep	
Prolong tailshock	
Horm/nonopiate	
Cold-water swims	
Brief tail shock	
Unknown/opiate	
SPA (PAG)	
SPA (VMM)	
Kindled seizure	
TNS-lo/freq-hi/in	
Vaginal probing	
DNIC & pain (xFS)	
Centrif rotation	
Placebo	
Anxiety (human)	
Sex (male)	
Spon hypertension	
Int cold water	
20 C swim (mice)	
Cold water	
Warm water (mice)	
Heat (40 C)	
Radiation	
Novelty (rat)	

(continued)

Table 2 (*Continued*)

	Opiate											Hormone				Circuitry				Neurochemistry								
	Sys. Nal	IT Nal	Mu Antag	Delta Ant	Kappa Ant	Dyn. Ant	Enk. Ant	Bend. Antis	X Tolerance	Plas. Level	CNS Level	Adrenal X	Ad: Demed	Hypox	Spinalize	DLF Les	NRA Les	PAG Les	Decereb.	5 HT CNS	Spin. 5 HT	CNS NE	Spinal NE	Dopamine	CNS ACh	CCK 8	Histamine	GABA
Unknown/nonopiate																												
SPA (pag)	o	x	o	x				o																				
SPA (PB)	o	x	x	x																				V				
TNS (Hi/f-lo/I)	o	x	x	x				o																				
Acupunc (hi freq)	o	x	x	x						o																		
Hypnosis	o	x	x	x																					o			
Vaginal probing	o	x	x	x																								
Centrif rotation	o	x	x	x																								
30°C swim	o	x	x	x																								
Firewalking	o	x	x	x																								
Vibration	o	x	x	x																								
Novelty (cat)	o	x	x	x																								
Feeding (cat)	o	x	x	x																								
Immobilization	o	x	x	x																								

Hormonal/unknown
  Insulin <
Unknown—no data cooling, ice massage, social isolation, laser, suggestion

Hyperalgesia

Unknown/opiate
  Mild footshock >
  21 day int FS >
Hormonal/unknown
  Novelty <
Unknown
  Holding; food deprivation (2021) >
  Ether, horizontal oscillation

Ineffective stressors: ether, horizontal oscillation, aversive noise, WW swim (rat)

[a] A review of the literature reveals that four classes of analgesic manipulations can be identified: neural/opiate, hormonal/opiate, neural/nonopiate, and hormonal/nonopiate. The criteria used to classify analgesia as opiate include naloxone reversibility and cross-tolerance with morphine. Hormonal analgesia is characterized as being attenuated by either adrenalectomy, adrenal demedullation, or hypophysectomy. These latter criteria were chosen, since all environmental stimuli that produce analgesia activate the pituitary–adrenal cortical and sympathetic–adrenal medullary axes. Regarding the neural substrates of these various analgesic responses, the most comprehensive data are available on the effect of dorsolateral funiculus (DLF) lesions, n. raphe alatus (NRA) lesions, and periaqueductal gray (PAG) lesions. As can be seen, DLF lesions attenuate all analgesic manipulations that have been tested, suggesting that the DLF may form a final common pathway for endogenous pain inhibitory systems. >, potentiation; <, attenuation; 0, no effect; ?, conflicting data exist indicating either no effect or attenuation; blank, no data are available; x, inappropriate category.

that the duration of footshock used by Hayes *et al.* (1978*a,b*) and Akil *et al.* (1976*a*) differed greatly and wondered whether this variable might explain the difference in their results. By comparing the effects of naloxone on analgesia produced by brief (3 min) versus prolonged (30 min) footshock, Lewis *et al.* (1980) showed that only the latter could be blocked by naloxone. This suggests that different analgesia systems are activated as the duration of footshock increases.

Concurrent with this work of Lewis *et al.* (1980), Watkins *et al.* (1982*a*) observed that brief shock restricted to the front paws produced analgesia, as measured by the tail-flick assay, which was antagonized by low doses (0.1 mg/kg) of naloxone. In contrast, even high doses (20 mg/kg) of naloxone failed to reduce analgesia produced by hind-paw shock. In addition, they showed that animals made tolerant to morphine showed cross-tolerance to front-paw but not to hind-paw footshock analgesia. Thus, it appears that front-paw shock activates an endogenous opiate analgesia system, whereas hind-paw shock activates an independent nonopiate analgesia system. In addition, this work showed again that stress is not a sufficient factor to activate opiate analgesia systems, since identical shock parameters were used for hind-paw and front-paw shock (Watkins *et al.*, 1982*a*).

Additional work has revealed the following important facts about front-paw and hind-paw footshock-induced analgesias (FSIA): (1) Front-paw FSIA is mediated by central nervous system opioids since elimination of extraneural opiates by hypophysectomy, adrenalectomy, or sympathetic blockade does not block the effects (Watkins *et al.*, 1982*d*). (2) Front-paw FSIA involves a neural circuit that ascends to the brain and then descends by way of the dorsolateral funiculus (DLF) to block pain transmission at the spinal level (Watkins *et al.*, 1982*c*). This descending DLF pathway originates in the nucleus raphe alatus (NRA) (Watkins *et al.*, 1983*b*). (3) The complete circuitry for the effect is caudal to the mesencephalon, since decerebration does not affect the analgesia (Watkins *et al.*, 1983*a*). (4) The critical opiate synapse for the system is situated in the spinal cord (see Fig. 6) at the segment of nociceptive input, since the intrathecal injection of 1 µg of naloxone in the lumbosacral but not the thoracic cord blocks the effect (Watkins and Mayer, 1982*a*). (5) Once the system is activated, continued opiate release is not needed, since naloxone blocks the effect only when given before footshock, not after (Watkins and Mayer, 1982*a*). (6) Spinal cord serotonin is critical for the expression of front-paw FSIA (Watkins *et al.*, 1984*e*). (7) Front-paw FSIA is blocked by small systemic or intrathecal doses of the peptide cholecystokinin (CCK) (Faris *et al.*, 1983) and potentiated by the putative CCK antagonists proglumide and benzotript (Watkins *et al.*, 1984*g*).

Hind-paw FSIA is also a CNS-mediated phenomenon (Watkins *et al.*, 1982*d*), which activates intraspinal and supraspinal pain inhibitory sys-

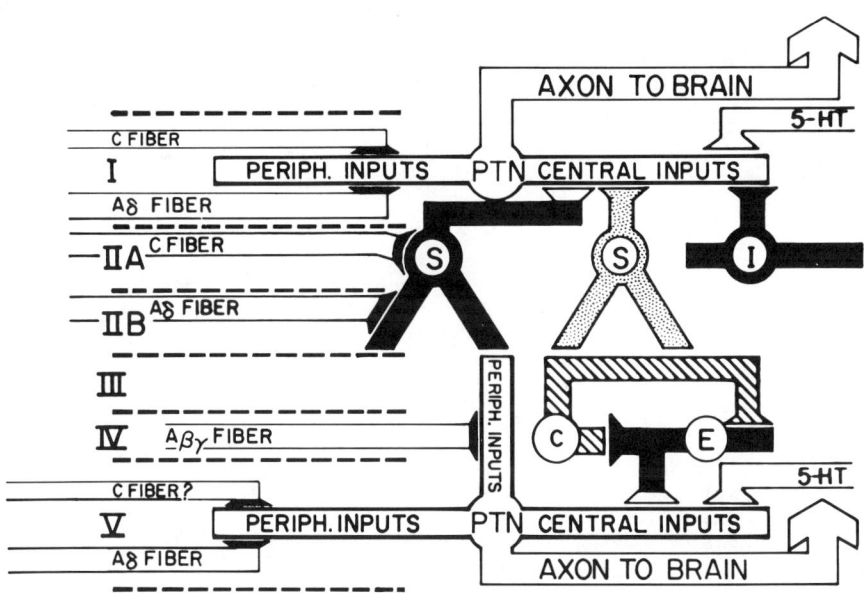

FIG. 6. Schematic diagram of the organization of the dorsal horn, including peripheral inputs, interneurons, and inputs originating from the central nervous system. Roman numerals, left of figure, Rexed's laminae I–V; filled terminals, excitatory connections; unfilled terminals, inhibitory connections. Filled cells indicate cells containing endogenous opioids. Note that an endorphinergic cell in laminae IV–V excites a cholecystokinin cell, which, in turn, inhibits an endorphinergic cell. C, cholecystokinin; E, endorphin; I, islet cell; S, stalked cell; PTN, pain transmission neuron.

tems (Watkins *et al.*, 1982c). The brain centers for hind-paw FSIA differ from those for front-paw FSIA, since NRA lesions do not eliminate the analgesia (Watkins *et al.*, 1983b). The neurochemical bases of hind-paw FSIA also differ from front-paw FSIA: (1) CCK, serotonin, and norepinephrine do not appear to be involved in hind-paw FSIA (Faris *et al.*, 1983; Watkins *et al.*, 1984e). (2) Brain, but not spinal cord, acetylocholine is necessary to the expression of hind-paw FSIA but does not appear to be involved in front-paw FSIA (Watkins *et al.*, 1984f).

Of considerable interest is that both hind-paw and front-paw FSIA can be classically conditioned by repeated pairings of a conditioned stimulus (CS) with footshock (Watkins *et al.*, 1982b). Regardless of whether hind-paw or front-paw shock is used as the unconditional stimulus (UCS), an opiate analgesia system in many ways similar to the one involved in front-paw FSIA is activated, since conditioned analgesia is eliminated by (1) systemic and intrathecal naloxone, (2) morphine tolerance, (3) DLF lesions, and (4) NRA lesions and is unaffected by hypophysectomy, adrenalectomy, or sympathetic blockade (Watkins and Mayer, 1982b). In addition, as would be expected, higher structures are involved in the conditioned analgesia, since it is eliminated by decerebration and reduced by periaqueductal gray lesions (Kinscheck *et al.*, 1984).

A circuit diagram of these systems is shown in Fig. 7. The details of the circuitry at the level of the spinal cord dorsal horn is given in Fig. 6. A few points are worthy of special note. As mentioned above, spinal cord

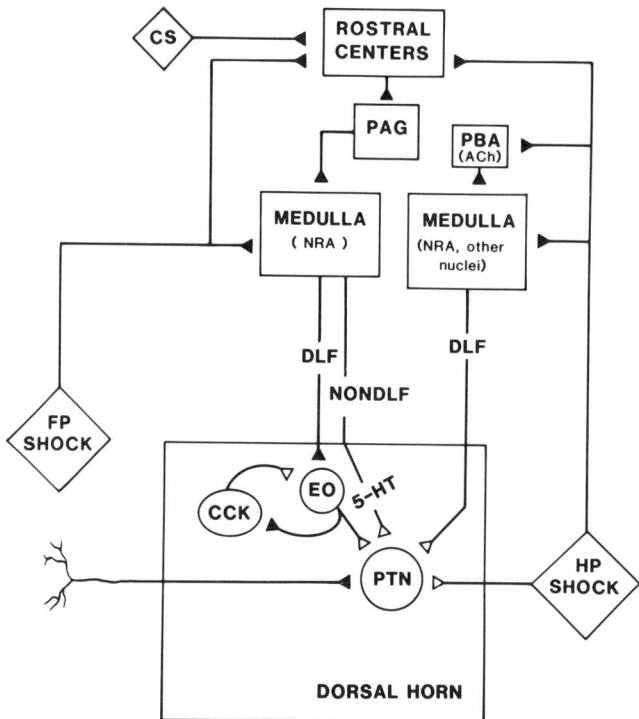

FIG. 7. Neural circuitry of opiate and nonopiate analgesia induced by front-paw and hind-paw shock. Front-paw shock activates the nucleus raphe alatus (NRA) within the ventral medulla. This nucleus sends a descending projection through the dorsolateral funiculus (DLF) to the dorsal horn of the spinal cord. A serotonergic pathway outside the DLF (non-DLF) is recruited as well. In turn, endogenous opioids are released, inhibiting pain transmission neurons (PTN). The activation of endogenous opiates stimulates a negative feedback loop that utilizes CCK to reduce activity of endogenous opioid systems. The hind-paw shock inhibits PTN via two nonopioid pathways: an intraspinal pathway and a descending DLF pathway. The latter originates from the NRA and from some other, as-yet-unidentified medullary area(s). Classically conditioned (opioid) analgesia seems to result from activation of the same DLF output pathway as front-paw (opioid) FSIA. After conditioning trials in which the conditioned stimulus is paired with either front-paw or hind-paw shock (the unconditioned stimulus), the conditioned stimulus becomes capable of activating rostral centers in the brain, which, in turn, activate the periaqueductal gray (PAG) and, subsequently, the nucleus raphe alatus. This results, via a descending DLF pathway, in the release of endogenous opioids within the dorsal horn to produce analgesia.

serotonin depletion attenuates analgesia elicited by front-paw FSIA. Lesions of the DLF also eliminate front-paw FSIA. Interestingly, mapping studies of the origin and course of encephalospinal serotonergic neurons indicate that cells of the ventral medulla, which contribute to the DLF, and medullary serotonin-containing cells constitute two completely separate populations (Johannessen et al., 1984). Thus, serotonin-containing neurons project to the spinal cord by way of a pathway other than the DLF. The significance of serotonin not projecting in the DLF is based on the following observations: (1) Front-paw FSIA, as well as other forms of analgesia, depend on the release of spinal cord serotonin; (2) they also depend on the integrity of the DLF. These suggest that if serotonin does not project in the DLF, more than one descending pathway (and more than one transmitter) is necessary for the expression of analgesia. In other words, the activation of synergistic systems is sometimes necessary. This would be a new and powerful explanation for understanding a number of perplexing aspects of the neural mechanisms of analgesia. Other lines of evidence also support such an explanation. First, as discussed above, Yeung and Rudy (1980a,b) have shown that such a synergy (or multiplicative effect) exists between spinal and supraspinal sites of morphine action. Second, although direct intrathecal application of serotonin can produce analgesia, inordinately high doses (200 μg) are necessary (Yaksh and Wilson, 1979). A third, more perplexing observation comes from unpublished work from my laboratory. We reasoned that since the integrity of the DLF is known to be necessary for the expression of virtually every encephalospinally mediated analgesia, direct stimulation of the DLF in the rat should produce analgesia. In no case, when stimulation was restricted to the DLF, did we observe inhibition of the tail-flick response. This supports the anatomical conclusion that the DLF is necessary, but not sufficient for analgesia. If this is the case, it is of importance, clinically, in that it suggests that small amounts of synergizing transmitters applied directly to the cord could produce potent analgesia.

A second important point is that the involvement of other neurotransmitters or neuromodulators at the spinal cord level may be quite complex. As shown in Figs. 6 and 7, CCK appears to modulate endogenous opioid systems. Intrathecal application of CCK antagonizes analgesia from exogenous opiate application as well as analgesia elicited by endogenous opiate activation (Faris et al., 1983). Also, CCK antagonists applied intrathecally potentiate these analgesias (Watkins et al., 1985a,b) as well as reverse opiate tolerance (Watkins et al., 1984g). These findings suggest that other transmitters and/or modulators may interact with opiates to form complex circuits. An understanding of these circuits should offer important opportunities to pharmacologically manipulate clinical pain syndromes, possibly without the drawbacks associated with opiate analgesia.

In addition to the work done by Liebeskind's group (see Terman et al., 1984, for a review) and our own, a number of other laboratories have now demonstrated that numerous environmental variables can be critical in determining the particular pain modulatory circuitry activated. For example, Maier's group has shown that inescapable tail shock results in opiate analgesia, but analgesia resulting from tail shocks with identical temporal and intensity characteristics is nonopiate if the shocks are escapable (Maier *et al.*, 1982). Table 2 summarizes the voluminous literature on environmental events now known to influence the transmission of pain. It is clear that numerous environmental manipulations modulate pain transmission. The literature in this field has become large, confusing, and, in many cases, seemingly irreconcilable. From Table 2, however, it can be seen that certain patterns of organization of analgesia systems are beginning to emerge. A number of facts now appear clear. (1) Even though quite diverse manipulations have been utilized to produce antinociception, the organizations of the neural systems underlying the effects have some striking similarities. Almost all the manipulations studied to date can activate multiple pain inhibitory pathways. When, however, the manipulation is refined, selective activation of more discrete components is usually possible. (2) When a supraspinal component is involved in the analgesia, it usually activates a neural circuit the basic components of which are situated no more rostral than the caudal brain stem. Even when more rostral components are involved, they seem to exert their effects by activating this more caudal circuitry (e.g., Kinscheck *et al.*, 1984). Thus, as with other behaviors such as feeding, a hierarchical organization appears to be involved in pain modulation. (3) A critical component of the caudal brain stem circuitry appears to involve all or part of the NRA (Watkins *et al.*, 1983*b*). (4) When the supraspinal pain modulatory circuitry is activated, the ultimate mechanism of pain modulation seems to result always, as far as I am aware, in the activation of encephalospinal inhibitory systems, since selective spinal lesions can always eliminate the analgesia (Watkins *et al.*, 1982*b*, 1983*a,b*). (5) In *all* descending pain modulatory systems studied to date, of which I am aware, the DLF is a necessary encephalospinal pathway. This is true when analgesia results from the application of systemic (Hayes *et al.*, 1978*b*) or intracerebrally microinjected (Murfin *et al.*, 1976) opiates, intracerebral microinjection of other chemicals (Hayes *et al.*, 1984), electrical stimulation of the brain (Basbaum *et al.*, 1975), as well as the various environmental manipulations discussed earlier (Kinscheck *et al.*, 1984; Watkins *et al.*, 1984*a,b*). These similarities seem to indicate that, although there may be great diversity in the manipulations and pathways producing analgesia, only a small number of final common-output pathways are present. We are, I feel, close to a relatively complete description of the details of this circuitry.

In sum, then, there appears to be strong evidence for the existence of multiple pain modulatory systems. Our knowledge of endogenous opiate analgesia systems probably represents the most detailed description of any opiate behavioral system available. Work of this sort has already begun to yield information with important implications for the problem of pain syndromes in humans. Further description of these systems is also likely to provide insights into mechanisms of opiate action and have important implications for treatment of drug abuse, another health care problem of immense proportions (Holden, 1985).

3. THE EFFECTS OF OPIATES ON REWARD

Opiates have long been used and abused because at least some human beings find them rewarding or reinforcing; that is, some people indicate that they enjoy opiates and will perform arbitrary behaviors in order to receive them. The problem of opiate abuse remains a difficult medical issue, not only because it is so entwined with political decisions but also because the neurobiology of the effects of opiates was, until recently, very poorly understood. In the last few years, considerable progress has been made in describing the neural mechanisms of opiate reinforcement. This information may prove useful in coping with opiate abuse. In addition, such knowledge may provide a model of drug abuse, in general, as well as shedding light on the reward process itself, which is so important in motivating a large variety of human behaviors. In this section, a discussion of the neural substrates involved in opiate self-administration will be followed by a discussion of the involvement of endogenous opioids in reward produced in other situations.

3.1. The Neural Substrate of Opiate Reward

Although it has long been known that humans and nonhuman animals will self-administer opiates via a systemic route (Jaffe and Martin, 1980), only recently has the site of opiate action within the central nervous system begun to be explored. As in the case of analgesia, the microinjection technique has proved critical for determining the locus of action for the rewarding effects of opiates. Rats will learn to self-administer small doses of opiates into the ventral tegmental area (Bozarth and Wise, 1981a). Importantly, injection into a number of areas showing high levels of endogenous opioids or opiate receptors will not support self-administration behavior. These areas include the mesencephalic periaqueductal gray matter, the lateral hypothalamic area, the nucleus accumbens, and the caudate nucleus (Wise, 1984). In a critical complementary experiment, it was demonstrated that injections of the narcotic antagonist naloxone into the ventral tegmental area, but not into the nucleus accumbens or caudate nucleus, blocked the rewarding effect of systemically administered heroin (Britt and Wise, 1983). Thus, it appears that opiate activation of the ventral tegmental area is both necessary and sufficient for opiate-induced reward.

It would certainly be of interest to know the type of opiate receptor and the endogenous ligand involved in opiate reward. Surprisingly little research has been done on these topics. The information that is available indicates that a different opiate receptor type is involved in opiate reward and in analgesia (Pollerberg et al., 1983). Given the complexity of this type of research, however, it is difficult to draw any firm conclusions at this time. It seems likely that considerably more work will be done on these issues in the near future.

This line of research has also begun to address the relationship of the rewarding property of opiates to opiate addiction. One general theory of addiction has been that animals and humans take opiates, at least in part, because they relieve the unpleasant symptoms of withdrawal; that is, physical dependence is the factor that initiates drug-taking behavior. Interestingly, prolonged infusion of opiates into the ventral tegmental area does not produce noticeable withdrawal symptoms when these animals are challenged with naloxone (Bozarth and Wise, 1984). On the other hand, animals will not self-administer opiates into the mesencephalic periaqueductal gray matter, but prolonged perfusion of opiates into that area does result in signs of physical dependence after naloxone challenge (Bozarth, 1982). Also, if, after a long period of abstinence, a priming injection of an opiate is made into the ventral tegmental area, animals will begin to self-administer opiates into this region (Wise, 1984). It appears, then, that addictive behavior can occur in the absence of withdrawal symptoms resulting from physical dependence. Thus, although physical dependence is not ruled out as the source of addictive behavior, the quest for opiate reward appears to be sufficient to initiate and maintain opiate self-administration.

3.2. The Opiate Reward and Other Forms of Reward

It is of considerable interest that the reward system activated by opiates may be, at least in part, the same system activated by other rewarding drugs, the positively reinforcing effects of electrical stimulation of the brain, and the reward derived from such natural reinforcers as food and water. Opiate reward appears to depend upon the integrity of a dopaminergic transmission system, since (1) haloperidol, a dopamine receptor blocker, eliminates the rewarding properties of opiates (Bozarth and Wise, 1981b; Spiraki et al., 1982); (2) opiates must be injected into a dopaminergic cell group (A-10) in the ventral tegmental area in order to be rewarding (Bozarth and Wise, 1981b; Phillips and LePiane, 1980); and (3) dopaminergic neurons in the ventral tegmental area are activated by opiates (Matthews and German, 1982; Ostrowski *et al.*, 1981). Increased dopaminergic synaptic effectiveness in the nucleus accumbens (the terminal field of A-10) appears to be critical for the rewarding action of amphetamine, cocaine, and phencyclidine to occur. Injection of these substances into the nucleus accumbens is rewarding (Wise, 1984), and dopamine antagonism in this area by neurotoxins (Lyness *et al.*, 1977a; Roberts *et al.*, 1977, 1980) or dopamine antagonists (Phillips and Broekkamp, 1980) blocks cocaine and amphetamine reward.

Again, the case of reward resulting from electrical stimulation of the brain, some of the same circuitry may be used. It has been shown that rewarding stimulation of the lateral hypothalamus depends on the activation of caudally directed axons that terminate in the dopaminergic areas of the ventral tegmentum (Bielajew and Shizgal, 1982; Corbett and Wise, 1980; Shizgal *et al.*, 1980). Also, dopaminergic integrity appears to be necessary for intracranial self-stimulation behavior to occur, since pharmacological disruption of dopaminergic transmission blocks this behavior. Figure 8 is a summary diagram of the neural circuitry described here (see

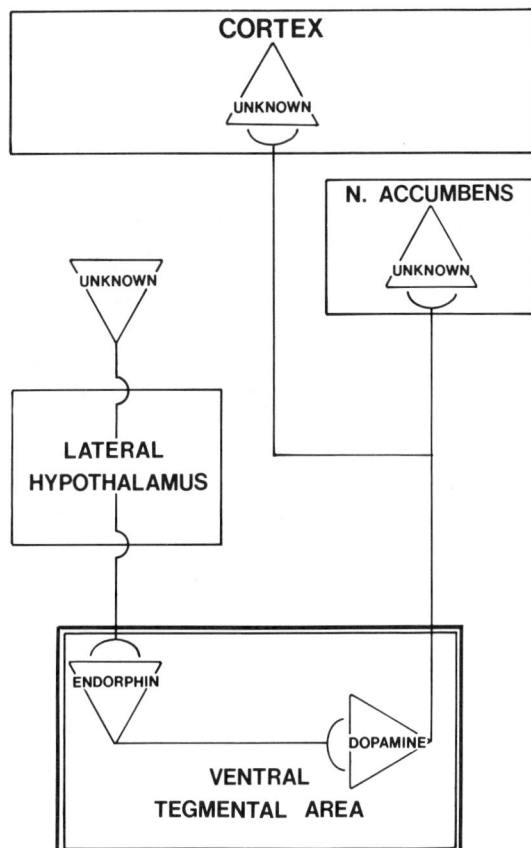

FIG. 8. Schematic diagram of the neural circuitry involved in reward. Opiate microinjection in the ventral tegmental area is rewarding and depends on dopamine release in the nucleus accumbens. See text for additional details.

Wise, 1984, for a more detailed treatment). A number of reports have indicated that the rewarding value of intracranial self-stimulation is reduced by the opiate antagonist naloxone (Belluzzi and Stein, 1977; Kelsey et al., 1984), although this effect has not been observed in some studies (Sanberg and Segal, 1978; Zvartau, 1977). Thus, it appears that dopamine is an important element in brain stimulation and opiate reward. Also, brain stimulation reward, at least under some circumstances, requires endogenous opiates for its expression.

Naturally occurring reward resulting from feeding and drinking may utilize portions of this neural circuit as well, although the literature on this point is extremely complex. It has been established that dopaminergic antagonists can reduce the reward value of food (Wise, 1978, 1984; Xenakis and Sclafani, 1982) and water (Gerber et al., 1981). The involvement of the mesolimbic (ventral tegmental–nucleus accumbens) dopaminergic system has not yet been verified but appears to be a likely possibility. A large literature exists on the role of endogenous opioids and feeding. Opioids are clearly and importantly involved, but in most cases, their reward value, as opposed to their ability to initiate motivated behaviors, is not clear. Some indication that the reward value of food is modulated by endogenous opioids in humans derives from a study by Cohen et al. (1985). They found that naloxone reduced food consumption in human subjects but did not reduce the amount of reported hunger. This literature is reviewed by Cooper and Sanger (1984), as well as by several other authors in the same reference. A summary of the recent literature in this field is given in Table 3.

That opioid-mediated reward is involved in euphoria elicited by nonconsummatory responses is supported by a recent study of "runner's high" (Janal et al., 1984). They found that euphoria and joy ratings on a visual analog scale were significantly increased after a 6.3-mile run at 85% of aerobic capacity. This effect was antagonized by naloxone. This study suggests that endogenous opioids may participate in subtle feelings of well-being, which can powerfully reinforce human behavior.

In summary, recent research has uncovered the following important facts about the elicitation of reward by opiates. (1) Opiates appear to produce reward, at least in the rat, by interacting with opiate receptors in the ventral tegmental area of the mesencephalon. At present, opiate action in this region seems both necessary and sufficient for reward. The involvement of other brain areas, however, cannot be ruled out until more extensive opiate microinjection mapping studies are performed. (2) The neural substrates of opiate reward and opiate physical dependence appear to be, to a considerable degree, independent. This observation should be important for our understanding and treatment of addiction. (3) Reward elicited by other drugs, consummatory responses, and other behaviors may activate at least some components of a common reward system. These results indicate the possibility of therapeutically modulating consummatory behaviors, such as eating, with selective opiate agonists and antagonists, as well as with other pharmacological manipulations.

4. THE EFFECTS OF OPIATES ON CARDIOVASCULAR FUNCTION

Opiates are known to have potent cardiovascular effects. These effects, as might be expected, are quite complex and vary with species, dose, route of administration, and state of consciousness. In spite of these complexities, this opiate action has been intensively studied, especially since the endogenous opioids were discovered. For an excellent, comprehensive review of cardiovascular effects of opiates, and a more detailed analysis of this topic, see Holaday (1983). This section follows the plan of previous sections; We will examine first the sites and mechanisms invoked by administration of exogenous opiates. Then, the involvement of endogenous opioids in cardiovascular perturbations produced by environmental manipulations will be discussed. Again, this section is not intended to be comprehensive but, rather, to provide the reader with an overview of the general approach that is utilized to examine the involvement of opiates in behavior.

4.1. Cardiovascular Effects of Exogenously Administered Opiates

As mentioned above, the effects of opiates on the cardiovascular system are quite complex. The systemic administration of opiates has the potential of modulating cardiovascular function at an extremely large number of sites. Holaday (1983) has reviewed the central nervous system, autonomic nervous system, peripheral nervous system, and extraneural structures both implicated in cardiovascular function and having opiate receptor sites and/or opioid immunoreactive cells. The central nervous system sites, for example, include the nucleus tractus solitarius, nucleus ambiguous, dorsal vagal nucleus, area postrema, numerous hypothalamic nuclei, preganglionic sympathetic and parasympathetic nuclei and limbic, cortical, and even cerebellar nuclei. From this example, it should be apparent that the effects of a systemically administered opiate are both varied and complex. The advent of opiate agonists and antagonists that are at least partially selective for particular receptors has somewhat simplified this problem, but the results of these studies are far from conclusive. Thus, in this section I shall emphasize studies in which the site of action of opiates is limited by the route of administration and receptor selectivity.

4.1.1. Cardiovascular Effects of CNS-Applied Opiates

Depending on a number of variables, opiates applied to the CNS can increase blood pressure (pressor effect, hypertension) or decrease blood pressure (depressor effect, hypotension) and increase heart rate (tachycardia) or decrease heart rate (bradycardia). The best general assertion that may be made about the effects of opiates on cardiovascular function is that naloxone-reversible effects are usually hypotension and bradycardia. For example, opiates applied to the cisterna magna (Laubie *et al.*, 1977) and the ventral brain stem (Florez and Mediavilla, 1977) produce naloxone-reversible hypotension and bradycardia, but application to the lateral ventricles produce tachycardia and hypertension that are not naloxone reversible (Feldberg and Wei, 1978*a*).

The application of opiates to specific nuclei within the brain has specific effects. For example, application to the hypothalamus typically produces hypotension and bradycardia (Feldberg and Wei, 1978*b*), although tachycardia and pressor effects sometimes occur (Feurstein and Faden, 1982). The application of opiates to brain stem parasympathetic nuclei, such as the nucleus ambiguous, typically produces bradycardia (Laubie *et al.*, 1979). As mentioned above, it should be remembered that many CNS nuclei are involved in cardiovascular control, so it would be expected that the microinjection of opiates at many sites would have varying effects. In addition, as in the case of analgesia, multiplicative effects cannot be ruled out. Thus, although some detail about the CNS substrates of opiate effects on the cardiovascular system are available, the picture probably is not complete.

4.1.2. Opiate Receptor Types and Cardiovascular Effects

The advent of relatively selective opiate receptor agonists and antagonists has led to a number of studies of the involvement of various receptor types in cardiovascular effects. These studies fall into two general categories: (1) animals are pretreated with a selective antagonist given systemically, and the effects of a systemically administered agonist are observed, and (2) selective agonists are applied to the brain.

A number of studies have examined the effect of pretreatment with systemic antagonists on the cardiovascular effects of general opiate agonists. A blockade of mu_1 receptors with naloxazone reduces morphine-induced hypotension but has little effect on morphine-induced bradycardia (Holaday, 1983). Other mu receptors, however, appear to be involved in morphine-induced bradycardia since β-funaltrexamine, a selective mu antagonist, can block the bradycardia (Holaday and Ward, 1982). This same study indicated that delta as well as mu receptors are involved in morphine-induced hypotension, since the hypotension was reduced not only by β-funaltrexamine but also by ICI 154,129, a selective delta antagonist.

The selective delta agonist d-Ala^2-d-Leu^5-enkephalin (DADLE), injected into the fourth ventricle, produces hypertension (Holaday, 1983). Injection of DADLE into the third ventricle, however, produces hypotension (Holaday, 1983). Mu agonists, on the other hand, produce bradycardia when injected into the fourth ventricle (Holaday and Faden, 1982). It appears, then, that brain sites mediating blood pressure and bradycardia are anatomically separable and depend, at least in part, on a different population of opiate receptors. In addition, it seems that the same receptor type can have opposing effects, depending on its location in the brain.

Progress in understanding the cardiovascular effects of opiates is being made, but it is still not clear in which nuclei different receptor populations mediate their effects, since only intraventricular injection studies have been performed in this area. It seems feasible at this point to microinject selective agonists and antagonists into discrete brain nuclei to address this question. Similarly, the type of receptor involved in the peripheral action of opiates could be examined with compounds that do not cross the blood–brain barrier.

4.2. Endogenous Opioids and Environmentally Produced Cardiovascular Effects

That administration of exogenous opiates results in substantial cardiovascular effects does not necessarily indicate that endogenous opioids constitute part of the neurochemical substrate of similar behaviors. As was the case with analgesia and reward, a number of environmental situations that modulate the cardiovascular system appear to utilize endogenous opioids. The general approach taken to a study of the involvement of endogenous opioids in cardiovascular regulation has been, again, similar to that utilized with analgesia and reward; perturbations of the system are introduced, and an attempt is made to reverse the effect with a narcotic antagonist. If this is successful, additional experiments, as described above are performed.

Interestingly, as is the case with analgesia and reward, opiate antagonists under normal circumstances have little, if any, effect on basic hemodynamic variables (Holaday and Loh, 1981). Thus, a general characteristic of endogenous opioid systems appears to be their low tonic levels of activity.

On the other hand, at least in the case of analgesia and the cardiovascular system, many situations invoke the activity of endogenous opioids. Holaday (1983) lists endotoxic shock, hemorrhagic shock, spinal shock, orthostatic hypotension, anesthetic hypotension, essential hypertension, and cerebral vascular disorders as involving endogenous opioids. Again, as is the case with analgesia, there appear to be numerous possible opioid systems, and only some such systems involve hormones. In this section, I shall briefly review the involvement of endogenous opioids in the hypotension resulting from endotoxic shock as an example of the pattern of research in this field. For more details on the conditions listed above, as well as other cardiovascular effects, the reader is referred to the excellent review by Holaday (1983).

Holaday and Faden (1978) were the first to report that naloxone antagonized endotoxin-induced hypotension. The effect appears to be mediated in the CNS, since ventriculocisternal administration of naloxone is effective (Janssen and Lutherer, 1980). Also, naloxone iodomethylate, a compound that does not cross the blood-brain barrier in significant amounts, is ineffective in antagonizing endotoxin-induced hypotension when administered peripherally but is effective when administered centrally (Rios and Jacob, 1981). As would be expected, administration of exogenous opiates increases endotoxic shock; this effect is reversed by naloxone (Holaday et al., 1982b). Delta receptors appear to be involved in the hypotensive effect of endotoxic shock, since ICI 154,129, a selective delta antagonist, reverses the hypotension, whereas naloxazone, a mu_1 antagonist, is without effect (Holaday, 1983). The effect of centrally acting opioids appears to be mediated by sympathetic outflow to the adrenal medulla, since adrenal demedullation prevents naloxone from antagonizing endotoxin-induced hypotension (Holiday et al., 1982a). The endogenous opioid ligand involved in endotoxin hypotension has not been identified.

Thus, there is a considerable amount of knowledge on the role of endogenous opioids in endotoxin-induced hypotension. This work is of practical significance, since it offers the potential of treatment in humans. There is still much work to be done to determine the precise sites of action and to identify the ligands involved. Also, the usual caveats, such as the possibility of multiplicative effects, should be observed. The research in this field, however, has come a long way in a short time, and it is continuing.

5. OTHER EFFECTS OF OPIATES ON BEHAVIOR

Table 3 lists some of the recent studies of the role of opiates in various behaviors. The table is not meant to be exhaustive, but rather it is an

TABLE 3
Partial Summary of Currently Available Literature on the Effects of Opiates on Behavior[a]

	Systemic		Microinjection		Antagonist		Mu, delta kappa		Cross tolerance	Release		Ligand antisera
Aggression					>	166						
					>	63						
					=	9						
					>	5						
Attention												
Autonomic eff												
Sympathetic	<	94	<	ICV 162						A	215	
Aversion	<	52	>	ICV 3						A	180	
	<	134	<	MH 105								
			<	ICV 93								
			=	ICV 134								
Drinking	R	124	>	ICV 6	>	159	<	42				
	R	38	<	LH 42	<	6	<	124				
			<	ICV 44	<	161	=	47				
			=	ICV 46	=	151	R	125				
					=	218						
					=	47						
					R	124						
Development	R	241	R	241	>	240	R	241		>	199	
					>	239				R	241	
					R	241						
EEG effects	<	223	<	CP 155								
	<	12	<	ICV 2								
	R	133										
Endocrine eff												
ACTH	<	65	>	PAG 100	<	64				=	115	
			<	PAG 99	=	170						

(continued)

TABLE 3 (*Continued*)

	Systemic	Microinjection	Antagonist	Mu, delta kappa	Cross tolerance	Release	Ligand antisera
Adrenal Function	> 127 <> 109 = 18	< ICV 109	< 92	A 55		< 121 < 39 A 55 A 79 A 58 A 186 R 219	
Growth hormone	> 194		> 194 > 1	> 194			
Insulin							
Oxytocin	> 119	R 140	> 183 > 196 > 34			< 34 < 196 A 146	= 18
Prolactin	> 90 > 194		< 183 < 209 = 129	> 90 > 194			
Thyrotropin		<> ICV 129					
TRH	< 62 R 87 R 86	> ICV 28 > PAG 224 < ICV 80 < ICV 110 R 87				> 13 < 200 A 21	
Vasopressin	> 148 < 217	< ICV 29 < ICV 118 R 140	= 118 = 196	< 29		< 95 < 34 < 217 = 196 A 146 A 227 A 222	< 19

Feeding	> 112	ICV 98	> 188	> 47		> 54	> 80
	> 113	ICV 46	> 12	> 98		> 131	> 187
	R 125	VMH 187	> 46	> 97			
	R 38	VMH 205	> 80	> 126			
	R 237	ICV 12	> 97	<> 150			
		ICV 80	> 137	R 125			
		ICV 136	> 138	R 237			
		ICV 6	> 150				
		HP 81	> 168				
			> 205				
			> 242				
			> 149				
			> 161				
			> 131				
			= 6				
			= 151				
			= 84				
			R 125				
			R 237				
GI effects	< 195	ICV 75	= 26	> 75	< 190	< 26	
	< 27	ICV 174		> 190		A 79	
	<> 181	ICV 190		> 41			
	= 74	ICV 195		<> 181			
		ICV 74		= 173			
		<> ICV 181					
		= IT 173					
Hibernation	> 172		< 132			> 158	
Immune system	> 147	R 31	R 31	R 31		R 31	
	R 31						
Learning	> 148						
	R 177		R 177				

(continued)

TABLE 3 (*Continued*)

	Systemic	Microinjection	Antagonist	Mu, delta kappa	Cross tolerance	Release	Ligand antisera
Memory	> 175		> 73				
	> 176		> 72				
			< 35				
			= 176				
Mood			< 103			> 103	
			< 185				
Motoric effects							
Akinesia		> VTA 25					
		> IT 61		> 61			
		> PAG 100					
		> ICV 8					
Catalepsy	> 69	> IT 70	< 16	> 220			
		> IT 67	< 67	> 70			
		> IT 220					
		> IT 221					
		> SN 206					
		> ICV 14					
		> PAG 229					
		> ICV 15					
		> AMY 40					
Grooming	> 211						
Hyperactivity		> ICV 8	< 143	<> 108			
		> PAG 100					
		> ICV 14					
		> NA 169					
		> ICV 225					
		<> ICV 108					

Category											
Convulsions	>	69	>	ICV 68	<	66	<>	208			
	>	130	<>	ICV 71			<>	71			
	<	208	<>	ICV 208			R	66			
	R	66	R	66							
Rotation			>	VTA 91	<	57					
			>	SN 206							
			>	PAG 100							
			>	MRF 102							
			<>	PAG 101							
Psychoactive drug											
Alcohol					<	182	>	32			
					<	10					
					<	49					
					<	152					
					<	17					
					<	104					
					<	193					
					<	11					
					<	51					
					<	80					
					R	37					
Barbiturates			<	PAG 160							
Benzodiazepines	<	85							<	192	< 80
									=	24	
									R	37	
Psychopathology											
Depression	>	116			>	36			=	153	
	R	139			=	48					
	R	56			=	202					
Schizophrenia	>	156	>	ICV 15	<	78			>	23	
	<	116			<	222			>	184	
	=	106			=	212			<>	154	
	R	139			=	43			=	154	
					=	144					
					=	216					
Other											
Psychotomimetic	R	237			>	114			=	114	= 20
											A 123

(continued)

TABLE 3 (continued)

	Systemic	Microinjection	Antagonist	Mu, delta kappa	Cross tolerance	Release	Ligand antisera
Punishment							
Pupillary response	R 133		R 133	R 133			
Reflexes	> 189	< ICV 203	> 231			> 59	
	> 96	< ICV 214	> 45				
	< 94		< 33				
	< 111		< 30				
	< 179		< 233				
	< 236		<> 232				
	< 117		= 234				
	< 198		R 53				
	< 230						
Renal function				< 191		> 191	
						< 217	
Respiratory effects	< 4	< ICV 167	> 120	< 167			
	R 133	< ICV 7	= 7	< 60			
		POM 60	R 133	< 107			
		< ICV 107		< 165			
		< AH 171		< 171			
		<> IT 83		<> 83			
				= 7			
				R 88			
				R 133			
Sexual behavior	> 210	< IT 228	> 228			< 197	
		< ICV 77	> 77				
		< ICV 142	< 141				
			< 197				

Sleep	>	50	>	ICV 207	
Social behavior	R	235			
Temperature	>	122	>	AH 163	> 22
	<	226	>	VTA 213	> 204
	>	109	>	ICV 164	= 163 > 164
	>	178	>	PAG 82	= 145 > 107
	<>	76	>	ICV 107	<> 76
	<>	110	>	VMH 201	
	<>	128	>	ICV 89	
			<	AH 128	
			<>	ICV 157	> 145
			<>	ICV 110	

[a]For each behavior, the effects of opiates are classified by the method of study. Numbers correspond to references below. >, potentiation of behavior; <, attenuation of behavior; <>, mixed effects; =, no effect; R, literature review; A, anatomical data; AH, anterior hypothalamus; AMY, amygdala; CP, caudate putamen; HP, hippocampus; ICV, intracerebroventricular injection; IT, intrathecal injection; LH, lateral hypothalamus; MH, medial hypothalamus; MRF, medial reticular formation; NA, nucleus accumbens; PAG, periaqueductal gray; POM, medial preoptic region of the hypothalamus; SN, substantia nigra; VMH, ventromedial hypothalamus; VTA, ventral tegmental area.

1. Ahren and Lundquist, 1984
2. Albus and Herz, 1972
3. Appel and Van Loon, 1983
4. Arndt et al., 1984
5. Arnstein et al., 1983
6. Baldwin and Parrott, 1985
7. Belenky, 1983
8. Beslin et al., 1982
9. Benton, 1984
10. Berman et al., 1984
11. Bernatzky et al., 1983
12. Bertiere et al., 1984
13. Bhargava, 1983
14. Blair et al., 1980
15. Bloom et al., 1976
16. Blum et al., 1984
17. Boada et al., 1981
18. Bodnar et al., 1982
19. Bodnar et al., 1984
20. Bouras et al., 1984
21. Bowker et al., 1983
22. Brain et al., 1984
23. Brambilla et al., 1984
24. Britton et al., 1983
25. Bunney et al., 1984
26. Burks and Grubb, 1974
27. Burleigh et al., 1981
28. Butler and Bodnar, 1984
29. Carter and Lightman, 1984
30. Cervero et al., 1981
31. Chang, 1984
32. Charness et al., 1983
33. Chung et al., 1983
34. Clarke and Patrick, 1983
35. Cohen et al., 1983
36. Cohen et al., 1984
37. Cooper, 1983
38. Cooper and Sanger, 1984
39. Costa et al., 1983
40. Costall and Naylor, 1974
41. Cowan and Gmerek, 1982
42. Czech et al., 1984
43. Davis et al., 1977
44. de Caro et al., 1979
45. Dehen et al., 1978
46. Deviche and Schepers, 1984
47. Deviche and Wohland, 1984
48. Devoize et al., 1984
49. DeWitte, 1984
50. Dick et al., 1983
51. Doi and Jurna, 1982
52. Domjan and Siegel, 1983
53. Duggan and North, 1983
54. Dum and Herz, 1984
55. Dumont and Lemaire, 1984
56. Emrich et al., 1983
57. Eshel and Korczyn, 1985
58. Evans et al., 1983
59. Facchinetti et al., 1984
60. Faden and Feurstein, 1983
61. Faden and Jacobs, 1983
62. Faden et al., 1983
63. Fanselow et al., 1980
64. Fekete et al., 1983
65. Fekete et al., 1984
66. Frenk, 1983
67. Frenk and Stein, 1984
68. Frenk et al., 1978
69. Frenk et al., 1982
70. Frenk et al., 1984a
71. Frenk et al., 1984b
72. Gallagher, 1982
73. Gallagher et al., 1983
74. Galligan and Burks, 1982
75. Galligan et al., 1984
76. Geller et al., 1983
77. Gessa et al., 1979
78. Gillman and Sandyk, 1985
79. Giraud et al., 1984
80. Gonzalez et al., 1984
81. Gosnell et al., 1985
82. Griffiths et al., 1983
83. Haddad et al., 1984
84. Hahn, 1984
85. Herling, 1983
86. Holaday, 1983
87. Holaday, 1984
88. Holaday and Tortella, 1984
89. Holaday et al., 1978
90. Holaday et al., 1984
91. Holmes and Wise, 1985
92. Hughes, 1984
93. Hunt et al., 1983
94. Ito et al., 1983
95. Iversen et al., 1978

(continued)

TABLE 3 (*continued*)

96. Iwata and Sakai, 1971
97. Jackson and Sewell, 1984
98. Jackson and Sewell, 1985
99. Jacquet, 1978
100. Jacquet, 1982
101. Jacquet and Wolf, 1981
102. Jacquet et al., 1976
103. Janal et al., 1984
104. Jeffcoate et al., 1979
105. Jenck et al., 1983
106. Jungkinz et al., 1984
107. Kamerling et al., 1983
108. Kameyama and Ukai, 1983
109. Kasson and George, 1983a
110. Kasson and George, 1983b
111. Kavaliers et al., 1983
112. Kavaliers et al., 1984
113. Kavaliers et al., 1985
114. Khazan et al., 1984
115. Kiser et al., 1983
116. Kline et al., 1977
117. Koll et al., 1963
118. Kordower and Bodnar, 1984
119. Kovacs et al., 1985
120. Kumazawa et al., 1985
121. LaGamma et al., 1984
122. Lal et al., 1976
123. Largent et al., 1984
124. Leander, 1984
125. Leander, 1985
126. Levine and Morley, 1983
127. Lewis et al., 1982
128. Lotti et al., 1965
129. Mannisto et al., 1984
130. Mansour and Valenstein, 1984
131. Margules et al., 1978
132. Margules et al., 1979
133. Martin, 1983
134. Martinez, 1985
135. McGinty and Bloom, 1983
136. McKay et al., 1981
137. McLaughlin and Baile, 1984a
138. McLaughlin and Baile, 1984b
139. McNicholas and Martin, 1984
140. Meisenberg and Simmons, 1983
141. Mendelson and Gorzalka, 1984
142. Meyerson and Terenius, 1977
143. Mickley and Stevens, 1983
144. Mielke and Gallant, 1977
145. Millan et al., 1981
146. Millan et al., 1984
147. Miller et al., 1983
148. Moore, 1983
149. Morley and Levine, 1980
150. Morley et al., 1984
151. Murphy et al., 1985
152. Myers et al., 1984
153. Naber et al., 1981
154. Naber et al., 1984
155. Neal and Keane, 1978
156. Nedopil and Ruther, 1979
157. Nemeroff et al., 1979
158. Oiltgen et al., 1982
159. Olson et al., 1981
160. Ossipov and Gebhart, 1984
161. Ostrowski et al., 1981
162. Owen et al., 1984
163. Pae et al., 1985
164. Pang et al., 1984
165. Pasternak et al., 1983
166. Paterson and Vickers, 1984
167. Pazos and Florez, 1984
168. Penicaud and Thompson, 1984
169. Pert and Sivit, 1977
170. Pertovaara et al., 1982
171. Pfeiffer et al., 1983
172. Plotnikoff and Miller, 1983
173. Porreca et al., 1983
174. Porreca et al., 1984
175. Rigter, 1978
176. Rigter et al., 1977
177. Riley et al., 1980
178. Ritzmann et al., 1983
179. Roby et al., 1983
180. Romangnano and Hamill, 1984
181. Ruckebusch et al., 1984
182. Samson and Doyle, 1985
183. Samson et al., 1985
184. Schoemaker et al., 1984
185. Schull et al., 1981
186. Schultzberg et al., 1978
187. Schulz et al., 1984
188. Simone et al., 1985
189. Sinclair, 1973
190. Sivam and Ho, 1984
191. Slizgi et al., 1984
192. Smith et al., 1984
193. Sorensen and Mattisson, 1978
194. Spiegel et al., 1982
195. Stewart and Curd, 1984
196. Summy-Long et al., 1984
197. Szechtman et al., 1981
198. Takagi et al., 1955
199. Tang et al., 1984
200. Tapia-Arancibia and Atier, 1983
201. Tepperman et al., 1981
202. Terenius et al., 1977
203. Teschemacher et al., 1973
204. Teskey et al., 1984
205. Thornhill and Saunders, 1984
206. Turski et al., 1983
207. Ukponmwan et al., 1984
208. Urca and Frenk, 1982
209. Vanvugt et al., 1978
210. Vathy et al., 1985
211. Veith et al., 1978
212. Verhoeven et al., 1984
213. Vezina and Stewert, 1985
214. Vigouret et al., 1973
215. Vincent et al., 1984
216. Volavka et al., 1977
217. Walker and Murphy, 1984
218. Wallace et al., 1984
219. Watkins and Mayer, 1982a
220. Watkins et al., 1984c
221. Watkins et al., 1984d
222. Watson et al., 1978
223. Wauquier et al., 1984
224. Webster et al., 1983
225. Wei et al., 1977
226. Weiss et al., 1984
227. Whitnall et al., 1983
228. Wiesenfeld-Hallin and Sodersten, 1984
229. Wilcox and Levitt, 1979
230. Wilker and Frank, 1948
231. Willer, 1983
232. Willer and Albe-Fessard, 1980
233. Willer et al., 1981
234. Willer et al., 1982
235. Wilson and Dorosz, 1984
236. Yaksh, 1978
237. Yim and Lowy, 1984
238. Young, 1980
239. Zagon and McLaughlin, 1983
240. Zagon and McLaughlin, 1984
241. Zagon et al., 1984
242. Zetler and Morsdorf, 1984

attempt to refer the reader to the more recent literature in the field, although older references that I consider of particular importance are included. The table is arranged around the primary experimental manipulations used to implicate opiates and endogenous opioid systems in behaviors. The value of the table lies not only in the data points presented but also in those that are missing. Missing data points tend to indicate either recently acquired technical and scientific facts or experiments that are technically difficult to perform. For example, almost all the behaviors listed have been challenged by systemic naloxone, since this simple procedure (although not without its pitfalls) can be performed inexpensively in almost any laboratory. However, intracerebral microinjections are technically quite difficult, resulting in less data collection. It is hoped that the table will provide the reader with a sense of organization for the field and perhaps inspire further experimentation in this exciting area of research.

6. REFERENCES

AHREN, B., and LUNDQUIST, I., 1984, Effects of naloxone on basal and stimulated insulin secretion in the mouse, *Eur. J. Pharmacol.* **102:**135–139.

AKIL, H., MAYER, D., and LIEBESKIND, J., 1972, Comparaison chez le rat entre l'analgesie induite par stimulation de la substance grise periaqueducale et l'analgesia morphinique, *C. R. Acad Sci.* **274:**3603–3605.

AKIL, H., MADDEN, J., PATRICK, R. L., and BARCHAS, J. D., 1976a, Stress-induced increase in endogenous opiate peptides: Concurrent analgesia and its partial reversal by naloxone, in: *Opiates and Endogenous Opioid Peptides* (H. W. Kosterlitz, ed.), Elsevier, North Holland, pp. 63–70.

AKIL, H., MAYER, D. J., and LIEBESKIND, J. C., 1976b, Antagonism of stimulation-produced analgesia by the narcotic antagonist, naloxone, *Science* **191:**961–962.

AKIL, H., WATSON, S. J., YOUNG, E., LEWIS, M. E., KHACHATURIAN, H., and WALKER, J. M., 1984, Endogenous opioids: Biology and function, *Annu. Rev. Neurosci.* **7:**223–256.

ALBUS, K., and HERZ, A., 1972, Inhibition of behavioural and EEG activation induced by morphine acting on lower brain-stem structures, *Electroencephalogr. Clin. Neurophysiol.* **33:**579–590.

ALBUS, K., SCHOTT, M., and HERZ, A., 1970, Interaction between morphine and morphine antagonists after systemic and intraventricular administration, *Eur. J. Pharmacol.* **12:**53–64.

APPEL, N. M., and VAN LOON, G. R., 1983, Activation of angiotensin II receptors in brain potentiates the stimulating effect of endogenous opioid neurons on central sympathetic outflow, *Peptides* **4:**59–62.

ARNDT, J. O., MIKAT, M., and PARASHER, C., 1984, Fentanyl's analgesic, respiratory, and cardiovascular actions in relation to dose and plasma concentration in unanesthetized dogs, *Anesthesiology* **61:**355–361.

ARNSTEN, A. F. T., SEGAL, D. S., NEVILLE, H. J., HILLYARD, S. A., JANOWSKI, D. S., JUDD, L. L., and BLOOM, F. E., 1983, Naloxone augments electrophysiological signs of selective attention in man, *Nature* **304:**725–726.

AZAMI, J., LLEWELYN, M. B., and ROBERTS, M. H. T., 1982, The contribution of nucleus reticularis paragigantocellularis and nucelus raphe magnus to the analgesia produced

by systemically administered morphine, investigated with the microinjection technique, *Pain* **12:**229–246.
BALDWIN, B. A., and PARROTT, R. F., 1985, Effects of intracerebroventricular injection of naloxone on operant feeding and drinking in pigs, *Pharmacol. Biochem. Behav.* **22:**37–40.
BARTON, C., BASBAUM, A. I., and FIELDS, H. L., 1980, Dissociation of supraspinal and spinal actions of morphine: A quantitative evaluation, *Brain Res.* **188:**487–498.
BASBAUM, A. I., MARLEY, N., and O'KEEFE, J., 1975, Effects of spinal cord lesions on the analgesic properties of electrical brain stimulation, in: *Advances in Pain Research and Therapy: Proceedings of the First World Congress on Pain* (J. J. Bonica and D. G. Albe-Fessard, eds.), Raven Press, New York, p. 268.
BEITEL, R. E., and DUBNER, R., 1976, Sensitization and depression of C-polymodal nociceptors by noxious heat applied to the monkey's face, in: *Proceedings of the First World Congress on Pain* (J. J. Bonica and D. Albefessard, eds.), Raven Press, New York, pp. 149–153.
BELENKY, G. L., GELINAS-SORELL, D., KENNER, J. R., and HOLADAY, J. W., 1983, Evidence for delta receptor involvement in the postictal antinociceptive responses to electroconvulsive shock in rats, *Life Sci.* **33:**585–586.
BELESLIN, D. B., SAMARDZIC, R., KRSTIC, S. K., and MICIC, D., 1982, Differences in central effects of β-endorphin and enkephalins: β-Endorphin a potent psychomotor stimulant, *Neuropharmacology* **21:**99–102.
BELLUZZI, J. D., and STEIN, L., 1977, Enkephalin may mediate euphoria and drive-reduction reward, *Nature* **266:**556–557.
BENTON, D., 1984, The long-term effects of naloxone, dibutyryl cyclic CMP, and chlorpromazine on aggression in mice monitored by an automated device, *Aggress. Behav.* **10:**79–90.
BERMAN, R. F., LEE, J. A., OLSON, K. L., and GOLDMAN, M. S., 1984, Effects of naloxone on ethanol dependence in rats, *Drug Alcohol Dependence* **13:**245–254.
BERNATSKY, G., DOI, T., and JURNA, I., 1983, Effects of intrathecally administered pentobarbital and naloxone on the activity evoked in ascending axons of the rat spinal cord by stimulation of afferent A and C fibres. Further evidence for a tonic endorphinergic inhibition in nociception, *Arch. Pharmacol.* **323:**211–216.
BERTIERE, M. C., SY, T. M., BAIGTS, F., MANDENOFF, A., and APFELBAUM, M., 1984, Stress and sucrose hyperphagia: Role of endogenous opiates, *Pharmacol. Biochem. Behav.* **20:**675–680.
BHARGAVA, H. N., 1983, Binding of (^{3}H)spiroperidol to striatal membranes of rats treated chronically with morphine. Influence of pro-leu-gly-NH2 and cyclo(leu-gly), *Neuropharmacology* **22:**1357–1362.
BIELAJEW, C., and SHIZGAL, P., 1982, Behaviorally derived measures of conduction velocity in the substrate for rewarding medial forebrain bundle stimulation, *Brain Res.* **237:**107–119.
BLAIR, R., CYTRYNIAK, H., SHIZGAL, P., and AMIT, Z., 1980, Heroin, but not levorphanol produces explosive motor behavior in naloxone-treated rats, *Psychopharmacology* **69:**313–314.
BLOOM, F., SEGAL, D., LING, N., and GUILLEMIN, R., 1976, Endorphins: Profound behavioral effects in rats suggest new etiological factors in mental illness, *Science* **194:**630–632.
BLUM, I., MUNITZ, H., SHALEV, A., and ROBERTS, E., 1984, Naloxone may be beneficial in the treatment of tardive dyskinesia, *Clin. Neuropharmacol.* **7:**265–267.
BOADA, J., FERIA, M., and SANZ, E., 1981, Inhibitory effect of naloxone on the ethanol-induced antinociception in mice, *Pharmacol. Res. Commun.* **13:**673–679.
BODNAR, R. J., SHARPLESS, N. S., KORDOWER, J. H., POTEGAL, M. and BARR, G. A., 1982, Analgesic responses following adrenal demedullation and peripheral catecholamine depletion, *Physiol. Behav.* **29:**1105–1109.

BODNAR, R. J., NILAVER, G., WALLACE, M. M., BADILLO-MARTINEZ, D., and ZIMMERMAN, E. A., 1984, Pain threshold changes in rats following central injection of beta-endorphin, met-enkephalin, vasopressin or oxytocin antisera, *Int. J. Neurosci.* **24:**149–160.

BONICA, J. J., 1980, Pain research and therapy: past and current status and future needs, in: *Pain Discomfort and Humanitarian Care* (L. K. Y. Ng and J. J. Bonica, eds.), Elsevier, New York, pp. 1–46.

BOURAS, C., TABAN, C. H., and CONSTANTINIDIS, J., 1984, Mapping of enkephalins in human brain. An immunohistofluorescence study on brains from patients with senile and presenile dementia, *Neuroscience* **12:**179–190.

BOWKER, R. M., WESTLUND, K. N., SULLIVAN, M. C., WILBER, J. F., and COULTER, J. D., 1983, Descending serotonergic, peptidergic and cholinergic pathways from the raphe nuclei: A multiple transmitter complex, *Brain Res.* **288:**33–48.

BOZARTH, M. A., 1982, Opiate reward mechanisms mapped by intracranial self-administration, in: *Neurobiology of Opiate Reward Mechanisms* (J. E. Smith and J. D. Lane, eds.), Raven Press, New York.

BOZARTH, M. A., and WISE, R. A., 1981a, Intracranial self-administration of morphine into the ventral tegmental area in rats, *Life Sci.* **28:**551–555.

BOZARTH, M. A., and WISE, R. A., 1981b, Heroin reward is dependent on a dopamingergic substrate, *Life Sci.* **29:**1881–1886.

BOZARTH, M., and WISE, R. A., 1984, Anatomically distant opiate receptor fields mediate reward and physical dependence, *Science* **224:**516–518.

BRAIN, P. F., JONES, S. E., BRAIN, S., and BENTON, D., 1984, Sequence analysis of social behavior illustrating the actions of 2 antagonists of endogenous opioids, in: *Ethopharmacological Aggression Behavior* (K. A. Miczek, M. R. Kruk, and B. Olivier, eds.), Liss, New York, pp. 43–58.

BRAMBILLA, F., FACCHINETTI, F., PETRAGLIA, F., VANZULLI, L., and GENAZZANI, A. R., 1984, Secretion pattern of endogenous opioids in chronic schizophrenia, *Am. J. Psychiatry* **141:**1183–1188.

BRITT, M. D., and WISE, R. A., 1983, Ventral tegmental site of opiate reward: Antagonism by a hydrophilic opiate receptor blocker, *Brain Res.* **258:**105–108.

BRITTON, K. T., STEWART, R. D., and RISCH, S. C., 1983, Benzodiazepines attenuate stimulated beta-endorphin release, *Psychopharmacol. Bull.* **19:**757–759.

BUNNEY, W. C., MASSARI, V. J., and PERT, A., 1984, Chronic morphine-induced hyperactivity in rats is altered by nucleus accumbens and ventral tegmental lesions, *Psychopharmacology* **82:**318–321.

BURKS, T. F., and GRUBB, M. N., 1974, Sites of acute morphine tolerance in intestine, *J. Pharmacol. Exp. Ther.* **191:**518–526.

BURLEIGH, D. E., GALLIGAN, J. J., and BURKS, T. F., 1981, Subcutaneous morphine reduces intestinal propulsion in rats partly by a central action, *Eur. J. Pharmacol.* **75:**283–287.

BUTLER, P. D., and BODNAR, R. J., 1984, Potentiation of foot shock analgesia by thyrotropin releasing hormone, *Peptides* **5:**635–640.

CARTER, D. A., and LIGHTMAN, S. L., 1984, Inhibition of vasopressin secretion by a kappa-opiate receptor agonist, *Neuroendocrinol. Lett.* **6:**95–100.

CERVERO, F., SCHOUENBORG, J., and SJOLUND, B. H., 1981, Effects of conditioning stimulation of somatic and visceral afferent fibres on viscero-somatic reflexes, *J. Physiol.* **317:**27–28.

CHANG, K-J., 1984, Opioid peptides have actions on the immune system, *Trends Neurosci.* **7:**234–235.

CHARNESS, M. E., GORDON, A. S., and DIAMOND, I., 1983, Ethanol modulation of opiate receptors in cultured neural cells, *Science* **222:**1246–1248.

CHUNG, J. M., FANG, Z. R., CARGILL, C. L., and WILLIS, W. D., 1983, Prolonged, naloxone-reversible inhibition of the flexion reflex in the cat, *Pain* **15:**35–54.

CLARKE, G., and PATRICK, G., 1983, Differential inhibitory action by morphine on the release of oxytocin and vasopressin from the isolated neural lobe, *Neurosci. Lett.* **39:**175–180.

COHEN, M. R., COHEN, R. M., PICKAR, D., WEINGARTNER, H., and MURPHY, D. L., 1983, High-dose naloxone infusions in normals, *Arch. Gen. Psychiatry* **40:**613–619.

COHEN, M. R., COHEN, R. M., PICKAR, D., SUNDERLAND, T., MUELLER, E. A., III, and MURPHY, D. L., 1984, High dose naloxone in depression, *Biol. Psychiatry* **19:**825–832.

COHEN, M. R., COHEN, R. M., PICKAR, D., and MURPHY, D. L., 1985, Naloxone reduces food intake in humans, *Psychosom. Med.* **47:**132–138.

COOPER, S. J., 1983, Benzodiazepine-opiate antagonist interactions in relation to anxiety and appetite, *Trends Pharmacol. Sci.* **4:**456–458.

COOPER, S. J., and SANGER, D. J., 1984, Endorphinergic mechanisms in food, salt and water intake—an overview, *Appetite* **5:**1–6.

CORBETT, D., and WISE, R. A., 1980, Intracranial self-stimulation in relation to the ascending dopaminergic systems of the midbrain: A moveable electrode mapping study, *Brain Res.* **185:**1–15.

COSTA, E., GUIDOTTI, A., HANBAUER, I., and SAIANI, L., 1983, Modulation of nicotinic receptor function by opiate recognition sites highly selective for met5-enkephalin-[arg6phe7]1, *Fed. Proc.* **42:**2946–2952.

COSTALL, B., and NAYLOR, R. J., 1974, A role for the amygdala in the development of the cataleptic and stereotypic actions of the narcotic agonists and antagonists in the rat, *Psychopharmacology* **35:**203–214.

COWAN, A., and GMEREK, D. E., 1982, In vivo studies with ICI 154, 129, a putative delta receptor antagonist, *Life Sci.* **31:**2213–2216.

CZECH, D. A., BLAKE, M. J., and STEIN, E. A., 1984, Drinking behavior is modulated by CNS administration of opioids in the rat, *Appetite* **5:**15–24.

DAVIS, G. C., BUNNEY, W., E. Jr., DEFRAITES, E. G., KLEINMAN, J. E., VAN KAMMEN, D. P., POST, R. M., and WYATT, R. J., 1977, Intravenous naloxone administration in schizophrenia and affective illness, *Science* **197:**74–77.

DE CARO, G., MICOSSI, L. G., and VENTURI, F., 1979, Drinking behaviour induced by intracerebroventricular administration of enkephalins to rats, *Nature* **277:**51–52.

DEHEN, H., WILLER, J. C., PRIER, S., BOUREAU, F., and CAMBIER, J., 1978, Congenital insensitivity to pain and the "morphinelike" analgesic system, *Pain* **5:**351–358.

DEVICHE, P., and SCHEPERS, G., 1984, Intracerebroventricular injection of ostrich beta-endorphin to satiated pigeons induces hyperphagia but not hyperdipsia, *Peptides* **5:**691–694.

DEVICHE, P., and WOHLAND, A., 1984, Opiate antagonists stereoselectively attenuate the consumption of food but not of water by pigeons, *Pharmacol. Biochem. Behav.* **21:**507–512.

DEVOIZE, J-L., RIGAL, F., ESCHALIER, A., TROLESE, J-F. and RENOUX, M., 1984, Influence of naloxone on antidepressant drug effects in the force swimming test in mice, *Psychopharmacology* **84:**71–75.

DEWEY, W. L., SNYDER, J. W., HARRIS, L. S., and HOWES, J. F., 1969, The effect of narcotics and narcotic antagonists on the tail-flick response in spinal mice, *J. Pharm. Pharmacol.* **21:**548–550.

DEWITTE, P., 1984, Naloxone reduces alcohol intake in a free-choice procedure even when both drinking bottles contain saccharin sodium or quinine substances, *Neuropsychobiology* **12:**73–77.

DICK, P., GRANDJEAN, M. E., and TISSOT, R., 1983, Successful treatment of withdrawal symptoms with delta sleep-inducing peptide, a neuropeptide with potential agonistic activity on opiate receptors, *Neuropsychobiology* **10:**205–208.

DOI, T., and JURNA, I., 1982, Intrathecal pentobarbital prevents naloxone-induced facilitation of the tail-flick response in the rat, *Neurosci Lett.* **32:**81–84.

DOMJAN, M., and SIEGEL, S., 1983, Attenuation of the aversive and analgesic effects of morphine by repeated adminsitration: Different mechanisms, *Physiol. Psychol.* **11:**155–158.

DOSTROVSKY, J. O., and DEAKIN, J. F. W., 1977, Periaqueductal grey lesions reduce morphine analgesia in the rat, *Neurosci. Lett* **4**:99–103.

DUGGAN, A. W., and NORTH, R. A., 1983, Electrophysiology of opioids. 3, *Pharmacol. Rev.* **35**:219–282.

DUM, J., and HERZ, A., 1984, Endorphinergic modulation of neural reward systems indicated by behavioral changes, *Pharmacol. Biochem. Behav.* **21**:259–266.

DUMONT, M., and LEMAIRE, S., 1984, Opioid receptors in bovine adrenal medulla, *Can. J. Physiol. Pharmacol.* **62**:1284–1291.

EMRICH, H. M., GUENTHER, R., and DOSE, M., 1983, Current perspectives in the pharmacopsychiatry of depression and mania, *Neuropharmacology* **22**:385–388.

ESHEL, Y., and KORCZYN, A. M., 1985, Circling behavior induced by phencyclidine in mice and its inhibition by naloxone, *Experientia* **41**:73–74.

EVANS, C. J., ERDELYI, E., WEBER, E., and BARCHAS, J. D., 1983, Identification of pro-opiomelanocortin-derived peptides in the human adrenal medulla, *Science* **221**:957–960.

FACCHINETTI, F., SANDRINI, G., PETRAGLIA, F., ALFONSI, E., NAPPI, G., and GENAZZANI, A. R., 1984, Concomitant increase in nociceptive flexion reflex threshold and plasma opioids following transcutaneous nerve stimulation, *Pain* **19**:295–304.

FADEN, A. I., and FEUERSTEIN, G., 1983, Hypothalamic regulation of the cardiovascular and respiratory systems: Role of specific opiate receptors, *Br. J. Pharmacol.* **79**:997–1002.

FADEN, A. I., and JACOBS, T. P., 1983, Dynorphin induces partially reversible paraplegia in the rat, *Eur. J. Pharmacol.* **91**:321–324.

FADEN, A. I., JACOBS, T. P., SMITH, G. P., GREEN, B., and ZIVIN, J. A., 1983, Neuropeptides in spinal cord injury: Comparative experimental models, *Peptides* **4**:631–634.

FANSELOW, M. S., SIGMUNDI, R. A., and BOLLES, R. C., 1980, Naloxone pretreatment enhances shock-elicited aggression, *Physiol. Psychol.* **8**:369–371.

FARIS, P., KOMISURAK, B., WATKINS, L., and MAYER, D. J., 1983, Evidence for the neuropeptide cholecystokinin as an antagonist of opiate analgesia, *Science* **219**:310–312.

FEKETE, M., DRAGO, F., VAN REE, J. M., BOHUS, B., WIEGANT, V. M., and DE WIED, D., 1983, Naltrexone-sensitive behavioral actions of the ACTH 4–9 analog (ORG 2766), *Life Sci.* **32**:2193–2204.

FEKETE, M. I. K., KANYICSKA, B., SZENTENDREI, T., and STARK, E., 1984, Loss of sensitivity to morphine induced by prolonged ACTH treatment, *Pharmacol. Biochem. Behav.* **20**:879–882.

FELDBERG, W., and WEI, E., 1978a, Central sites at which morphine acts when producing cardiovascular effects, *J. Physiol.* **275**:57.

FELDBERG, W., and WEI, E., 1978b, Central cardiovascular effects of enkephalins and C-fragment of lipotropin, *J. Physiol.* **280**:18.

FEURSTEIN, G., and FADEN, A. I., 1982, Hypothalamic sites for cardiovascular regulation by mu, delta, or kappa opioid agonists, *Life Sci.* **31**:2197–2200.

FLOREZ, J., and MEDIAVILLA, A., 1977, Respiratory and cardiovascular effects of met-enkephalin applied to the ventral surface of the brain stem, *Brain Res.* **138**:585–590.

FRENK, H., 1983, Pro- and anticonvulsant actions of morphine and the endogenous opioids: Involvement and interactions of multiple opiate and non-opiate systems, *Brain Res. Rev.* **6**:197–210.

FRENK, H., and STEIN, B. E., 1984, Endogenous opioids mediate ECS-induced catalepsy at supraspinal levels, *Brain Res.* **303**:109–112.

FRENK, H., URCA, G., and LIEBESKIND, J. C., 1978, Epileptic properties of leucine- and methionine-enkephalin: Comparison with morphine and reversibility by naloxone, *Brain Res.* **147**:327–337.

FRENK, H., LIBAN, A., BALAMUTH, R., and URCA, G., 1982, Opiate and non-opiate aspects of morphine induced seizures, *Brain Res.* **253**:253–261.

FRENK, H., WATKINS, L. R., and MAYER, D. J., 1984a, Differential behavioral effects induced by intrathecal microinjection of opiates: Comparison of convulsive and cataleptic effects produced by morphine, methadone, and D-Ala2-methionine-enkephalinamide, *Brain Res.* **299:**31–42.

FRENK, H., WATKINS, L. R., MILLER, J., and MAYER, D. J., 1984b, Nonspecific convulsions are induced by morphine but not D-Ala2-methionine-enkephalinamide at cortical sites, *Brain Res.* **299:**51–59.

GALLAGHER, M., 1982, Naloxone enhancement of memory processes: Effects of other opiate antagonists, *Behav. Neural. Biol.* **35:**375–382.

GALLAGHER, M., KING, R. A., and YOUNG, N. B., 1983, Opiate antagonists improve spatial memory, *Science* **221:**975–976.

GALLIGAN, J. J., and BURKS, T. F., 1982, Opioid peptides inhibit intestinal transit in the rat by a central mechanism, *Eur. J. Pharmacol.* **85:**61–68.

GALLIGAN, J. J., MOSBERG, H. I., HURST, R., HRUBY, V. J., and BURKS, T. F., 1984, Cerebral delta-opioid receptors mediate analgesia but not the intestinal motility effects of intracerebroventricularly administered opioids, *J. Pharmacol. Exp. Ther.* **229:**641–648.

GELLER, E. B., HAWK, C., KEINATH, S. H., TALLARIDA, R. J., and ADLER, M. W., 1983, Subclasses of opioids based on body temperature change in rats—acute subcutaneous administration, *J. Pharmacol. Exp. Ther.* **225:**391–398.

GERBER, G. J., SING, J., and WISE, R. A., 1981, Pimozide attenuates lever pressing for water reinforcement in rats, *Pharmacol. Biochem. Behav.* **14:**201–205.

GESSA, G. L., PAGLIETTI, E., and QUARANTOTTI, B. P., 1979, Induction of copulatory behavior in sexually inactive rats by naloxone, *Science* **204:**203–205.

GILLMAN, M. A., and SANDYK, R., 1985, Reversal of captopril-induced psychosis with naloxone, *Am. J. Psychiatry* **142:**270.

GIRAUD, A. S., DOCKRAY, G. J., and WILLIAMS, R. G., 1984, Immunoreactivity met-enkephalin arg6 in rat brain, and bovine brain, gut and adrenal, *J. Neurochem.* **43:**1236–1242.

GONZALEZ, Y., FERNANDEZ-TOME, M. P., SANCHEZ-FRANCO, F., and DEL RIO, J., 1984, Antagonism of diazepam-induced feeding in rats by antisera to opioid peptides, *Life Sci.* **35:**1423–1430.

GOSNELL, B. A., WAGGONER, D. W., MORLEY, J. E., and LEVINE, A. S., 1985, The pineal gland and opiate-induced feeding, *Physiol. Behav.* **34:**1–6.

GRIFFITHS, E. C., SLATER, P., and WIDDOWSON, P. S., 1983, Effects of opioids, neurotensin and thyrotrophin releasing hormone on rectal temperature after application to periaqueductal grey region of rat brain, *J. Physiol. (London)* **342:**38P.

HADDAD, G. G., SCHAEFFER, J. I., and CHANG, K. J., 1984, Opposite effect of the δ- and μ-opioid receptor agonists on ventilation in conscious adult dogs, *Brain Res.* **323:**73–82.

HAHN, E. F., 1984, Interaction of naloxone and sodium chloride intake on body weight gain in WKY and SHR rats, *Res. Commun. Chem. Pathol. Pharm.* **44:**339–346.

HAIGLER, H. J., and SPRING, D. D., 1978, Comparison of analgesic and behavioral effects of [D-Ala2] met-enkephalinamide and morphine in mesencephalic reticular formation of rats, *Life Sci.* **23:**1229–1240.

HAMMOND, D. L., and PROUDFIT, H. K., 1980, Effects of locus coeruleus lesions on morphine-induced antinociception, *Brain Res.* **188:**79–91.

HARDY, J. D., WOLFF, H. G., and GOODELL, H., 1952, *Pain Sensations and Reactions*, Williams & Wilkins, Baltimore.

HAYES, R. L., BENNETT, G. J., NEWLON, P., and MAYER, D. J., 1976, Analgesic effects of certain noxious and stressful manipulations in the rat, *Soc. Neurosci Abstr.* **2:**939.

HAYES, R. L., BENNETT, G. J., NEWLON, P. G., and MAYER, D. J., 1978a, Behavioral and physiological studies on non-narcotic analgesia in the rat elicited by certain environmental stimuli, *Brain Res.* **155:**69–90.

HAYES, R. L., PRICE, D. D., BENNETT, G. J., WILCOX, G. L., and MAYER, D. J., 1978b, Differential effects of spinal cord lesions on narcotic and non-narcotic suppression of nociceptive reflexes: Further evidence for the physiologic multiplicity of pain modulation, *Brain Res.* **155:**91–101.

HAYES, R. L., KATAYAMA, Y., WATKINS, L. R., and BECKER, D. P., 1984, Bilateral lesions of the dorsolateral funiculus of the cat spinal cord: Effects on basal nociceptive reflexes and nociceptive suppression produced by cholinergic activation of the pontine parabrachial region, *Brain Res.* **311**:267–280.

HERLING, S., 1983, Naltrexone blocks the response-latency increasing effects but not the discriminative effects of diazepam in rats, *Eur. J. Pharmacol.* **88**:121–124.

HILLER, J. M., PEARSON, J., and SIMON, E. J., 1973, Distribution of stereospecific binding of the potent narcotic analgesic etorphine in the human brain: Predominance in the limbic system, *Res. Commun. Chem. Pathol. Pharm.* **6**:1052–1062.

HOLADAY, J. W., 1983, Cardiovascular effects of endogenous opiate systems, *Annu. Rev. Pharmacol. Toxicol.* **23**:541–594.

HOLADAY, J. W., 1984, Neuropeptides in shock and traumatic injury—sites and mechanisms of action, in: *Neuroendocrine Perspectives* (E. E. Muller and R. M. MacLeod, eds.), Elsevier Scientific Publishing, New York, pp. 161–200.

HOLADAY, J. W., and FADEN, A. I., 1978, Naloxone reversal of endotoxin hypotension suggests role of endorphins in shock, *Nature* **275**:450–451.

HOLADAY, J. W., and FADEN, A. I., 1982, Selective cardiorespiratory differences between third and fourth ventricular injections on "mu" and "delta" opiate agonists, *Fed. Proc.* **41**:1468.

HOLADAY, J. W., and LOH, H. H., 1981, Neurobiology of beta-endorphin and related peptides, in: *Hormonal Proteins and Peptides* (C. H. Li, ed.), Academic Press, New York, pp. 202–290.

HOLADAY, J. W., and TORTELLA, F. C., 1984, Multiple opioid receptors: Possible physiological functions of mu and delta binding sites *in vivo*, in: *Central and Peripheral Endorphins: Basic and Clinical Aspects* (E. E. Mueller and A. R. Genazzani, eds.), Raven Press, New York, pp. 237–250.

HOLADAY, J. W., and WARD, S. J., 1982, Morphine-induced bradycardia is predominantly mediated at mu sites, whereas morphine-induced hypotension may involve both mu and delta opioid receptors, *Soc. Neurosci. Abst.* **8**:389.

HOLADAY, J. W., LOH, H. H., and LI, C. H., 1978, Unique behavioral effects of beta-endorphin and their relationship to thermoregulation and hypothalamic function, *Life Sci.* **22**:1525–1536.

HOLADAY, J. W., D'AMATO, R. J., RUVIO, B. A., and FADEN, A. I., 1982a, Action of naloxone and TRH on the autonomic regulation of circulation, in: *Advances in Biochemical Psychopharmacology* (E. Costa and M. Trabucchi, eds.), Raven Press, New York, pp. 353–362.

HOLADAY, J. W., RUVIO, B. A., and SICKEL, J., 1982b, Morphine exacerbates the cardiovascular pathophysiology of endotoxic shock in rats, *Circ. Shock* **9**:169.

HOLADAY, J. W., GILBEAU, P. W., SMITH, C. G., and PENNINGTON, L. L., 1984, Multiple opioid receptors in the regulation of neuroendocrine responses in the conscious rat and monkey, in: *Opioid Modulation of Endocrine Function* (G. Delitala, M. Motta, and M. Serio, eds.), Raven Press, New York, pp. 21–32.

HOLDEN, D., 1985, ADAMHA funding pressed, *Science* **227**:147–149.

HOLMES, L. J., and WISE, R. A., 1985, Contralateral circling induced by tegmental morphine: Anatomical localization, pharmacological specificity, and phenomenology, *Brain Res.* **326**:19–26.

HUGHES, G. S., Jr., 1984, Naloxone and methylprednisolone sodium succinate enhance sympathomedullary discharge in patients with septic shock, *Life Sci.* **35**:2319–2326.

HUGHES, J., 1975, Search for the endogenous ligand of the opiate receptor, *Neurosci. Res. Program Bull.* **13**:55–58.

IRWIN, S., HOUDE, R. W., BENNETT, D. R., HENDERSHOT, L. C., and SEEVERS, M. H., 1951, The effects of morphine, methadone and meperidine on some reflex responses of spinal animals to nociceptive stimulation, *J. Pharmacol. Exp. Ther.* **101**:132–143.

ITO, K., NAKAMURA, H., SATO, A., and SATO, Y., 1983, Depressive effect of morphine on the sympathetic reflex elicited by stimulation of unmyelinated hindlimb afferent nerve fibers in anesthetized cats, *Neurosci Lett.* **39:**169–174.

IVERSEN, L. L., IVERSEN, S. D., BLOOM, F. E. VARGO, T., and GUILLEMIN, R., 1978, Release of enkephalin from rat globus pallidus *in vitro*, *Nature* **271:**679–680.

IWATA, N., and SAKAI, Y., 1971, Effects of some narcotic analgesics and related compounds upon the extensor monosynaptic reflex inhibition from cutaneous nerve and high threshold muscle afferent, *Jpn. J. Pharmacol.* **21:**447–454.

JACKSON, H. C., and SEWELL, R. D. E., 1984, The involvement of mu- and kappa- but not delta-opioid receptors in the body weight gain of suckling rats, *Psychopharmacology* **84:**143–144.

JACKSON, H. D., and SEWELL, R. D. E., 1985, Involvement of endogenous enkephalins in the feeding response to diazepam, *Eur. J. Pharmacol.* **107:**389–392.

JACQUET, Y. F., 1978, Opiate effects after adrenocorticotropin or beta-endorphin injection in the periaqueductal gray matter of rats, *Science* **201:**1032–1034.

JACQUET, Y. F., 1982, Dual actions of morphine on the central nervous system: parallel action of beta-endorphin and ACTH, *Ann. NY Acad. Sci.* **398:**272–290.

JACQUET, Y. F., and LAJTHA, A., 1973, Morphine action at central nervous system sites in rat: Analgesia or hyperalgesia depending on site and dose, *Science* **182:**490–491.

JACQUET, Y. F., and LAJTHA, A., 1974, Paradoxical effects after microinjection of morphine in the periaqueductal gray matter in the rat, *Science* **185:**1055–1057.

JACQUET, Y. F., and WOLF, G., 1981, Morphine and ACTH1-24: Correlative behavior excitation following microinjection in rat periaqueductal gray, *Brain Res.* **219:**214–219.

JACQUET, Y. F., CAROL, M. and RUSSELL, I. S., 1976, Morphine-induced rotation in naive, nonlesioned rats, *Science* **192:**261.

JAFFE, J. H., and MARTIN, W. R., 1980, Opioid analgesics and antagonsits, in: *The Pharmacological Basis of Therapeutics* (A. G. Gilman, L. S. Goodman, and A. Gilman, eds.), Macmillan, New York, pp. 494–534.

JANAL, M. N., COLT, E. W. D., CLARK, W. C., and GLUSMAN, M., 1984, Pain sensitivity, mood and plasma endocrine levels in man following long-distance running: Effects of naloxone, *Pain* **19:**13–26.

JANSSEN, H. F., and LUTHERER, L. O., 1980, Ventriculocisternal administration of naloxone protects against severe hypotension during endotoxin shock, *Brain Res.* **194:**608–612.

JEFFCOATE, W. J., HERBERT, M., CULLEN, M. H., HASTINGS, A. G., and WALDER, C. P., 1979, Prevention of effects of alcohol intoxication by naloxone, *Lancet* **ii:**1157–1159.

JENCK, F. P., SCHMITT, P., and KARLI, P., 1983, Morphine applied to the mesencephalic central gray suppresses brain stimulation induced escape, *Pharmacol. Biochem. Behav.* **19:**301–308.

JOHANNESSEN, J. N., WATKINS, L. R., and MAYER, D. J., 1984, Nonserotonergic origins of the dorsolateral funiculus in the rat ventral medulla, *J. Neurosci.* **4:**757–766.

JUNGKINZ, G., NEDOPIL, N., and RUTHER, E., 1984, Acute effects of the synthetic analogue of methionine enkephalin FK 33-824 in schizophrenic patients. A double blind trial, *Pharmacopsychiatry* **17:**76–78.

KAMERLING, S. G., MARTIN, W. R., WU, K. M., and WETTSTEIN, J. C., 1983, Medullary kappa hyperalgesia mechanisms II. The effects of ethylketazocine administered into the fourth cerebral ventrical of the conscious dog, *Life Sci.* **33:**1839–1843.

KAMEYAMA, T., and UKAI, M., 1983, Multi-dimensional analyses of behavior in mice treated with morphine, endorphins and (des-tyrosine1)-gamma-endorphin, *Pharmacol Biochem. Behav.* **19:**671–677.

KASSON, B. G., and GEORGE, R., 1983a, Endocrine influences on the actions of morphine. I. Alteration of target gland hormones, *J. Pharmacol. Exp. Ther.* **224:**273–281.

KASSON, B. G., and GEORGE, R., 1983b, Endocrine influences on the actions of morphine. III. Responses to hypothalamic hormones, *Neuroendocrinology* **37:**416–420.

KAVALIERS, M., HIRST, M., and TESKEY, G. C., 1983, A functional role for an opiate system in snail thermal behavior, *Science* **220**:99–101.
KAVALIERS, M., HIRST, M., and TESKEY, G. C., 1984, Opioid-induced feeding in the slug, *Limax maximus, Physiol. Behav.* **33**:765–768.
KAVALIERS, M., HIRST, M., and TESKEY, G. C., 1985, Nocturnal feeding in the mouse—opiate and pineal influence, *Life Sci.* **36**:973–980.
KELSEY, J. N., BELLUZZI, J. D., and STEIN, L., 1984, Does naloxone suppress self-stimulation by decreasing reward or by increasing aversion? *Brain Res.* **307**:55–60.
KHAZAN N., YOUNG, G. A., EL-FAKANY, E. E., HONG, O., and CALLIGARO, D., 1984, Sigma receptors mediate the psychotomimetic effects of n-allylnormetazocine (SKF-10,047), but not its opioid agonistic-antagonistic properties, *Neuropharmacology* **23**:983–988.
KINSCHECK, I. G., WATKINS, L. R., and MAYER, D. J., 1984, Fear is not critical to classically conditioned analgesia: The effects of periaqueductal gray lesions and administration of chlordiazepoxide, *Brain Res.* **298**:33–44.
KISER, R. S., JACKSON, S., SMITH, R., REES, L. H., LOWRY, P. J., and BESSER, G. M., 1983, Endorphin-related peptides in rat cerebrospinal fluid, *Brain Res.* **288**:187–192.
KISHIOKA, A., IGUCHI, Y., OZAKI, M., and YAMAMOTO, H., 1983, Effect of electrical lesioning of nucleus reticularis gigantocellularis of rat medulla oblongata on morphine analgesia, *Folia Pharmacol Jpn.* **82**:475–484.
KLINE, N. S., LI, C. H., LEHMANN, H. E., LAJTHA, A., LASKI, E., and COOPER, T., 1977, Beta-endorphin-induced changes in schizophrenic and depressed patients, *Arch. Gen. Psychiatry* **34**:1111–1115.
KOLL, W., HAASE, J., BLOCK, G., and MUHLBERG, B., 1963, The predilective action of small doses of morphine on nociceptive spinal reflexes of low spinal cats, *Int. J. Neuropharmacol.* **2**:57–65.
KORDOWER, H. H., and BODNAR, R. J., 1984, Vasopressin analgesia: Specificity of action and non-opioid effects, *Peptides* **5**:747–756.
KOVACS, G. L., VESCERNYES, M., LACZI, F., FALUDI, M., TELEGDY, G., and LASZLO, F. A., 1985, Acute morphine treatment and morphine tolerance/dependence alter immunoreactive oxytocin levels in the mouse hippocampus, *Brain Res.* **328**:158–160.
KRUGER, L., and LIEBESKIND, J. C., 1984, *Advances in Pain Research and Therapy: Neural Mechanisms of Pain*, Raven Press, New York.
KUMAZAWA, T., EGUCHI, K., and TADAKI, E., 1985, Naloxone-reversible respiratory inhibition induced by muscular thin-fiber afferents in decerebrated cats, *Neurosci Lett.* **53**:81–86.
LAGAMMA, E. F., ADLER, J. E., and BLACK, I. B., 1984, Impulse activity differentially regulates [Leu]enkephalin and catecholamine characters in the adrenal medulla, *Science* **224**:1102–1104.
LAI, Y., and CHAN, S. H. H., 1982, Antagonization of clonidine- and morphine-promoted antinociception by kainic acid lesion of nucleus reticularis gigantocellularis in the rat, *Exp. Neurol.* **78**:38–45.
LAL, H., MIKSIC, S., and SMITH, N., 1976, Naloxone antagonism of conditioned hyperthermia: An evidence for release of endogenous opioid, *Life Sci.* **18**:971–976.
LARGENT, B. L., GUNDLACH, L., and SNYDER, S. H., 1984, Psychotomimetic opiate receptors labeled and visualized with (+)-[^{3}H]3-(3-hydroxyphenyl)-N-(1-propyl)piperidine, *Proc. Natl. Acad. Sci. USA* **81**:4983–4987.
LAUBIE, M., SCHMITT, H., VINCENT, M., and REMOND, G., 1977, Central cardiovascular effects of morphinominetic peptides in dogs, *Eur. J. Pharmacol.* **46**:67–71.
LAUBIE, M., SCHMITT, H., and VINCENT, M., 1979, Vagal bradycardia produced by microinjections of morphine-like drugs into the nucleus ambiguus in anesthetized dogs, *Eur. J. Pharmacol.* **59**:287–291.
LEANDER, J. D., 1984, Kappa-opioid agonists and antagonists—effects on drinking and urinary output, *Appetite* **5**:7–14.

LEANDER, J. D., 1985, Behavioral effects of agonist and antagonist actions at kappa-opioid receptors, in: *Behavioral Pharmacology: The Current Status: Neurology and Neurobiology* (L. S. Seiden and R. L. Balster, eds.), Liss, New York, pp. 93–110.

LEVINE, A. S., and MORLEY, J. E., 1983, Adrenal modulation of opiate induced feeding, *Pharmacol. Biochem. Behav.* **19**:403–406.

LEWIS, J. W., CANNON, J. T., and LIEBESKIND, J. K., 1980, Opioid and nonopioid mechanisms of stress analgesia, *Science* **208**:623–625.

LEWIS, J. W., TORDOFF, M. G., SHERMAN, J. E., and LIEBESKIND, J. C., 1982, Adrenal medullary enkephalin-like peptides may mediate opioid stress analgesia, *Science* **217**:557–559.

LIM, R. K. S., 1966, A revised concept of the mechanism of analgesia and pain, in: *Pain* (R. S. Knighton and P. R. Dumke, eds.), Little, Brown, Boston, pp. 117–154.

LOTTI, V. J., LOMAX, P., and GEORGE, R., 1965, Temperature responses in the rat following intracerebral microinjection of morphine, *J. Pharmacol. Exp. Ther.* **150**:135–139.

LYNESS, W. H., FRIEDLE, N. M., and MOORE, K. E., 1979, Destruction of dopaminergic nerve terminals in nucleus accumbens: Effect on *d*-amphetamine self-administration, *Pharmacol. Biochem. Behav.* **11**:553–556.

MACHT, D. I., 1915, The history of opium and some of its preparations and alkaloids, *JAMA* **64**:477–481.

MAIER, S. F., DRUGAN, R. C., and GRAU, J. W., 1982, Controllability, coping behavior, and stress-induced analgesia in the rat, *Pain* **12**:47–56.

MANNISTO, P. T., RAUHALA, P., TUOMINEN, R., and MATTILA, J., 1984, Dual action of morphine on cold-stimulated thyrotropin secretion in male rats, *Life Sci.* **35**:1101–1108.

MANSOUR, A., and VALENSTEIN, E. S., 1984, Morphine responsiveness and seizure proneness, *Exp. Neurol.* **85**:346–357.

MARGULES, D. L., LEWIS, M. J., SHIBUYA, H., and PERT, C. B., 1978, Beta-endorphin is associated with overeating in genetically obese mice (ob/ob) and rats (fa/fa), *Science* **202**:988–991.

MARGULES, D. L., BOLDMAN, B., and FINCK, A., 1979, Hibernation: An opioid-dependent state? *Brain Res. Bull.* **4**:721–724.

MARTIN, W. R., 1983, Pharmacology of opioids. 4, *Pharmacol. Rev.* **35**:283–323.

MARTINEZ, J. L., JR., 1985, Central versus peripheral actions of Leu-enkephalin on acquisition of a one-way active avoidance response in rats, *Brain Res.* **327**:37–44.

MATTHEWS, R. T., and GERMAN, D. C., 1982, Electrophysiological evidence for morphine excitation of ventral tegmental area dopamine neurons, *Soc. Neurosci. Abstr.* **8**:777.

MAYER, D. J., and HAYES, R., 1975, Stimulation-produced analgesia: Development of tolerance and cross tolerance to morphine, *Science* **188**:941–943.

MAYER, D. J., and PRICE, D. D., 1976, Central nervous system mechanisms of analgesia, *Pain* **2**:379–404.

MAYER, D. J., and PRICE, D. D., 1982, A physiological and psychological analysis of pain: A potential model of motivation, in: *The Physiological Mechanisms of Motivation* (D. W. Pfaff, ed.), Springer-Verlag, New York, pp. 433–471.

MAYER, D. J., and WATKINS, L. R., 1984, Multiple endogenous opiate and nonopiate analgesia systems, in: *Advances in Pain Research and Therapy* (L. Kruger and J. C. Liebeskind, eds.), Raven Press, New York, pp. 253–276.

MAYER, D. J., WOLFLE, T. L., AKIL, H., CARDER, B., and LIEBESKIND, J. C., 1971, Analgesia from electrical stimulation in the brainstem of the rat, *Science* **174**:1351–1354.

MAYER, D. J., PRICE, D. D., and BECKER, D. P., 1975, Neurophysiological characterization of the anterolateral spinal cord neurons contributing to pain perception in man, *Pain* **1**:51–58.

MCGINTY, J. F., and BLOOM, F. E., 1983, Double immunostaining reveals distinctions among opioid peptidergic neurons in the medial basal hypothalamus, *Brain Res.* **278**:145–154.

MCKAY, L. D., KENNEY, N. J., EDENS, N. K., WILLIAMS, R. H., and WOODS, S., 1981, Intra-

cerebroventricular beta-endorphin increases food intake of rats, *Life Sci.* **29:**1429–1435.
MCLAUGHLIN, C. L., and BAILE, C. A., 1984a, Feeding behavior responses of Zucker rats to naloxone, *Physiol. Behav.* **32:**755–762.
MCLAUGHLIN, C. L., and BAILE, C. A., 1984b, Increased sensitivity of Zucker obese rats to naloxone is present at weaning, *Physiol. Behav.* **32:**929–934.
MCNICHOLAS, L. F., and MARTIN, W. R., 1984, New and experimental therapeutic roles for naloxone and related opioid antagonists, *Drugs* **27:**81–93.
MEISENBERG, G., and SIMMONS, W. H., 1983, Centrally mediated effects of neurohypophyseal hormones, *Neurosci. Biobehav. Rev.* **7:**263–280.
MELZACK, R., 1973, *The Puzzle of Pain,* Basic Books, New York.
MELZACK, R., and CASEY, K. L., 1968, Sensory, motivational and central control determinants of pain: A new conceptual model, in: *The Skin Senses* (D. Kenshalo, ed.) Charles C Thomas, Springfield, IL, pp. 423–439.
MELZACK, R., and WALL, P. D., 1965, Pain mechanisms: A new theory, *Science* **150:**971–979.
MENDELSON, S. D., and GORZALKA, B. B., 1984, Cholecystokinin–octapeptide produces inhibition of lordosis in the female rat, *Pharmacol. Biochem. Behav.* **21:**755–760.
MEYERSON, B. J., and TERENIUS, L., 1977, Beta-endorphin and male sexual behavior, *Eur. J. Pharmacol.* **42:**191.
MICKLEY, G. A., and STEVENS, K. E., 1983, Endogenous opiates mediate radiogenic behavioral change, *Science* **220:**1185–1187.
MILKE, D. H., and GALLANT, D. M., 1977, Oral opiate antagonist in chronic schizophrenic—pilot study, *Am. J. Psychiatry.* **134:**1430.
MILLAN, M. J., PRZEWLOCKI, R., JERLICZ, M., GRAMSCH, C., HOLLT, V., and HERZ, A., 1981, Stress-induced release of brain and pituitary beta-endorphin: Major role of endorphins in generation of hyperthermia, not analgesia, *Brain Res.* **208:**325–338.
MILLAN, M. H., MILLAN, M. J., and HERZ, A., 1984, The hypothalamic paraventricular nucleus: Relationship to brain and pituitary pools of vasopressin and oxytocin as compared to dynorphin, beta-endorphin and related opioid peptides in the rat, *Neuroendocrinology* **38:**108–116.
MILLER, G. C., MURGO, A. J., and PLOTNIKOFF, N. P., 1983, Enkephalins-enhancement of active t-cell rosettes from lymphoma patients, *Clin. Immunol. Immunopathol.* **26:**446–451.
MOORE, J. E., 1983, Arginine vasopressin enhances retention of morphine tolerance, *Pharmacol. Biochem. Behav.* **19:**561–566.
MORLEY, J. E., and LEVINE, A. S., 1980, Stress-induced eating is mediated through endogenous opiates, *Science* **209:**259–1261.
MORLEY, J. E., LEVINE, A. S., NIZIELSKI, S., GOSNELL, B. A., PLOTKA, E., BILLINGTON, C. J., and SEAL, U. S., 1984, Species diversity and opioid feeding systems, in: *Central and Peripheral Endorphins: Basic and Clinical Aspects, Physiopathological Aspects* (E. E. Muller and A. R. Genazzani, eds.) Raven Press, New York, pp. 279–284.
MURFIN, R., BENNETT, G. J., and MAYER, D. J., 1976, The effects of dorsolateral spinal cord (DLF) lesions on analgesia from morphine microinjected into the periaqueductal gray matter (PAG) of the rat, *Soc. Neurosci. Abstr.* **2:**946.
MURPHY, E. A., PORTER, J. H., and HEATH, G. F., 1985, Suppression of schedule-induced drinking and food-reinforced bar pressing by tail-pinch is not reversed by naloxone, *Behav. Neural. Biol.* **43:**86–99.
MUSTO, D. F., 1973, *The American Disease,* Yale University Press, New Haven, CT.
MYERS, W. D., NG, K. T., and SINGER, G., 1984, Effects of naloxone and buprenorphine on intravenous acetaldehyde self-injection in rats, *Physiol. Behav.* **33:**449–456.
NABER, D., PICKAR, D., POST, R. M., VANKAMMEN, D. P., WATERS, R. N., BALLENGER, J. C., GOODWIN, F. K., and BUNNEY, W. E., 1981, Endogenous opoid activity and beta-endor-

phin immunoreactivity in CSF of psychiatric patients and normal volunteers, *Am. J. Psychiatry* **138:**1457–1462.
NABER, D., NEDOPIL, N., and EBEN, E., 1984, No correlation between neuroleptic-induced increase of beta-endorphin serum level and therapeutic efficacy in schizophrenia, *Br. J. Psychiatry* **144:**651–653.
NATHAN, P. W., and SMITH, M. C., 1979, Clinico-anatomical correlation in anterolateral cordotomy, in: *Advances in Pain Research and Therapy* (J. J. Bonica, J. C. Liebeskind, and N. G. Albe-Fessard, eds.), Raven Press, New York, pp. 921–926.
NEAL, H., and KEANE, P. E., 1978, The effects of local micro injections of opiates and enkephalins into the forebrain on the electrocorticogram of the rat, *Electroencephalogr. Clin. Neurophysiol.* **45:**655–665.
NEDOPIL, N., and RUTHER, E., 1979, Effects of the synthetic analogue of methionin enkephalin FK 33 824 on psychotic symptoms, *Pharmakopsychiat. Neuro-Psych.* **12:**277–280.
NEMEROFF, C. B., OOSBAHR, A. J., MANBERG, P. J., ERVIN, G. N., and PRANGE, A. J., 1979, Alterations in nociception and body temperature after intra-cisternal administration of neurotensin, beta-endorphin, other endogenous peptides and morphine, *Proc. Natl. Acad. Sci. U.S.A.* **76:**5368–5371.
NOORDENBOS, W., 1959, *Pain,* Elsevier, North Holland, Amsterdam.
OILTGEN, P. R., WALSH, J. W., HAMANN, S. R., RANDALL, D. C., SPURRIER, W. A., and MYERS, R. D., 1982, Hibernation "trigger": Opioid-like inhibitory action on brain function of the monkey, *Pharmacol. Biochem. Behav.* **17:**1271–1274.
OLEY, N., CORDOVA, C., KELLY, M. L., and BRONZINO, J. D., 1982, Morphine administration to the region of the solitary tract nucleus produces analgesia in rats, *Brain Res.* **236:**511–515.
OLSON, R. D., FERNANDEZ, R. C., KASTIN, A. J., OLSON, G. A., DELATTE, S. W., VON ALMEN, T. K., ERICKSON, D. G., and HASTINGS, D. C., 1981, Low doses of naloxone and MIF-1 peptides increase fluid consumption in rats, *Pharmacol. Biochem. Behav.* **15:**921–924.
OSSIPOV, M. H., and GEBHART, G. F., 1984, Light pentobarbital anesthesia diminishes the antinociceptive potency of morphine administered intracranially but not intrathecally in the rat, *Eur. J. Pharmacol.* **97:**137–140.
OSTROWSKI, N. L., ROWLAND, N., FOLEY, T. L., NELSON, J. L., and REID, L. D., 1981, Morphine antagonists and consummatory behaviors, *Pharmacol. Biochem. Behav.* **14:**549–559.
OWEN, M. D., GISOLFI, C. V., REYNOLDS, D. G., and GURLL, N. J., 1984, Autonomic effects of central injections of d-Ala2-metenkephalinamide (DAME) in the conscious monkey, *Peptides* **5:**737–742.
PAE, Y. S., LAI, H., and HORITA, A., 1985, Hyperthermia in the rat from handling stress blocked by naltrexone injected into the preoptic–anterior hypothalamus, *Pharmacol. Biochem. Behav.* **22:**337–340.
PANG, I. H., BERNARDINNI, G. L., and CLARK, W. G., 1984, Hyperthermic response of the cat to intraventricular injection of the opioid delta-receptor agonist D-Ala2-D-Leu5-enkephalin, *Brain Res. Bull.* **13:**263–268.
PASTERNAK, G. W., GINTZLER, A. R., HOUGHTEN, R. A., LING, G. S. F., GOODMAN, R. R., SPIEGEL, K., NISHIMURA, S., *et al.,* 1983, Biochemical and pharmacological evidence for opioid receptor multiplicity in the central nervous system, *Life Sci.* **33:**167–174.
PATERSON, A. T., and VICKERS, C., 1984, Saline drinking and naloxone: Light cycle dependent effects on social behaviour in male mice, *Pharmacol. Biochem. Behav.* **21:**495–500.
PAZOS, A., and FLOREZ, J., 1984, A comparative study in rats of the respiratory depression and analgesia induced by mu- and delta-opioid agonists, *Eur. J. Pharmacol.* **99:**15–22.
PENICAUD, L., and THOMPSON, D., 1984, Effects of systemic intracerebroventricular naloxone injection on basal and 2-deoxy-D-glucose-induced ingestive behavior, *Life Sci.* **35:**2297–2302.
PERT, A., and SIVIT, C., 1977, Neuroanatomical focus for morphine and enkephalin-induced hypermotility, *Nature* **265:**645–646.

PERT, C. B., and SNYDER, S. H., 1973, Opiate receptor: Demonstration in nervous tissue, *Science* **179**:1011–1013.
PERT, A., and YAKSH, T., 1974, Sites of morphine induced analgesia in the primate brain: Relation to pain pathways, *Brain Res.* **80**:135–140.
PERT, C. B., SNOWMAN, A. M., and SNYDER, S. H., 1974, Localization of opiate receptor binding in synaptic membranes of rat brain, *Brain Res.* **70**:184–188.
PERT, C. B., KUHAR, M. J., and SNYDER, S. H., 1975, Autoradiographic localization of the opiate receptor in rat brain, *Life Sci.* **16**:1849–1854.
PERTOVAARA, A., KEMPPAINEN, P., JOHANSSON, G., and KARONEN, S. L., 1982, Ischemic pain nonsegmentally produces a predominant reduction of pain and thermal sensitivity in man: A selective role for endogenous opioids, *Brain Res.* **251**:83–92.
PFEIFFER, A., FEUERSTEIN, G., KOPIN, I. J., and FADEN, A. I., 1983, Cardiovascular and respiratory effects of mu-opiate and kappa-opiate agonists microinjected into the anterior hypothalmic brain area of awake rats, *J. Pharmacol. Exp. Ther.* **225**:735–741.
PHILLIPS, A. G., and BROEKKAMP, C. L. E., 1980, Inhibition of intravenous cocaine self-administration by rats after microinjection of spiroperidol into the nucleus accumbens, *Soc. Neurosci. Abstr.* **6**:105.
PHILLIPS, A. G., and LEPIANE, F. G., 1980, Reinforcing effects of morphine microinjection into the ventral tegmental area, *Pharmacol. Biochem. Behav.* **12**:965–968.
PLOTNIKOFF, N. P., and MILLER, G. C., 1983, Enkephalins as immunomodulators, *Int. J. Immunopharmacol.* **5**:437–442.
POLLERBERG, G. E., COSTA, T., SHEARMAN, G. T., HERZ, A., and REID, L. D., 1983, Opioid antinociception and positive reinforcement are mediated by different types of opioid receptors, *Life Sci.* **33**:1549–1560.
PORRECA, F., FILLA, A., and BURKS, T. F., 1983, Studies *in vivo* with dynorphin-(1-9): Analgesia but not gastrointestinal effects following intrathecal administration to mice, *Eur. J. Pharmacol.* **91**:291–294.
PORRECA, F., MOSBERG, H. I., HURST, R., HRUBY, V. J., and BURKS, T. F., 1984, Roles of mu-receptors, delta-receptors and kappa-opioid receptors in spinal and supraspinal mediation of gastrointestinal transit effects and hot-plate analgesia in the mouse, *J. Pharmacol. Exp. Ther.* **230**:341–348.
POTTOFF, P., VALENTINO, D., and LAL, H., 1979, Attenuation of morphine analgesia by lesions of the preoptic forebrain region in the rat, *Life Sci.* **24**:421–424.
PRICE, D. D., and DUBNER, R., 1977, Neurons that subserve the sensory-discriminative aspects of pain, *Pain* **3**:307–338.
PRICE, D. D., and MAYER, D. J., 1975, Neurophysiological characterization of the anterolateral quadrant neurons subserving pain in *M. mulatta*, *Pain* **1**:59–72.
PRICE, D. D., HU, J. W., DUBNER, R., and GRACELY, R., 1977, Peripheral suppression of first pain and central summation of second pain evoked by noxious heat pulses, *Pain* **3**:57–68.
PRICE, D. D., HAYES, R. L., RUDA, M., and DUBNER, R., 1978, Spatial and temporal transformation of input to spinothalamic tract neurons and their relation to somatic sensation, *J. Neurophysiol.* **41**:933–947.
PROUDFIT, H. K., and ANDERSON, E. G., 1975, Morphine analgesia: Blockade by raphe magnus lesions, *Brain Res.* **98**:612–618.
REYNOLDS, D. V., 1969, Surgery in the rat during electrical analgesia induced by focal brain stimulation, *Science* **164**:444–445.
RIGTER, H., 1978, Attenuation of amnesia in rats by systemically administered enkephalins, *Science* **200**:83–85.
RIGTER, H., GREVEN, H., and VANRIEZEN, H., 1977, Failure of naloxone to prevent reduction of amnesia by enkephalins, *Neuropharmacology* **16**:545–547.
RILEY, A. L., ZELLNER, D. A., and DUNCAN, H. J.., 1980, The role of endorphins in animal learning and behavior, *Neurosci. Biobehav. Rev.* **4**:69–76.
RIOS, L. and JACOB, J., 1981, Comparisons des effets du chlorhydrate et de l'iodomethylate

de naloxone sur le choc endotoxinique chez le rat anesthisie, *Arch. Inst. Pasteur Tunis.* **58:**313–327.

RITZMANN, R. F., LEE, J. M., and FIELDS, J. Z., 1983, Effect of peptides on morphine-induced tolerance and physical dependence, *Psychopharmacol. Bull.* **19:**321–324.

ROBERTS, D. C. S., CORCORAN, M. E., and FIBIGER, H. C., 1977, On the role of ascending catecholaminergic systems in intravenous self-administration of cocaine, *Pharmacol. Biochem. Behav.* **6:**615–620.

ROBERTS, D. C. S., KOOB, G. F., KLONOFF, P., and FIBIGER, H. C., 1980, Extinction and recovery of cocaine self-administration following 6-hydroxy-dopamine lesions of the nucleus accumbens, *Pharmacol. Biochem. Behav.* **12:**781–787.

ROBY, A., WILLER, J-C., and BUSSEL, B., 1983, Effect of a synthetic enkephalin analogue on spinal nociceptive messages in humans, *Neuropharmacology* **22:**1121–1136.

RODGERS, R. J., 1977, Elevation of aversive threshold in rats by intra-amygdaloid injection of morphine sulphate, *Pharmacol. Biochem. Behav.* **6:**385–390.

RODGERS, R. J., 1978, Influence of intra-amygdaloid opiate injections on shock thresholds, tail-flick latencies and open field behaviour in rats, *Brain Res.* **153:**211–216.

ROMANGNANO, M. A., and HAMILL, R. W., 1984, Spinal sympathetic pathway: An enkephalin ladder, *Science* **225:**737–739.

RUKEBUSCH, Y., BARDON, T. H., and PAIRET, M., 1984, Opioid control of the ruminant stomach motility: Functional importance of mu, kappa and delta receptors, *Life Sci.* **35:**1731–1738.

SAMANIN, R., and VALZELLI, L., 1971, Increase of morphine-induced analgesia by stimulation of the nucleus raphe dorsalis, *Eur. J. Pharmacol.* **16:**298–302.

SAMSON, H. H., and DOYLE, T. F., 1985, Oral ethanol self-administration in the rat: Effect of naloxone, *Pharmacol. Biochem. Behav.* **22:**91–100.

SAMSON, W. K., MCDONALD, J. K., and LUMPKIN, M. D., 1985, Naloxone-induced dissociation of oxytocin and prolactin releases, *Neuroendocrinology* **40:**68–71.

SANBERG, D. E., and SEGAL, M., 1978, Pharmacological analysis of analgesia and self-stimulation elicited by electrical stimulation of catacholamine nuclei in the rat brain, *Brain Res.* **151:**529–542.

SATOH, M., and TAKAGI, H., 1971, Effect of morphine on the pre- and postsynaptic inhibitions in the spinal cord, *Eur. J. Pharmacol.* **14:**150–154.

SCHOEMAKER, H., and DAVIS, T. P., 1984, Differential *in vitro* metabolism of beta-endorphin in schizophrenia, *Peptides* **5:**1049–1054.

SCHULL, J., KAPLAN, H., and O'BRIEN, C. P., 1981, Naloxone can alter experimental pain and mood in humans, *Physiol. Pharmacol.* **9:**245–251.

SCHULTZBERG, M., LUNDBERG, J. M., HOKFELT, T., TERENIUS, L., BRANDT, J., ELDE, R. P., and GOLDSTEIN, M., 1978, Enkephalinlike immunoreactivity in gland cells and nerve terminals of the adrenal medulla, *Neuroscience* **3:**1169–1186.

SCHULZ, R., WILHEIM, A., and DIRLICH, G., 1984, Intracerebral injection of different antibodies against endogenous opioids suggests alpha-neoendorphin participation in control of feeding behaviour, *Naunyn Schmied Arch. Pharmacol.* **326:**222–226.

SHIZGAL, P., BIELAJEW, C., CORBETT, D., SKELTON, R., and YEOMANS, J., 1980, Behavioral methods for inferring conduction velocity and anatomical linkage: I. Pathways connecting rewarding brain stimulation sites, *J. Comp. Physiol. Psychol.* **94:**227–237.

SIMONE, D. A., BODNAR, R. J., GOLDMAN, E. J., and PASTERNAK, G. W., 1985, Involvement of opioid receptor subtypes in rat feeding behavior, *Life Sci.* **36:**829–834.

SINCLAIR, J. G., 1973, Morphine and meperidine on bulbospinal inhibition of the monosynaptic reflex, *Eur. J. Pharmacol.* **21:**111.

SIVAM, S. P., and HO, I. K., 1984, Antinociceptive and gastrointestinal effects of opiates: an analysis of the nature of the involvement of mu and delta receptors of the central nervous system in morphine-tolerant and non-tolerant mice, *Neuropharmacology* **23:**105–108.

SLIZGI, G. R., TAYLOR, C. J., and LUDENS, J. H., 1984, Effects of the highly selective kappa-opioid, U-50,488, on renal function in the anesthetized dog, *J. Pharmacol. Exp. Ther.* **230**:641–645.

SMITH, J. E., CO, C., and LANE, J. D., 1984, Limbic muscarinic cholinergic and benzodiazepine receptor changes with chronic intravenous morphine and self-administration, *Pharmacol. Biochem. Behav.* **20**:443–450.

SORENSEN, S. C., and MATTISSON, K., 1978, Naloxone as an antagonist in severe alcohol intoxication, *Lancet* **ii**:688–689.

SPIEGEL, K., KOURIDES, I. A., and PASTERNAK, G. W., 1982, Different receptors mediate morphine-induced prolactin and growth hormone release, *Life Sci.* **31**:2177–2180.

SPIRAKI, C., FIBIGER, H. C., and PHILLIPS, A. G., 1982, Attenuation by haloperidol of place preference conditioning using food reinforcement, *Psychopharmacology* **77**:379–382.

STEWART, J. J., and CURD, C. D., 1984, Antipropulsive effects of central and peripheral morphine in the rat gastrointestinal tract, *J. Pharm. Pharmacol.* **36**:476–477.

SUMMY-LONG, J. Y., MILLER, D. S., ROSELLA-DAMPMAN, L. M., HARTMAN, R. D., and EMMERT, S. E., 1984, A functional role for opioid peptides in the differential secretion of vasopressin and oxytocin, *Brain Res.* **309**:362–366.

SZECHTMAN, H., SIMANTOV, R., and HERSHKOWITZ, M., 1981, Sexual behavior decreases pain sensitivity and stimulates endogenous opioids in male rats, *Eur. J. Pharmacol.* **70**:279–286.

TAKAGI, H., 1980, The nucleus reticularis paragigantocellularis as a site of analgesic action of morphine and enkephalin, *Trends Pharmacol. Sci.* **1**:182–184.

TAKAGI, H., MATSUMURA, M., YANAI, A., and OGIU, K., 1955, The effect of analgesics on the spinal reflex activity of the cat, *Jpn. J. Pharmacol.* **4**:176–187.

TAKAGI, H., DOI, T., and AKAIKE, A., 1976, Microinjection of morphine into the medial part of the bulbar reticular formation in rabbit and rat: Inhibitory effects on lamina V cells of spinal dorsal horn and behavioral analgesia, in: *Opiates and Endogenous Opioid Peptides* (H. W. Kosterlitz, ed.), North Holland, Amsterdam, pp. 191–198.

TANG, F., TANG, J., CHOU, J., and COSTA, E., 1984, Age-related and diurnal changes in met5-enk-arg6-phe7 and met5-enkephalin contents of pituitary and rat brain structures, *Life Sci.* **35**:1005–1014.

TAPIA-ARANCIBIA, L., and ASTIER, H., 1983, Opiate inhibition of K^+-induced TRH release from superfused mediobasal hypothalami in rats, *Neuroendocrinology* **37**:166–168.

TEPPERMAN, F. S., HIRST, M., and GOWDEY, C. W., 1981, Hypothalamic injection of morphine: Feeding and temperature responses, *Life Sci.* **28**:2459–2468.

TERENIUS, L., 1973, Stereospecific interaction between narcotic analgesics and a synaptic plasma membrane fraction of rat cerebral cortex, *Acta Pharmacol. Toxicol.* **32**:317–320.

TERENIUS, L., WASHLSTROM, A., and AGREN, H., 1977, Naloxone (NarcanR) treatment in depression: Clinical observations and effects on CSF endorphins and monoamine metabolites, *Psychopharmacology* **54**:31–33.

TERMAN, G. W., SHAVIT, Y., LEWIS, J. W., CANNON, J. T., and LIEBESKIND, J. C., 1984, Intrinsic mechanisms of pain inhibition: activation by stress, *Science* **226**:1270–1277.

TESCHEMACHER, H. J., SCHUBERT, P., and HERZ, A., 1973, Autoradiographic studies concerning the supraspinal site of the antinociceptive action of morphine when inhibiting the hindleg flexor reflex in rabbits, *Neuropharmacology.* **12**:123–132.

TESKEY, G. C., KAVALIERS, M., and HIRST, M., 1984, Social conflict activates opioid analgesic and ingestive behaviors in male mice, *Life Sci.* **35**:303–316.

THORNHILL, J. A., and SAUNDERS, W., 1984, Ventromedial and lateral hypothalamic injections of naloxone or naltrexone suppress the acute food intake of food-deprived rats, *Appetite* **5**:25–30.

TOREBJORK, H. E., 1974, Afferent C units responding to mechanical, thermal and chemical stimuli in human nonglabrous skin, *Acta Physiol. Scand.* **92**:374–390.

Tsou, K., 1963, Antagonism of morphine analgesia by the intracerebral microinjection of nalorphine, *Acta Physiol. Sin.* **26**:332–337.

Tsou, K., and Jang, C. S., 1964, Studies on the site of analgesic action of morphine by intracerebral micro-injection, *Scientia Sinica* **13**:1099–1109.

Türski, L., Havemann, U., and Kuschinsky, K., 1983, The role of substantia nigra in motility of the rat. Muscular rigidity, body asymmetry and catalepsy after injection of morphine into the nigra, *Neuropharmacology* **22**:1039–1048.

Ukponmwan, O. E., Rupreht, J., and Dzoljic, M. R., 1984, REM sleep deprivation decreases the antinociceptive property of enkephalinase-inhibition, morphine and cold-water swim, *Gen. Pharmacol.* **15**:255–258.

Urca, G., and Frenk, H., 1982, Systemic morphine blocks the seizures induced by intracerebroventricular (i.c.v.) injections of opiates and opioid peptides, *Brain Res.* **246**:121–126.

Van Ree, J. M., 1977, Multiple brain sites involved in morphine antinociception, *J. Pharm. Pharmacol.* **29**:765–766.

Vanvugt, D. A., Bruni, J. F., and Meites, J., 1978, Naloxone inhibition of stress-induced increase in prolactin secretion, *Life Sci.* **22**:85–90.

Vathy, I. U., Etgen, A. M., and Barfield, R. J., 1985, Effects of prenatal exposure to morphine on the development of sexual behavior in rats, *Pharmacol. Biochem. Behav.* **22**:227–232.

Veith, J. L., Sandman, C. A., Walker, J. M., Coy, D. H., and Kastin, A. J., 1978, Systemic administration of endorphins selectively alters open field behavior of rats, *Physiol. Behav.* **20**:539–542.

Verhoeven, W. M. A., van Praag, H. M., and van Ree, J. M., 1984, Repeated naloxone administration in schizophrenia, *Psychiatr. Res.* **12**:297–312.

Vezina, P., and Stewart, J., 1985, Hyperthermia induced by morphine administration to the VTA of the rat brain: An effect dissociable from morphine-induced reward and hyperactivity, *Life Sci.* **36**:1095–1106.

Vigouret, J., Teschemacher, H. J., Albus, K., and Herz, A., 1973, Differentiation between spinal and supraspinal sites of action of morphine when inhibiting the hindleg flexor reflex in rabbits, *Neuropharmacology* **12**:111–121.

Vincent, S. R., Dalsgaard, C. J., Schultzberg, M., Holkfelt, T., Christensson, I., and Terenius, L., 1984, Dynorphin-immunoreactive neurons in the autonomic nervous system, *Neuroscience* **11**:973–988.

Volavka, J., Mallya, A., Baig, S., and Perez-Cruet, J., 1977, Naloxone in chronic schizophrenia, *Science* **196**:1227–1228.

Walker, L. A., and Murphy, J. C., 1984, Antinatriuretic effect of acute morphine administration in conscious rats, *J. Pharmacol. Exp. Ther.* **229**:404–408.

Wallace, M., Willis, G., and Singer, G., 1984, The effect of naloxone on schedule-induced and other drinking, *Appetite* **5**:39–44.

Watkins, L. R., and Mayer, D. J., 1982a, Involvement of spinal opioid systems in foot-shock-induced analgesia: Antagonism by naloxone is possible only before induction of analgesia, *Brain Res.* **242**:309–316.

Watkins, L. R., and Mayer, D. J., 1982b, Organization of endogenous opiate and nonopiate pain control systems, *Science* **216**:1185–1192.

Watkins, L. R., Griffin, G., Leichnetz, G. R., and Mayer, D. J., 1980, The somatotopic organization of the nucleus raphe magnus and surrounding brainstem structures as revealed by HRP slow-release gels, *Brain Res.* **181**:1–15.

Watkins, L. R., Cobelli, D. A., Faris, P., Aceto, M. D., and Mayer, D. J., 1982a, Opiate vs non-opiate footshock-induced analgesia: The body region shocked is a critical factor, *Brain Res.* **242**:299–308.

Watkins, L. R., Cobelli, D. A., and Mayer, D. J., 1982b, Classical conditioning of front paw and hind paw footshock-induced analgesia (FSIA): Naloxone reversibility and descending pathways, *Brain Res.* **243**:119–132.

WATKINS, L. R., COBELLI, D. A., and MAYER, D. J., 1982c, Opiate vs non-opiate footshock-induced analgesia (FSIA): Descending and intraspinal components, *Brain Res.* **245:**97–106.
WATKINS, L. R., COBELLI, D. A., NEWSOME, H. H., and MAYER, D. J., 1982d, Footshock-induced analgesia is dependent neither on pituitary nor sympathetic activation, *Brain Res.* **245:**81–96.
WATKINS, L. R., KINSCHECK, I. B., and MAYER, D. J., 1983a, The neural basis of footshock analgesia: The effect of periaqueductal gray lesions and decerebration, *Brain Res.* **276:**317–324.
WATKINS, L. R., YOUNG, E. G., KINSCHECK, I. B., and MAYER, D. J., 1983b, The neural basis of footshock analgesia: The role of specific ventral medullary nuclei, *Brain Res.* **276:**305–315.
WATKINS, L. R., DRUGAN, R., HYSON, R. L., MOYE, T. B., RYAN, S. M., MAYER, D. J., and MAIER, S. F., 1984a, Opiate and non-opiate analgesia induced by inescapable tailshock: Effects of dorsolateral funiculus lesions and decerebration, *Brain Res.* **291:**325–336.
WATKINS, L. R., FARIS, P. L., KOMISURAK, B. R., and MAYER, D. J., 1984b, Dorsolateral funiculus and intraspinal pathways mediate vaginal stimulation-induced suppression of nociceptive responding in rats, *Brain Res.* **294:**59–65.
WATKINS, L. R., FRENK, H., MILLER, J., and MAYER, D. J., 1984c, Cataleptic effects of opiates following intrathecal administration, *Brain Res.* **299:**43–49.
WATKINS, L. R., FRENK, H., MILLER, J., and MAYER, D. J., 1984d, Effect of spinal cord lesions on convulsive activity induced by intrathecal morphine, *Brain Res.* **310:**337–340.
WATKINS, L. R., JOHANNESSEN, J. N., KINSCHECK, I. B., and MAYER, D. J., 1984e, The neurochemical basis of footshock analgesia: The role of spinal cord serotonin and norepinephrine, *Brain Res.* **290:**107–117.
WATKINS, L. R., KATAYAMA, Y., KINSCHECK, I. B., MAYER, D. J., and HAYES, R. L., 1984f, Muscarinic cholinergic mediation of opiate and nonopiate environmentally induced analgesias, *Brain Res.* **300:**231–242.
WATKINS, L. R., KINSCHECK, I. B., and MAYER, D. J., 1984g, Potentiation of opiate analgesia and apparent reversal of morphine tolerance by proglumide, *Science* **224:**395–396.
WATKINS, L. R., KINSCHECK, I. B., KAUFMAN, E. F. S., MILLER, J., FRENK, H., and MAYER, D. J., 1985a, Cholecystokinin antagonists selectively potentiate analgesia induced by endogenous opiates, *Brain Res.* **327:**181–190.
WATKINS, L. R., KINSCHECK, I. B., and MAYER, D. J., 1985b, Potentiation of morphine analgesia by the cholecystokinin antagonist proglumide, *Brain Res.* **327:**169–180.
WATSON, S. J., BERGER, P. A., AKIL, H., and BARCHAS, J. D., 1978, Effects of naloxone on schizophrenia: Reduction in hallucinations in a subpopulation of subjects, *Science* **201:**73–76.
WAUQUIER, A., BOVILL, J. G., and SEBEL, P. S., 1984, Electroencephalographic effects of fentanyl-, sulfentanil-, and alfentanil anaesthesia in man, *Neuropsychobiology.* **11:**203–206.
WEBSTER, V. A. D., GRIFFITHS, E. C., and SLATER, P., 1983, Antinociceptive effects of thyrotrophin-releasing hormone and its analogues in the rat periaqueductal grey region, *Neurosci. Lett.* **42:**67–70.
WEI, E. T., TSENG, L. F., LOH, H. H., and LI, C. H., 1977, Comparison of the behavioral effects of beta-endorphin and enkephalin analogs, *Life Sci.* **21:**321–328.
WEISS, J., THOMPSON, M. L., and SHUSTER, L., 1984, Effects of naloxone and naltrexone on drug-induced hypothermia in mice, *Neuropharmacology* **23:**483–490.
WHITNALL, M. H., GAINER, H., COX, B. M., and MOLINEAUX, C. J., 1983, Dynorphin-A-(1-8) is contained within vasopressin neurosecretory vesicles in rat pituitary, *Science* **222:**1137–1139.
WIESENFELD-HALLIN, Z., and SODERSTEN, P., 1984, Spinal opiates affect sexual behaviour in rats, *Nature* **309:**257–258.

WIKLER, A., and FRANK, K., 1948, Hindlimb reflexes of chronic spinal dogs during cycles of addiction to morphine and methadone, *J. Pharmacol. Exp. Ther.* **94**:382–400.
WILCOX, R. E., and LEVITT, R. A., 1979, Naloxone reversal of morphine catatonia: Role of caudate and periaqueductal gray, *Pharmacol. Biochem. Behav.* **9**:425–428.
WILLER, J. C., 1983, Nociceptive flexion reflexes as a tool for pain research in man, in: *Motor Control Mechanisms in Health and Disease* (J. E. Desmedt, ed.), Raven Press, New York, pp. 809–828.
WILLER, J. C., and ALBE-FESSARD, D., 1980, Electrophysiological evidence for a release of endogenous opiates in stress-induced analgesia in man, *Brain Res.* **198**:419–426.
WILLER, J. C., DEHEN, H., and CAMBIER, J., 1981, Stress-induced analgesia in humans: Endogenous opioids and naloxone-reversible depression of pain reflexes, *Science* **212**:689–690.
WILLER, J. C., ROBY, A., BOULU, P., and ALBE-FESSARD, D., 1982, Depressive effect of high frequency peripheral conditioning stimulation upon the nociceptive component of the human blink reflex. Lack of naloxone effect, *Brain Res.* **239**:322–326.
WILSON, L., and DOROSZ, L., 1984, Possible role of the opioid peptides in sleep, *Med. Hypoth.* **14**:269–280.
WISE, R. A., 1984, Neural mechanisms of the reinforcing action of cocaine, in: *NIDA Research Monograph Cocaine: Pharmacology, Effects, and Treatment of Abuse* (J. Grabowski, ed.), NIDA, Rockville, MD, pp. 15–33.
WISE, R. A., SPINDLER, J., DEWIT, H., and GERBER, G. J., 1978, Neuroleptic-induced "anhedonia" in rats: Pimozide blocks the reward quality of food, *Science* **201**:262–264.
XENAKIS, S., and SCLAFANI, A., 1982, The dopaminergic mediation of a sweet reward in normal and VMH hyperphagic rats, *Pharmacol. Biochem. Behav.* **16**:293–302.
YAKSH, T. L., 1978, Opiate receptors for behavioral analgesia resemble those related to the depression of spinal nociceptive neurons, *Science* **199**:1231–1233.
YAKSH, T. L., and RUDY, T. A., 1976, Chronic catheterization of the spinal subarachnoid space, *Physiol. Behav.* **17**:1031–1036.
YAKSH, T. L., and RUDY, T. A., 1977, Studies on the direct spinal action of narcotics in the production of analgesia in the rat, *J. Pharmacol. Exp. Ther.* **202**:411–428.
YAKSH, T. L., and WILSON, P. R., 1979, Spinal serotonin terminal system mediates antinociception, *J. Pharmacol. Exp. Ther.* **208**:446–453.
YAKSH, T. L., YEUNG, J. C., and RUDY, T. A., 1976, Systematic examination in the rat of brain sites sensitive to the direct application of morphine: Observation of differential effects within the periaqueductal gray, *Brain Res.* **114**:83–104.
YEUNG, J. C., and RUDY, T. A., 1980a, Sites of antinociceptive action of systemically injected morphine—involvement of supraspinal loci as revealed by intracerebroventricular injection of naloxone, *J. Pharmacol. Exp. Ther.* **215**:626–632.
YEUNG, J. C., and RUDY, T. A., 1980b, Multiplicative interaction between narcotic agonisms expressed at spinal and supraspinal sites of antinociceptive action as revealed by concurrent intrathecal and intracerebroventricular injections of morphine, *J. Pharmacol. Exp. Ther.* **215**:633–642.
YEUNG, J. C., YAKSH, T. L., and RUDY, T. A., 1975, Effects of brain lesions on the antinociceptive properties of morphine in rats, *Clin. Exp. Pharm. Physiol.* **2**:261–268.
YIM, G. K. W., and LOWY, M. T., 1984, Opioids, feeding, and anorexias, *Fed. Proc.* **43**:2893–2896.
YOUNG, E. G., WATKINS, L. R., and MAYER, D. J., 1984, Comparison of the effects of ventral medullary lesions on systemic and microinjection morphine analgesia, *Brain Res.*, **290**:119–129.
YOUNG, G. A., 1980, Naloxone enhancement of punishment in the rat, *Life Sci.* **26**:1787–1792.
ZAGON, I. S., and MCLAUGHLIN, P. J., 1983, Increased brain size and cellular content in infant rats treated with an opiate antagonist, *Science* **221**:1179–1180.

ZAGON, I. S., and McLAUGHLIN, P. J., 1984, Naltrexone modulates body and brain development in rats: A role for endogenous opioid systems in growth, *Life Sci.* **35**:2057–2064.

ZAGON, I. S., McLAUGHLIN, P. J., and ZAGON, E., 1984, Opiate, endorphins, and the developing organism: A comprehensive bibliography, 1982–1983, *Neurosci. Biobehav. Rev.* **8**:387–404.

ZETLER, G., and MORSDORF, K. H., 1984, Effects of ceruletide and cholecystokinin octapeptide on eating in mice. Interactions with naloxone and the enkephalin analogue, FK33-824, *Naunyn Schmied Arch. Pharmacol.* **325**:209–213.

ZORMAN, G., BELCHER, G., ADAMS, J. E., and FIELDS, H. L., 1982, Lumbar intrathecal naloxone blocks analgesia produced by microstimulation of the ventromedial medulla in the rat, *Brain Res.* **236**:77–89.

ZVARTAU, E. E., 1977, Action of naloxone on emotionally positive and antinociceptive effects of hypothalamic stimulation in rats, *Bull. Exp. Biol. Med.–Engl. Tr.* **88**:1306–1308.

9

NEUROPEPTIDES AND MEMORY

George F. Koob

1. NEUROPEPTIDES

Some of the earliest evidence suggesting a behavioral role for peptides came from studies of pituitary–adrenal function. For example, De Wied and others demonstrated that the behavioral effects produced by removal of the pituitary could be reversed by adrenocorticotropin hormone (ACTH) and other peptides, such as vasopressin (AVP) (De Wied, 1980). Later work established that these peptides could produce profound effects on extinction of learned responses in normal animals even with synthetic analogs reputedly devoid of endocrinological activity. Variously interpreted as actions on attention (ACTH) or on memory consolidation (AVP), these effects were hypothesized to be mediated via some neural substrate. Where this substrate is located and how these pituitary-derived peptides normally interact with it remain largely unknown.

In the last decade the identification of an ever-increasing number of peptides localized within neurons of the central nervous system (CNS) has given new impetus to the search for their functional significance. One general hypothesis, described largely from the earlier work on pituitary peptides, has been that these peptides in the CNS have an important role in adaptive behavior. This implies, at some level, a role in learning, the acquisition of new information, and memory, the retention of this new information for future use. This chapter will discuss, first, the animal models used to characterize memory effects, their advantages and disad-

---

George F. Koob • Division of Preclinical Neuroscience and Endocrinology, Scripps Clinic and Research Foundation, La Jolla, California 92037.

TABLE 1
Neuropeptides Implicated in Memory Function

Neuronal peptide	Structure
Hypophyseal hormones	
Vasopressin	Cys-Tyr-Phe-Glu-Arg-Cys-Pro-Arg-Gly-NH$_2$ (S–S bridge between Cys residues)
Oxytocin	Cys-Tyr-Ile-Glu-ARG-Cys-Pro-Leu-Gly-NH$_2$ (S–S bridge between Cys residues)
Opioid peptides	
Leucine-enkephalin	Try-Gly-Gly-Phe-Leu-OH
Methionine-enkephalin	Try-Gly-Gly-Phe-Met-OH
β-Endorphin	Try-Gly-Gly-Phe-Met-Thr-Ser-Glu-Lys-Ser-Gln-Thr-Pro-Leu-Val-Thr-Leu-Phe-Lys-Asn-Ala-Ile-Val-Lys-Asn-Ala-His-Lys-Gly-Gln-OH
Adrenocorticotropic (human ACTH 1-39)	H-Ser-Tyr-Ser-Met-Glu-His-Phe-Arg-Trp-Gly-Lys-Pro-Val-Gly-Lys-Arg-Arg-Pro-Val-Lys-Val-Tyr-Pro-Asn-Gly-Ala-Glu-Asp-Glu-Ser-Ala-Glu-Ala-Phe-Pro-Leu-Glu-Phe-OH
ACTH$_{4-10}$	Met-Glu-His-Phe-Arg-Try-Gly
ORG 2766	H-Met(O)-Glu-His-Phe-D Lys-Phe-OH
Somatostatin	H-Ala-Gly-Cys-Lys-Asn-Phe-Phe-Trp-Lys-Thr-Ser-Thr-Ser-Cys-OH (S–S bridge between Cys residues)
Nonhypophyseal hormones	
Substance P	Arg-Pro-Lys-Pro-Gln-Gln-Phe-Phe-Gly-Leu-Met-NH$_2$
Neurotensin	<Glu-Leu-Tyr-Glu-Asn-Lys-Pro-Arg-Arg-Pro-Tyr-Ile-Leu-COOH
Angiotensin II	Asp-Arg-Val-Tyr-Ile-His-Pro-Phe
Cholecystokinin octapeptide (CCK8)	Asp-Tyr-HSO$_3$-Met-Gly-Trp-Met-Asp-Phe-NH$_2$

vantages, and their functional significance. Next, specific experimental findings relating peptides to memory will be reviewed with special emphasis on mechanism and site of action. Finally, some attempt will be made to synthesize and integrate these purported memory effects with other known functions of these peptides and to discuss their significance in terms of the processing and retention of information.

Neuropeptides implicated in memory function are numerous (see Table 1). From the hypothalamic–pituitary–adrenal system they include vasopressin, oxytocin, ACTH, and endorphins; other gut peptides such as angiotensin and cholecystokinin have recently been studied. All these peptides now have been localized within the CNS using immunocytochemical techniques and thus can be considered as possible neurotransmitters or neuromodulators (for a recent review, see Emson, 1979).

2. CONCEPTUAL AND METHODOLOGICAL CONSIDERATIONS

2.1. Conceptual Model

To date, with the exception of a few studies, the evidence implicating neuropeptides in memory function is derived from studies using animal models, usually rats or mice. *Learning* here is defined as the acquisition of new or different information; *memory* is defined as the preservation of the learned information (Heise, 1981). These animal models are based on a conceptual model in which four stages of memory are assumed: sensory registration, storage or consolidation, maintenance, and retrieval; the same considerations that have been discussed for pharmacological effects on memory (Hunter *et al.*, 1977) are equally important for the study of the role of neuropeptides in memory. In fact, they become particularly relevant with peptides, given that the molecular and cellular mechanisms of action for peptides are largely unknown.

Drugs or neuropeptides are typically administered during one of three of the phases of the associative process (see Fig. 1). Treatment can occur before acquisition (A), after training (B), before retention (C), or any combination of the above. Treatments before acquisition and retention are confounded easily by nonspecific, i.e., nonassociative, perfor-

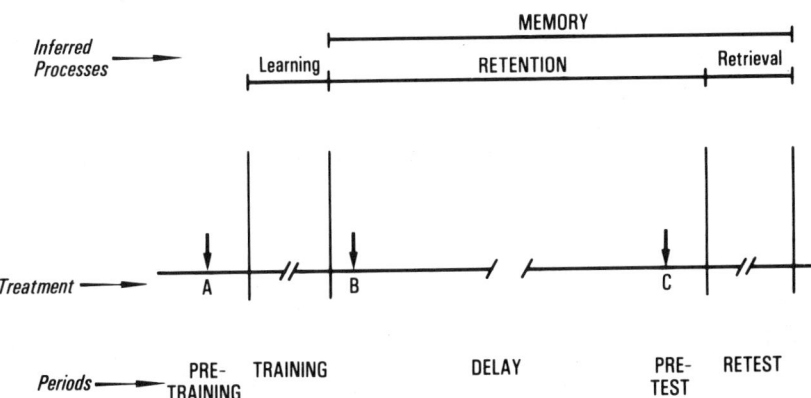

FIG. 1. Schematic representation of the different time periods, treatments, and inferred cognitive processes occurring during a drug or peptide trial in a learning experiment (redrawn from Heise, 1981). (A) Injection during the pretraining period or preacquisition; (B) injection after training or postconsolidation or during consolidation; (C) injection pretest or before retention.

mance effects, e.g., ataxia. One of the most popular approaches in animal models has been to examine treatment effects immediately after training (B) when memory consolidation processes are assumed to be maximally susceptible to alteration (McGaugh, 1966). Susceptibility to treatment effects is thought to decline as a time-dependent process after this critical period, and treatment during this memory maintenance phase is often used as a control for possible long-acting proactive effects of a treatment.

Thus, the major means of exploring the role of a given peptide has been to inject either the peptide or its antagonist into the animal during the consolidation, maintenance, or retrieval of memory. The assumption presumably made here is that the normal endogenous function of the peptide will be exaggerated. For an antagonist, the opposite would be the case. This "top-down" approach lends itself to phenomena, and it is hoped that it will reveal mechanisms or structures necessary or even important for normal memory. However, this approach for exposing the role of endogenous substances in memory is based on neurobiological assumptions that may or may not be true. For example, the concept that more agonist (putative peptide neurotransmitter or neuromodulator) facilitates function may not be valid, and the ubiquitous nature of inverted U-shaped dose–effect curves in the work to be reviewed here suggests that this is, indeed, the case.

2.2. Animal Tests

By far the most common procedure used to date to assess peptide function has been the inhibitory or passive avoidance response. Here the rat or mouse is placed on a platform or in a small, lighted compartment for one or several training trials, and when the animal invariably steps down from the platform or enters an adjacent dark compartment, it is given a painful footshock. At least 24 hr later, the animal receives a second trial (retest), and if it is given an appropriate amount of shock, its latency to reenter on the retest trial is longer than the trial where shock was given. This latency is the "memory" effect that can be modified by the appropriate pretraining, posttraining, or preretention treatment.

Two other procedures have been commonly used to assess the potential role of a drug or neurotransmitter in memory: the antiamnesia model and extinction behavior. The antiamnesia model traditionally is based on the observation that some disturbance to the animal can disrupt the transfer of information from memory, i.e., can disrupt consolidation. This consolidation process, as mentioned earlier, is seen as a time-dependent process, and thus amnesia should be maximal for experiences immediately before a disturbance and less for experiences more remote in time. In animal studies many disturbances, such as electroconvulsive shock, hypoxia produced by carbon dioxide, and administration of protein synthesis inhibitors, have been used as amnesic agents. The drug or peptide treatment is observed as an attempt to reverse this disturbance-induced amnesia (Rigter and van Riezen, 1978), and the treatment either precedes the acquisition trial (consolidation) or is given before the test trial (retrieval).

The third animal model that has been used extensively is extinction behavior and is similar to the other two tests in that it involves aversively motivated behavior and treatment presumably during consolidation of the presumed association or prior to retrieval. Here rats are trained to avoid shock by jumping on a pole or moving to another compartment, and once acquisition is complete, undergo a series of extinction trials (De Wied, 1966). Drug or peptide treatment again can be given prior to acquisition, after acquisition, or during extinction. Treatments during extinction are confounded by the addition of nonreward, but most tests suggest that a given treatment that prolongs extinction of active avoidance of an aversive event also increases memory when used in the inhibitory (passive) avoidance test (see Section 3.1), which, in a sense, is also a prolongation of extinction.

3. HYPOPHYSEAL PEPTIDES AND MEMORY

3.1. Vasopressin

The primary physiological action of vasopressin is to conserve body water by acting on the kidney (for review see Sawyer, 1964). The pathological or congenital loss of vasopressin-secreting neurons from the hypothalamus produces a pronounced and chronic diuresis (diabetes insipidus) (Hays, 1980). Vasopressin also has potent pressor actions, and although this pressor effect requires significantly higher doses than the antidiuretic action, this vasoconstrictor action of vasopressin may be physiologically significant during hypovolemic or hypotensive rises (Zerbe et al., 1982).

In early behavioral work, De Wied and associates (De Wied, 1965) found that hypophysectomized rats were deficient in a number of behavioral situations, especially the acquisition and extinction of aversively motivated tasks. These deficiencies were reversible by the administration of a crude pituitary extract, pitressin, and, in later work, by lysine vasopressin (LVP) in microgram amounts injected subcutaneously (Bohus et al., 1973). Vasopressin also reversed the behavioral deficits observed in Brattleboro-strain rats with congenital diabetes insipidus (Bohus et al., 1975; De Wied et al., 1975a).

Further, LVP injected subcutaneously delayed extinction in an active avoidance task in intact animals (De Wied, 1971) and in a passive (inhibitory) avoidance task (Ader and De Wied, 1972), as did intracerebroventricular injection of nanogram quantities of AVP (De Wied, 1976). These same investigators reported that AVP enhanced retention of the passive avoidance response when injected subcutaneously either just after the training test (shock) or just before the retention test, but not at times in between (Bohus et al., 1978b), suggesting that AVP enhanced both consolidation and retrieval of memory.

Evidence to support the hypothesis that vasopressin produces its behavioral effects independently of its classic renal or pressor effects came from the work of De Wied and associates with different analogs of vasopressin. For example, desglycinamide–lysine vasopressin, a vasopressin analogy with minimal pressor and renal activity, reverses the behavioral deficits associated with diabetes insipidus (De Wied et al., 1975a) and has effects similar to those of vasopressin in active avoidance tests (Walter et al., 1978). Desglycinamide–lysine vasopressin, or lysine vasopressin, also has a vasopressin effect in counteracting several drug-induced disruptions of consolidation, including diethyldithiocarbamate, pentylenetetrazol, puromycin, and CO_2-induced amnesia (Asin, 1980; Bookin and Pfeifer, 1977; Lande et al., 1972; Rigter et al., 1974). The relative behavioral potencies of these analogs suggests that the ring structure of vasopressin may be most important for the "consolidation" of acquired avoidance responses, whereas the C-terminal appears to be more important for reversing the effects of amnesia treatments (Van Ree et al., 1978).

With few exceptions, the data regarding a role for vasopressin, itself, in memory came from studies employing aversively motivated tasks. Obviously, this limits the nature of the behavioral conclusions that can be drawn from such data. If vasopressin does have memory-enhancing properties, this effect should also be demonstrable with positively motivated tasks. Several reports have now shown an effect with vasopressin analogs. In rats trained to discriminate sides of a T maze using a sex reward, desglycinamide–lysine vasopressin facilitated retention (Bohus, 1977). In rats receiving vasopressin during acquisition training in a black–white discrimination T-maze task extinction was prolonged, but only on the side using the black discriminative stimulus (Hostetter et al., 1977). Desglycinamide arginine vasopressin has been shown to facilitate the acquisition of an autoshaping response and to prolong extinction of this response (Messing and Sparber, 1983). In one of the only observations to date of an effect of the endogenous peptide itself, posttraining administration of arginine vasopressin facilitated subsequent test performance in a one-trial water-finding task (Ettenberg et al., 1983a).

However, recent findings with vasopressin antagonists have addressed some questions raised by this earlier work of De Wied and associates. A pressor antagonist analog of arginine vasopressin, 1-deamino-penicillamine, 2-(O-methyl)tyrosine AVP (dPTyr(Me)AVP), which prevented the AVP pressor response (Bankowski *et al.*, 1978), blocked the effects of both subcutaneously and intraventricularly injected AVP on prolongation of extinction of active avoidance (Le Moal *et al.*, 1981) (see Fig. 2). The antagonist had little effects on its own except at high doses, when it facilitated extinction of active avoidance (Koob *et al.*, 1981b). This antagonist also blocked the effects of AVP on passive avoidance and the effects of AVP on an appetitive task (Ettenberg *et al.*, 1983a), but at a somewhat higher doses (Lebrun *et al.*, 1984). (See Figs. 3 and 4.) For that matter, all behavioral effects of vasopressin investigated to date have been reversed by the V-1 AVP antagonist (Le Moal *et al.*, 1984; De Wied *et al.*, 1984). These effects may indicate either that signals from peripheral visceral sources play an important role in subsequent behavioral changes or that the receptors at which AVP elicits its pressor effect are similar to those in the CNS leading to its behavioral action.

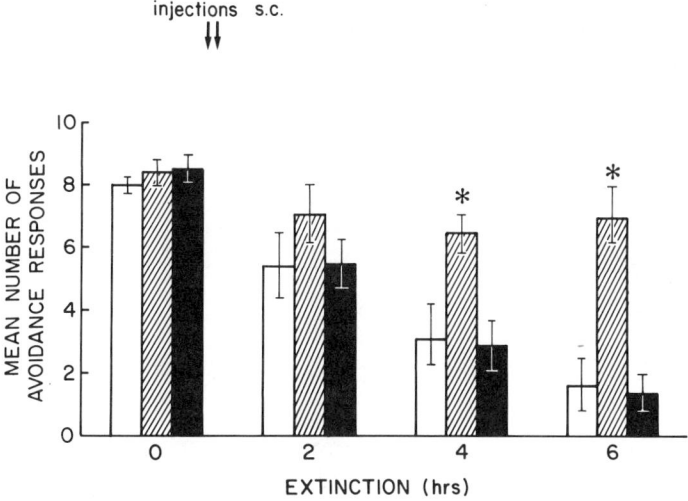

FIG. 2. Effects of AVP and AVP plus dPTyr(Me)AVP on extinction of active avoidance behavior. After three days of training, rats were injected subcutaneously with saline (twice at 2.0-min intervals) or AVP plus saline or AVP plus dPTyr(Me)AVP immediately after the first set of 10 extinction trials on day 4. Rats receiving AVP showed persistent avoidance throughout the 6 hr of observation, when tested on 10 trials at each of the next three 2-hr intervals, whereas rats receiving either saline with no peptide or both peptides extinguished this active avoidance behavior at similar rates. Saline + saline (□) (N = 9); saline + AVP, 6 µg/kg (▨) (N = 9); dPTyr(Me)AVP, 30 µg/kg + AVP, 6 µg/kg (■).*Significantly different from both the saline with no peptide and both peptide groups; $p < .05$, Newman-Keuls test following analysis of variance. (From Le Moal *et al.*, 1984, with permission from *Nature*.)

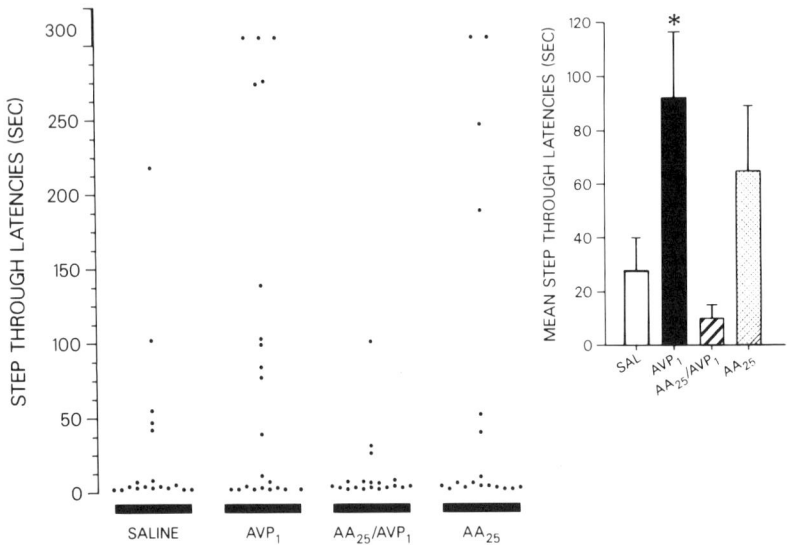

FIG. 3. Effects of AVP, dPTyr(Me)AVP (AA), and AVP plus dPTyr(Me)AVP on retention of an inhibitory avoidance task. The peptides were injected subcutaneously immediately after the acquisition trial. Data represent the individual scatter diagram of latency scores during the retention test, 24 hr after the acquisition trial. Saline ($N = 18$); AVP, 1 μg/rat ($N = 22$); dPTyr(Me)AVP, 25 μg/rat + AVP, 1 μ/rat ($N = 19$); dPTyr(Me)AVP, 25 μg/rat ($N = 18$). Insert shows the mean latency score ($\pm$ SEM) produced by each group during the retention test. *Significantly different from saline group ($p < .05$ t test). (From Lebrun et al., 1984, with permission from Life Sciences.)

These observations have prompted a significant effort to distinguish between these two hypotheses, and some controversy still exists as to the final resolution. For example, in two recent studies, De Wied and associates have shown that a new analog of vasopressin [pGlu4,Cyt6] AVP 4-8(AVP4-8) is much more active than AVP itself in facilitating passive avoidance when injected peripherally posttraining (Burbach et al., 1983). This analog has no pressor activity, and these effects can be produced by an even more potent AVP pressor antagonist (De Wied et al., 1984), even when the antagonist is injected in nanogram amounts intracerebroventricularly. Similar results were obtained using AVP itself (De Wied et al., 1984), leading De Wied and associates to conclude that both peripherally and centrally derived AVP act via a common action on CNS receptors.

Work in our laboratory using the pressor antagonist dPtyr(Me)AVP and extinction of active avoidance supports precisely the opposite conclusion. The pressor antagonist reverses the effects of AVP administered subcutaneously (s.c.) only at doses sufficient to reverse the peripheral pressor effects, i.e., 5000 nanograms intracerebroventricularly (i.c.v.) (Lebrun et al., 1985). Similar effects have been observed for the facilitation of performance in the water-finding task (Ettenberg, 1985). Peripheral administration of this antagonist also readily reverses the central effects of nonpressor-enhancing doses of AVP in active avoidance, suggesting that the antagonist readily crosses the blood–brain barrier (Le Moal et al., 1982). Thus, our conclusion is dramatically different from that of De Wied and associates, and we hypothesize that there are two AVP systems, one central and the other peripheral, and that although these systems may ultimately act on a similar behavioral substrate, they do so by different and independent mechanisms.

Another area of some controversy in vasopressin research centers on the divergent results obtained using Brattleboro rats, which are genetically devoid of vasopressin in both the CNS and pituitary. Whereas the early reports claimed that Brattleboro rats were impaired in retention of active and passive avoidance (De Wied et al., 1975a; Bohus et al., 1975b), several studies have demonstrated that non-Utrecht Brattleboro rats are unimpaired in a variety of learning tests (Celestian et al., 1975; Bailey and Weiss, 1979; Brito et al., 1980; Carey and Miller, 1982). Indeed, in other laboratories, Brattleboro rats often show longer retention latencies for shock avoidance, i.e., better memory than non-Brattleboro rats, and some controversy exists as to the proper control groups (for point/counterpoint, see Gash and Thomas, 1983, 1984; De Wied, 1984a,b).

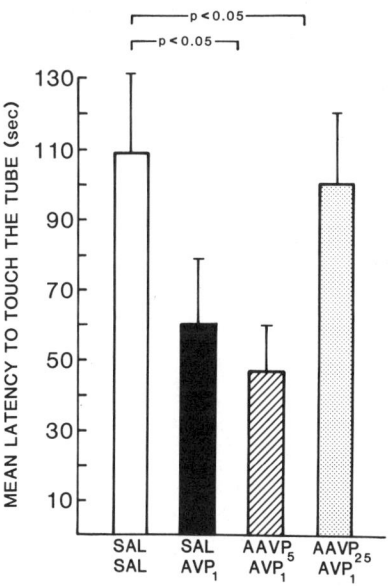

FIG. 4. Mean (± SEM) and median latencies to contact a dry drinking tube on test day. Vasopressin potentiated the learned performance of treated animals compared to control animals. This effect was reversed by a 25 µg (but not a 5 µg) dose of the V-1 AVP antagonist peptide dPTyr(Me)AVP (AAVP). (From Ettenberg et al., 1983, with permission from *Pharmacology, Biochemistry, and Behavior*.)

Clinical studies with vasopressin and vasopressin analogs have shown mixed results. Lysine vasopressin improved performance in tests involving attention, concentration, and memory in a double-blind study involving aged subjects (Legros *et al.*, 1978). Other researchers have reported improvements in retrograde and anterograde amnesia in an open preliminary study with lysine vasopressin (Oliveros *et al.*, 1978) and in the amnesia associated with Korsakoff's syndrome in a double-blind study on one patient (LeBoeuf *et al.*, 1978). More recently, in a double-blind study, a synthetic analog of vasopressin, 1-desamino-8-D-arginine vasopressin (DDAVP), produced consistent improvements in tests to measure long-term memory in patients suffering from affective illness; DDAVP also produced improvements in serial learning and prompted free recall and recall of semantically related words in both cognitively impaired and unimpaired adults (Weingartner *et al.*, 1981). In another double-blind study, DDAVP enhanced learning in a concept-shift task in normal healthy males (Beckwith *et al.*, 1982). Curiously, in animal studies, the replacement of the L-arginine in arginine vasopressin by D-arginine markedly decreased AVP's ability to alter extinction of pole-jump avoidance (Walter *et al.*, 1978). Whether this reflects species differences in response to vasopressin or the difference in the nature of the behavioral tests remains to be determined. Chronic intranasal DGAVP improved short-term and long-term memory in both normal and diabetes insipidus patients in a double-blind trial (Laczi *et al.*, 1983). Positive effects for DDAVP have also been observed in learning in Lesch–Nyhan children in an open, within-subjects experiment (Anderson *et al.*, 1979).

Other studies have not been so positive. Failures have been reported for lysine vasopressin, DDAVP, and DGAVP in open trials in posttraumatic amnesia (Koch-Hendriksen and Nielsen, 1981; Jenkins *et al.*, 1979, 1981), and a failure has been reported with Korsakoff patients in an open trial (Blake *et al.*, 1978). DDAVP also failed to improve cognitively impaired patients in a double-blind trial (Tinklenberg *et al.*, 1981), and lysine vasopressin failed to produce any improvements in memory or learning in seven head-injured patients in double-blind trials (Fewtrell *et al.*, 1982).

Hypotheses for the mechanism of action of these behavioral effects of AVP vary to some extent with the aforementioned position regarding a peripheral versus a central site. For example, the "peripheralists" can list a series of unconditioned effects of AVP that ultimately could contribute to a behavioral state sufficient to prolong or augment stress-motivated behavior (see Sahgal, 1984). AVP produces pressor actions, aversive effects (acts as an unconditioned stimulus for conditioned taste and place aversion), and motor effects (Ettenberg *et al.*, 1983). However, AVP also has behavioral effects when injected directly into the brain in nanogram doses (De Wied, 1971; Koob *et al.*, 1986; Kovacs *et al.*, 1979*a,b*), doses

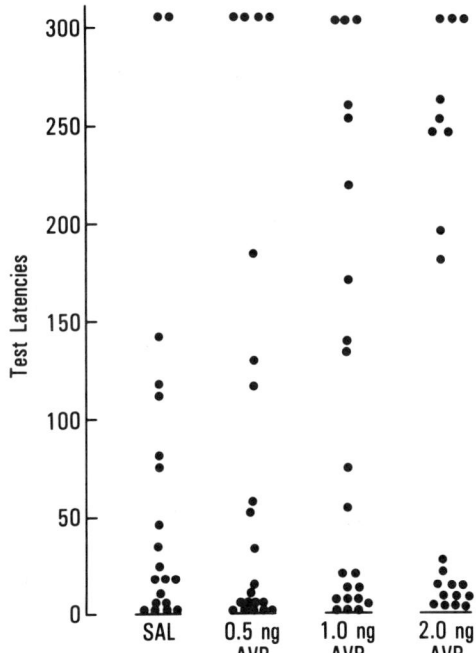

FIG. 5. Individual scatter diagram of latency scores during retention for rats receiving saline 0.5, 1.0, or 2.0 ng of AVP (i.c.v.) immediately posttraining (shock) in an inhibitory avoidance test. Scores over 300 sec represent rats that never reentered. Nonparametrical statistical analyses revealed a significant difference between the groups in that rats in the 1.0- and 2.0-ng groups showed significantly more scores above 120 sec. (Information Statistic; Kullback, 1968; $2I = 11.4764$, $df = 6$, $p < .05$.)

that do not increase systemic blood pressure (Koob et al., 1986) (see Fig. 5).

Others have argued that AVP is physiologically involved in memory processes via direct action on the CNS, since a specific vasopressin antiserum injected i.c.v. posttraining in passive avoidance produced deficits in subsequent retention trials (van Wimersma Greidanus and De Wied, 1979b; van Wimersma Greidanus et al., 1975). Also, AVP accelerated the disappearance of norepinephrine in the dorsal septal nucleus, dorsal hippocampus, and parafascicular nucleus, among other places (Tanaka et al., 1977a,b). Injection of AVP into these areas facilitated consolidation in passive avoidance (Kovacs et al., 1979b), and destruction of these structures, as well as the noradrenergic projections to them, blocked the facilitatory effects of AVP on avoidance behavior (van Wimersma Greidanus and De Wied, 1976a; van Wimersma Greidanus et al., 1975, 1979; Kovacs et al., 1979a).

Of course, for this latter hypothesis to be correct, one must assume that AVP crosses the blood–brain barrier after peripheral injection. Most of the data in the literature suggest that this is not the case (see Le Moal et al., 1984, and Deyo et al., 1985 for reviews) (see Fig. 6). However, a recent study using a large dose of AVP (5 µg/rat) suggests that a small amount of vasopressin, i.e., 0.002%, may reach the cerebrospinal fluid

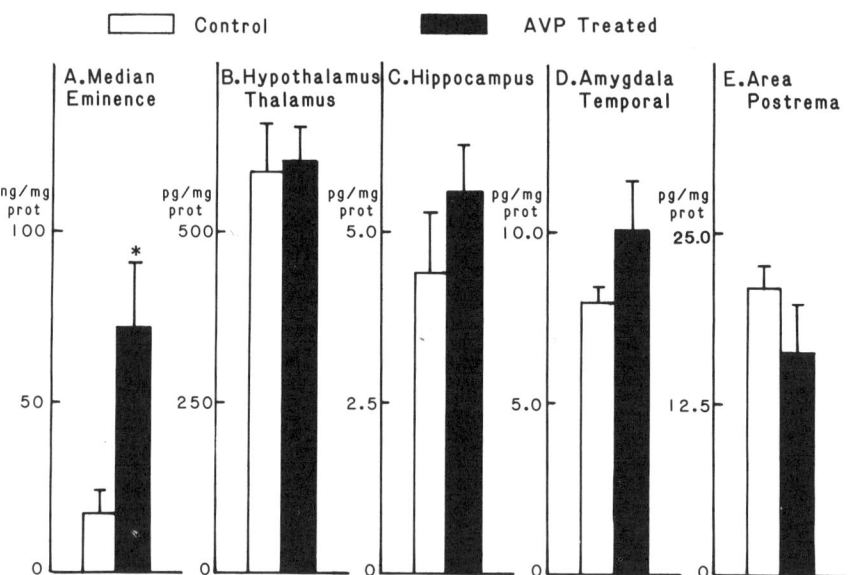

FIG. 6. The concentrations of AVP in (A) the median eminence of the hypothalamus, (B) the hypothalamus–thalamus, (C) the hippocampus, (D) the amygdala–temporal cortex, and (E) the area postrema from perfused brains from rats injected, subcutaneously, with vehicle or with 5000 ng AVP/kg 20 min after injection of AVP. The perfusion procedure is described in Deyo et al. (1986). The values are means ± SEM's expressed as nanogram AVP/mg protein (A and B) or picogram AVP/mg protein (C–E). *$p < .05$; $n = 6$/bar. (From Deyo et al., 1986, with permission from *Neuroendocrinology*.)

(CSF) 10 min postinjection (Mens et al., 1983). This enormous dose, which raises blood AVP levels to 9700 pg/ml at 10 min [(i.e., 1000 times higher than the maximum dose observed in our laboratory even following severe water deprivation (Deyo et al., 1985)], only raises CSF levels by 20 pg/ml. Thus, it is not clear that peripherally administered AVP acts to alter behavior by directly acting on brain receptors. Nor is it likely that these treatments involving such high doses of vasopressin mimic the kind of blood levels of AVP generated physiologically, leaving the question of AVP penetration into the CNS unresolved (see Section 5.5 for more discussion of this general issue).

3.2. Oxytocin

The primary physiological action of oxytocin in mammals is to hasten parturition and to stimulate lactation by the myoepithelial cells of the mammary gland. Oxytocin is released after suckling and may also facilitate nursing and maternal behavior after intraventricular administration to females (Pedersen and Prange, 1979). Oxytocin also causes uterine contraction, although it is not thought to induce labor but rather to augment intrinsic contractile activity and thus accelerate delivery (Chard, 1972). Curiously, oxytocin is also found in male rats. Oxytocin is structurally related to AVP, both being nonapeptides (see Table 1), and in fact, oxytocin has some antidiuretic activity and AVP has some ability to produce uterine contractions.

Studies implicating a role for oxytocin in learning and memory are much less extensive than those for vasopressin, and those studies with peripheral injections are somewhat contradictory. In earlier work, oxytocin injected s.c. either delayed extinction of active avoidance, but was less active than vasopressin (De Wied and Gispen, 1977), facilitated extinction (Schultz *et al.*, 1974, 1976), or had no effect (Bohus *et al.*, 1978a). Yet intraventricular administration of 1 ng of oxytocin after each acquisition session did facilitate extinction of active avoidance (Bohus *et al.*, 1978a).

The results with inhibitory (passive) avoidance are more consistent. Oxytocin injected s.c. after training impaired retention (Bohus *et al.*, 1978b; Kovacs *et al.*, 1978). Oxytocin injected intraventricularly also produced an effect opposite to that of AVP in passive avoidance, leading De Wied and associates to hypothesize that oxytocin has amnesic properties (De Wied and Bohus, 1979). Apparently, virtually the whole molecule of oxytocin is required for this action, since removal of anything but the C-terminal amino acid glycinamide residue causes a significant loss of activity (van Wimersma Greidanus *et al.*, 1983). A possible site of action for oxytocin is the central noradrenergic system, since local injection of oxytocin into the pathway of the dorsal noradrenergic bundle also impairs retention of passive avoidance (Kovacs *et al.*, 1978). Particularly intriguing is the fact that most of the studies with oxytocin and learning involve male rats, for whom there is no obvious physiological (hormonal) function for oxytocin.

3.3. Adrenocorticotropic Hormone

Adrenocorticotropic hormone (ACTH) has long been associated with the chain of events required to preserve homeostasis in an organism adapting to a dynamically changing environment. Activation of ACTH release from the pituitary by corticotropin-releasing factor and the subsequent elevation of plasma corticosteroids is, for many, a critical factor in the definition of a stress response, and ACTH has been considered important not only for the endocrine and metabolic responses to stress but also for behavioral responses to stress. For example, early work showed that completely hypophysectomized rats were severely handicapped in the acquisition of active and passive avoidance (Applezweig and Baudry, 1955; Anderson *et al.*, 1968; De Wied, 1964). Also, ACTH administered during acquisition of an avoidance task delayed extinction of the learned response in normal rats (Murphy and Miller, 1955).

Later, De Wied demonstrated that the rapid extinction produced by removal of the posterior and intermediate lobe of the pituitary could be reversed by ACTH and related peptides (De Wied, 1965). However, injection of corticosteroids or dexamethasone did not restore learning capacity to normal, but ACTH analogs lacking endocrine activity were effective (De Wied, 1980). In fact, synthetic steroids can facilitate extinction (Bohus and Lissak, 1968), and ACTH also delayed extinction in adrenalectomized rats (Miller and Ogawa, 1962). Subsequent work has shown that ACTH and ACTH analogs without endocrine activity can prolong extinction of learned responses in both aversively and appetitively motivated tasks (De Wied, 1966, 1969, 1974; Greven and De Wied, 1973; Levine and Jones, 1965; Lissak and Bohus, 1972; Kastin *et al.*, 1973; Guth *et al.*, 1971; Gray, 1971; Garrud *et al.*, 1974; Bohus *et al.*, 1973, 1975a; Rigter and Popping, 1976; Levine *et al.*, 1977; Sandman *et al.*, 1972, 1973a,b, 1974, 1980), but have little effect on the acquisition of learned responses in normal animals (Guth *et al.*, 1971; Bohus *et al.*, 1968; Hennessy *et al.*, 1973; Miller and Caul, 1973). The whole ACTH molecule is not required, since ACTH 4-10 is active (Greven and De Wied, 1973). Indeed, there is significant evidence that the ACTH 4-9, ORG 2766 (H-Met(O)-Glu-His-Phe-D-Lys-Phe-OH), is more potent than the well-studied ACTH analog, ACTH 4-10, that is virtually devoid of endocrine activity (Rigter *et al.*, 1976; Greven and De Wied, 1973). Also, the relationship of the size of the molecule and its effectiveness may be related to the complexity of the task involved. Rats showed an inverse linear relationship between molecular size and improvement in learning in a simple black–white discrimination task but a U-shaped function in a more complex reversal learning task (Sandman *et al.*, 1980a).

ACTH has been implicated in retrieval processes, since systemic administration of ACTH 4-10 prior to retention reversed carbon dioxide-induced amnesia (Rigter and Van Riezen, 1975; Rigter *et al.*, 1974), and ACTH 4-10 administration prior to testing can enhance retrieval in a number of tasks, particularly passive (inhibitory) avoidance (Greven and De Wied, 1973; McGaugh, 1983; de Almeida and Izquierdo, 1984). ACTH has also been shown to be effective when given immediately after the conditioning trial in passive (inhibitory) avoidance (Gold and van Buskirk, 1976). In that study, a U-shaped dose–effect function was observed in a given experiment. Rats treated with 0.03 or 0.3 IU of ACTH showed enhanced performance on the retrieval test 24 hr later, but rats treated with 3.0 IU showed impaired performance (Gold and van Buskirk, 1976).

However, ACTH 4-10 was ineffective in reversing amnesia when injected prior to acquisition in the carbon dioxide amnesia test (Rigter et al., 1974). In a systematic series of tests, Rigter and colleagues established that the threshold for ACTH 4-10 to reverse amnesia was between 0.1 and 1 µg/rat injected subcutaneously, and that ACTH 11-24 was virtually inactive (Rigter et al., 1976).

This enhancement of retrieval and prolongation of extinction has been interpreted in several different ways but generally is interpreted as an effect on attentional processes (De Wied, 1974) or as "temporary increases in the motivational significance of environmental cues" (De Wied, 1980); others have suggested that ACTH produces "a more general change in the ability of an animal to alter its behavior in response to unpredictable changes in reinforcement contingencies" (Gray and Garrud, 1977); or that ACTH produces "enhanced fear-motivated responding" (Weiss et al., 1969) or that "ACTH improves selective attention" (Sandman et al., 1981). Indeed, there are reports of increases in emotionality with ACTH 4-10 administration (File, 1978, 1979).

An extensive series of studies has been performed with human subjects using ACTH 4-10 and ACTH analogs (usually ORG 2766), and although improvements in performance have been observed, there is little evidence to support a direct effect on learning or memory processes (Gaillard, 1981). ACTH 4-10 has been shown to improve pattern discrimination (Sandman et al., 1977) and to increase performance in a visual retention test (Miller et al., 1974; Sandman et al., 1975). Others have observed improvements in reaction time of motor performance in a continuous skill-learning task with ACTH 4-10 and ORG 2766, but this improvement was restricted largely to the slow reaction time associated with fatigue and lapses of attention (Miller et al., 1976; Gaillard and Sanders, 1975; Gaillard and Varey, 1979). Similar changes in retention time have been observed in cognitively impaired elderly subjects (Ferris et al., 1976; Branconnier et al., 1979).

The results with ACTH analogs in more cognitive tasks are not so consistent. In a series of studies, Sandman and co-workers have obtained improvements in learning in mentally retarded subjects with ACTH 4-10 (Sandman et al., 1976, 1981; Walker and Sandman, 1979). These included improvements in learning intradimensional and extradimensional shifts, visual retention, spatial localization, and matching auditory patterns. However, others have reported inconsistent results (Ferris et al., 1976; Gaillard and Varey, 1979; see Gaillard, 1981), and Sandman and co-workers regard their effects as an ACTH-induced improvement in selective attention rather than an increase in learning capacity. The results of studies of short-term and long-term memory in humans with ACTH have been largely negative (Gaillard, 1981). In summary, ACTH analogs appear to have their most pronounced beneficial effects on long duration tasks, and these data indicate that ACTH is most likely to improve performance in situations of fatigue or distraction and to help a subject maintain task concentration. Thus, the hypotheses derived from the human studies regarding the psychological processes mediating the behavioral effects of ACTH are not unlike those derived from the animal studies with ACTH.

However, an even more difficult question centers on the site and physiological mechanism of action of these behavioral effects. One hypothesis has been that ACTH acts directly on some neural substrate in the brain, even after peripheral injection. Indeed, consistent with this hypothesis is the observation that intracerebral injection of ACTH 4-10 into the parafascicular nucleus of the thalamus can also prolong extinction of active avoidance (van Wimersma Greidanus and De Wied, 1971), and lesions of this region (the amygdala, the septum, and the dorsal hippocampus) can block the delay in extinction produced by peripherally administered ACTH analogs (Bohus and De Wied, 1967; van Wimersma Greidanus *et al.*, 1975, 1979; van Wimersma Greidanus and De Wied, 1976*a*). Also, there is at least one report that a potent ACTH analog can pass the blood–brain barrier in low concentrations (Verhoef and Witter, 1976) (see Section 5.5 for more discussion of this general question of peptides entering the CNS). Consistent with this hypothesis is the observation that 100 times less ACTH 4-10 is needed to prolong extinction after i.c.v. administration (De Wied *et al.*, 1978*a*).

The alternative hypothesis that ACTH produces its action through some peripheral mechanism has been suggested by some authors (de Almeida and Izquierdo, 1984) who found central injections to be ineffective. However, little evidence exists to show where or how such an action takes place, particularly since the ACTH analogs ACTH 4-10 and ORG 2766 have markedly reduced adrenocorticotropic activity. Thus, in the absence of a definitive adrenal link, any hypotheses regarding a peripheral action for ACTH face the same problem as that for central hypothesis: i.e., identification of a receptor or an endogenous substrate or both.

3.4. Endorphins

The effects of opioid peptides on learning and memory can easily be related to the classic effects of opiates on pain perception (analgesia) and on changes in "mood" (hedonic actions), particularly since most memory tasks imploy aversive events as the unconditioned stimulus. Morphine injected pretest or posttraining disrupts learning and performance of conditioned avoidance responses (see Koob and Bloom, 1983). Morphine also produces significant retrograde amnesia in passive avoidance (Messing *et al.*, 1981). Similar effects have been observed with opioid peptides injected directly into the CNS, where they are known to have an opiatelike action (Lucion *et al.*, 1982).

Naloxone, the opiate antagonist, facilitates memory, as one would predict if endogenous opioid peptides have a role in memory. Naloxone facilitated performance with pre- and posttraining injection s.c. in active and passive avoidance (Messing et al., 1979, 1981; Gallagher, 1982) or posttraining injection directly into the amygdala (Gallagher and Kapp, 1978). Other researchers have demonstrated facilitatory effects of naloxone injected posttraining in shuttle box avoidance behavior (Izquierdo, 1979), habituation (Izquierdo, 1980a), shock-induced fighting (Tazi et al., 1983), and schedule-induced polydipsia (Tazi et al., 1984). Much more compelling has been evidence showing that naloxone injected posttraining can facilitate subsequent retention in a appetitively motivated task (Gallagher et al., 1983). These studies regarding central sites of action for endogenous opioid peptides and the peripheral administration of drugs known to interact with them are straightforward and logical; however, the data regarding peripheral administration of microgram quantities of rapidly inactivated opioid peptides are much more complicated.

Opioid peptides (methionine and leucine enkephalin) injected intraperitoneally (i.p.) immediately before acquisition of active avoidance impaired acquisition of an active avoidance task, but produced no effect when injected 15 min before training (Rigter et al., 1980a,b). Others have observed impairment in retention of shuttlebox avoidance with leucine enkephalin and β-endorphin given intraperitoneally immediately posttraining (Izquierdo, 1980a,b; Izquierdo et al., 1980a,b,c; Martinez and Rigter, 1980). Similar results were observed with methionine enkephalin and des-try-methionine enkephalin (Izquierdo et al., 1980c; Izquierdo and Dias, 1981). This facilitatory effect of opioid peptides was dose dependent, describing an inverted U-shaped curve when moderate doses caused "amnesia," but lower and higher doses were ineffective (Martinez and Rigter, 1980; Izquierdo, 1980b; Izquierdo et al., 1980a,b).

In contrast to these results, other researchers have observed exactly opposite results with opioid peptides injected during extinction of active avoidance (De Wied et al., 1978a,b; Koob et al., 1981a; Le Moal et al., 1979) or injected 1 hr prior to retention of passive avoidance (Koob et al., 1981b; Kovacs and De Wied, 1981). Also, similar 1-hr pretreatment with opioid peptides attenuates amnesia produced by carbon dioxide (Rigter et al., 1977; Rigter, 1978). Curiously, however, certain analogs of β-endorphins, such as γ-endorphin and des-tyrosine γ-endorphin, facilitated extinction of active avoidance or disrupted passive avoidance when injected 1 hr prior to testing (De Wied et al., 1978a, 1980; Koob et al., 1981a; Kovacs et al., 1981b). Clearly, the time course of injection relative to training and testing protocols appears critical in determining the direction of the observed change in peripherally administered endorphins on memory. Indeed, the complete reversal of effects by changing one amino acid (γ- versus α-endorphin, see De Wied et al., 1978a,b) suggests that some metabolism following injection could play a role in modifying any initial effects of an endorphin release. Also, this may form one basis for the ubiquitous U-shaped dose–response relationships observed with these peptide/memory interactions.

Evidence that suggests a peripheral site of action for the memory effects of opioid peptides comes from a series of studies by Martinez and colleagues. Leucine enkephalin administered shortly before training impairs acquisition of avoidance tasks in rats and mice (Rigter et al., 1980a,b, 1981; Martinez and Rigter, 1982; Martinez et al., 1981, 1984b). These effects could be reversed by adrenal demedullation (Martinez and Rigter, 1982), nor were these effects observed with central administration of leucine enkephalin (Martinez et al., 1985). Also, administration of methyl naloxonium, a quarternary derivative of naloxone that does not cross the blood–brain barrier, or leucine enkephalin antiserum, enhanced acquisition of avoidance and escape learning when injected intraperitoneally in mice (Martinez et al., 1984a). These studies together suggest that peripheral leucine enkephalin systems are, in some way, part of an endogenous modulation of memory function.

3.5. Somatostatin

A hypothalamic pituitary peptide that inhibits the release of growth hormone was first isolated by Brazeau and colleagues (1973) and named somatostatin. This tetradecapeptide has potent physiological effects in inhibiting growth hormone release from the pituitary (Vale et al., 1975). Somatostatin is found in high concentrations in the basal hypothalamus but also has been found extrahypothalamically in the CNS. In fact, it is estimated that 90% of the somatostatin of the brain is found outside the hypothalamus (see Emson, 1979). Immunohistochemical studies show somatostatin-positive neurons in such regions as the amygdala, midbrain, neocortex, and hippocampus. Terminals have been seen in the extrapyramidal system as well as the cortex, amygdala, and spinal cord (see Emson, 1979).

Somatostatin also has behavioral actions when injected directly into the brain. In rats, somatostatin injected into the amygdala increases motor activation (Rezek et al., 1977) and scratching behavior (Dobry et al., 1981). Somatostatin also induced barrel rotation (Cohn and Cohn, 1975) and prolonged pentobarbital sleeping time (Brown and Vale, 1975) and decreased self-stimulation behavior (Vecsei et al., 1982).

Somatostatin also has effects on learned behavior. Somatostatin injected i.c.v. delayed extinction of active avoidance (Bollok et al., 1983; Vecsei et al., 1983a) and also attenuated electroconvulsive shock-induced amnesia in rats (Vecsei et al., 1983b, 1984). Interestingly, this antiamnesia effect and the prolongation of active avoidance by somatostatin can be blocked by phenoxybenzamine, the α-adrenergic antagonist, suggesting a role for central noradrenergic mechanisms in the antiamnesic effect (Vecsei *et al.*, 1983a, 1984).

Somatostatin brain levels have been shown to decrease dramatically in patients with senile dementia of the Alzheimer's type (Davies *et al.*, 1980; Rossor *et al.*, 1980), but to date no dramatic link has been found between somatostatin and learning in aged subjects. In one study in primates, somatostatin injected s.c. had no systematic effects on a delayed-response procedure (Bartus *et al.*, 1982). Somatostatin improved performance at only one dose (0.1 mg/kg) in one of three aged cebus monkeys.

4. NONHYPOPHYSEAL PEPTIDES AND MEMORY

4.1. Neurotensin

Neurotensin, a tridecapeptide with vasoactive properties, was originally characterized by Carraway and Leeman (1973). Neurotensin is found in high concentration in the gastrointestinal system, and when administered systemically, it produces a marked hyperglycemia and inhibits gastric acid secretion (see Nemeroff *et al.*, 1983).

Neurotensin is also found in the CNS, with the highest concentrations in the hypothalamus (35% of total neurotensin in the brain), but significant amounts have also been found in the midbrain, brain stem, cortex, and extrapyramidal system (see Emson, 1979; Nemeroff *et al.*, 1983). High concentrations of neurotensin as measured by radioimmunoassay have been reported in such extrahypothalamic structures as the nucleus accumbens, septum, amygdala, and interpeduncular region (Kobayashi *et al.*, 1977).

Neurotensin injected directly into the CNS produces a variety of behavioral effects, including decreases in locomotor behavior, decreases in food intake, decreases in active avoidance behavior, and potentiation of the sedative properties of barbiturates and ethanol (see Nemeroff *et al.*, 1983). These effects are similar to some of the actions of antipsychotic drugs, and neurotensin has been proposed as a possible endogenous modulator of central dopamine function (Nemeroff, 1980).

The effects of neurotensin in learning situations are somewhat inconsistent. Neurotensin injected i.c.v. in rats previously trained (90% correct) in a two-way active avoidance task significantly decreased avoidance responding but failed to alter escape behavior (Luttinger *et al.*, 1982). However, others have observed a prolongation of extinction of one-way active avoidance with similar doses injected i.c.v. during extinction, and an increase in passive avoidance latencies with similar doses injected i.c.v. immediately posttraining or preretention (van Wimersma Greidanus et al., 1982). The basis for this difference is not clear at this time but may be related to the response requirements in the two tasks and the earlier observations that neurotensin is potent in reducing the activation induced by stimulant drugs (Nemeroff et al., 1983).

4.2. Angiotensin

Angiotensin II (A-II), an octapeptide, is derived from plasma angiotensinogen via an action of renin and angiotensin converting enzyme. It has potent physiological and behavioral effects when injected systemically, increasing blood pressure and drinking behavior (see Prange et al., 1978). Angiotensin-immunoreactive neurons have been demonstrated in the hypothalamus, and immunoreactive terminals have been reported in the periventricular gray, median eminence, the region surrounding the locus ceruleus, amygdala, brain stem, and spinal cord (Emson, 1979). All the metabolic aspects of the renin–angiotensin system appear to be present in the brain, with the highest concentrations of angiotensin converting enzyme being found in the striatum (Roth et al., 1975).

A few studies have implicated brain angiotensin in learning and memory. A-II (0.1–1 µg) injected directly into the neostriatum immediately after training in passive avoidance disrupted retention 24 hr later (Morgan and Routtenberg, 1977). In another study, i.c.v. administration of renin, which produces low amounts of A-II in CSF, also disrupted passive avoidance (Koller et al., 1979). In a more recent study using shuttle box avoidance, angiotensin injected i.c.v. at higher doses facilitated acquisition, but failed to alter extinction (Baranowska et al., 1983). Curiously, [SAR 1, IIe 8]-angiotensin, a specific A-II antagonist, produced a facilitatory effect similar to that of angiotensin and failed to reverse the effects of angiotensin. These studies suggest that the effects of angiotensin on learning may depend on dose, and further work will be required to determine whether high dose effects are specific to an action on angiotensin receptors.

4.3. Cholecystokinin

Cholecystokinin (CCK) is a 33-amino-acid peptide that was originally isolated from the gut. The C-terminal octapeptide, CCK-8, appears to possess the full biological activity of the parent compound. Systemically administered CCK produces a contraction of the gallbladder and stimulates insulin and glucagon secretion (Frame et al., 1975).

CCK is also found in the CNS predominantly in the form of CCK-8. CCK-8 is found in significant amounts in forebrain areas, particularly in the cerebral cortex (Emson, 1979), and appears to coexist with dopamine in a subpopulation of dopaminergic neurons within the mesolimbic system (Hokfelt et al., 1980).

CCK has been reported to have numerous behavioral actions, most notably decreasing food intake when injected systematically (Gibbs et al., 1973). It has also been proposed as a satiety signal (Gibbs et al., 1973), but this interpretation for the antifeeding action is controversial (Deutsch and Hardy, 1977). Other effects of CCK include analgesic, sedative, anticonvulsant, and antipsychoticlike (see Zetler, 1981).

CCK also affects learning and memory. Both cholecystokinin octapeptide sulfate ester (CCK-8-SE) and the nonsulfated cholecystokinin octapeptide (CCK-8-NS), injected intraperitoneally (i.p.), improved performance in passive avoidance (Fekete et al., 1981a); i.c.v. administration of cholecystokinin antiserum had the opposite effects (Fekete et al., 1981b). Similar results were obtained for CCK-8-SE and CCK-8-NS injected i.c.v. either pretraining, posttraining, or preretention (Kadar et al., 1981). Doses here ranged from fmole to pmole. Opposite effects were obtained upon i.c.v. administration of CCK-8-SE and CCK-8-NS in one-way active avoidance, in which CCK-8 impaired acquisition and facilitated extinction (Fekete et al., 1981c). CCK-8-SE administered systemically (i.p.) also attenuated performance of two-way active avoidance and facilitated extinction in doses of 160–3840 µg/kg (Cohen et al., 1982). CCK-8-SE also possesses significant sedative and antipsychoticlike activity (Cohen et al., 1982; Schneider et al., 1983; Vaccarino and Koob, 1984), suggesting that the effects observed on passive avoidance described earlier may be secondary to these motivational/motor actions.

4.4. Substance P

Substance P was originally identified in the gut and the brain as a substance with potent hypotensive properties (Von Euler and Gaddum, 1931). It was subsequently identified as a unadecapeptide (Chang and Leeman, 1970), with numerous nonneural actions, such as producing hypotension, stimulating histamine release, producing smooth muscle contraction, and inducing the production of saliva (see Prange et al., 1978). Substance P has subsequently been mapped in the CNS and appears to be localized in primary sensory neurons, the hypothalamus, caudate nucleus, bed nucleus of the stria terminals, and amygdala and in various regions of the midbrain and the pons, notably the periaqueductal central gray (Emson, 1979). Much physiological data have been generated to suggest that substance P is an excitatory neurotransmitter in a variety of physiological pathways, in addition to the originally proposed primary sensory neurons (Emson, 1979).

Substance P injected either systemically or directly into the CNS produces analgesia (Frederickson *et al.*, 1978; Stewart *et al.*, 1976). Substance P also increases locomotor behavior, when injected centrally (Kelley and Iversen, 1979; Stinus *et al.*, 1978), and induces grooming (Katz, 1979). Injected systemically, substance P decreases spontaneous activity and blocks amphetamine activity (Starr *et al.*, 1978).

The effects of substance P on learning and memory are equally difficult to categorize simply. Substance P injected into the substantia nigra or the amygdala immediately posttraining in passive avoidance impairs retention (Huston and Staubli, 1978, 1979). However, injections into the lateral hypothalamus or septum facilitate retention of passive avoidance (Staubli and Huston, 1979, 1980). As elaborated by these investigators, this pattern of response parallels the response observed from direct electrical stimulation of the brain. Other work with peripheral injections (s.c.) in mice has shown that posttrial administration of substance P facilitated retention of passive avoidance and increased resistance to extinction in an active avoidance task when injected before or after training (Schlesinger *et al.*, 1983*a*). Subcutaneous posttrial injection of substance P in mice also reversed the amnestic effects of both electroconvulsive shock and cycloheximide (Schlesinger *et al.*, 1983*b*). Substance P injected i.p. in rats restored the avoidance deficit usually observed in spontaneously hypertensive rats (Hecht *et al.*, 1982) and significantly improved retention of a footshock-motivated brightness discrimination task after pre- and posttraining injection (Wetzel and Matthies, 1982).

Finally, it appears that N-terminal and C-terminal fragments of substance P can have different effects on behavior. The N-terminal SP(1-7) reduced fighting and decreased grooming behavior when injected i.p. (Hall and Stewart, 1982); however, pyroglutamyl SP(7-11) had opposite effects (Hall and Stewart, 1982). In a recent study, similar differences were observed in passive avoidance retention following injection of substance P analogs in picogram amounts into the nucleus accumbens (Gaffori *et al.*, 1984). Substance P(1-11) and the C-terminal fragment pyroglutamyl SP(7-11) attenuated passive avoidance retention when injected 1 hr prior to retention, but the N-terminal fragment SP(1-7) had the opposite effect and facilitated passive avoidance behavior. These results with substance P suggest that its action on learning and memory may be determined not only by the anatomical location of the substance P receptors in the central nervous system but also by how the substance P molecule is biotransformed. The possibility that peripherally administered substance

P accesses CNS sites directly adds yet another dimension. These three factors—anatomical site of action, relative access to the central nervous system, and the active site or sites within the peptide molecule—may be common factors important for determining functional significance of all the peptides discussed earlier.

5. SYNTHESIS

5.1. Hypophyseal Peptides—Summary

This chapter has considered the possible role of both hypophyseal and nonhypophyseal peptides in the neurobiology of memory. The hypophyseal peptides (vasopressin, oxytocin, ACTH, endorphins, and somatostatin) are all produced by the pituitary, and thus have clearly identifiable hormonal roles. The are also found in the CNS outside the hypothalamic pituitary system, where they have been hypothesized to have a neurotropic function. Their role in memory processing has largely been deduced from studies of exogenously administered peptide or, in some cases, by the use of antagonists or antisera. Vasopressin, ACTH and somatostatin, in general, facilitate memory, whereas endorphins and oxytocin, in general, impair memory (see Table 2). With all these peptides, systemic as well as central administration is effective, although the doses employed with systemic injections are usually much greater than those used with

TABLE 2
Memory Effects of Neuropeptides

Neuropeptide	Summary of effects on "memory"
Hypophyseal hormones	
Vasopressin	Facilitation
Oxytocin	Inhibition
Leucine-enkephalin	Inhibition
Methionine-enkephalin	Inhibition
β-endorphin	Inhibition
Adrenocorticotropic (human ACTH 1-39)	Facilitation
$ACTH_{4-10}$	Facilitation
ORG 2766	Facilitation
Somatostatin	Facilitation
Nonhypophyseal hormones	
Substance P	Inhibition
Neurotensin	Inhibition
Angiotensin II	Inhibition
Cholecystokinin octapeptide (CCK-8)	Inhibition

direct intracerebroventricular or intracerebral injections. However, controversy exists as to the ability of these peptides to cross readily the blood–brain barrier, calling into question the site and mechanism of action for these memory effects of systemically administered peptide (see Section 5.5).

5.2. Nonhypophyseal Peptides—Summary

These peptides are found generally in both the gut and the brain and have a variety of physiological actions, upon systemic administration, that appear unrelated per se to any specific memory action. Their action on memory varies considerably with dose and site of administration within the CNS. Neurotensin, angiotensin, cholecystokinin, and substance P, all at some doses or injection sites, disrupt memory when injected directly into the CNS. However, other researchers have observed a facilitation of memory in certain tests with neurotensin, at higher doses of angiotensin, in certain tests with cholecystokinin, and at certain sites or routes of administration with substance P. The basis for this diversity of action is not clear at this time and may simply reflect the paucity of information available. With some of these peptides (cholecystokinin and substance P), peripheral injections were effective, but in the case of substance P, systemic injections produced effects opposite to those observed following injection into many CNS sites.

5.3. Site and Mechanism of Action

The argument for a simple central site of action for peptides is usually based on the previously mentioned difference in potency of the peptide centrally versus peripherally and on the observation that endocrinologically inactive analogs are still active in altering behavior. Still unexplained, however, is how even these analogs penetrate to an active site in the CNS, and, perhaps more important, whether such analogs are ever formed naturally or interact with the same receptor as the parent compound. And if peripherally derived peptides do act directly in the CNS, the question remains as to how these peripheral sources modulate the normal CNS activity of neurons containing these peptides.

The mechanism of action of these peptides is largely unknown. Even if the most extensively studied peptides vasopressin and ACTH are used as examples, the picture is less than clear. Vasopressin has been hypothesized to act directly in the CNS through noradrenergic mechanisms. Even if this hypothesis were correct, the role of noradrenergic systems themselves in memory function is controversial. In a recent excellent review, Sahgal (1984) discusses in depth the vasopressin memory hypothesis and concludes that its central action may involve arousal mechanisms but that peripheral administration may be aversive. This is similar to our view that AVP may produce behavioral effects via separate, but possibly homologous mechanisms, a central neurotropic action and a peripheral hormonal action (Koob et al., 1985). In this view, the peripheral visceral signals produced by peripherally acting vasopressin may mimic the signals occurring naturally during learning of aversive contingencies (Koob et al., 1985). The mechanism and substrate for the central actions remain to be determined.

For ACTH, the site and mechanism of action are even less well defined. There is substantial evidence to suggest that ACTH and ACTH analogs devoid of endocrinological activity have behavioral actions variously described as a facilitation of "attentional processes" (see Section 3.3). There is some evidence for the presence of immunoreactive ACTH in the CNS (Krieger et al., 1977), but some controversy as to whether the antibodies in these studies are actually measuring ACTH (Bayon et al., 1983). A few lesion studies have suggested a central action for ACTH in limbic midbrain structures (De Wied et al., 1975b). However, firm evidence for the penetration of these peptides into the CNS and evidence for ACTH receptors and/or neurons would go far toward elucidating an important role for this peptide.

5.4. U-Shaped Dose–Effect Functions

A ubiquitous characteristic of dose–effect relationships in behavioral pharmacology and, in particular, in the behavioral pharmacology of peptides is the U-shaped function. Typically, peptides alter memory measures in a dose-dependent monotonic function up to some optimum dose, and then the effectiveness of the peptide declines in a similar monotonic function with ever-increasing doses. The basis for this phenomenon is not obvious, although several different hypotheses can be considered, none of which are necessarily exclusive.

First, with natural peptides that have clear physiological effects, such as vasopressin, when high doses greatly increase blood pressure, one could easily consider the descending part of the dose–effect curve as a nonspecific effect superimposed upon the normal facilitatory effect of AVP acting on a memory substrate. However, in many cases U-shaped functions are evident even after peripheral injections of very small amounts of what appear to be endocrinologically inert analogs of neuropeptides (see Sections 3.3 and 3.4). Clearly, other explanations are necessary. Another behavioral explanation centers on the relationship between performance and arousal, which is classically also a U-shaped function. Here, poor performance is observed at low levels of arousal and at very high states of arousal. The best performance is generated at some optimal arousal state in between. For a recent discussion of this point with regard to vasopressin, see Sahgal (1984). However, this explanation begs the question of the actual mechanism by which these peptides alter memory processes (see Section 5.6).

The more physiological explanations for these U-shaped functions include such cellular phenomena as recurrent inhibition. One could imagine, in a given receptor system, that a super excess of transmitter available might ultimately shut off transmission as inhibition from recurrent collaterals increased, to produce, ultimately, a mixed or opposite effect on behavior. Evidence for this type of response may be forthcoming upon the identification of neurochemically specific synapses. An alternative explanation, which to some extent includes the first hypothesis given above, is that of multiple sites of action for the same neuropeptide. Low doses may act at certain sites with receptors of high affinity or high accessibility to exogenously administered peptides, whereas high doses may access low-affinity receptors or distant sites that produce opposite effects. Certainly, the evidence for dramatically opposite effects with substance P injected intracerebrally at different sites supports this kind of hypothesis.

These U-shaped functions thus not only have important implications for the physiological mechanism of action for the memory-altering effects of neuropeptides, they also have important implications for future clinical applications. Their ubiquitousness clearly limits the interpretability of single-dose studies. Finally, they may provide important clues as to the very behavioral nature of these neuropeptide effects.

5.5. Blood–Brain Barrier

Whether the neuropeptides discussed in this chapter cross the blood–brain barrier is very controversial. In the case of most of the hypophyseal peptides, memory effects have been observed following both central and peripheral administration. Yet, most of the data in the literature support a negative conclusion (Pardridge, 1983); i.e., the permeability of the blood–brain barrier to peptides is low and not significantly different from that for other putative transmitters in the circulation. Those studies that do purport to show extraction into the brain from systemic injection either use very high concentrations or report first-pass extraction of only 1–2%. For example, intravenous infusions of oxytocin and vasopressin do not raise CSF levels of these peptides except when very high doses are injected (Wood, 1982), and the first-pass extraction of enkephalins or thyrotropin-releasing hormone is only 1–2%, similar to that for monoamines (Olendorf, 1974).

The ability of a neuropeptide molecule in the plasma to penetrate into the brain is a function of either its lipid solubility or the presence of a specific transport system. Since most peptides, with the exception of some new analogs, such as the vasopressin antagonist peptides (see Section 3.1), are not lipophilic, it is unlikely that this could be a possible mechanism. The apparent lack of an identifiable carrier transport mechanism (Zaidi and Heller, 1974; Pardridge, 1983) makes it unclear as to how even 1–2% brain extraction can occur. One possibility is that the peptides gain access to the CNS via circumventricular organs for which the blood–brain barrier is significantly reduced. Further work will be necessary to support this hypothesis and to determine whether such a mechanism could explain the behavioral effects of systemically administered peptides.

5.6. Is It Memory?

The role of neuropeptides in learning and memory is as difficult to define at this stage as the role of drugs and other more classic neurotransmitters (Zornetzer, 1978; Heise, 1981). Clearly, these neuropeptides have significant effects on the retention of learned behavior, most notably retention of active and/or passive (inhibitory) avoidance. However, as noted by Heise (1981) referring to a point raised by Weissman (1967), there is no "comparison standard" by which to validate a role for peptides in "memory." Heise argues strongly for more research into this essential problem, research that would benefit any putative role for peptides as well as drugs in general.

Neuropeptide studies have met some of the major criteria for considering a substance as critically involved in memory [see Squire and Davis (1981) and Table 3]. In general, the facilitation or disruption observed

TABLE 3
Criteria Useful in Considering Whether a Particular Brain System Is Critically Involved in Memory Modulation[a]

A. Drugs affecting the brain system should be time and dose dependent
B. Facilitation as well as disruption of memory should occur with appropriate manipulation of the system
C. Removal of the system should affect memory
D. There should be a correlation between learning and some measure of physiological or neurochemical activity of the system
E. Effects of manipulating the system should be obtainable across a variety of tasks, not just aversive or appetitive tasks or tasks requiring movement

[a]Taken from Squire and Davis, 1981.

varies inversely with the time elapsed between training and drug administration. There is dose dependency. There also is some evidence for a few of the peptides that removal of the system will affect memory, such as with the use of antisera or peptide antagonists. No lesion studies *specific* to a given neuropeptide system have been performed to date. The fourth criterion of Table 3, that there should be some correlation between learning and some measure of physiological or neurochemical activity of the system, is only now being explored with the advent of more sensitive and specific neuropeptide assays. This is an area of important future growth. Finally, the fifth criterion, of manipulating the system across a variety of tasks, is only now being explored.

In general, studies of the effects of neuropeptides on anything but aversive tasks have been limited. Recent work has shown significant effects with neurohypophyseal peptides on appetitively motivated tasks, i.e., naloxone effects in radial arm maze, vasopressin effects in a water-finding task and appetitive discriminations, and ACTH effects on extinction of appetitively motivated behavior. Nevertheless, there are many reports of negative results with appetitive tasks (for vasopressin see Sahgal, 1984), and the overall picture is largely of numerous peptides altering passive (inhibitory) avoidance behavior.

As discussed extensively by others (Heise, 1981; Sahgal, 1984), the interpretation of results from avoidance tasks is difficult at best. Shock as an unconditioned stimulus has major effects on other behavioral variables, such as motivation and arousal, that can dramatically alter performance. In a series of studies with vasopressin, Sahgal and co-workers found little evidence of a consistent and reliable improvement in passive avoidance in all rats treated with AVP (i.e., no exclusion criteria were used to make the population sample more homogeneous) but instead significant bimodal scores, i.e., scores clustered at the low end of the distribution, where the rats reenter quickly, or scores clustered at the high end (scores in excess of 300s) (Sahgal et al., 1982; Sahgal and Wright, 1983) (see also Lebrun et al., 1984, for similar results). These authors suggest that AVP acts on the inverted U-shaped relationship where poor performance is observed if the subject is in a low arousal state; but at very high levels of arousal, performance is impaired. According to this hypothesis, AVP given immediately after the shock trial will increase arousal, and this, in turn, will improve consolidation in underaroused rats but disrupt consolidation in overaroused animals, thus producing the bimodal distribution described above (Sahgal and Wright, 1983). This motivational hypothesis of Sahgal and associates may point to a possible explanation for many of the previously reported effects of AVP, including those reported for appetitive tasks.

In addition, as discussed by Sahgal (1984) in some detail, tests employing discriminated passive avoidance in which the subject is required to remember which of two distinctly colored boxes delivered the shock showed that treatments such as electroconvulsive shock (Carew, 1970) or neuropeptide administration (Sahgal, 1984) altered reentry latencies appropriately, but did *not* change the correct choice; i.e., the animals remembered normally which box delivered the shock. This, plus the elaborate procedures necessary to observe a facilitation of memory with certain peptides (Rigter, 1982), calls into question exactly what behavioral constructs are being measured by passive (inhibitory) avoidance. However, perhaps of equal importance is to turn the question around and ask exactly what is a rat learning in such a task and how sensitive is that learning to alteration? Obviously, there is a definite need to develop and utilize other animal memory paradigms, including some of those used in neuropsychology, such as delayed response and delayed matching to sample. It also would be of some interest to use more species-specific tasks, such as olfactory discriminations in rats.

Thus, the answer to the question "Is it memory?" is for the moment probably "no" or at least "too early to tell." The ubiquitousness of the alterations in passive avoidance (nearly all neuropeptides have some effect), the conceptual problems discussed earlier, and previously established mobilization of many of these neuropeptides with stress suggest to this writer that more motivational variables should be considered.

5.7. James–Lange Theory of Memory

A motivational analysis of neuropeptide effects on memory has been proposed by Gold and McGaugh (1977) and elaborated by Martinez (1985). James and Lange postulated that an emotional experience is the result of the biological changes that follow an environmental event and that the feeling of these same changes *is* the emotion (James, 1961). The extrapolation of this theory to memory would simply be that memory of an environmental event is the result of the biological changes that follow such an event. A corollary of this view is that the representation of the experience remains labile for a period of time during which the biological changes (including, presumably, modulatory neuropeptides) can affect this experience. This forms the basis for the first criteria elaborated in Table 3 of a time-dependent treatment effect, and considerable evidence supports such a proposition (Martinez, 1985). A further corollary of this position is that factors of the training situations, such as the strength of unconditioned stimulus (usually shock), may determine whether a modulatory neuropeptide will enhance or impair retention performance. Furthermore, Martinez (1985) has proposed that, following an environmental event, endogenous substances, most likely hormones, will be released that influence learning, and these substances have been labeled *learning modulatory hormones* (McGaugh and Martinez, 1981). The neuropeptides discussed earlier would fall into that category.

5.8. State Dependency

The view cited in Section 5.7 holds that endogenous substances are released following an environmental event that can function to influence learning. How exactly these substances influence learning is not clear. One of the assumptions here, however, is that there is some "memory" system that ultimately can be modulated. A possibly more radical view of the James–Lange theory of memory is that the biological response following an environmental event is made up of a panoply of hormonal/neuropeptide changes that serve to act as discriminative stimuli for the "recall" of that environmental event. Under this scheme, the blood pressure associated with the learning of an avoidance response can be mimicked by addition of a vasopressor neuropeptide, such as vasopressin. Thus, instead of vasopressin actually influencing a "memory" system, vasopressin acts to trigger some of the conditions under which a memory would most likely be recalled.

Whereas this state-dependent hypothesis could easily explain the prolongation of extinction associated with injection *during* extinction or improved retention following injection immediately prior to retention, it does not easily explain the posttraining facilitation of passive (inhibitory) avoidance, an experimental protocol explicitly designed to obviate this problem (Zornetzer, 1978; McGaugh, 1973). Here, one has to postulate that such a state-dependent cue has anterograde actions in that it helps prolong or extend the strength of unconditioned stimulus. Thus, stimulant drugs and "stress" or "arousal" neuropeptides would be expected to facilitate memory, whereas sedative drugs or "stress"-alleviating neuropeptides would be expected to attenuate memory, which indeed appears to be the case. Even more intriguing, however, is the fact that the recent suggestions of a peripheral site of action for some neuropeptides (Martinez, 1985) may involve peripheral visceral cues that act in a "motivational" or state-dependent fashion.

A version of this state-dependency hypothesis has been adopted by Izquierdo and colleagues (Izquierdo *et al.*, 1980*b*) to explain the effects of opioid peptides on learning and memory. The authors hypothesize that there is a CNS physiological, amnesic mechanism mediated by opioid peptides that is triggered by environmental events, and that the action of a given opioid peptide or antagonist administered systemically will depend on the relative state of activity of this central system. The authors use this model to explain why naloxone facilitates memory when injected posttraining and endorphins attenuate memory when injected posttraining, but when given prior to retention, endorphins enhance retrieval (Izquierdo *et al.*, 1980*b*). Problems with these results and the model rest with questions as to whether peripherally administered endorphins actually penetrate the CNS. Thus, it is not clear how peripherally administered endorphins match a state induced by centrally released endorphins. Indeed, the observation that opioid peptides are actually released in the CNS during training needs to be carefully evaluated. Nevertheless, the hypothesis that state dependency to an endogenously released substance occurs with an exogenously administered substance is an intriguing one that merits further exploration.

5.9. Homology of Function

Finally, from a biological perspective it is worth speculating as to whether the function of these neuropeptides in memory may somehow be related to their classic hormonal action. For example, the hypophyseal neuropeptides, all along hypothesized to maintain body homeostasis by the regulation of body organ systems, may also regulate central states in an integrative fashion (Iversen, 1981). One could speculate that opioid peptides have a role in pain perception and in reducing the memory of pain as well. Vasopressin and ACTH may not only mobilize peripheral mechanisms to environmental challenge and stress, but also have a role in the behavioral response to stress. As hypothesized by others, this activating property may be the basis for the role of vasopressin in facilitating memory. Although this homology of function hypothesis is intriguing, the evidence to support such a hypothesis with the nonneurohypophyseal neuropeptides is much more difficult to document, but then the hormonal function for these peptides is also less well defined.

In summary, neuropeptides clearly can modulate learning and memory, and the effects described to date meet some of the criteria for brain systems critically involved in memory modulation. Other criteria have yet to be evaluated. The site and biological mechanism of action for these memory effects are still largely unknown, and controversy still exists as to the relative importance of central versus peripheral mechanisms. Finally, even the proposition of whether these neuropeptides have a true memory-modulating function is being questioned upon experimental, biological, and theoretical grounds. Nevertheless, one cannot help but speculate that knowledge of how these endogenous substances contribute to the retention for future use of the representation of an environmental event may be a key ultimately to the nature of the memory process itself.

6. REFERENCES

ADER, R., and DE WIED, D., 1972, Effects of lysine vasopressin on passive avoidance learning, *Psychon. Sci.* **29**:46–48.

ANDERSON, D. C., WINARD, W., and TAM, T., 1968, Adrenocorticotrophic hormone and acquisition of a passive avoidance response, *J. Comp. Physiol. Psychol.* **66**:497–499.

ANDERSON, L. T., DAVID, R., BONNET, K., and DANCIS, J., 1979, Passive avoidance learning in Lesch–Nyhan disease: Effect of 1-Desamino-8-Arginine-vasopressin, *Life Sci.* **24**:905–910.

APPLEZWEIG, M. H., and BAUDRY, F. D., 1955, The pituitary–adrenocortical system in avoidance learning, *Psychol. Rep.* **1:**417–420.
ASIN, K. E., 1980, Lysine vasopressin attenuation of diethylidithiocarbamate-induced amnesia, *Pharmacol. Biochem. Behav.* **12:**343–46.
Bailey, W. H., and Weiss, J. M., 1979, Evaluation of a 'memory deficit' in vasopressin-deficient rats, *Brain Res.* **162:**174–178.
BANKOWSKI, K., MANNING, M., HALDAR, J., and SAWYER, W. H., 1978, Design of potent antagonists of the vasopressor response to arginine-vasopressin, *J. Med. Chem.* **21:**850–53.
BARANOWSKA, D., BRASZKO, J. J., and WISNIENSKI, K., 1983, Effect of angiotensin II and vasopressin on acquisition and extinction of conditioned avoidance in rats, *Psychopharmacology* **81:** 247–251.
BARTUS, R. T., DEAN, R. G., and BEER, B., 1982, Neuropeptide effects on memory in aged monkeys, *Neurobiol. Aging* **3:**61–68.
BAYON, A., SHOEMAKER, W. J., MCGINTY, J. F., and BLOOM, F., 1983, Immunodetection of endorphins and enkephalins: A search for reliability, *Int. Rev. Neurobiol.* **24:**51–92.
BECKWITH, B. E., PETROS, T., KANAAN-BECKWITH, S., COUK, D. I., and HAUGE, R. J., 1982, Vasopressin analog (DDAVP) facilitates concept learning in human males, *Peptides* **3:**627–630.
BLAKE, D. R., DODD, M. J., and EVANS, J. G., 1978, Vasopressin in amnesia, *Lancet* **1:**608.
BOHUS, B., 1977, Effect of desglycinamide-lysine vasopressin (DG-LVP) on sexually motivated T-maze behavior of the male rat, *Hormones Behav.* **8:**52–61.
BOHUS, B., and DE WIED, D., 1967, Failure of α-MSH to delay extinction of conditioned avoidance behavior in rats with lesions in the parafascicular nuclei of the thalamus, *Physiol. Behav.* **2:**221–223.
BOHUS, B., and LISSAK, K., 1968, Adrenocortical hormones and avoidance behavior in rats, *Int. J. Neuropharmacol.* **7:**301–306.
BOHUS, B., NYAKAS, C. S., and ENDROCZI, E., 1968, Effects of adrenocorticotrophic hormone on avoidance behavior of intact and adrenalectomized rats, *Int. J. Neuropharmacol.* **7:**307–314.
BOHUS, B., Gispen, W. H., and De Wied, D., 1973, Effect of lysine vasopressin and $ACTH_{4-10}$ on conditioned avoidance behavior of hypophysectomized rats, *Neuroendocrinology* **11:**137–143.
BOHUS, B., HENDRIX, H. H. L., VAN KOLFSCHOTEN, A. A., and KREDIET, T. G., 1975a, Effect of $ACTH_{4-10}$ on copulatory and sexually motivated approach behavior in the male rat, in: *Sexual Behavior: Pharmacology and Biochemistry* (M. Sandler and G. L. Gessa, eds.), Raven Press, New York, pp. 269–275.
BOHUS, B., VAN WIMERSMA GREIDANUS, Tj. B., and DE WIED, D., 1975b, Behavioral and endocrine responses of rats with hereditary hypothalamic diabetes insipidus (Brattleboro strain), *Physiol. Behav.* **14:**609–615.
BOHUS, B., URBAN, I., VAN WIMERSMA GREIDANUS, Tj. B., and DE WIED, D., 1978a, Opposite effects of oxytocin and vasopressin on avoidance behavior and hippocampal theta rhythm in the rat, *Neuropharmacology* **17:**239–247.
BOHUS, B., KOVACS, G. L., and DE WIED, D., 1978b, Oxytocin, vasopressin and memory: Opposite effects on consolidation and retrieval processes, *Brain Res.* **157:**414–17.
BOLLOK, I., VECSEI, L., and TELEGDY, G., 1983, The effects of interaction between propranol and somatostatin on the active avoidance behavior, open-field activity and electroconvulsive-shock-induced amnesia of rats, *Neuropeptides* **3:**263–270.
BOOKIN, H. B., and PFEIFER, W. D., 1977, Effect of lysine vasopressin on pentylenetetrazol-induced retrogade amnesia in rats, *Pharmacol. Biochem. Behav.* **7:**51–54.
BRANCONNIER, R. J., COLE, J. O., and GARDOS, G., 1979, $ACTH_{4-10}$ in amelioration of neuropsychological symptomatology associated with senile organic syndrome, *Psychopharmacology* **61:**161–165.

Brazeau, P., Vale, W., Burgus, R., Ling, N., Butcher, M., Rivier, J., and Guillemin, R., 1973, Hypothalamic polypeptide that inhibits the secretion of immunoreactive pituitary growth hormone, *Science* **179:**77–79.

Brito, G. N. O., Thomas, G. J., Gingold, S. I., and Gash, D. M., 1980, Behavioral characteristics of vasopressin-deficient rats (Brattleboro strain), *Brain Res. Bull.* **6:**71–75.

Brown, M., and Vale, W., 1975, Central nervous system effects of hypothalamic peptides, *Endocrinology* **96:**1333–1336.

Burbach, J. P. H., Kovacs, G. L., De Wied, D., van Gispen, J. W., and Greven, H. M., 1983, A major metabolite of arginine vasopressin in the brain is a highly potent neuropeptide, *Science* **221:**1310–1312.

Carew, T. J., 1970, Do passive avoidance tasks permit assessment of retrograde amnesia in rats? *J. Comp. Physiol. Psychol.* **72:**267–271.

Carey, R. J., and Miller, M., 1982, Absence of learning and memory deficits in the vasopressin deficient rat (Brattleboro strain), *Behav. Brain Res.* **6:**1–13.

Carraway, R., and Leeman, S. E., 1973, The isolation of a new hypotensive peptide, neurotensin, from bovine hypothalami, *J. Biol. Chem.* **248:**6854–6861.

Celestian, J. F., Carey, R. J., and Miller, M., 1975, Unimpaired maintenance of a conditioned avoidance response in the rat with diabetes insipidus, *Physiol. Behav.* **15:**707–711.

Chang, M. M., and Leeman, S. E., 1970, Isolation of a gialogic peptide from bovine hypothalamus and its characterization as substance P, *J. Biol. Chem.* **245:**4784–4790.

Chard, T., 1972, The posterior pituitary in human and animal parturition, *J. Reprod. Fertil.* (Suppl 16):121–138.

Cohen, S. L., Knight, M., Tamminga, C. A., and Chase, T. N., 1982, Cholecystokinin-octapeptide effects on conditioned avoidance behavior, stereotype and catalepsy, *Eur. J. Pharmacol.* **83:**213–22.

Cohn, M. L., and Cohn, M., 1975, "Barrel rotation" induced by somatostatin in the nonlesioned rat, *Brain Res.* **96:**138–141.

Davies, P., Katzman, R., and Terry, R. D., 1980, Reduced somatostatin-like immunoreactivity in the cerebral cortex from cases of Alzheimer disease and Alzheimer senile dementia, *Nature* **288:**279–280.

de Almeida, M. A., and Izquierdo, M. R., 1984, Effect of intraperitoneal and intracerebroventricular administration of ACTH, epinephrine, or β-endorphin on retrieval of an inhibitory avoidance task in rats, *Behav. Neural. Biol.* **40:**119–122.

Deutsch, J. A., and Hardy, W. T., 1977, Cholecystokinin produces bait shyness in rats, *Nature* **266:**196.

De Wied, D., 1964, Influence of anterior pituitary on avoidance learning and escape behavior, *Am. J. Physiol.* **207:**255–259.

De Wied, D., 1965, The influence of the posterior and intermediate lobe of the pituitary and pituitary peptides on the maintenance of a conditioned avoidance response in rats, *Int. J. Neuropharmacol.* **4:**157–67.

De Wied, D., 1966, Inhibitory effect of ACTH and related peptides on extinction of conditioned avoidance behavior in rats, *Proc. Soc. Exp. Biol. Med.* **122:**28–32.

De Wied, D., 1969, Effects of peptide hormones on behavior, in: *Frontiers in Neuroendocrinology* (W. E. Ganong and L. Martini, eds.), Oxford University Press, New York/London, pp. 97–140.

De Wied, D., 1971, Long term effect of vasopressin on the maintenance of a conditioned avoidance response in rats, *Nature* **232:**58–60.

De Wied, D., 1974, Pituitary-adrenal system hormones and behavior, in: *The Neurosciences. Third Study Program* (F. G. Schmitt and F. G. Worden, eds.), MIT Press, Cambridge, MA, pp. 653–666.

De Wied, D., 1976, Behavioral effects of intraventricularly administered vasopressin and vasopressin fragments, *Life Sci.* **19:**685–690.

DE WIED, D., 1980, Pituitary-adrenal system hormones and behavior, in: *Selye's Guide to Stress Research,* Vol. 1 (H. Selye, ed.), Van Nostrand Reinhold Co., New York, pp. 252–279.
DE WIED, D., 1984a, The importance of vasopressin in memory, *Trends Neurosci.* **7:**62–64.
DE WIED, D., 1984b, The importance of vasopressin in memory, *Trends Neurosci.* **7:**109.
DE WIED, D., and BOHUS, B., 1979, Modulation of memory processes by neuropeptides of hypothalamic-neurophypophyseal origin, in: *Brain Mechanism in Memory and Learning: From the Single Neuron to Man* (M. A. B. Brazier, ed.), Raven Press, New York, pp. 139–149.
DE WIED, D., and GISPEN, W. H., 1977, Behavioral effects of peptides, in: *Peptides in Neurobiology* (H. Gainer, ed.), Plenum Press, New York, pp. 397–448.
DE WIED, D., BOHUS, B., and VAN WIMERSMA GREIDANUS, Tj. B., 1975a, Memory deficit in rats with hereditary diabetes insipidus, *Brain Res.* **85:**152–156.
DE WIED, D., WITTER, A., and GREVEN, H. M., 1975b, Behaviourally active ACTH analogs, *Biochem. Pharmacol.* **24:**1463–1468.
DE WIED, D., BOHUS, B., VAN REE, J. M., and URBAN, I., 1978a, Behavioral and electrophysiological effects of peptides related to lipotropin (β-LPH), *J. Pharmacol. Exp. Ther.* **204:**570–580.
DE WIED, D., KOVACS, G. L., BOHUS, B., VAN REE, J. M., and GREVEN, H. M., 1978b, Neuroleptic activity of the neuropeptide β-LPH 62–77, *Eur. J. Pharmacol.* **49:**427–436.
DE WIED, D., VAN REE, J. M., and GREVEN, H. M., 1980, Neuroleptic-like activity of peptides related to [Des-Tyr 1] β-endorphin: Structure activity studies, *Life Sci.* **26:**1575–1579.
DE WIED, D., GAFFORI, O., VAN REE, J. M., and DEJONG, W., 1984, Central target for the behavioral effects of vasopressin neuropeptides, *Nature* **305:**276–278.
DEYO, S. N., SHOEMAKER, W. J., ETTENBERG, A., BLOOM, F. E., and KOOB, G. F., 1986, Subcutaneous administration of behaviorally effective doses of arginine vasopressin results in brain uptake in only the median eminence, *Neuroendocrinology* **42:**260–266.
DOBRY, P. J. K., PIERCEY, M. F., and SCHROEDER, L. A., 1981, Pharmacological characterization of scratching behavior induced by intracranial injection of substance P and somatostatin, *Neuropharmacology* **20:**267–272.
EMSON, P. C., 1979, Peptides as neurotransmitter candidates in the mammalian CNS, *Prog. Neurobiol.* 13:61–116.
ETTENBERG, A., 1984, Intracerebroventricular application of a pressor antagonist of vasopressin prevents both the "memory" and "aversive" actions of vasopressin, *Behav. Brain Res.* **14:**201–211.
ETTENBERG, A., LE MOAL, M., KOOB, G. F., and BLOOM, F. E., 1983a, Vasopressin potentiation in performance of a learned appetitive task: Reversal by a pressor antagonist analog of vasopressin, *Pharmacol. Biochem. Behav.* **18:**645–647.
ETTENBERG, A., VAN DER KOOY, D., LE MOAL, M., KOOB, G. F., and BLOOM, F. E. 1983b, Can aversive properties of (peripherally-injected) vasopressin account for its putative role in memory? *Behav. Brain Res.* **7:**331–350.
VON EULER, U. S., and GADDUM, J. H., 1931, An unidentified depressor substance in certain tissue extracts, *J. Physiol. London* **72:**74–87.
FEKETE, M., KADAR, T., PENKE, B., and TELEGDY, G., 1981a, Modulation of passive avoidance behaviour by cholecystokinin octapeptides in rats, *Neuropeptides* **1:**301–304.
FEKETE, M., LONOVICS, J., and TELEGDY, G., 1981b, Modulation of passive avoidance behaviour of rats by intracerebroventricular administration of cholecystokinin antiserum, *Neuropeptides* **1:**363–369.
FEKETE, M., SZABO, A., BALAZO, M., and TELEGDY, G., 1981c, Effects of intraventricular administration of cholecystokinin octapeptide sulfate ester and unsulfated cholecystokinin octapeptide on active avoidance and conditioned feeding behaviour of rats, *Acta Physiol. Acad. Sci. Hung.* **58:**39.

FERRIS, S. H., SATHANATHAN, G., GERSHON, S., CLARK, C., and MOSKINSKY, J., 1976, Cognitive effects of ACTH$_{4-10}$ in the elderly, *Pharmacol. Biochem. Behav.* **5**:73–78.
FEWTRELL, W. D., HOUSE, A. O., JAMIE, P. F., OATES, M. R., and COOPER, J. E., 1982, Effects of vasopressin on memory and new learning in a brain-injured population, *Psychol. Med.* **12**:423–425.
FILE, S. E., 1978, ACTH but not corticosterone impairs habituation and reduces exploration, *Pharmacol. Biochem. Behav.* **9**:161–166.
FILE, S., 1979, Effects of ACTH$_{4-10}$ in the social interaction test of anxiety, *Brain Res.* **171**:157–160.
FRAME, C. M., DAVIDSON, M. B., and STURDEVANT, R. A. L., 1975, Effects of the octapeptide of cholecystokinin on insulin and glucagon secretion in the dog, *Endocrinology* **97**:549–553.
FREDERICKSON, R. C. A., BURGIS, V., HARRELL, C. E., and EDWARDS, J. D., 1978, Dual action of substance P on nociception: Possible role of endogenous opioids, *Science* **199**:1359–1362.
GAFFORI, O., STEWART, J. M., and DE WIED, D., 1984, Influence of substance P and fragments on passive avoidance behavior, *Experientia* **40**:89–91.
GAILLARD, A. W. K., 1981, ACTH analogs and human performance, in: *Endogenous Peptides and Learning and Memory Processes* (J. L. Martinez, Jr., R. A. Jensen, R. B. Messing, H. Rigter, and J. L. McGaugh, eds.), Academic Press, New York, pp. 181–196.
GAILLARD, A. W. K., and SANDERS, A. F., 1975, Some effects of ACTH$_{4-10}$ on performance during a serial reaction task, *Psychopharmacologia* **42**:201–208.
GAILLARD, A. W. K., and VAREY, C. A., 1979, Some effects of an ACTH$_{4-10}$ analog (ORG 2766) on human performance, *Physiol. Behav.* **23**:79–84.
GALLAGHER, M., 1982, Naloxone enhancement of memory processes, effects of other opiate antagonists, *Behav. Neural. Biol.* **35**:375–382.
GALLAGHER, M., and KAPP, B. S., 1978, Manipulation of opiate activity in the amygdala alters memory processes, *Life Sci.* **23**:1973–1978.
GALLAGHER, M., KING, R. A., and YOUNG, N. B., 1983, Opiate antagonists improve spatial memory, *Science* **221**:975–976.
GARRUD, P., GRAY, J. A., and DE WIED, D., 1974, Pituitary-adrenal hormones and extinction of rewarded behavior in the rat, *Physiol. Behav.* **12**:109–119.
GASH, D. M., and THOMAS, G. J., 1983, What is the importance of vasopressin in memory processes? *Trends Neurosci.* **6**:197–198.
GASH, D. M., and THOMAS, G. J., 1984, Reply from Don M. Gash and Garth J. Thomas, *Trends Neurosci.* **7**:64–65.
GIBBS, J., YOUNG, R. C., and SMITH, G. P., 1973, Cholecystokinin elicits satiety in rats with open gastric fistulas, *Nature* **245**:323–325.
GOLD, P. E., and McGAUGH, J. L., 1977, Hormones and memory, in: *Neuropeptide Influences on the Brain and Behavior* (L. H. Miller, C. A. Sandman, and A. J. Kastin, eds.), Raven Press, New York, pp. 127–143.
GOLD, P. E., and VAN BUSKIRK, R. B., 1976, Enhancement and impairment of memory processes with posttrial injections of adrenocorticotrophic hormone, *Behav. Biol.* **16**:387–400.
GRAY, J. A., 1971, Effect of ACTH on extinction of rewarded behaviour is blocked by previous administration of ACTH, *Nature* **119**:52–54.
GRAY, J. A., and GARRUD, P., 1977, Adrenopituitary hormones and frustrative nonreward, in: *Neuropeptides Influences on the Brain and Behavior. Advances in Biochemical Psychopharmacology*, Vol. 17 (L. H. Miller, C. A. Sandman, and A. J. Kastin, eds.), Raven Press, New York, pp. 201–212.
GREVEN, H. M., and DE WIED, D., 1973, The influence of peptides derived from corticotrophin (ACTH) on performance. Structure-activity studies, in: *Drug Effects on Neu-*

roendocrine Regulation, Progress in Brain Research, Vol. 39 (E. Zimmerman, W. H. Gispen, B. H. Marks, and D. De Wied, eds.), Elsevier, Amsterdam, pp. 429–442.

GUTH, S., LEVINE, S., and SEWARD, J. P., 1971, Appetitive acquisition and extinction effects with exogenous ACTH, Physiol. Behav. **7:**195–200.

HALL, M. E., and STEWART, J. M., 1982, Opposite behavioral effects of N- and C-terminal fragments of substance P, Soc. Neurosci. Abstr. **8:**369.

HAYS, R. M., 1980, Agents affecting the renal conservation of water, in: The Pharmacological Basis of Therapeutics, 6th ed. (A. G. Gilman, L. S. Goodman, and A. Gilman, eds.), Macmillan, New York, pp. 916–934.

HECHT, K., OEHME, P., and POPPEL, M., 1982, Action of substance P and SP-hexapeptide analogue on avoidance learning in rats, Pharmazie **37:**791–792.

HEISE, G. A., 1981, Learning and memory facilitators: Experimental definition and current status, Trends Pharmacol. Sci. **2:**158–160.

HENNESSY, J. W., COHEN, M. E., and ROSEN, A. J., 1973, Adrenocortical influences upon the extinction of an appetitive runway response, Physiol. Behav. **11:**767–770.

HOKFELT, T., REHFELD, J. F., SKIRBOLL, L., IVEMARK, B., GOLDSTEIN, M., and MARKEY, K., 1980, Evidence for coexistence of dopamine and CCK in mesolimbic neurones, Nature **285:**476–478.

HOSTETTER, G., JUBB, S. L. and KOZLOWSKI, G. P., 1977, Vasopressin affects the behavior of rats in a positively-rewarded discrimination task, Life Sci. **21:**1323–1328.

HUNTER, B., ZORNETZER, S. F., JARVIK, M. E., and MCGAUGH, J. L., 1977, Modulation of learning and memory: Effects of drugs influencing neurotransmitters, in: Handbook of Psychopharmacology, Vol. 18 (L. L. Iversen, S. D. Iversen, and S. H. Snyder, eds.), Plenum Press, New York, pp. 531–577.

HUSTON, J. P., and STAUBLI, U., 1978, Retrograde amnesia produced by post-trial injection of substance P into substantia nigra, Brain Res. **159:**468–472.

HUSTON, J. P., and STAUBLI, U., 1979, Post-trial injection of substance P into lateral hypothalamus and amygdala, respectively facilitates and impairs learning, Behav. Neural. Biol. **27:**244–248.

IVERSEN, S. A., 1981, Neuropeptides: Do they integrate body and brain? Nature **291:**454.

IZQUIERDO, I., 1979, Effect of naloxone and morphine on various forms of memory in the rat: Possible role of endogenous opiate mechanisms in memory consolidation, Psychopharmacology **66:**199–203.

IZQUIERDO, I., 1980a, Effect of beta-endorphin and naloxone on acquisition, memory and retrieval of shuttle avoidance and habituation learning in rats, Psychopharmacology **69:**111–115.

IZQUIERDO, I., 1980b, Effect of a low and high dose of Beta-endorphin on acquisition and retention in the rat, Behav. Neural. Biol. **30:**460–464.

IZQUIERDO, I., and DIAS, R. D., 1981, Retrograde amnesia caused by Met-Leu- and Des Tyr-Met enkephalin in the rat and its reversal by naloxone, Neurosci. Lett. **22:**189–193

IZQUIERDO, I., SOUZA, D. O., CARRASCO, M. A., DIAS, R. D., PERRY, M. L., EISINGER, S., ELISABETSKY, E., and VENDITE, D. A., 1980a, Beta-endorphin causes retrograde amnesia and is released from the rat brain by various forms of training and stimulation, Psychopharmacology **39:**460–464.

IZQUIERDO, I., DIAS, R. D., SOUZA, D. O., CARRASCO, M. A., ELISABETSKY, E., and PERRY, M. L., 1980b, The role of opioid peptides in memory and learning, Behav. Brain Res. **1:**451–468.

IZQUIERDO, I., DIAS, R. D., SOUZA, D. O., CARRASCO, M. A., ELISABETSKY, and PERRY, M. L., 1980c, The role of opioid peptides in memory and learning, Behav. Brain Res. **1:**451–468.

IZQUIERDO, I., PAIVA, A. C. M., and ELISABETSKY, E., 1980c, Post-training intraperitoneal administration of leu-enkaphalin and beta-endorphin causes retrograde amnesia for two different tasks in rats, Behav. Neural Biol. **28:**246–250.

JAMES, W. J., 1961, *Psychology: The Briefer Course* (G. Allport, ed.), Harper and Brothers, New York, pp. 240–257.

JENKINS, J. S., MATHER, H. M., CAUGHLAN, A. K., and JENKINS, D. G., 1979, Desmopressin in posttraumatic amnesia, *Lancet* **2:**1245–1246.

JENKINS, J. S., MATHER, H. M., CAUGHLAN, A. K., and JENKINS, D. G., 1981, Desmopressin and desglycinamide vasopressin in post traumatic amnesia, *Lancet* **1:**39.

KADAR, T., FEKETE, M., and TELEGDY, G., 1981, Modulation of passive avoidance behaviors of rats by intracerebroventricular administration of cholecystokinin in octapeptide sulfate ester and nonsulfated cholecystokinin octapeptide, *Acta Physiol. Acad. Sci. Hung.* **58:**269–274.

KASTIN, A., MILLER, L., NOCKTON, R., SANDMAN, C. SCHALLY, A., and STRATTON, L., 1973, Behavioral aspects of melanocyte stimulating hormone (MSH), in: *Drug Effect on Neuroendocrine Regulation, Progress in Brain Research* (E. Zimmerman, W. Gispen, B. Marks, and D. De Wied, eds.), Elsevier Scientific Pub. Co., Amsterdam, pp. 461–470.

KATZ, R. J., 1979, Central injection of substance P elicits grooming behavior and motor inhibition in mice, *Neurosci. Lett.* **12:**133–136.

KELLEY, A. E., and IVERSEN, S. D., 1979, Behavioral activation induced in the rat by substance P infusion into ventral tegmental area: Implication of dopaminergic A10 neurons, *Neurosci. Lett.* **11:**335–339.

KOBAYASHI, R. M., BROWN, M. R., and VALE, W., 1977, Regional distribution of neurotensin and somatostatin in rat brain, *Brain Res.* **126:**584–588.

KOCH-HENDRIKSEN, N., and NIELSEN, H., 1981, Vasopressin in posttraumatic amnesia, *Lancet* **2:**38–39.

KOLLER, M., KRAUSE, H. P., HOFFMEISTER, F., and GARTEN, D., 1979, Endogenous brain angiostensin II disrupts passive avoidance behavior in rates, *Neurosci. Lett.* **14:**71–75.

KOOB, G. F., and BLOOM, F. E., 1983, Behavioural effects of opioid peptides, *Br. Med. Bull.* **39:**89–94.

KOOB, G. F., LE MOAL, M., and BLOOM, F. E., 1981*a*, Enkephalin and endorphin influences on appetitive and aversive conditioning, in: *Endogenous Peptides and Learning and Memory Processes* (J. L. Martinez, Jr., R. A. Jensen, R. B. Messing, H. Rigter, and J. L. McGaugh, eds.), Academic Press, New York, pp. 305–324.

KOOB, G. F., LE MOAL, M., GAFFORI, O., MANNING, M., SAWYER, W. H., RIVIER, J., and BLOOM, F. E., 1981*b*, Arginine vasopressin and a vasopressin antagonist peptide: Opposite effects on extinction of active avoidance in rats, *Reg. Peptide* **2:**153–163.

KOOB, G. F., DANTZER, R., BLUTHÉ, R.-M., LEBRUN, C., BLOOM, F. E., and LE MOAL, M., 1986, Central injections of arginine vasopressin prolong extinction of active avoidance, *Peptides* **7:**213–218.

KOOB, G. F., LEBRUN, C., MARTINEZ, J. L., JR., DANTZER, R., LE MOAL, M., and BLOOM, F. E., 1985, Arginine vasopressin, stress and memory, in: *Vasopressin* (R. Schrier, ed.), Raven Press, New York, pp. 195–201.

KOVACS, G. L., VESCEI, L., and TELEGDY, G., 1978, Opposite action of oxytocin to vasopressin in passive avoidance in rates, *Physiol. Behav.* **20:**801–802.

KOVACS, G. L., BOHUS, B., and VERSTEEG, D. H. G., 1979*a*, Facilitation of memory consolidation by vasopressin: Mediation by terminals of the dorsal noradrenergic bundle? *Brain Res.* **172:**73–85.

KOVACS, G. L., BOHUS, B., VERSTEEG, D. H. G., DE KLOET, E. R., and DE WIED, D., 1979*b*, Effect of oxytocin and vasopressin on memory consolidation sites of action and catecholaminergic correlates after micro injection into limbic-midbrain structures, *Brain Res.* **175:**303–314.

KOVACS, G. L., BOHUS, B., and DE WIED, D., 1981*a*, Retention of passive avoidance behavior in rats following alpha and gamma endorphin administration: Effects of postlearning treatments, *Neurosci. Lett.* **22:**79–82.

KOVACS, G. L., and DE WIED, D., 1981*b*, Endorphin influences on learning and memory, in: *Endogenous Peptides and Learning and Memory Processes* (J. L. Martinez, Jr., R. A. Jensen, R. B. Messing, H. Rigter, and J. L. McGaugh, eds.), Academic Press, New York, pp. 231–247.

KREIGER, D. J., LIOTTA, A., and BROWNSTEIN, M. J., 1977, Presence of corticotropin in limbic system of normal and hypophysectomized rats, *Brain Res.* **128**:575–579.

KULBACK, S., 1968, *Information Theory and Statistics*, Dover, New York.

LACZI, F., VAN REE, J. M., WAGNER, A., VALKUSZ, Z., JARDANHAZY, T., KOVACS, G. L., TELEGDY, G., SZILARD, J., LASZLO, F. A., and DE WIED, D., 1983, Effects of desglycinamidearginine vasopressin (DG-AVP) on memory processes in diabetes insipidus patients and non diabetic subjects, *Acta Endocrinol.* **102**:205–212.

LANDE, S., FLEXNER, T. B., and FLEXNER, L. L., 1972, Effects of corticotrophin and desglycinamide lysine vasopressin on suppression of memory by puromycin, *Proc. Natl. Acad. Sci. USA* **69**:558–60.

LEBOEUF, A., LODGE, J., and EAMES, P. G., 1978, Vasopressin and memory in Korsakoff syndrome, *Lancet* **2**:1370.

LEBRUN, C. J., RIGTER, H., MARTINEZ, J. L., JR., KOOB, G. F., LE MOAL, M., and BLOOM, F. E., 1984, Antagonism of effects of vasopressin (AVP) on inhibitory avoidance by a vasopressin antagonist peptide [dPTyr (Me) AVP], *Life Sci.* **35**:1505–1512.

LEBRUN, C., LE MOAL, M. KOOB, G. F., and BLOOM, F. E., 1985, Vasopressin pressor antagonist injected centrally reverses peripheral behavioral effects of vasopressin but only at doses that reverse increases in blood pressure, *Reg. Peptides* **11**:173–181.

LEGROS, J. J., GILOT, P., SERON, X., CLAESSENS, J., ADAM, A., MOEGLEN, J. M., AUDIBERT, A., and BERCHIER, P., 1978, Influence of vasopressin on learning and memory, *Lancet* **1**:41–42.

LE MOAL, M., KOOB, G. F., and BLOOM, F. E., 1979, Endorphins and extinction differential actions on appetitive and aversive tasks, *Life Sci.* **24**:1631–1636.

LE MOAL, M., KOOB, G. F., KODA, L. Y., BLOOM, F. E., MANNING, M., SAWYER, W. H., and RIVIER, J., 1981, Vasopressin antagonist peptide: Blockade of pressor receptor prevents behavioral action of vasopressin, *Nature* **291**:491–493.

LE MOAL, M., KOOB, G. F., MORMEDE, P., DANTZER, R., and BLOOM, F. E., 1982, Vasopressin pressor antagonist reverses central behavioral effects of vasopressin, *Neurosci. Abstr.* **8**:368.

LE MOAL, M., DANTZER, R., MORMEDE, P., BADUEL, A., LEBRUN, C., ETTENBERG, A., VAN DER KOOY, D., WENGER, J., DEYO, S., KOOB, G. F., and BLOOM, F. E., 1984, Behavioral effects of peripheral administration of arginine vasopressin: A review of our search for a mode of action and a hypothesis, *Psychoneuroendocrinology* **9**:319–341.

LEVINE, S., and JONES, L. E., 1965, Adrenocorticotrophic hormone (ACTH) and passive avoidance learning, *J. Comp. Physiol. Psychol.* **59**:357–360.

LEVINE, S., SMOTHERMAN, W. P., and HENNESSY, J. W., 1977, Pituitary-adrenal hormones and learned taste aversion, in: *Neuropeptide Influences on the Brain and Behavior* (L. H. Miller, C. A. Sandman, and A. J. Kastin, eds.), Raven Press, New York, pp. 163–177.

LISSAK, K., and BOHUS, B., 1972, Pituitary hormones and avoidance behavior of the rat, *Int. J. Psychobiol.* **2**:103–115.

LUCION, A. B., ROSITO, G., SAPPER, D., PALMINI, A. L., and IZQUIERDO, I., 1982, Intracerebroventricular administration of nanogram amounts of α-endorphin and methionine enkephalin causes retrograde amnesia in rats, *Behav. Brain Res.* **4**:111–115.

LUTTINGER, D., NEMEROFF, C. B., and PRANGE, A. J., JR., 1982, The effects of neuropeptides on discrete-trial conditioned avoidance responding, *Brain Res.* **237**:183–192.

MARTINEZ, J. L., JR., 1985, Endogenous modulators of learning and memory to be published, in: *Theory in Psychopharmacology*, Vol. 2 (S. Cooper, ed.), Academic Press, London.

MARTINEZ, J. L., JR., and RIGTER, H., 1980, Endorphins alter acquisition and consolidation of an inhibitory avoidance response in rats, *Neurosci. Lett.* **19**:197–201.

MARTINEZ, J. L., JR., and RIGTER, H., 1982, Enkephalin actions on avoidance conditioning may be related to adrenal medullary function, *Behav. Brain Res.* **6:**289–299.
MARTINEZ, J. L. JR., RIGTER, H., JENSEN, R. A., MESSING, R. B., VASQUEZ, B. J., and MCGAUGH, J. L., 1981, Endorphin and enkephalin effects on avoidance conditioning, the other side of the pituitary-adrenal axis, in: *Endogenous Peptides and Learning and Memory Processes* (J. L. Martinez, Jr., R. A. Jensen, R. B. Messing, H. Rigter, and J. L. McGaugh, eds.), Academic Press, New York, pp. 395–324.
MARTINEZ, J. L., JR., CONNER, P., DANA, R. C., CHAVKIN, C., BLOOM, F., and DE GRAFF, J., 1984a, Endogenous modulation of peripheral leu-enkephalin systems affects avoidance conditioning, *Neurosci. Abstr.* **10:**176.
MARTINEZ, J. L., JR., OLSON, K., and HILSTON, C., 1984b, Opposite effects of met-enkephalin and leu-enkephalin on a discriminated shock-escape task, *Behav. Neurosci.* **98:**487–495.
MARTINEZ, J. L., JR., CONNER, P., and DANA, R. C., 1985, Central versus peripheral actions of leu-enkephalin on acquisition of a one-way active avoidance response in rats, *Brain Res.* **327:**37–43.
MCGAUGH, J. L., 1966, Time-dependent processes in memory storage, *Science* **153:**1351–1358.
MCGAUGH, J. L., 1973, Drug facilitation of learning and memory, *Annu. Rev. Pharmacol.* **13:**1351–1358.
MCGAUGH, J. L., 1983, Preserving the presence of the past: Hormonal influences on memory storage, *Am. Psychologist* **38:**161–174.
MCGAUGH, J. L., and MARTINEZ, J. L., JR., 1981, Learning modulatory hormones: An introduction to endogenous peptides and learning and memory processes, in: *Endogenous Peptides and Learning and Memory Processes* (J. L. Martinez, Jr., R. A. Jensen, R. B. Messing, H. Rigter, and J. L. McGaugh, eds.), Academic Press, New York, pp. 1–3.
MENS, W. B., WIHER, A., and VAN WIMERSMA GREIDANUS, Tj. B., 1983, Penetration of neurohypophyseal hormones from plasma into cerebrospinal fluid (CSF): Half-times of disappearance of these neuropeptides from CSF, *Brain Res.* **262:**143–149.
MESSING, R. B., and SPARBER, S. R., 1983, Des-Gly-vasopressin improves acquisition and slows extinction of autoshaped behavior, *Eur. J. Pharmacol.* **89:**43–51.
MESSING, R. B., JENSEN, R. A., MARTINEZ, J. L. JR., SPIEHLER, V. R., VASQUEZ, B. J., SOUMIREU-MOURAT, B., LIANG, D. C., and MCGAUGH, J. L., 1979, Naloxone enhancement of memory, *Behav. Neural. Biol.* **27:**266–275.
MESSING, R. B., JENSEN, R., VASQUEZ, B. J., MARTINEZ, J. L., SPIEHLER, V. R., and MCGAUGH, J. L., 1981, in: *Endogenous Peptides and Learning and Memory Processes* (J. L. Martinez, Jr., R. A. Jensen, R. B., Messing, H. Rigter, and J. L. McGaugh, eds.), Academic Press, New York, pp. 431–444.
MILLER, R. E., and OGAWA, N., 1962, The effect of adrenocorticotrophic hormone (ACTH) on avoidance conditioning in the adrenalectomized rat, *J. Comp. Physiol. Psychol.* **55:**211–213.
MILLER, R. E., and CAUL, W. F., 1973, Effect of adrenocorticotropic hormone on appetitive discrimination learning in the rat, *Physiol. Behav.* **10:**141–143.
MILLER, L. H., HARRIS, L. C., VAN RIEZEN, H., and KASTIN, A. J., 1976, Neuroheptapeptide influence on attention and memory in man, *Pharmacol. Biochem. Behav.* **5** (Suppl. 1):17–21.
MILLER, L. H., KASTIN, A. J., SANDMAN, C. A., FINK, M., and VAN VEEN, W. J., 1974, Polypeptide influences on attention, memory, and anxiety in man, *Pharmacol. Biochem. Behav.* **2:**663–668.
MORGAN, J. M., and ROUTTENBERG, A., 1977, Angiotensin injected into the neostriatum after learning disrupts retention performance, *Science* **196:**87–89.
MURPHY, J. V., and MILLER, R. E., 1955, The effect of adrenocorticotrophic hormone (ACTH) on avoidance conditioning in the rat, *J. Comp. Physiol. Psychol.* **48:**47–49.

NEMEROFF, C. B., 1980, Neurotensin: Perhaps an endogenous neuroleptic? *Biol. Psychiatry* **15**:283–302.
NEMEROFF, C. B., LUTTINGER, D., and PRANGE, A. J., JR., 1983, Neurotensin and bombesin, in: *Handbook of Psychopharmacology*, Vol. 16 (L. H. Iversen, S. D. Iversen, and S. H. Snyder, eds.), Plenum Press, New York, pp. 363–466.
OLENDORF, W. H., 1974, Blood–brain barrier permeability to drugs, *Annu. Rev. Pharmacol.* **14**:239–248.
OLIVEROS, J. C., JANDALI, M. K., TIMSIT-BERTHIER, M., REMY, R., BENGHEZAL, A., AUDIBERT, A., and MOEGLEN, J. H., 1978, Vasopressin in amnesia, *Lancet* **1**:42.
PARDRIDGE, W. M., 1983, Neuropeptides and the blood–brain barrier, *Annu. Rev. Physiol.* **45**:73–82.
PEDERSON, C. A., and PRANGE, A. J., 1979, Induction of maternal behaviour in virgin rats after intracerebroventricular administration of oxytocin, *Proc. Natl. Acad. Sci. USA* **76**:661–665.
PRANGE, A. J., JR., NEMEROFF, C. B., LIPTON, M. A., BREESE, G. R., and WILSON, I. C., 1978, Peptides and the central nervous system, in: *Handbook of Psychopharmacology* (L. L. Iversen, S. D. Iversen, and S. H. Snyder, eds.), Plenum Press, New York, pp. 1–106.
REZEK, M., HAVLICEK, V., HUGHES, K. R., and FRIESEN, H., 1977, Behavioural and motor excitation and inhibition induced by the administration of small and large doses of somatostatin into amygdala, *Neuropharmacology* **16**:157–162.
RIGTER, H., 1978, Attenuation of amnesia in rats by systemically administered enkephalin, *Science* **200**:83–85.
RIGTER, H., 1982, Vasopressin and memory: The influence of prior experience with the training situation, *Behav. Neural. Biol.* **34**:337–351.
RIGTER, H., and POPPING, A., 1976, Hormonal influences on the extinction of conditioned taste aversion, *Psychopharmacologia (Berlin)* **46**:255–261.
RIGTER, H., and VAN RIEZEN, H., 1975, Anti-amnesic effect of $ACTH_{4\text{-}10}$: Its independence of the nature of the amnesic agent and the behavioral test, *Physiol. Behav.* **14**:563–566.
RIGTER, H., and VAN RIEZEN, H., 1978, Hormones and Memory, in: *Psychopharmacology: A Generation of Progress* (M. A. Lipton, A. Di Masco, and K. F. Killam, eds.), Raven Press, New York, pp. 677–689.
RIGTER, H., VAN RIEZEN, H., and DE WIED, D., 1974, The effects of ACTH and vasopressin-analogues on CO_2-induced retrograde amnesia in rats, *Physiol. Behav.* **13**:381–388.
RIGTER, H., JANSSENS-ELBERTSE, R., and VAN RIEZEN, H., 1976, Reversal of amnesia by an orally active $ACTH_{4\text{-}9}$ analog (Org 2766), *Pharmacol. Biochem. Behav.* **5**(Suppl. 1):53–58.
RIGTER, H., SHUSTER, S., and THODY, A. J., 1977, ACTH αMSH and β-LPH: Pituitary hormone with similar activity in an amnesia test in rats, *J. Pharm. Pharmacol.* **29**:110–111.
RIGTER, H., HANNAN, T. J., MESSING, R. B., MARTINEZ, J. L., JR., VASQUEZ, B. J., JENSEN, R. A., VELIQUETTE, J., and MCGAUGH, J. L., 1980a, Enkephalins interfere with acquisition of an active avoidance response, *Life Sci.* **26**:337–345.
RIGTER, H. JENSEN, R. A., MARTINEZ, J. L., JR., MESSING, R. B., VASQUEZ, B. J., LIANG, K. C., and MCGAUGH, J. L., 1980b, Enkephalin and fear-motivated behavior, *Proc. Natl. Acad. Sci. USA* **77**:3729–3732.
RIGTER, H., DEKKER, I., and MARTINEZ, J. L., JR., 1981, A comparison of the ability of opioid peptides and opiates to affect active avoidance conditioning in rats, *Reg. Peptides* **2**:317–322.
ROSSOR, M. N., EMSON, P. C., MOUNTJOY, C. Q., ROTH, M., and IVERSEN, L. L., 1980, Reduced amounts of immunoreactive somatostatin in the temporal cortex in senile dementia of Alzheimer type, *Neurosci. Lett.* **20**:373–377.
ROTH, M. M., HEATH, R. G., and WARD, M., 1975, Angiotensin-converting enzyme in human brain, *J. Neurochem.* **25**:83–85.

SAHGAL, A., 1984, A critique of the vasopressin memory hypothesis, *Psychopharmacology* **83**:215-228.
SAHGAL, A., and WRIGHT, C., 1983, A comparison of the effects of vasopressin and oxytocin with amphetamine and chlordiazepoxide on passive avoidance behaviour in rats, *Psychopharmacology* **80**:88-92.
SAHGAL, A., KEITH, A. B., WRIGHT, C., and EDWARDSON, J. A., 1982, Failure of vasopressin to enhance memory in a passive avoidance task in rats, *Neurosci. Lett.* **28**:87-92.
SANDMAN, C. A., MILLER, L. H., KASTIN, A. J., and SCHALLY, A. V., 1972, A neuroendocrine influence on attention and memory, *J. Comp. Physiol. Psychol.* **80**:54-58.
SANDMAN, C. A., ALEXANDER, W. D., and KASTIN, A. J., 1973a, Neuroendocrine influences on visual discrimination and reversal learning in the albino and hooded rat, *Physiol. Behav.* **11**:613-617.
SANDMAN, C., KASTIN, A., and SCHALLY, A., 1973b, Melanocyte-stimulating hormone and learned appetitive behavior, *Experientia* **92**:372-379.
SANDMAN, C. A., BECKWITH, B. E., GIDDIS, M. M., and KASTIN, A. J., 1974, Melanocyte stimulating hormone (MSH) and overtraining effects on extradimensional shift (EDS) learning, *Physiol. Behav.* **13**:163-166.
SANDMAN, C. A., GEORGE, J. M., NOLAN, J., VAN RIEZEN, H., and KASTIN, A. J., 1975, Enhancement of attention in man with ACTH/MSH$^{4\text{-}10}$, *Physiol. Behav.* **15**:427-431.
SANDMAN, C. A., GEORGE, J., WALKER, B. B., and NOLAN, J. D., 1976, Neuropeptide MSH–ACTH$^{4\text{-}10}$ enhances attention in the mentally retarded, *Pharmacol. Biochem. Behav.* **5** (Suppl. 1):23-28.
SANDMAN, C. A., GEORGE, J., MCCANNE, T. R., NOLAN, J. D., KASWAN, J., and KASTIN, A. J., 1977, MSH/ACTH$^{4\text{-}10}$ influences behavioral and physiological measures of attention, *J. Clin. Endocrinol. Metab.* **44**:884-890.
SANDMAN, C. A., BECKWITH, B. G., and KASTIN, A. J., 1980, Are learning and attention related to the sequence of amino acids in ACTH/MSH peptides? *Peptides* **1**:277-280.
SANDMAN, C. A., KASTIN, A. J., and SCHALLY, A. V., 1981, Neuropeptide influences on the central nervous system, A psychobiological perspective, in: *Neuroendocrine Regulation and Altered Behaviour* (P. D. Hrdina and R. L. Singhal, eds.), Croom Helm Ltd., London, pp. 3-28.
SAWYER, W. H., 1964, Vertebrate neurophypophysial principles, *Endocrinology* **75**:981-990.
SCHLESINGER, K., LIPSITZ, D. U., PECK, P. L., PELLEYMOUNTER, M. A., STEWART, J. M., and CHASE, T. N., 1983a, Substance P enhancement of passive and active avoidance conditioning in mice, *Pharmacol. Biochem. Behav.* **19**:655-661.
SCHLESINGER, K., LIPSITZ, D. U., PECK, P. L., STEWART, J. M., and CHASE, T. N., 1983b, Substance P reversal of electroconvulsive shock and cycloheximide-induced retrograde amnesia, *Behav. Neural. Biol.* **39**:30-39.
SCHNEIDER, L. H., ALPERT, J. E., and IVERSEN, S. D., 1983, CCK 8 modulation of mesolimbic dopamine: Antagonism of amphetamine stimulated behaviors, *Peptides* **4**:749-753.
SCHULZ, H., KOVACS, G. L., and TELEGDY, G., 1974, Effects of doses of vasopressin and oxytocin on avoidance behavior in rats, *Acta Physiol. Acad. Sci. Hun.* **45**:211-215.
SCHULZ, H., KOVACS, G. L., and TELEGDY, G., 1976, The effect of vasopressin and oxytocin on avoidance behavior in rats, in: *Cellular and Molecular Bases of Neuroendocrine Processes* (E. Endroczi, ed.), Akademia, Kindo, Budapest, pp. 555-564.
SQUIRE, L. R., and DAVIS, H. P., 1981, The pharmacology of memory: A neurobiological perspective, *Annu. Rev. Pharmacol. Toxicol.* **21**:323-356.
STARR, M. S., JAMES, T. A., and GAYTTEN, D., 1978, Behavioral depressant and antinociceptive properties of substance P in the mouse: Possible implication of brain monamines, *Eur. J. Pharmacol.* **48**:203-212.
STAUBLI, U., and HUSTON, J. P., 1979, Differential effects on learning by ventromedial vs. lateral hypothalamic injection of substance P, *Pharmacol. Biochem. Behav.* **10**:783-786.

STAUBLI, U., and HUSTON, J. P., 1980, Facilitation of learning by post-trial injection of substance P into the medial septal nucleus, *Behav. Brain Res.* **1:**245–255.

STEWART, J. M., GETTO, C. J., NELDER, K., REEVE, E. B., KRIVOY, W. A., and ZIMMERMAN, E., 1976, Substance P and analgesia, *Nature* **262:**784–785.

STINUS, L., KELLEY, A. E., and IVERSEN, S. D., 1978, Increased spontaneous activity following substance P infusion into A10 dopaminergic area, *Nature* **276:**616–618.

TANAKA, M., DE KLOET, E. R., DE WIED, D., and VERSTEEG, D. H. G., 1977a, Arginine^8–vasopressin affects catecholamine metabolism in specific brain nuclei, *Life Sci.* **20:**1799–1808.

TANAKA, M., VERSTEEG, D. H. G., and DE WIED, D., 1977b, Regional effects of vasopressin on rat brain catecholamine metabolism, *Neurosci. Lett.* **4:**321–325.

TAZI, A., DANTZER, R., MORMEDE, P., and LE MOAL, M., 1983, Effects of posttrial administration of naloxone and β-endorphin on shock induced fighting in rats, *Behav. Neural. Biol.* **39:**192–202.

TAZI, A., DANTZER, R., NORMEDE, P., and LE MOAL, M., 1985, Effects of naloxone, β-endorphin and ACTH on acquisition of schedule-induced polydipsia, *Psychopharmacology* **85:**87–91.

TINKLENBERG, J. R., PFEFFERBAUM, A., and BERGER, P. A., 1981, 1-Desamino-D-arginine vasopressin (DDAVP) in cognitively impaired patients, *Psychopharmacol. Bull.* **17:**206–207.

VACCARINO, F. J., and KOOB, G. F., 1984, Microinjections of nanogram amounts of sulfated cholecystokinin octapeptide into the rat nucleus accumbens attenuates brain stimulation reward, *Neurosci. Lett.* **52:**61–66.

VALE, W., BRAZEAU, P., RIVIER, C., BROWN, M., ROSS, B., RIVER, J., BURGUS, R., LING, N., and GUILLEMIN, R., 1975, Somatostatin recent progress, *Hormone Res.* **31:**365–397.

VECSEI, L., SCHWARZBERG, H., and TELEGDY, G., 1982, The effect of somatostatin on the self-stimulation of rats, *Neuroendocrinol. Lett.* **4:**37–41.

VECSEI, L., BOLLOK, I., and TELEGDY, G., 1983a, Intracerebroventricular somatostatin attenuates electroconvulsive-shock-induced amnesia in rats, *Peptides* **4:**293–295.

VECSEI, L., BOLLOK, I., and TELEGDY, G., 1983b, The effect of linear somatostatin on the active avoidance behaviour and open-field activity on haloperidol, phenoxybenzamine, and atropine pretreated rats, *Acta Physiol. Hung.* **62:**205–211.

VECSEI, L., BOLLOK, I., and TELEGDY, G., 1984, Phenoxybenzamine antagonizes somatostatin-induced anti-amnesia in rats, *Eur. J. Pharmacol.* **99:**325–328.

VAN REE, J. M., BOHUS, B., VERSTEEG, D. H., and DE WIED, D., 1978, Neurohypophyseal principles and memory processes, *Biochem. Pharmacol.* **27:**1793–1800.

VAN WIMERSMA GREIDANUS, Tj. B., and DE WIED, D., 1971, Effects of systemic and intracerebral administration of two opposite acting ACTH-related peptides on extinction of conditioned avoidance behaviour, *Neuroendocrinology* **7:**291–301.

VAN WIMERSMA GREIDANUS, Tj. B., DOGTEROM, J., and DE WIED, D., 1975, Intraventricular administration of antivasopressin serum inhibits memory consolidation in rats, *Life Sci.* **16:**637–644.

VAN WIMERSMA GREIDANUS, Tj. B., and DE WIED, D., 1976a, Dorsal hippocampus: A site of action of neuropeptides on avoidance behavior? *Pharmacol. Biochem. Behav.* **5**(Suppl. 1):29–33.

VAN WIMERSMA GREIDANUS, Tj. B., and DE WIED, D., 1976b, Modulation of passive avoidance behavior of rats by intracerebroventricular administration of antivasopressin serum, *Behav. Biol.* **18:**325–333.

VAN WIMERSMA GREIDANUS, Tj. B., CROISET, G., BAKKER, I., and BOUMAN, H., 1979, Amygdaloid lesions block the effect of neuropeptides (vasopressin, ACTH$^{4\text{-}10}$) on avoidance behavior, *Physiol. Behav.* **22:**291–295.

VAN WIMERSMA GREIDANUS, Tj. B., VAN PRAAG, M. C., KALMANN, R., RINKEL, G. J., CROISET, G., HOEKE, E. C., VAN EGMOND, M. A., and FEKETE, M., 1982, Behavioral effects of neurotensin, *Ann. NY Acad. Sci.* **400:**319–29.

van Wimersma Greidanus, Tj. B., Bohus, B., and De Wied, D., 1983, Vasopressin and oxytocin in learning and memory, in: *Endogenous Peptides and Learning and Memory Processes* (J. L. Martinez, Jr., R. A. Jensen, R. B. Messing, H. Righter, and J. L. McGaugh, eds.), Academic Press, New York, pp. 413–427.

Verhoef, J., and Witter, A., 1976, In vivo fate of a behaviorally active ACTH$^{4-9}$ analog in rats after systemic administration, *Pharmacol. Biochem. Behav.* **4**:583–590.

Walker, B. B., and Sandman, C. A., 1979, Influences of an analog of the neuropeptide ACTH$^{4-9}$ on mentally retarded adults, *Am. J. Ment. Defic.* **83**:346–352.

Walter, R., van Ree, J. M., and De Wied, D., 1978, Modification of conditioned behavior of rats by neurohypophyseal hormones and analogs, *Proc. Natl. Acad. Sci. USA* **75**:2493–2496.

Weingartner, H., Gold, P., Ballenger, J. C., Smallberg, S. A., Summers, R., Rubinow, D. R., Post, R. M., and Goodwin, F. K., 1981, Effects of vasopressin on human memory functions, *Science* **211**:601–603.

Weiss, J. M., McEwen, B. S., Silva, M. T. A., and Kalkut, M. F., 1969, Pituitary–adrenal influences on fear responding, *Science* **163**:197–199.

Weissman, A., 1967, Drugs and memory and learning, *Annu. Rep. Med. Chem.* **3**:279–289.

Wetzel, W., and Matthies, H., 1982, Effect of substance P on the retention of a brightness discrimination task in rats, *Acta Biol. Med. Germ.* **41**:647–652.

Wood, J. H., 1982, Neuroendocrinology of cerebrospinal fluid: Peptides, steroids and other hormones, *Neurosurgery* **11**:293–305.

Zaidi, S. M. A., and Heller, H., 1974, Can neurohypophysial hormones cross the blood–cerebrospinal fluid barrier? *J. Endocrinol.* **60**:195–196.

Zerbe, R. L., Bayorh, M. A., and Feuerstein, G., 1982, Vasopressin: An essential pressor factor for blood pressure recovery following hemorrhage, *Peptides* **3**:509–514.

Zetler, G., 1981, Central depressant effects of caerulein and cholecystokinin octapeptide (CCK 8) differ from those of diazepam and haloperidol, *Neuropharmacology* **20**:277–283.

Zornetzer, S. F., 1978, Neurotransmitter modulation and memory: A new neuropharmacological phrenology, in: *Psychopharmacology: A Generation of Progress* (M. A. Lipton, A. Di Mascio, and K. F. Killan, eds.), Raven Press, New York, pp. 637–649.

10

THE ACTIONS OF NEUROLEPTIC DRUGS ON APPETITIVE INSTRUMENTAL BEHAVIORS

John D. Salamone

1. INTRODUCTION

Scientific study of the behavioral effects of neuroleptic drugs involves many different disciplines. Psychiatric treatment of psychoses has been revolutionized by the use of these agents to combat schizophrenia. The common pharmacological ground that most neuroleptic drugs share is an opposition to the action of dopamine (DA), usually by blockade of DA receptors. In this regard, pharmacologists have utilized the reliable behavioral sequelae of neuroleptic action to serve as "behavioral assays" for evaluating the potency of known neuroleptic drugs and identifying new ones. To the physiological psychologist, neuroleptics are a tool—a means of investigating the behavioral processes in which DA is involved. Although any substantial review of this area must employ views obtained from the different disciplines involved, it is largely from the latter perspective that the present chapter is derived.

Concepts of the behavioral functions of brain DA systems have undergone considerable revision over the last several years. Research into the behavioral results of neuroleptic administration has been one of the major factors in these changes. In part, neuroleptic studies have contrib-

---

John D. Salamone • Department of Behavioral Neuroscience, University of Pittsburgh, Pittsburgh, Pennsylvania 15260.

uted so much because researchers have begun to ask more complicated behavioral questions. For many years, scientists collected basic data on neuroleptics, which included identifying which behaviors were affected by the drugs, the direction of those effects, and at what doses they occurred. One conclusion based upon such data, which still enjoys considerable credence today, is that neuroleptic drugs generally suppress a number of different behaviors by interfering with movement (see, for example, Janssen et al., 1965). Subsequently, scientists began to question a strict motoric interpretation of neuroleptic effects and began to implicate such complex psychological processes as reinforcement or incentive motivation (Wise et al., 1978a; Wise, 1982).

The present chapter will examine these and other hypotheses and will attempt to develop principles with which to evaluate the action of neuroleptic drugs on conditioned appetitive behaviors.

2. HYPOTHESES ON THE BEHAVIORAL ACTIONS OF NEUROLEPTICS

Pharmacologists or neuroscientists who are not behaviorally oriented might question the need for generating hypotheses on the behavioral mechanisms interfered with by neuroleptic drugs. A strict behaviorist could argue similarly and suggest that all that is really necessary is to obtain a detailed description of DA antagonist effects. Indeed, the whole question of whether neuroleptics interfere with "motor performance," "reward," or "motivation" could at times appear too theoretical and too esoteric to be of any practical utility. However, I would like to submit that such hypotheses are central to the progress of physiological psychology and psychopharmacology. Biochemists and pharmacologists do not simply describe how one drug inhibits another drug's action or some enzyme. Rather, they attribute specific types of relationships to various kinds of mechanisms. So, too, should behavioral scientists continue to move beyond description into the realm of generating hypotheses and suggesting mechanisms.

2.1. Behavioral Profile of Neuroleptic Effects

Of course, the first stage in any attempt to advance hypotheses is to examine the basic data being considered. In this instance, the field is so large that only a brief summary can be given here. Following this, a more detailed review of specific areas is provided.

2.1.1. Spontaneous Activities

A number of spontaneous activities have been tested for their sensitivity to DA antagonist drugs. In general, it has been found that neuroleptic drugs suppress these behaviors in a dose-dependent manner. Rearing and ambulation in rats are suppressed by a variety of neuroleptics (Janssen *et al.*, 1965). Inhibition of mouse climbing is also reliably obtained from DA antagonists (Costall *et al.*, 1982). Male sexual behavior (Tagliamonte *et al.*, 1974), feeding (Janssen *et al.*, 1965; Rolls *et al.*, 1974), and drinking (Rowland and Engle, 1977; Xenakis and Sclafani, 1981) decrease with neuroleptic administration.

2.1.2. Drug-Induced Activities

As one might expect, behavioral consequences of injection of drugs that enhance activity in the dopaminergic system are typically blocked by neuroleptics. Dopamine antagonists oppose the increase in locomotor activity (Schlecter and Butcher, 1972) and stereotyped behaviors (Janssen *et al.*, 1965; Munkuad and Randrup, 1966) induced by amphetamine. Apomorphine stereotypy is blocked by neuroleptics (Janssen *et al.*, 1965), as is the rotation produced by amphetamine in rats lesioned unilaterally with 6-OHDA (Pycock *et al.*, 1975; Ungerstedt, 1971*b*).

2.1.3. Aversively Motivated Instrumental Behaviors

Performance of active avoidance responses is interfered with by DA antagonists (Posluns, 1962; Janssen *et al.*, 1965; Niemgeers *et al.*, 1970). The inhibition of avoidance responses can occur at doses that leave the escape response unimpaired (Herz, 1960; Posluns, 1962; Fibiger *et al.*, 1975). Passive avoidance is only minimally impaired by neuroleptics, compared to the rather profound interference with active avoidance responses (Morpurgo, 1965).

2.1.4. Appetitively Motivated Instrumental Behaviors

Data on the effects of neuroleptics upon appetitive tasks will form the bulk of this chapter and, as such, will only be briefly mentioned here. Suffice it to say that DA antagonists impair a variety of instrumental behaviors sustained by a broad range of reinforcers (Monti and Hance, 1967; Rolls *et al.*, 1974; Fibiger *et al.*, 1976; Wise *et al.*, 1978*a,b*; Phillips and Fibiger, 1979; Mason *et al.*, 1980; Tombaugh *et al.*, 1979, 1980, 1982; Beninger, 1982).

2.2. Early Motor Hypotheses

To summarize, neuroleptics generally have a suppressant effect upon a wide variety of behaviors. Janssen *et al.* (1965) observed that the potencies of various DA antagonists (of the phenothiazine and butyrophenone types) in reducing jumping, rearing, ambulation, and food intake and in inducing cataleptic immobility were all highly intercorrelated. They concluded that these effects all reflect the same basic process—inhibition of behavioral responses at relatively low doses and complete cataleptic immobility at higher doses. It is plausible that such a conclusion could also be drawn regarding effects of neuroleptics upon instrumental behaviors. Fibiger *et al.* (1976) attributed the decreased operant responding for food resulting from haloperidol or pimozide injection to an impairment in the initiation and maintenance of movement. Rolls *et al.* (1974) found that lever pressing for food could be suppressed at drug doses lower than those necessary for reducing food intake. This led Fibiger *et al.* (1976) to suggest that motivation for food was not reduced by these low doses and bolstered their conclusion that a motor impairment underlay the operant deficit.

The motoric interpretation of neuroleptic effects on behavior is consistent with views on DA function obtained from other lines of study. One of the major recipients of dopaminergic innervation in the brain is the striatum (Ungerstedt, 1971c; Beckstead *et al.*, 1979). The striatum is traditionally considered to be a part of the "extrapyramidal" motor system (Wilson, 1914). Areas of striatum receive inputs from motor cortex (Kemp and Powell, 1970; Kunzle, 1975), and striatal output, via globus pallidus, projects to thalamic nuclei that have connections to motor cortex (Szabo, 1962; Cowan and Powell, 1966; Nauta and Mehler, 1966). The activity of some striatal neurons is associated with movement (Delong and Strick, 1974). Nucleus accumbens, another DA terminal area, also projects to the area of the globus pallidus and has been implicated in the control of motor activity (Mogenson *et al.*, 1980).

Depletion of DA from striatum leads to a syndrome of akinesia, aphagia (Ungerstedt, 1971a; Marshall *et al.*, 1974), and sensorimotor disturbances (Marshall *et al.*, 1974). Lesions that reduce DA from the nucleus accumbens decrease spontaneous and amphetamine-induced locomotion (Kelly *et al.*, 1975; Koob *et al.*, 1978). Parkinson's disease, which is characterized by muscle rigidity, resting tremor, and akinesia, is conclusively linked to a depletion of nigrostriatal DA (reviewed by Hornykiewicz, 1972). As a reference to this finding, motor effects of DA antagonists are sometimes labeled "parkinsonian." By the mid-1970s, a picture of DA function had emerged that suggested that, at least in some brain areas, DA is involved in the regulation of movement. Interference with DA transmission by administration of DA antagonists results in a suppression of movement, which will manifest itself in the inhibition of a variety of conditioned and unconditioned behaviors. Since the development of this classic description of DA function, a considerable amount of research has been done, which suggests a much more complicated picture of dopaminergic function.

2.3. Anhedonia and the Link between Dopamine and Reinforcement

2.3.1. Historical Development of the Anhedonia Concept

During the 1970s, the idea gradually evolved that dopamine was critically involved in the process of reinforcement. This offered an explanation of the effects of neuroleptics in terms of interference with reward rather than motor dysfunction. Research into intracranial self-stimulation (ICSS) did much to help this development. For years, it had been hoped that ICSS research would yield insights into the brain mechanisms of reinforcement. Eventually, evidence was uncovered that pointed to an important role for DA in ICSS.

Mapping studies indicated a correspondence between anatomical loci in the DA (and noradrenaline) systems and positive ICSS sites (Crow, 1972; German and Bowden, 1974). Destruction of DA neurons by injection of 6-hydroxydopamine impaired ICSS responding (Cooper *et al.*, 1974; Fibiger *et al.*, 1976). Injection of DA antagonists decreased ICSS response rates (Lippa *et al.*, 1973; Fibiger *et al.*, 1976). Although these data did not conclusively demonstrate that DA manipulations effect reinforcement rather than movement (Fibiger *et al.*, 1976; Ornstein and Huston, 1975), they could be seen as consistent with a reinforcement hypothesis.

Fouriezos and Wise (1976) investigated the possible reinforcement-suppressing effects of pimozide by examining the pattern of ICSS responding following the drug. It was observed that rats responded normally or near-normally at the beginning of the test session, but responding declined across the test period. This pattern resembled that seen with extinction. In addition, a rat that had stopped responding under pimozide was separated from the lever by a barrier and showed "spontaneous recovery" when allowed access to the barrier again.

Wise (1978) reviewed the literature on DA and ICSS and suggested that DA may play an important role in the reward produced by brain stimulation. He noted that such drugs as amphetamine, which enhance activity in the DA system, produce euphoria in humans. This euphoria can be blocked by pimozide (Gunne *et al.*, 1972). Wise (1978) also suggested that research should be undertaken on the effects of neuroleptics on the rewarding properties of natural reinforcers, such as food.

2.3.2. Anhedonia as Blunting of Primary Reinforcement

In the late 1970s, Wise began to study whether pimozide could reduce the rewarding impact of stimuli other than ICSS (Wise *et al.*, 1978*a,b*). The progressive decline in responding that was reported in the Fouriezos and Wise (1976) study was also observed in lever pressing on a continuous-reinforcement schedule (CRF) for food or saccharin reinforcement (Wise *et al.*, 1978*a,b*). Rats running in an alleyway for food reinforcement showed a progressive increase in run time (Wise *et al.*, 1978*a*). Animals tested on a CRF and receiving pimozide on successive days showed greater decreases in responding each day (Wise *et al.*, 1978*a,b*). Besides the fact that these patterns resemble those seen under extinction, it was also reported that there was a transfer of the decline in responding on successive days between extinction and pimozide (Wise *et al.*, 1978*a,b*).

These data have been used as the basis for the formulation of the anhedonia hypothesis of neuroleptic effects (Wise *et al.*, 1978*a,b*; Wise, 1982). According to this hypothesis, as originally formulated, neuroleptic drugs attenuate responding for a number of different primary reinforcers because the drugs reduce the "rewarding impact" of the stimulus. It was suggested that a motor explanation of neuroleptic effects was untenable because, in the beginning of a test session, a neuroleptic-treated rat will respond at near-normal levels. This is thought to reflect the preservation of response capacity in the animal (Wise, 1978*a,b*, 1982). In addition, "spontaneous recovery" effects, such as those obtained by Fouriezos and Wise (1976) and Franklin and McCoy (1979), demonstrate response capacity in the subject at a time when responding would normally have ceased or been severely reduced. Thus, a neuroleptic-treated animal is capable of responding, but does not do so because the reinforcer does not exert its effect in sustaining the response.

2.3.3. Anhedonia as Interference with Incentive Motivation

Within a few years of the introduction of the anhedonia hypothesis, some experimental results emerged that led to a modification of the original proposal. Phillips and Fibiger (1979) investigated the effects of 0.1 mg/kg haloperidol on variable-interval (VI) performance for ICSS in rats. They reported that simultaneously exposing animals to both extinction and haloperidol caused greater response reduction than did haloperidol alone. It is difficult to see how this could be, if the effect of haloperidol was merely to induce an extinctionlike effect. Moreover, they observed that responding began to slow even before the presentation of the first reinforcer. Surely, if extinction of primary reinforcement was the only result of haloperidol administration, then responding could not slow down until the reinforcer had been encountered.

Work from Wise's own laboratory also yielded results inconsistent with the original anhedonia hypothesis (Gray and Wise, 1980). Studying the effects of 1.0 mg/kg pimozide on VI 2.5-min performance, Gray and Wise (1980) also found that response decrements preceded presentation of the first reinforcer. As did Phillips and Fibiger (1979), Gray and Wise (1980) observed that pimozide plus extinction led to greater decreases in response rate than extinction alone. These results led to an amending of the original anhedonia hypothesis (Gray and Wise, 1980). In addition to blunting primary reinforcing effects of food, neuroleptics were also said to reduce the effectiveness of incentive–motivational cues present in the test environment. These are cues that, because of their association with primary reinforcers, can elicit and sustain appetitive behaviors (Bindra, 1974). The more recent formulations of the anhedonia hypothesis (i.e., Wise, 1982) have used both primary reinforcer and incentive–motivational interpretations.

3. EVALUATION OF EXPERIMENTS ON DOPAMINERGIC INVOLVEMENT IN REINFORCEMENT

Since the initial proposal of the anhedonia hypothesis, a voluminous literature on the topic of neuroleptic drugs and reinforcement processes has accumulated. The purpose of this section is to evaluate whether the two tenets of the anhedonia hypothesis have been supported by subsequent experimentation. Moreover, some of the conceptual and theoretical issues incited by this hypothesis are discussed.

3.1. On the Proposed Similarity between Neuroleptics and Extinction

In general, little support has been found for the suggestion that the effects of neuroleptic drugs resemble extinction. Tombaugh et al. (1980) reported that, although repeated exposure to pimozide and extinction following intermittent reinforcement both resulted in progressive decreases in lever pressing over several days, the cumulative decrease with

1.0 mg/kg pimozide was considerably larger. Faustman and Fowler (1981) recorded the duration of lever depression times in rats and found that haloperidol significantly increased lever depression time, while extinction did not. The same researchers also failed to observe the repeated-exposure extinction effect with clozapine (Faustman and Fowler, 1982). Studies have failed to replicate the "transfer" effect between extinction and neuroleptics (Beninger, 1982; Mason et al. 1980; Tombaugh et al., 1980).

Haloperidol and extinction produced dissimilar effects on a lever-pressing task that used different force requirements (Asin and Fibiger, 1984). Mason et al. (1980) failed to observe a partial reinforcement effect when pimozide was periodically given during alleyway training. In a comparison of responding on a fixed-ratio 20 schedule following 0.1 mg/kg haloperidol with extinction treatment, extinction subjects emitted proportionately more ratios that were faster than the previous baseline response rate than did haloperidol subjects (Salamone, 1986). Evenden and Robbins (1983a) observed that α-flupenthixol and extinction had different effects on a win–stay choice paradigm. Whether a neuroleptic drug produces "extinction" depends importantly upon the particular operant that is being reinforced. Mason et al. (1980) failed to observe "extinction" of responding on a DRL schedule of food reinforcement at 1.0 mg/kg pimozide—a dose frequently used in anhedonia experiments. Administration of 0.4 mg/kg haloperidol, a dose that essentially eliminates operant lever pressing, did not affect performance of an instrumental response in which the subject merely had to be in proximity to the food dish on an FI 30-sec schedule (Salamone, 1986). Ettenberg et al. (1981) observed that a dose of pimozide that "extinguishes" lever pressing for brain stimulation did not alter nose poking for brain-stimulation reinforcement.

Wise (1982) has dismissed studies such as that of Ettenberg et al. (1981), suggesting that they are irrelevant to the question of animal lever pressing for reinforcement. According to Wise (1982, p. 48), these experiments "tell us nothing very convincing about the ability of a rat to lever-press under neuroleptic conditions." However, according to Wise's own theory, "the ability of an animal to lever-press" is *not* what is affected by DA antagonists. Instead, what is supposedly altered is the effect of the reinforcer. Whereas experiments utilizing operants other than lever pressing do not say anything about the ability of an animal to press a lever, they do say something about the ability of a reinforcer to maintain some behavior. They say that this ability is still intact.

It seems clear that the sensitivity of a behavior to neuroleptic intervention depends to a great extent on the specific behavior in question. Despite Wise's claim (Wise, 1982, p. 48) that "the different dose sensitivity has no clear implication at all for the question of whether neuroleptics interfere with motivational or motor processes," this finding remains a robust one, and requires an explanation. Doses of neuroleptics that impair operant lever pressing leave feeding on pellets intact (Rolls et al., 1974); doses of DA antagonists that suppress some operants leave others unimpaired (Ettenberg et al., 1981; Mason et al., 1980). These findings should not be obfuscated or ignored. Rather, they represent one of the most salient characteristics of the effect of neuroleptics on the broad spectrum of behavior. Response requirement is an important determinant of neuroleptic action. Although response requirement is also a determinant of performance in extinction, it is evident that the effects of response requirement upon extinction and upon neuroleptic actions do not covary.

3.2. The Response Capacity Argument

According to Wise (Wise et al., 1978a; Wise, 1982), another line of evidence supporting the anhedonia hypothesis is that the capacity of neuroleptic-treated animals to respond remains intact. Wise et al. (1978a) observed that animals exposed to pimozide treatment for the first time showed normal response rates while responding on a CRF schedule for food reinforcement. It was only on subsequent exposures to the drug that response rates decreased. According to Wise et al. (1978a, p. 262), "the fact that pimozide treated animals responded as often as did the normally rewarded control group on the first test shows that there was no significant impairment of normal lever-pressing capacity. . . ." Wise (1982) also points out that neuroleptic-treated animals can show periods of normal or near-normal responding in the initial part of their test sessions.

Additional support for this argument has been drawn from studies involving operant responding for brain stimulation. Fouriezos and Wise (1976) investigated the effect of pimozide on responding in a chamber in which the lever was in an alcove that could be closed off from the subject. During drug administration tests, the door was closed after 10 min, in the time period when responding had ceased. It was observed that reopening the door after 10 additional minutes led the animal to reinitiate responding. In another study, Franklin and McCoy (1979) demonstrated that responding extinguished by pimozide treatment was temporarily reinstated by presentation of a light previously paired with reinforcement. They maintained that this phenomenon did not reflect a general arousal effect, since a light impaired with reward had no such effect; shaking the animals did not increase responding.

The interpretation by Wise (Wise et al., 1978a; Wise, 1982) of these data is that they demonstrate a retained capacity for operant responding under neuroleptic treatment. However, I feel that this is not a necessary, or even viable, conclusion. The major fault with this interpretation is that it assumes that there is a static, unifaceted entity—"response capacity"—which, when demonstrated to exist under one environmental condition, must necessarily exist under all environmental conditions. A study demonstrating normal response rate in the beginning of a session only conclusively indicates response capacity in the beginning of that session! It does not prove the existence of response capacity throughout the session, or on another test day. If presentation of a stimulus paired with reinforcement restores operant responding, it only proves that the animal is capable of responding with that stimulus present. It is entirely possible that, rather than being absolutely static, the "capacity" to respond is labile and is mitigated by various environmental stimuli. Thus, one interpretation of the finding that a stimulus paired with reinforcement can reinstate responding is that that stimulus restores response capacity.

This argument, although possible, is not a very strong scientific hypothesis. It is, in fact, just as weak as Wise's statement that response capacity is left intact by neuroleptics. These are both assertions that do not readily lend themselves to scientific analysis. It would be as difficult to prove the absence of response capacity while an animal is not responding as it would be to demonstrate its presence. For these reasons, this author feels that the response capacity issue as described by Wise (1982) is not a particularly useful avenue to pursue; it is, instead, a cul-de-sac.

3.3. The Use of Paradigms Purported to Dissociate Reinforcement from Performance

In most of the studies cited earlier, a putative deficit in reward processes or preservation of response capacity was inferred from changes in response rates or patterns. Alternative methodologies have been suggested to provide independent measurements of the rewarding impact of stimuli and also motor performance. Some of these methodologies have been used to study the effects of neuroleptic drugs, including response–intensity relationships, reward summation functions, and response–reinforcement matching. Despite the apparent differences of these methods, they all share a common conceptual framework, as illustrated in Fig. 1. The X axis of this figure represents some dimension of reinforcement value, such as ICSS current, number of ICSS pulses, or density of food reinforcement. The Y axis is a performance measure, such as rate of responding or run speed. In each instance, instrumental performance increases with increasing reinforcement value, up to some stable maximum level. Increasing ICSS current yields increasing response rate, up to maximum responding. In the reward summation test, increasing the number of ICSS pulses leads to a relatively rapid rise in alleyway run speed, up to maximum speed. With the matching equation of Herrnstein (1970), the same basic pattern is described, which is greater response rate with increases in reinforcement density up to asymptotic response rates.

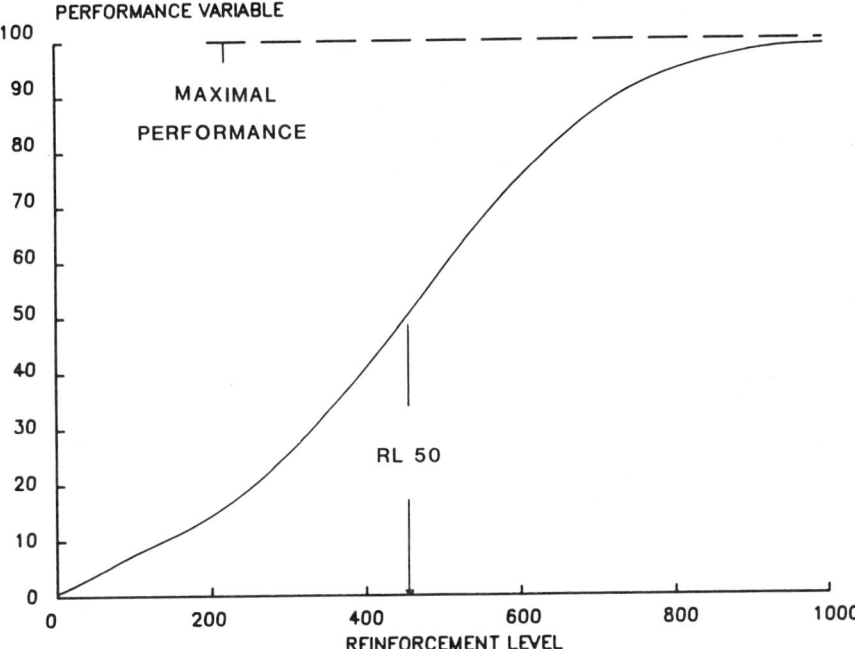

FIG. 1. A representation of the general relationship between level of reinforcement (in frequency or magnitude) and response output. The specific response measure will vary from test to test but could include such measures as response rate or speed. This type of relationship generally yields at least two parameters, one for asymptotic responding and the other for the level of reinforcement that yields half-maximal responding. Drug effects are assessed in terms of their actions on these parameters.

These functions can be used to calculate indices of motor performance and rewarding impact (Fig. 1). The level of maximal responding is usually identified as the index of motor performance. The degree of displacement of the curve along the X axis is interpreted as indicative of reinforcement impact. Often this index is obtained by recording the level of reinforcement that gives a response output that is half maximal (RL_{50}). In this way, the rewarding impact of a reinforcing stimulus can be analogous to the potency (using an ED_{50}) of a pharmacological stimulus.

3.3.1. Response–Intensity Studies on ICSS

Investigations of response–intensity relations in ICSS have usually been undertaken to measure ICSS thresholds and typically used indices other than the RL_{50}. It has been demonstrated that neuroleptics raise ICSS thresholds (Esposito *et al.*, 1979; Leith and Barrett, 1980; Schaefer and Holtzman, 1979; Schaefer and Michael, 1980). Esposito *et al.* (1979)

showed increases in ICSS thresholds at doses of neuroleptics that did not increase response latencies. However, very few studies on ICSS thresholds measured performance across the wide range of currents, including those that yield maximal responding. It is not at all clear that a threshold measurement in the absence of maximum response rate data is a clear measure of reinforcement that is independent of motor capabilities. Thus, studies that extend the range of currents to those yielding near-maximal performance are useful to examine. Leith and Barrett (1980) chronically administered reserpine to rats responding for ICSS at 15 intensities in a descending order. Their definition of threshold was the RL_{50} current and the current range extended up to the point at or near maximal responding. Over the first several days, the deficit obtained reflected mostly an increase in the RL_{50}. Although the effects upon maximal responding were not reported, it appears that there was a decrease in maximal responding after 17–19 days of treatment (Leith and Barrett, 1980, Fig. 1). Wise (1982, Fig. 4) also presented response–intensity data following neuroleptic administration. Here again, a shift in the RL_{50} was also accompanied by a decrease in maximal responding.

Another way of measuring ICSS thresholds is the two-lever autotitration procedure of Stein and Ray (1960). In this procedure, responding on an ICSS lever leads to the delivery of ICSS reinforcement to the rat and, also, to stepwise decrements in the ICSS current. The rat can reset the current level to maximum by pressing the second lever. Thus, the point at which the rat repeatedly resets is taken to be the intensity threshold. Schaefer and Holtzman (1979) and Schaefer and Michael (1980) demonstrated that haloperidol and loxapine produced dose-related increases in ICSS reset levels. However, there is no evidence that most drugs induced a relatively pure change in the reinforcing impact of the ICSS current. Response rates also decreased with these drugs in the same dose range as the increases in threshold. It is particularly interesting to examine the effects of pimozide on this paradigm (Schaefer and Michael, 1980), since pimozide is the prototypical drug for the induction of the anhedonia effect (Wise et al., 1978a,b). Pimozide induced a graded, dose-related decrease in response rate from 0.3 to 1.75 mg/kg. An increase in threshold intensity was observed only at 1.75 mg/kg, a dose that is considerably higher than the 1.0 mg/kg typically used in anhedonia studies. Moreover, three of eight rats at this dose showed disruption of behavior (Schaefer and Michael, 1980, p. 12). Of all the drugs tested, only clozapine showed an increase in threshold at doses that did not yield decreases in response rates (Schaefer and Michael, 1980).

Despite the intuitive appeal of the two-lever autotitration procedure, one should exercise caution in interpreting results from this paradigm. It might be true that some drugs show selective effects on threshold rather than rate measures and that this could signify a relative independence of the two effects. However, performance on this task could never be considered as independent from effects upon the processes regulating the organization of complex behaviors. DA systems have been implicated in the control of switching between behaviors and perseveration (Evenden and Robbins, 1983b; Koob et al., 1978; Lyon and Robbins, 1975; Robbins and Watson, 1981). It is possible that drug-induced changes in two-lever autotitration represent a reorganization of the two sets of responses, rather than a change in threshold per se.

3.3.2. Reward Summation Effects

The reward summation function was defined by Edmonds and Gallistel (1974) as the function relating running speed in a runway to the number of ICSS pulses a rat receives as reinforcement for running. This function roughly follows a sigmoidal shape (see Fig. 1), and the "locus of rise" in the function is the level of current at which an abrupt increment in speed is observed. This value is sometimes calculated as the log pulse number yielding half-maximal run speed (RL_{50}). A considerable number of studies have been published on the effects of neuroleptics upon reward summation (Edmonds and Gallistel, 1977; Franklin, 1978; Gallistel and Karras, 1984; Stellar et al., 1983). Each of these rely upon the earlier work of Gallistel (Edmonds and Gallistel, 1974; Edmonds et al., 1974) to provide the rationale as well as the methodology for this area. Thus, a detailed critique of the Edmonds and Gallistel (1974) experiments is warranted.

Edmonds et al. (1974) demonstrated that reducing ICSS current intensity shifted the summation curve to the right, as signified by an increase in the locus of rise. Since a decreased current intensity represents a lower reinforcement value, an X-axis shift to the right was interpreted to indicate a decrease in the reinforcing impact of the stimulation (as in Fig. 1). The purpose of the Edmonds and Gallistel (1974) study was to investigate whether certain "performance variables" could selectively alter asymptotic run speed without affecting the locus of rise. In this way, a dissociation of reward and performance effects could be achieved.

A thorough examination of the Edmonds and Gallistel (1974) article leads me to be skeptical as to whether such a dissociation was actually achieved. These researchers utilized a number of performance variables, including priming, the grade of the runway, the presence of disease, curare, methocarbamol, and atropine. They concluded that "performance factors affected the height (asymptotic speed) of the function but not the location of the sharp rise in the function" (p. 876). Yet this conclusion was based on results obtained from very few rats (often one or two rats per condition) and was not supported by any inferential statistics. Such an important negative conclusion should require testing of large numbers of rats with an absence of any statistical effect. In this case, all that was done was that individual data from a few rats were presented and reported to be "within the range of day-to-day instability of the curves" (p. 879). It is interesting to note that much of the performance data expressed in the figures of the Edmonds and Gallistel (1974) article show slight shifts of the locus of rise toward the right. For example, increasing task difficulty by increasing the grade of the runway or imposing hurdles shifted the locus of rise in two of three rats (Edmonds and Gallistel, 1974, Fig. 4). Similarly, *Pseudomonas* pneumonia also produced a slight increase in the locus of rise (Edmonds and Gallistel, 1974, Fig. 6). Although these were shifts toward an increase in locus of rise, one should consider that "day-to-day variability" would involve shifts in both directions. The authors pointed out that these shifts are small compared to the shifts produced by reducing stimulating current. However, one has much more control over current intensity than severity of pneumonia. It is possible that more systematic variation of these performance variables in large numbers of rats would yield greater, more consistent shifts in the locus of rise.

These difficulties with the reward summation paradigm should lead one to be cautious in interpreting neuroleptic effects on this test. Nevertheless, reward summation experiments do provide an interesting look at performance in a novel behavioral situation. α-Methyl-para-tyrosine, which inhibits catecholamine synthesis, increased the locus of rise and also decreased the maximum run speed (Edmonds and Gallistel, 1977). Similarly, pimozide increased locus of rise and decreased maximum run speed (Franklin, 1978; Stellar *et al.*, 1983). α-Flupenthixol injected directly into the nucleus accumbens raised the locus of rise in three of five rats and decreased asymptotic run speed in four of five animals (Stellar *et al.*, 1983). Gallistel and Karras (1984) gave pimozide to rats performing on a lever-pressing version of the reward summation test. Small increases in the locus of rise were obtained, but no data on maximum response rate were reported.

The results from the studies just cited indicate that neuroleptics produce both X-axis displacement effects and maximum response effects. Stellar *et al.* (1983) suggested that the locus of rise shift may occur at relatively low doses that do not decrease maximum run speed. At 0.25 mg/kg pimozide, four of four rats had increases in the LR_{50} that were outside the 95% confidence limits, whereas only one rat had a decrease in maximum run speed that was considered significant (though, in fact, two of the other three rats did have slight decreases). At 0.5 mg/kg, all four rats showed an effect on both parameters. However, this dose-related dissociation of effects has not been consistently observed. Franklin (1978) reported that, at 0.1 mg/kg of pimozide, asymptotic run speed was significantly reduced, but locus of rise was unaffected. Thus, a clear demonstration of a selective effect of neuroleptics upon locus of rise has not materialized. The most that can be claimed is that the alterations in asymptotic speed and locus of rise are not correlated across subjects (Edmonds and Gallistel, 1977; Franklin, 1978).

3.3.3. Neuroleptics and Response–Reinforcement Matching

Response–reinforcement matching is an area that is now widely studied by behavioral scientists (Baum, 1974; Herrnstein, 1961, 1970; see also review by deVilliers, 1977). Neuroleptic effects in these paradigms would yield results of considerable interest. Moreover, reinforcers other than ICSS are typically used in matching experiments, so that these results would have a generality not offered by the methodologies described above.

To date, only two experiments have been reported on neuroleptic administration in matching paradigms (Heyman, 1983; Morely et al., 1984). Each of these used a paradigm derived from the work of Herrnstein (1970), who demonstrated that the relationship between reinforcement density and response rate in VI schedules could be described by a hyperbolic equation. This equation is

$$R = \frac{kr}{r + r_e}$$

where R is the response rate, r is the reinforcement rate, k is a constant signifying maximum response rate, and r_e is the reinforcement rate yielding half-maximal responding (RL_{50}; see Fig. 1).

Heyman (1983) studied the effect of pimozide on a five-component multiple schedule (VI 160, 80, 40, 20, 10 sec). Doses of 0.2, 0.3, and 0.6 mg/kg were given four rats, three times for each treatment. The results of these sessions were averaged, and hyperbolae were constructed for each rat at each dose. Heyman (1983) observed increases in the RL_{50} (r_e) and decreases in maximum response rate (k). However, it was stated that k was less affected by pimozide than was r_e. It was only at 0.6 mg/kg that k was decreased in all four subjects, whereas r_e was increased at each dose in a dose-related manner.

A different conclusion was reached by Morely et al. (1984), who used a behavioral test designed from mathematical manipulation of Herrnstein's (1970) hyperbola. According to their view, a drug that elevates r_e would have a greater suppressant effect on responding at high reinforcement densities than low ones, whereas a drug that decreases k would have an effect independent of reinforcement frequency. Morely et al. (1984) injected pimozide in doses of 0.125–0.5 mg/kg, while rats were responding on a high-reinforcement-frequency schedule (VI 10 sec) and a low-frequency schedule (VI 100 sec).

In terms of percent suppression of responding, there was no difference in pimozide's effect upon VI 10 or VI 100 responding, as shown by a lack of a significant dose × schedule interaction (Morely et al., 1984). Thus, it was concluded that pimozide suppressed k but had no effect upon r_e.

It is interesting that the Morely et al. (1984) and Heyman (1983) experiments yielded such different outcomes. Although the rationale behind the Morely et al. (1984) experiment is clear, testing for effects at two different VI schedules does not offer the analytical power that using a range of VI values would. Heyman (1983) did utilize a multiple schedule with five VI values. However, some important problems with this study must be discussed before any weight is given to its findings.

The major difficulty with the Heyman (1983) study is that the results of the curve-fitting analyses are not consistent with the individual subject data presented. In particular, the assertion that changes in maximum response rate were small and inconsistent, except at 0.6 mg/kg pimozide, was somewhat dubious. Although it is true that estimates of k changed less with pimozide than r_e, a close inspection of Heyman's (1983) Table 1 suggests that these calculations do not capture the essence of the data observed. At 0.2 mg/kg pimozide, three of the four rats had maximum *obtained* (not estimated) response rates that were lower than during baseline testing. In the VI 10 component of the schedule, which gave the highest response rates for all subjects, average response rate following 0.2 mg/kg pimozide was 79.5% (± SEM 8.0) of base line.

At the two higher doses, responding in the VI 10 was severely reduced relative to base line. Yet, these reductions were not always manifested in a reduction in k. One example will illustrate this point clearly. Rat 901 had a calculated base line k of 132.6 responses/min (Heyman, 1983, Table 2). The calculated k for this same rat at 0.6 mg/kg pimozide was 130.3 responses/min, which one could interpret as essentially no decrease in maximum response rate. However, this estimate of k is noticeably different from the data shown in his Table 1. Here one sees that responding under the VI 10 component, which was the highest reinforcement density and which gave the maximum *obtained* response rate, was reduced to 12.3% of the base-line response rate! Somehow, the equations led Heyman (1983) to conclude that the maximum response rate for rat 901 at 0.6 mg/kg pimozide was a rate that was more than 13 times the fastest rate the animal exhibited in the test sessions. The way in which the matching equations accounted for this was to utilize an extremely high r_e value—2671 reinforcements per hour. This r_e value was more than seven times the highest programmed density of reinforcement in the experiment. There is no evidence to suggest that the rat would increase its response rate with increased reinforcement to the extent predicted by Heyman (1983). In fact, it is entirely likely that at 2671 reinforcements

TABLE 1
Recalculation of Matching Parameters, Standard Errors, and t Values from Rat 21 of Heyman (1983)

Dose	Parameter	Parameter value	Standard error	t value	Probability
Baseline	k	149.4	19.1	7.80	0.004
	r_e	167.4	45.6	3.67	0.035
0.2 mg/kg pimozide	k	143.8	42.2	3.41	0.042
	r_e	368.4	174.7	2.10	0.125
0.3 mg/kg pimozide	k	121.8	37.6	3.24	0.048
	r_e	652.9	279.3	2.33	0.101
0.6 mg/kg pimozide	k	90.7	94.6	0.958	0.409
	r_e	1187.1	1439.4	0.825	0.470

per hour (one reinforcement per 1.35 sec on average) the response rate would be considerably lower than the rate at 360 reinforcements per hour, since the rat would probably perceive this schedule as close to a CRF.

One could say that, despite the points raised above, the matching equations did provide a good fit of the rats' performance for base-line conditions and following pimozide administration. However, the most important point is not the degree of fit of the curves to the observed data points but rather the accuracy of the parameters themselves. To analyze the determination of the parameters in the Heyman (1983) study, I recalculated the curves with a computer program that also listed the standard errors for the parameters r_e and k.* The data were obtained from Table 1 of Heyman (1983).

Parameters r_e and k, which were calculated for rat 21 at each treatment, were identical to those obtained by Heyman. However, it was also observed that there was an increase in the standard errors with increasing dose (see Table 1 of this chapter). For example, the standard error for k at 0.6 mg/kg pimozide was 94.6 responses/min, which is greater than the k value itself. The parameter r_e did not significantly differ from zero on any of the drug tests. It is difficult to draw any firm conclusions based on such variability in parameter estimation. The wide variability of the parameters probably stems from the fact that maximum response rate had to be extrapolated from well out of the range of the schedules used and response rates obtained. The use of more schedule components with high

---

* This analysis was provided with the assistance of Dr. Andy Richardson, the computer and curve-fitting specialist in our laboratory, and was performed using an RS1 curve-fitting program. The program calculated a t value (parameter/standard error) to test whether the parameter differed from 0.

reinforcement density would allow the researcher to make a more accurate estimate of the maximum response rate.

Another difficulty with the Heyman (1983) article is the use of obtained rather than programmed reinforcement rates as the X-axis variable. In this way, the Heyman (1983) article differs from the Morely *et al.* (1984) study. The use of obtained reinforcement frequencies in matching equations is quite common. In undrugged animals, there is usually considerable agreement between the two systems. However, it is questionable whether one can legitimately use obtained reinforcement rates from an animal that has received a drug that lowers response and reinforcement rates. Rather than being an independent variable, the obtained reinforcement rate is a dependent variable, which is itself affected by drug dose.

The use of these drug-reduced obtained reinforcement rates shifted the data points even further to the left, away from reinforcement rates close to r_e. One should also question whether it is appropriate, as Heyman (1983) did, to average three different obtained reinforcement rates at the same programmed reinforcement level and then to express them as the mean obtained reinforcement. It is possible that an obtained reinforcement rate from one schedule component might be close to an obtained reinforcement rate from another component schedule, yet the two would not have been averaged.

In addition to the empirical problems just described, there are important theoretical considerations in the use of matching equations for describing drug effects on reinforcing stimuli. According to Herrnstein (1974), response rate for food reinforcement was a function of relative rather than absolute reinforcement. Thus, response rate should be seen as affected by the reinforcement level of other stimuli in the test environment, as well as the primary reinforcer. A shift in r_e could be consistent with a change in the reinforcing value of other stimuli. Thus, it is possible that a neuroleptic would cause sniffing in a corner to be relatively more reinforcing, instead of rendering food relatively less reinforcing. Another difficulty is the suggestion of Wise (1982) that neuroleptics impair the rewarding impact of many different reinforcers. If this occurred to an equal extent with all stimuli, then one would predict that the relative reinforcement value of food or water would remain unchanged following neuroleptic treatment.

3.4. Conclusions

Upon detailed critical examination of the relevant literature, there appears to be little conclusive support for the hypothesis that neuroleptic drugs block the primary reinforcing effects of stimuli. Detailed comparison of neuroleptic effects with extinction reveals a lack of equivalence. Paradigms that are suggested to provide independent measures of motor performance and reward reveal that neuroleptics interfere with measures of both these processes.

There have been suggestions of a relatively selective effect of pimozide on reward-related parameters at low doses (Stellar *et al.*, 1983; Heyman, 1983). However, this has not been a consistent finding (Franklin, 1978) and is not supported in all instances by a close examination of the data (Heyman, 1983).

Evaluations of paradigms such as reward summation and matching hinge upon two related and important questions: (1) Are the measures of motor performance and reward independent? (2) Are the measures used selective indicators of the process they are designed to reflect?

Edmonds and Gallistel (1977) and Franklin (1978) maintained that asymptotic run speed and RL_{50} are uncorrelated and that this demonstrates an independent effect of neuroleptics on reward processes. Such a proposition should be viewed skeptically. Even if, in some experiments, maximum run speed is uncorrelated with RL_{50}, it does not mean that motor performance is independent of RL_{50}. Surely, motor performance is a complex process that has several key indicators, of which maximum response rate is only one. It is not certain to what extent the various indices of motor performance would correlate with each other, let alone with some other variable. In an undrugged rat, it is possible to demonstrate an independence between asymptotic speed and RL_{50} under some conditions, such as reduced current intensity in ICSS, but this does not mean that this independence extends to all conditions. If a drugged rat shows changes in both RL_{50} and maximum responding, it does not necessarily mean that "reward" and "motor performance" are both affected. It is entirely possible that the drug is acting on some other process and that this effect is responsible for changes in both measures.

The important issue of whether the indices used actually reflect the constructs or processes they were designed to measure is one that has not been discussed to a great extent. It is typically an assumed feature of most of the studies cited earlier. At this point, it cannot be concluded that an effect on some measure of asymptotic performance is the only valid criterion for demonstrating a motor impairment. As was pointed out by Leibman (1983) in his review of ICSS methodology, subtle motor impairments might well escape detection in reward summation studies. The presumption of functional equivalence between "maximum response rate" and "motor performance" is a gross conceptual oversimplification. Nor is it clear why RL_{50} measures should be viewed as "pure" measures of reinforcing impact of stimuli. Facets of motor performance, or even such variables as incentive, could contribute to the RL_{50} measure.

4. INCENTIVE EXPLANATION OF NEUROLEPTIC ACTIONS

As stated above, Wise (1982; Wise *et al.*, 1978a,b) has posited that DA antagonists blunt the "hedonic impact" of primary reinforcers. In addition, it has been hypothesized that neuroleptics also impair "incentive-motivation" and the reinforcing properties of secondary reinforcers (Gray and Wise, 1980; Wise, 1982). This explanation was originally put forth to explain the results of Gray and Wise (1980) that 1.0 mg/kg pimozide, a dose that causes an extinctionlike effect on CRF responding, has a much more powerful effect on VI responding. Moreover, responding of animals treated with DA antagonists on VI schedules is slower than normal, even before the first encounter with reinforcement (Phillips and Fibiger, 1979; Gray and Wise, 1980). Wise (1982; Gray and Wise, 1980) has stated that this occurs because responding on intermittent schedules of reinforcement is also maintained by secondary reinforcers and incentive–motivational stimuli, such as the click of the lever microswitch. The position was taken that as well as blunting the "hedonic impact" of the primary reinforcer, neuroleptics also blunt the impact of incentives.

Although this position has several advantages over a pure "anhedonia" hypothesis, there are still several problems with this interpretation of data. First, this view is intended to be an extension of the "reward" explanation of neuroleptic effects. Yet, some incentive theorists have considered incentive and reinforcement to represent different processes. In the hypotheticodeductive system of Spence (1956), each mediating process was reflected by a different parameter. Habit or associative strength was signified by "sHr," whereas incentive was labeled "k." According to Cofer (1972), although the same stimulus could function as both a reinforcer and an incentive, these two functions are, in fact, separate. Reinforcement refers to a strengthening of specific responses followed by a reinforcer; incentives are said to "induce states of arousal in organisms" (Cofer, 1972, p. 89). According to reviews by Bolles (1972) and Bindra (1974, 1978), this view of reinforcement and incentive as two distinct processes was the traditional, dominant conception of the time. If reinforcement and incentive are separate processes, then the incentive explanation of neuroleptic effects should not be considered an extension of a reinforcement explanation. It is, in fact, a different hypothesis.

The conceptualization of incentive offered by Wise (1982) appears to be similar to that proposed by Bindra (1974, 1978). However, it should be emphasized that Bindra (1974) and other incentive theorists, such as Bolles (1972) and Killeen (1975), intended incentive–motivation to *replace* the concept of reinforcement, and they attempted to discard the response–reinforcement principle. Wise (1982), on the other hand, employs both a hedonic-based reinforcement principle and an incentive–motivation principle and claims that neuroleptics block both processes. There is no empirical support for the validity of this particular system.

It is important to ponder what is meant by the terms *incentive* or *incentive–motivation*. Unfortunately, there is no standard lexicon from which all psychologists draw their terms. There are as many different definitions of incentive as there are incentive theorists. Yet, despite the array of different definitions, most descriptions have one feature in common. Most definitions of incentive are grounded in some observable heightening of motor activity, induced by the incentive stimulus. For Spence (1956), incentive modulated the vigor and strength of the instrumental behavior. Cofer and Appley (1964) related incentive to the existence of an "anticipation–invigoration" mechanism. Killeen (1975) stated that arousal or incentive was a state characterized by nonspecific activation of a number of behaviors, analogous to the gain-control of an amplifier. In Killeen's (1975, 1981; Killeen *et al.*, 1978) mathematical system, incentive effects are quantified by measuring increases in various motor activities. According to Bindra (1972), incentive–motivation is characterized by the fact that certain stimuli have "action–instigational" effects. In a subsequent article, Bindra (1974) defined the incentive–motivational state as a "hypothetical set of neural processes that promotes goal-directed actions in relation to particular classes of incentive stimuli" (p. 201).

The inextricable link between "incentive" and such constructs as arousal, activation, invigoration, and motor activity virtually negates any dichotomy between Wise's (1982) incentive hypothesis and so-called motor explanations of DA antagonist effects. The statement that DA antagonists impair incentive–motivation is logically equivalent to saying that those drugs block the increased motor activity induced by various stimuli. How different is it to say that neuroleptics block the instigation of action from saying that they impair the initiation of movement? The link between putative incentive–motivational systems in the brain and the motor system was emphasized by Broekkamp *et al.* (1977), who stated that "it is arbitrary to define exactly the line between the two systems. [For example] the incentive stimulation can be considered either as the last part of the motivational system or the first part of the motor system" (p. 70).

Stricker and Zigmond (1976) previously had implicated brain DA systems in arousal and motivation. Wise (1982) cited their work as support for the anhedonia hypothesis. Yet a close inspection of the Stricker and Zigmond (1976) paper reveals that these researchers acknowledged the relationship between motivation and motor activity. In the context of describing the rise of brain catecholamine levels in motivation, they explicitly state that brain DA systems are involved in "locomotor activity" and "behavioral responsiveness" (p. 140).

The studies of Fouriezos and Wise (1976) and Franklin and McCoy (1979) are consistent with the interpretation that DA systems are involved in mediating responsiveness to the environment. Similar findings were obtained by Marshall *et al.* (1976), who demonstrated that immersion in a water or an ice bath or exposure to other animals could temporarily reverse sensorimotor impairments due to DA lesions. The akinesia of Parkinson's patients is also temporarily reversable under some stimulus conditions (Schwab and Zeiper, 1965).

The interpretation offered for these data by Marshall *et al.* (1976) was that arousal or activation could restore performance following DA lesion. Franklin and McCoy (1979) and Wise (1982) argued against this interpretation for neuroleptic studies, although their basis for doing so was rather weak. Supposedly, one control for the "arousing" effects of presenting a stimulus paired with reinforcement was to present to another group of subjects a stimulus that was randomly presented relative to reinforcement. This stimulus did not reinstate responding (Franklin and McCoy, 1979). Yet how could one conclusively argue that such an insignificant stimulus was equally as arousing as a stimulus that was paired with reinforcement? Moreover, Franklin and McCoy (1979) tried to control for the arousal effect by shaking the test chamber; they observed that this manipulation did not increase responding. However, there are conceptual and methodological problems with this. In the first place, there is no indication that "shaking the apparatus" (p. 72) would provide the degree or type of activation to even serve as a valid comparison. How many times was it shaken? How vigorously was it shaken? Also, shaking the apparatus was only done to animals that were not responding (p. 72); thus this was not an unbiased subject population. In short, there has not been a valid refutation of the hypothesis that the activation produced by certain environmental conditions modulates the efficacy of DA-related manipulations.

Another difficulty with the hypothesis that DA antagonists block incentive motivation is the ambiguous relationship between incentive stimuli and secondary reinforcers. Wise (1982) asserts that responding on VI schedules is maintained by secondary reinforcers. Yet one must be very stringent in using the term *secondary reinforcement*. There are instances when stimuli that have been paired with reinforcers do not have secondary reinforcing properties (Skinner, 1938; Weissman and Crossman, 1966). One cannot simply affirm that secondary reinforcement is in action. Rather, this must be demonstrated by following rigorous criteria.

A study has demonstrated that DA antagonists attenuate the acquisition of secondary reinforcement (Beninger and Phillips, 1980). In addition, DA agonists facilitate the acquisition of secondary reinforcement (Hill, 1970; Robbins, 1975). In the Beninger and Phillips study, these data were interpreted as providing direct, important support for the anhedonia hypothesis. However, the overriding fact remains that researchers know even less about secondary reinforcement than they do about primary reinforcement. Despite a large number of theories, there is no general, accepted explanation of the process that underlies secondary reinforcement. The fact that neuroleptics attenuate acquisition of secondary reinforcement is interesting, yet it is not at all clear what the relevance of this finding is. It is possible that the elicitation of approach responses or increased activity is a part of the process that underlies conditioned reinforcement and that this effect is blocked by neuroleptic drugs.

In general, most authors who discuss the concept of incentive define an incentive stimulus in much broader terms than "a secondary reinforcer." For Bolles (1972) and Bindra (1974), conditioned incentive stimuli are those stimuli that have been associated with the primary incentive stimulus, such as food. Bindra (1974) used the term *conditioned incentive–discriminative stimulus* to describe such stimuli. The concepts of stimulus–stimulus association and discriminative stimuli as manifestations of incentive motivation are extremely relevant to Wise's (1982) incentive hypothesis of neuroleptic action. However, numerous studies have shown that, despite a diminished response output, the responding of neuroleptic-treated subjects is still under the control of discriminative stimuli (Franklin and McCoy, 1979; Tombaugh et al., 1980; Tombaugh, 1981; Szostak and Tombaugh, 1981; Beninger, 1982). It is difficult to see how "conditioned incentive–discriminative stimulus" effects could be so greatly impaired when stimulus control is still maintained.

To summarize, my review of the hypothesis that DA antagonists blunt the impact of incentive–motivational stimuli leads me to conclude that much depends upon the definition of incentive. If one refers to discriminative properties of stimuli, then these properties do not seem to be disrupted by neuroleptics. A definition of incentive that involves "motor activities," "action-instigation," and "elicitation of approach responses" is consistent with much of the available data. However, such an interpretation is not incompatible with an explanation in terms of some aspects of motor function.

5. AN ALTERNATIVE EXPLANATION OF DOPAMINE ANTAGONIST EFFECTS ON OPERANT BEHAVIOR

As stated in Sections 3 and 4, some of the difficulties with the anhedonia hypothesis stem from conceptual and definitional problems. One might consider that the particular definition of *reinforcement* or *incentive* used is relatively unimportant. However, there is a strong argument to be made for specifying exactly what is meant by the use of such constructs as reinforcement. In particular, if one is trying to suggest involvement of DA in certain behavioral mechanisms, then one should adequately describe what functions these mechanisms are performing. For this reason the next section of this chapter introduces a model of appetitive behavior that can be used to account for many of the actions of neuroleptic drugs.

5.1. A Multiprocess Model for Describing Control of Operant Response Output

The effects of neuroleptics on instrumental behavior are not strictly consistent with an impairment in incentive–motivation as proposed by Bindra (1974, 1978). One possible problem is that incentive–motivation incorporates too many mechanisms. Various aspects of incentive–motivation, such as approach to and consumption of food and discrimination, are spared at doses of neuroleptics that severely impair the operant response rate (Beninger, 1982; Fibiger et al., 1976; Franklin and McCoy, 1979; Rolls et al., 1974; Tombaugh et al., 1980; Tombaugh, 1981; Szostak and Tombaugh, 1981). This indicates some degree of dissociation among elements of what was thought to be a global process.

A model that distinguishes between some of the different processes involved in instrumental responding might prove to be more useful in accounting for the effects of neuroleptics on these behaviors. A multiprocess model for control of instrumental responding is depicted in Fig. 2. In this model, the process that controls selection of the specific appetitive instrumental response is considered as distinct from the mechanism that generally regulates response output. The appetitive response selection

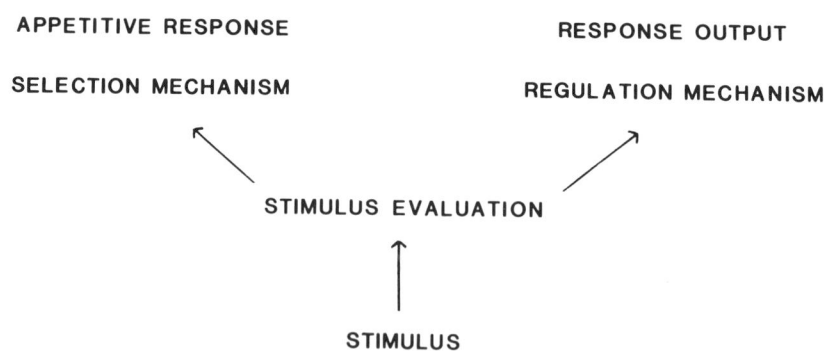

FIG. 2. A multiprocess model for the control of appetitive instrumental responding. The model implies a possible dissociability between the response selection and response output regulation mechanisms. Stimulus evaluation is meant to include processes, such as sensation, which are necessary for stimuli to act upon the organism and lead to a change in response output and choice.

mechanism (ARSM) is involved in the selection of specific instrumental responses and the modulation of instrumental response topography. This function is related to a "reinforcement" process. The response output regulation mechanism (RORM) controls quantitative aspects of responsiveness to the reinforcing stimulus, including the rate, amplitude, and duration of movements. This is not dissimilar from the traditional concept of *incentive*. The responses controlled by the RORM include the appetitive response itself, as well as aspects of the consummatory response and other activities present in the instrumental learning situation.

Normally, the two mechanisms jointly act to control instrumental responding. However, it is suggested that systemic administration of moderate-to-low doses of neuroleptics can dissociate the ARSM and the RORM by producing relatively selective impairment of the RORM. This dissociation is apparent only in behavioral paradigms that have separate measures related to the two mechanisms. Tombaugh *et al.* (1983) conducted such an experiment when they studied the effects of pimozide on the performance of rats in a T-maze, light–dark discrimination task. Although pimozide-treated rats were able to perform the discrimination and execute the correct reinforced response, the rate of running in the maze was significantly reduced. Using a two-lever win–stay paradigm, Evenden and Robbins (1983a) showed that α-flupenthixol decreased the response rate but did not impair the response choice measure. Pimozide reliably decreased response rate but not response choice accuracy in a two-hole discrimination task with ICSS in mice (Bowers *et al.*, 1985). Salamone (1986) studied the effects of haloperidol on rats performing a simple place location response for food in an apparatus that also measured locomotor activity. Haloperidol did not reduce time spent on the reinforced floor panel, but it did reduce locomotor activity. These experiments represent evidence that neuroleptics can impair quantitative features of instrumental response output at doses that do not disrupt the selection of the appropriate instrumental response. This suggests that DA systems are involved in the function of the RORM.

The major function of the RORM is to control such quantitative aspects of response output as response frequency and duration. Changes in these features of response output resulting from neuroleptic administration have been reported. Tombaugh *et al.* reported that local frequencies of lever pressing on both a fixed-ratio and a variable-interval schedule were decreased by pimozide. Treatment with neuroleptics decreases the rate of feeding behavior (Blundell, 1981). The duration of individual lever-press responses increased following neuroleptic injection (Faustman and Fowler, 1981). However, another important aspect of response duration is the duration of periods of responding. In many situations, animals emit "bursts" of responses that are separated by periods of no responses. Baum and Rachlin (1969) considered the duration of periods of responding a useful measure for operant experiments. Moreover, animals can sustain performance over large units of time so that, depending upon the task, animals will continue to emit periods of responding throughout a long test session. It is felt that neuroleptic drugs interfere with the ability of rats to maintain responding through time. This deficit would be manifested in several ways, including increases in postreinforcement pause, decreases in time spent lever pressing or feeding, and a difficulty in maintaining responding throughout the test session. Thus, the decline in responding over the test session that is produced by neuroleptics is thought to reflect an impairment in response maintenance. The terms *response maintenance* and *duration* are intended to be used as more than merely empirical descriptions of the fact that responding declines. Rather, it is suggested that the sustained emission of responses through time is one of the important effects of significant stimuli upon an animal and that maintenance of responses is one of the significant dimensions of motor control.

As well as controlling instrumental response output, the RORM is involved in the regulation of activities induced by presentation of such reinforcing stimuli as food. It has been suggested that stimuli that act as reinforcers also have response-activating characteristics (Cofer and Appley, 1964; Killeen, 1975, 1981; Killeen *et al.*, 1978). Killeen has demonstrated that periodic presentation of food to rats or pigeons increase a variety of activities related to the rate of food delivery. DA antagonists or DA lesions have consistently been shown to impair performance of schedule- or food-induced behaviors (Keehn *et al.*, 1976; Keehn and Riusech, 1977; Robbins and Koob, 1980; Wallace *et al.*, 1983). These studies constitute further evidence that DA is importantly involved in the process whereby the activity of the organism in relation to significant environmental stimuli is controlled.

5.2. On the Role of Brain Dopamine Systems in Appetitive Instrumental Behavior

In the first section of this chapter, it was suggested that research into the behavioral effects of neuroleptics would yield information relevant to the question of what role DA systems play in controlling behavior. It is interesting to consider what neuroleptic research does or does not tell us about the behavioral functions of DA. Although systemic administration of neuroleptics does not appear to interfere with the posited response selection process, it is nevertheless not possible to conclude that DA has no involvement whatsoever in this process. Systemically administered neuroleptics block DA receptors throughout the CNS and do not really indicate what functions DA in each isolated regions is performing. It is possible that DA manipulations in discrete areas will produce in deficits in response selection measures.

One should also be cautious in prematurely interpreting deficits resulting from neuroleptics solely in terms of DA systems. Most of these drugs also act on other neurotransmitter systems, which cannot be lightly discounted. However, in most instances, additional evidence can be used to support the putative dopaminergic role in mediating neuroleptic effects. For example, Gallistel and Davis (1983) demonstrated that the potencies of neuroleptics in blocking ICSS are correlated with the affinities of these drugs for the DA D_2 receptor. In addition, a vast amount of anatomical, pharmacological, neurophysiological, and behavioral data all support the contention that DA systems are involved with some aspects of movement.

The suggested involvement of DA systems in the regulation of response output is supported by studies involving behaviors other than appetitive responses. Morpurgo (1965) concluded that the effects of neuroleptics upon response initiation in active avoidance were greater than the effects on response choice as shown in passive avoidance or discrimination tests. Based upon studies of neuroleptic effects on escape and shock-induced behavior, Anisman (Anisman and Zacharko, 1982; Anisman et al., 1979) concluded that neuroleptics impair the maintenance of movement. This hypothesis had previously been offered by Gaddy and Neill (1977) to explain the fact that 6-OHDA applied to striatum affected behaviors requiring sustained activity (feeding, ICSS) more than those characterized by brief movement (muricide, female lordosis). It is possible that there are common mechanisms that regulate the output of a number of different responses, including aversive and "spontaneous" activities as well as appetitive ones.

One aspect of appetitive behavior that has recently been emphasized is how such variables as "response costs," "constraints," or "amplitude" of the operant response affect output (McDowell and Kessell, 1979; Staddon, 1979; Rachlin, 1981; Kaufman, 1980; Kaufman et al., 1980). According to theories of animal foraging, the profitability of a food source, in terms of the ratio of food gained to the expenditure of resources necessary to obtain it, is an important determinant of foraging patterns (Krebs, 1978). Neill and Justice (1981) offered a hypothesis of dopaminergic function related to such concepts, in which the DA in the nucleus accumbens is seen as involved in the evaluation of reinforcing stimuli relative to how much effort is necessary to obtain them. Increasing DA release in the nucleus accumbens by injecting amphetamine was said to increase the "willingness" of the animal to exert effort for a given level of reinforcement (Neill and Justice, 1981).

In the opinion of this researcher, the position that nucleus accumbens DA is involved in the "evaluation" of reinforcement/effort is somewhat premature. Nevertheless, it is felt that DA in accumbens and striatum is involved in the exertion of "effort." Such a capacity enables animals to obtain access to food or other significant stimuli, even if a high behavioral output is required. An interesting line of experimentation would be to offer an animal "choices" between various reinforcers that are associated with operants of varying difficulty. Baum (1974) developed a parameter for "response bias" in matching experiments, to account for deviations from matching when one response may require more effort than the other. Using such a paradigm, DA-related drugs could be given to see whether the allocation of response output could be biased toward or away from more or less effortful responses.

According to the biochemist Albert Lehninger, "the cell is a nonequilibrium open system, a machine for extracting free energy from the environment" (1975, p. 8). Organisms obtain free energy from the environment by ingesting nutritive substances. However, obtaining nutritive substances typically involves some work. Thus, complex organisms must expend energy in the form of muscle contractions in order to obtain the energy necessary for survival. In fact, organisms also expend energy to obtain access to or in response to a variety of significant stimuli. It is suggested here that DA systems are involved in the regulation of much of the energy output, in terms of muscle activity, of complex organisms. The idea that DA is involved in the regulation of various activities should not be viewed as incompatible with an involvement in subtle and interesting features of instrumental behavior. Indeed, many definitions of *incentive* or *motivation* acknowledge the importance of control of activity in these concepts. Young (1961) defined motivation as "the process of arousing actions, sustaining the activity in progress, and regulating the pattern of activity." It is probably more useful to integrate the two views of DA as being involved in movement and motivation than to postulate an artificial dichotomy between them.

ACKNOWLEDGMENTS

Many thanks to D. B. Neill, T. W. Robbins, and S. D. Iversen for their helpful comments.

6. REFERENCES

ANISMAN, H., and ZACHARKO, R., 1982, Stimulus change influences escape performance: Deficits induced by uncontrollable stress by haloperidol, *Pharmacol. Biochem. Behav.* **17**:263–269.

ANISMAN, H., REMINGTON, G., and SKLAR, L. S., 1979, Effect of inescapable shock on subsequent escape performance: Catecholaminergic and cholinergic mediation of response initiation and maintenance, *Psychopharmacology*, **61**:107–124.

ASIN, K. E., and FIBIGER, H. C., 1984, Force requirements in lever-pressing and responding after haloperidol, *Pharmacol. Biochem. Behav.* **20**:323–326.

BAUM, W. M., 1974, On two types of deviation from the matching law: Bias and undermatching, *J. Exp. Anal. Behav.* **22**:231–242.

BAUM, W. M., and RACHLIN, H. C., 1969, Choice as time allocation, *J. Exp. Anal. Behav.* **12**:861–874.

BECKSTEAD, R. M., DOMESICK, V. B., and NAUTA, W. J., 1979, Efferent connections of the substantia nigra and ventral tegmental area in the rat, *Brain Res.* **175**:191–217.

BENINGER, R. J., 1982, A comparison of the effects of pimozide and non-reinforcement on discriminated operant responding in rats, *Pharmacol. Biochem. Behav.* **16**:667–669.

BENINGER, R. J., and PHILLIPS, A. G., 1980, The effects of pimozide on the establishment of conditioned reinforcement, *Psychopharmacology* **68**:147–153.

BINDRA, D., 1972, Neuropsychological interpretation of the effects of drive and incentive-motivation on general and instrumental behavior, *Psychol. Rev.* **75**:1–22.

BINDRA, D., 1974, A motivation view of learning, performance and behavior modification, *Psychol. Rev.* **81**:199–213.

BINDRA, D., 1978, How adaptive behavior is produced: A perceptual–motivational alternative to response–reinforcement, *Behav. Brain Sci.* **1**:41–91.

BLUNDELL, J. E., 1981, Bio-grammar of feeding: Pharmacological manipulations and their interpretations, in: *Theory in Psychopharmacology* (S. J. Cooper, ed.), Academic Press, London.

BOLLES, R. C., 1972, Reinforcement, expectancy and learning, *Psychol. Rev.* **79**:394–409.

BOWERS, W., HAMILTON, M., ZACHARKO, R. M., and ANISMAN, H., 1985, Differential effects of pimozide on response-rate and choice accuracy in a self-stimulation paradigm in mice, *Pharmacol. Biochem. Behav.* **22**:521–526.

BROEKKAMP, C. L., VAN DONGEN, P. A., and VAN ROSSUM, 1977, Neostriatal involvement in reinforcement and motivation, in: *Psychobiology of the Striatum* (A. R. Cools, A. M. Lohman, and J. H. van den Bercken, eds.), North-Holland, Amsterdam.

COFER, C. N., 1972, *Motivation and Emotion*, Scott, Foresman, Glenview, IL.

COFER, C. N., and APPLEY, M. H., 1964, *Motivation: Theory and Research*, Wiley, New York.

COOPER, B., COTT, J., and BREESE, G., 1974, Effects of catecholamine-depleting drugs and amphetamine on self-stimulation of the brain following various 6-hydroxydopamine treatments, *Psychopharmacologia* **37**:235–246.

COSTALL, B., ENIOJUKAN, J. F., and NAYLOR, R. J., 1982, Spontaneous climbing behaviour in mice, its measurement and dopaminergic involvement, *Eur. J. Pharmacol.* **85**:125–132.

COWAN, W. M., and POWELL, T. P., 1966, Strio-pallidal projection in the monkey, *J. Neurol. Neurosurg. Psychiatry* **29**:426–439.

CROW, T. J., 1972, Catecholamine-containing neurones and electrical self-stimulation: A review of some data, *Psychol. Med.* **2**:414–421.

DELONG, M. R., and STRICK, P. L., 1974, Relation of basal ganglia, cerebellum, and motor cortex units to ramp and ballistic movements, *Brain Res.* **71**:327–335.

DEVILLIERS, P. A., 1977, Choice in concurrent schedules and a quantitative formulation of the law of effect, in: *Handbook of Operant Behavior* (W. K. Honig and J. E. R. Staddon, eds.), Prentice-Hall, Englewood Cliffs, NJ.

EDMONDS, P. E., and GALLISTEL, C. R., 1974, Parametric analysis of brain stimulation reward in the rat: Effect of performance variables on the reward summation function, *J. Comp. Physiol. Psychol.* **87**:876–883.

EDMONDS, D. E., and GALLISTEL, C. R., 1977, Reward versus performance in self-stimulation: Electrode specific effects of methyl-*p*-tyrosine on reward in the rat, *J. Comp. Physiol. Psychol.* **91**:962–974.

EDMONDS, D. E., STELLAR, J. R., and GALLISTEL, C. R., 1974, Parametric analysis of brain stimulation reward in the rat: II. Temporal summation in the reward system, *J. Comp. Physiol. Psychol.* **87**:860–869.

ESPOSITO, R. V., FAULKNER, W., and KORNETSKY, C., 1979, Specific modulation of brain stimulation reward of haloperidol, *Pharmacol. Biochem. Behav.* **10**:937–940.

ETTENBERG, A., KOOB, G. F., and BLOOM, F., 1981, Response artifact in the measurement of neuroleptic-induced anhedonia, *Science* **209**:357–359.

EVENDEN, J. L., and ROBBINS, T. W., 1983a, Dissociable effects of d-amphetamine, chlordiazepoxide and α-flupenthixol on choice and rate measures of reinforcement in the rat, *Psychopharmacology* **79**:180–186.

EVENDEN, J. L., and ROBBINS, T. W., 1983b, Increased response switching, perseveration and perseverative switching following d-amphetamine in the rat, *Psychopharmacology* **80**:67–73.

FAUSTMAN, W. O., and FOWLER, S. C., 1981, Use of operant response duration to distinguish the effects of haloperidol from non-reward, *Pharmacol. Biochem. Behav.* **15**:327–329.

FAUSTMAN, W. O., and FOWLER, S. C., 1982, An examination of methodological refinements, clozapine and fluphenazine in the antedonia paradigm, *Pharmacol. Biochem. Behav.* **17**:987–993.

FIBIGER, H. C., ZIS, A., and PHILLIPS, A. G., 1975, Haloperidol-induced disruption of conditioned avoidance responding: Attenuation by prior training or by anticholinergic drugs, *Eur. J. Pharmacol.* **30**:309–314.

FIBIGER, H. C., CARTER, D. A., and PHILLIPS, A. G., 1976, Decreased intracranial self-stimulation after neuroleptics or 6-hydroxydopamine: Evidence for mediation by motor deficits rather than by reduced reward, *Psychopharmacology* **47**:21–27.

FOURIEZOS, G., and WISE, R. A., 1976, Pimozide-induced extinction of intracranial self-stimulation; response patterns rule out motor performance deficits, *Brain Res.* **103**:377–380.

FRANKLIN, K. B., 1978, Catecholamines and self-stimulation: Reward and performance deficits dissociated, *Pharmacol. Biochem. Behav.* **9**:813–820.

FRANKLIN, K. B. T., and MCCOY, S. H., 1979, Pimozide-induced extinction in rats: Stimulus control of responding rules out motor deficit, *Pharmacol. Biochem. Behav.* **11**:71–75.

GADDY, T. R., and NEILL, D. B., 1977, Differential behavioral changes following intrastriatal applications of 6-hydroxydopamine, *Brain Res.* **119**:439–446.

GALLISTEL, C. R., and DAVIS, A. J., 1983, Affinity for the dopamine D_2 receptor predicts neuroleptic potency in blocking the reinforcing effect of MFB stimulation, *Pharmacol. Biochem. Behav.* **19**:867–872.

GALLISTEL, C. R., and KARRAS, D., 1984, Pimozide and amphetamine have opposing effects on the reward summation function, *Pharmacol. Biochem. Behav.* **20**:73–77.

GERMAN, D. C., and BOWDEN, D. M., 1974, Catecholamine systems as the neural substrate for intracranial self-stimulation: A hypothesis, *Brain Res.* **73**:381–419.

GRAY, T., and WISE, R. A., 1980, Effects of pimozide on lever-pressing behavior maintained on an intermittent reinforcement schedule, *Pharmacol. Biochem. Behav.* **12**:931–935.

GUNNE, L. M., ANGGARD, E., and JONSSON, L. E., 1972, Clinical trials with amphetamine-blocking drugs, *Psychiatr. Neurol. Neurochir.* **75**:225–226.

HERRNSTEIN, R., 1961, Relative and absolute strength of response as a function of frequency of reinforcement, *J. Exp. Anal. Behav.* **4**:267–272.

HERRNSTEIN, R. J., 1970, On the law of effect, *J. Exp. Anal. Behav.* **13**:243–266.

HERRNSTEIN, R. J., 1974, Formal properties of the matching law, *J. Exp. Anal. Behav.* **21**:159–164.

HERZ, A., 1960, Drugs and the conditioned avoidance response, *Int. Rev. Neurobiol.* **2**:229–277.

HEYMAN, G. M., 1983, A parametric evaluation of the hedonic and motoric effects of drugs: Pimozide and amphetamine, *J. Exp. Anal. Behav.* **40**:113–122.

HILL, R. T., 1970, Facilitation of conditioned reinforcement as a mechanism of psychomotor stimulation, in: *Amphetamine and Related Compounds* (E. Costa and S. Garattini, eds.), Raven Press, New York.

HORNYKIEWICZ, O., 1972, Dopamine and its physiological significance in brain function, in: *The Structure and Function of Nervous Tissue* (G. H. Browne, ed.), Academic Press, New York.
JANSSEN, P. A. J., NIEMEGEERS, C. J. E., and SCHELLEKENS, K. H. L., 1965, Is it possible to predict the clinical effects of neuroleptic drugs (major tranquillisers) from animal data? *Arzneim.-Forsch.* **15**:104–117.
KAUFMAN, L. W., 1980, Foraging cost and meal patterns in ferrets, *Physiol. Behav.* **25**:139–141.
KAUFMAN, L. W., COLLIER, G., HILL, W. L., and COLLINS, K., 1980, Meal cost and meal patterns in an uncaged domestic cat, *Physiol. Behav.* **25**:135–137.
KEEHN, J. D., and RIUSECH, R., 1977, Schedule-induced water and saccharin polydipsia under haloperidol, *Bull. Psychonom. Soc.* **9**:413–414.
KEEHN, J. D., COULSON, G. E., and KLIEB, J., 1976, Effects of haloperidol on schedule-induced polydipsia, *J. Exp. Anal. Behav.* **25**:105–112.
KELLY, P. H., SEVIOUR, P. W., and IVERSEN, S. D., 1975, Amphetamine and apomorphine responses in the rat following 6-OHDA lesions of the nucleus accumbens septi and corpus striatum, *Brain Res.* **94**:507–522.
KEMP, J., and POWELL, T. P., 1970, The cortico-striate projection in the monkey, *Brain* **93**:525–546.
KILLEEN, P., 1975, On the temporal control of behavior, *Psychol. Rev.* **82**:89–115.
KILLEEN, P., 1981, Incentive theory, in: *Response Structure and Organization* (D. Bernstein, ed.), University of Nebraska Press, Lincoln.
KILLEEN, P., HANSON, S., and OSBOURNE, S., 1978, Arousal: Its genesis and manifestation as response rate, *Psychol. Rev.* **85**:571–581.
KOOB, G. F., RILEY, S. J., SMITH, S. C., and ROBBINS, T. W., 1978, Effects of 6-hydroxydopamine lesions of the nucleus accumbens septi and olfactory tubercle on feeding, locomotor activity, and amphetamine anorexia in the rat, *J. Comp. Physiol. Psychol.* **92**:917–927.
KREBS, J. R., 1978, Optimal foraging: Decision rules for predators, in: *Behavioral Ecology* (J. R. Krebs and W. B. Davise, eds.), Sinauer Associates, Sunderland, MA.
KUNZLE, H., 1975, Bilateral projection from precentral motor cortex to the putamen and other parts of the basal ganglia. An autoradiographic study in *Macaca dascicularis, Brain Res.* **88**:195–210.
LEHNINGER, A., 1975, *Biochemistry*, Worth Publishers, New York.
LEIBMAN, J. M., 1983, Discriminating between reward and performance: A critical review of intracranial self-stimulation methodology, *Neurosci. Biobehav. Rev.* **7**:45–72.
LEITH, N. J., and BARRETT, R. J., 1980, Effects of chronic amphetamine or reserpine on self-stimulation responding: Animal model of depression? *Psychopharmacology* **72**:9–15.
LIPPA, A. S., ANTELMAN, S., FISHER, A., and CANFIELD, D., 1973, Neurochemical mediation of reward: A significant role for dopamine, *Pharmacol. Biochem. Behav.* **1**:25–28.
LYON, M., and ROBBINS, T., 1975, The action of central nervous stimulant drugs: A general theory concerning amphetamine effects, in: *Current Developments in Psychopharmacology*, Vol. 2 (W. Essman and L. Valzelli, eds.), Spectrum, New York.
MARSHALL, J. F., RICHARDSON, J. S., and TEITELBAUM, P., 1974, Nigrostriatal damage and the lateral hypothalamic syndrome, *J. Comp. Physiol. Psychol.* **87**:808–830.
MARHSALL, J. F., LEVITAN, D., and STRICKER, E. M., 1976, Activation-induced restoration of sensorimotor functions in rats with dopamine-depleting brain lesions, *J. Comp. Physiol. Psychol.* **90**:536–546.
MASON, S. T., BENINGER, R. J., FIBIGER, H. C., and PHILLIPS, A. G., 1980, Pimozide-induced suppression of responding: Evidence against a block of food reward, *Pharmacol. Biochem. Behav.* **12**:917–923.
MCDOWELL, J. J., and KESSELL, R., 1979, A multivariate rate equation for variable-interval performance, *J. Exp. Anal. Behav.* **31**:267–283.

Mogensen, G., Jones, D., and Yim, C. Y., 1980, From motivation to action: Function interface between the limbic system and the motor system, *Prog. Neurobiol.* **14**:69–97.

Monti, J. M., and Hance, A. J., 1967, Effects of haloperidol and trifluperidol on operant behavior in the rat, *Psychopharmacologia* **12**:34–43.

Morely, M. J., Bradshaw, C. M., and Szabadi, E., 1984, The effect of pimozide on variable-interval performance: A test of the "anhedonia" hypothesis of the mode of action of neuroleptics, *Psychopharmacology* **84**:531–536.

Morpurgo, C., 1965, Drug-induced modifications of discriminated avoidance behavior in rats, *Psychopharmacologia* **8**:91–99.

Munkvad, I., and Randrup, A., 1966, The persistence of amphetamine stereotypies in spite of strong sedation, *Acta Psychiatr. Scand.* **42**(Suppl. 191):178.

Nauta, W., and Mehler, W. R., 1966, Projections of the lentiforme nucleus in the monkey, *Brain Res.* **1**:3–42.

Neill, D. B., and Justice, J. B., Jr., 1981, An hypothesis for a behavioral function of dopaminergic transmission in nucleus accumbens, in: *The Neurobiology of Nucleus Accumbens* (R. B. Chronister and J. F. Defrance, eds.), Huer Institute, Brunswick.

Niemgeers, C. J. E., Verbruggen, F. J., and Janssen, P. A. J., 1970, The influence of various neuroleptic drugs on shock avoidance responding in rats, *Psychopharmacologia* **17**:151–159.

Ornstein, K., and Huston, J., 1975, Influence of 6-hydroxydopamine injection in the substantia nigra on lateral hypothalamic reinforcement, *Neurosci. Lett.* **1**:339–347.

Phillips, A. G., and Fibiger, H. C., 1979, Decreased resistance to extinction after haloperidol: Implications for the role of dopamine in reinforcement, *Pharmacol. Biochem. Behav.* **10**:751–761.

Posluns, D., 1962, An analysis of chlorpromazine-induced suppression of the avoidance response, *Psychopharmacologia* **3**:361–373.

Pycock, C. J., Tarsy, P., and Marsden, C. D., 1975, Inhibition of circling behavior by neuroleptic drugs in mice with unilateral 6-hydroxydopamine lesions of the striatum, *Psychopharmacologia* **45**:211–219.

Rachlin, H., 1981, Absolute and relative consumption space, in: *Response Structure and Organization* (D. Bernstein, ed.), University of Nebraska Press, Lincoln.

Robbins, T. W., 1975, The potentiation of conditioned reinforcement by psychomotor stimulant drugs: DA test of Hill's hypothesis, *Psychopharmacology* **45**:103–114.

Robbins, T. W., and Koob, G. F., 1980, Selective disruption of displacement behaviour by lesions of the mesolimbic dopamine system, *Nature* **285**:409–412.

Robbins, T. W., and Watson, B. A., 1981, Effects of d-amphetamine on response repetition and win-stay behavior in the rat, in: *Quantification of Steady-State Operant Behavior* (C. M. Bradshaw, E. Szabadi, and C. F. Lowe, eds.), Elsevier/North Holland, pp. 441–444.

Rolls, E. T., Rolls, B. J., Kelly, P. H., Shaw, S. G., Wood, R. J., and Dale, R., 1974, The relative attenuation of self-stimulation, eating and drinking produced by dopamine-receptor blockade, *Psychopharmacologia* **38**:219–230.

Rowland, H., and Engle, D. J., 1977, Feeding and drinking interaction after acute butyrophenome administration, *Pharmacol. Biochem. Behav.* **7**:295–301.

Salamone, J. D., 1986, Different effects of haloperidol and extinction on instrumental behaviours, *Psychopharmacology* **88**:18–23.

Schaefer, G. J., and Holtzman, S. G., 1979, Free-operant and autotitration brain self-stimulation procedures in the rat: A comparison of drug effects, *Pharmacol. Biochem. Behav.* **10**:127–135.

Schaefer, G. P., and Michael, R., 1980, Acute effects of neuroleptics on brain self-stimulation thresholds in rats, *Psychopharmacology* **67**:9–15.

Schlecter, J. M., and Butcher, L. L., 1972, Blockade by pimozide of (+)amphetamine-induced hyperkinesia in mice, *J. Pharm. Pharmacol.* **24**:408–409.

Schwab, R. S., and Zieper, I., 1965, Effects of mood, motivation, stress and alertness on the performance in Parkinson's disease, *Psychiat. Neurol.* **150**:345–357.

SKINNER, B. F., 1938, *Behavior of Organisms,* Appleton-Century-Crofts, New York.
SPENCE, K., 1956, *Behavior Theory and Conditioning,* Yale University Press, New Haven, CT.
STADDON, J. E., 1979, Operant behavior as adaption to constraint, *J. Exp. Psychol. Gen.* **108**:48–67.
STEIN, L., and RAY, O. S., 1960. Brain stimulation reward "thresholds" self-determined in rats, *Psychopharmacologia* **1**:251–256.
STELLAR, J. R., KELLEY, A. E., and CORBETT, D., 1983, Effects of peripheral and central dopamine blockade on lateral hypothalamic self-stimulation: Evidence for both reward and motor deficits, *Pharmacol. Biochem. Behav.* **18**:433–442.
STRICKER, E. M., and ZIGMOND, M. J., 1976, Recovery of function after damage to central catecholamine-containing neurons: A neurochemical modal for the lateral hypothalamic syndrome, in: *Progress in Psychobiology and Physiological Psychology,* Vol. 6 (J. M. Sprague and A. N. Epstein, eds.), Academic Press, New York.
SWANSON, L. W., and COWAN, W. M., 1975, A note on the connection and development of nucleus accumbens, *Brain Res.* **92**:324–330.
SZABO, J., 1962, Topical distribution of the striatal efferents in the monkey, *Exp. Neurol.* **5**:21–36.
SZOSTAK, C., and TOMBAUGH, T. N., 1981, Use of a fixed consecutive number schedule of reinforcement to investigate the effects of pimozide on behavior controlled by internal and external stimuli, *Pharmacol. Biochem Behav.* **15**:609–617.
TAGLIAMONTE, A., FRATTA, W., DEL FIACCO, M., and GESSA, G. L., 1974, Possible stimulatory role of brain dopamine in the copulatory behavior of male rats, *Pharmacol. Biochem. Behav.* **2**:257–260.
TOMBAUGH, T. N., 1981, Effects of pimozide on non-discriminated and discriminated control in the pigeon, *Psychopharmacology* **73**:137–141.
TOMBAUGH, T. N., TOMBAUGH, J., and ANISMAN, H., 1979, Effects of dopamine receptor blockade on alimentary behaviors: Home cage food consumption, magazine training, operant acquisition and performance, *Psychopharmacology* **66**:219–225.
TOMBAUGH, T. N., ANISMAN, H., and TOMBAUGH, J., 1980, Extinction and dopamine receptor blockade after intermittent reinforcement training: Failure to observe functional equivalence, *Psychopharmacology* **70**:19–28.
TOMBAUGH, T. N., SZOSTAK, C., VOORNEVELD, P., and TOMBAUGH, J. W., 1982, Failure to obtain functional equivalence between dopamine receptor blockade and extinction: Evidence supporting a sensorimotor conditioning hypothesis, *Pharmacol. Biochem. Behav.* **1**:67–72.
TOMBAUGH, T. N., SZOSTAK, C., and MILLS, P., 1983, Failure of pimozide to disrupt the acquisition of light-dark and spatial discrimination problems, *Psychopharmacology* **79**:161–168.
UNGERSTEDT, U., 1971a, Adipsia and aphagia after 6-hydroxydopamine induced degeneration of the nigro-striatal dopamine system, *Acta Physiol. Scand.* **83**(Suppl. 367):95–122.
UNGERSTEDT, U., 1971b, Striatal dopamine release after amphetamine or nerve degeneration revealed by rotational behavior, *Acta Physiol. Scand.* **83**(Suppl. 367):49–68.
UNGERSTEDT, U., 1971c, Stereotaxic mapping of the monoamine pathways in the rat brain, *Acta Physiol. Scand.* **83**(Suppl. 367):1–48.
WALLACE, M., SINGER, G., FINLAY, J., and GIBSON, S., 1983, The effect of 6-OHDA lesions of the nucleus accumbens septum on schedule-induced drinking, wheelrunning and corticosterone levels in the rat, *Pharmacol. Biochem. Behav.* **18**:129–136.
WEISSMAN, N. W., and CROSSMAN, E. K., 1966, A comparison of two types of extinction following fixed-ratio training, *J. Exp. Anal. Behav.* **9**:41–46.
WILSON, S. A., 1914, An experimental research into the anatomy and physiology of corpus striatum, *Brain* **36**:427–492.
WISE, R. A., 1978, Catecholamine theories of reward: A critical review, *Brain Res.* **152**:215–247.

WISE, R. A., 1982, Neuroleptics and operant behavior: The anhedonia hypothesis, *Behav. Brain Sci.* **5**:39–87.
WISE, R. A., SPINDLER, J., DE WITT, H., and GERBER, G. J., 1978a, Neuroleptic-induced "anhedonia" in rats: Pimozide blocks reward quality of food, *Science* **201**:262–264.
WISE, R. A., SPINDLER, J., and LEGULT, L., 1978b, Major attenuation of food reward with performance-sparing doses of pimozide in the rat, *Can. J. Psychol.* **32**:77–85.
XENAKIS, S., and SCLAFANI, A., 1981, The effects of pimozide on the consumption of a palatable saccharin-glucose solution in the rat, *Pharmacol. Biochem. Behav.* **15**:435–442.
YOUNG, P. T., 1961, *Motivation and Emotion*, John Wiley and Sons, New York.

11

SECOND-GENERATION ANTIDEPRESSANTS

S. J. Enna and Michael S. Eison

1. INTRODUCTION

Drug therapy for depression was introduced in the 1950s. Two distinct chemical classes—hydrazines and dibenzazepines—were originally found useful for the treatment of this disorder. The hydrazines are relatively potent inhibitors of a variety of enzymes, including monoamine oxidase (MAO), which participates in the metabolism of catecholamines and serotonin. The dibenzazepines inhibit the neuronal reaccumulation of monoamines, and in particular, norepinephrine and serotonin. Both groups elevate mood in individuals suffering from endogenous depression, a disorder that, up to that time, could only be effectively reversed with shock therapy. This discovery revolutionized the treatment of affective illness and contributed significantly to the establishment of psychopharmacology.

Subsequent years witnessed the synthesis and testing of a host of related agents, most of which had pharmacological characteristics virtually identical to those of the original compounds (Usdin, 1978). The monoamine uptake inhibitors were so similar in structure that this class became known as tricyclic antidepressants because they all possessed a trio of fused rings (Fig. 1). In addition to inhibiting norepinephrine and sero-

---

S. J. Enna • Nova Pharmaceutical Corporation, Baltimore, Maryland 21224.   *Michael S. Eison* • Central Nervous System Research, Pharmaceutical Research and Development Division, Bristol-Myers Company, Wallingford, Connecticut 06429.

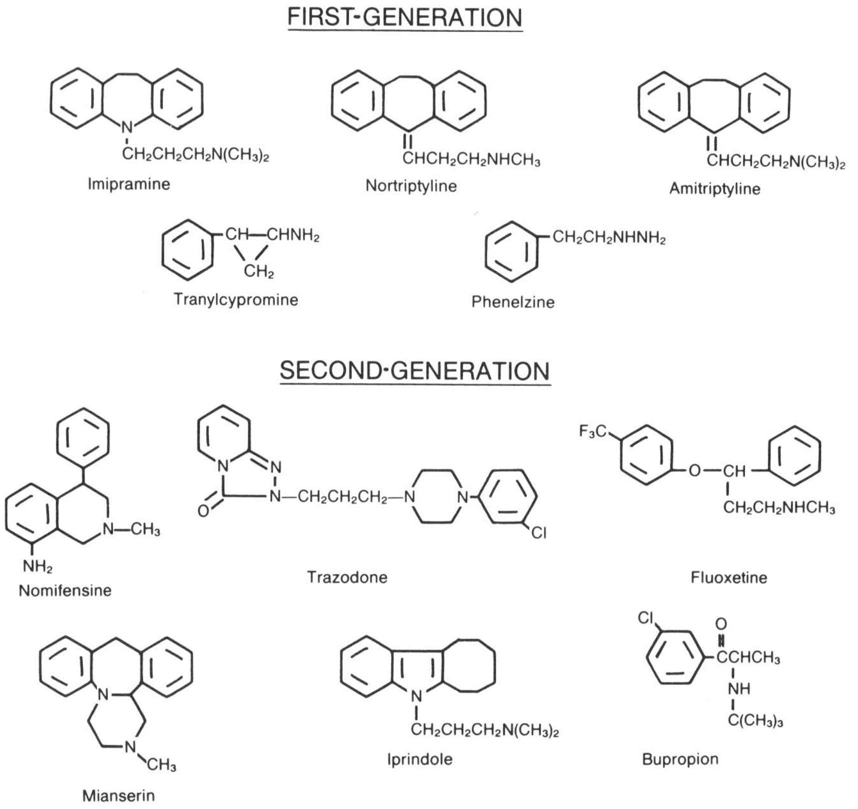

FIG. 1. Chemical structures of some first- and second-generation antidepressants.

tonin reuptake, tricyclic antidepressants display antihistaminic, anticholinergic, and α-adrenergic blocking activities (Enna and Kendall, 1981; Richelson, 1984).

The discovery that both the tricyclic antidepressants and MAO inhibitors increase monoaminergic transmission contributed to the monoamine hypothesis of affective illness. This theory holds that depression results from an underactivity in central noradrenergic or serotonergic transmission (Baldessarini, 1975; Schildkraut, 1978). The MAO inhibitors and tricyclic antidepressants were thought to normalize behavior by redressing this imbalance. Accordingly, this theory was based on the assumption that enhancement in central nervous system (CNS) monoaminergic transmission was responsible for the therapeutic action, whereas the other properties of these agents mediated side effects (Peroutka and Snyder, 1981). For example, the anticholinergic action of tricyclic antidepressants is undoubtedly responsible for the dry mouth and constipation that are commonly encountered with these drugs. A possible consequence of the nonselective nature of the MAO inhibitors includes hypertensive crisis, which results from inhibition of hepatic enzymes responsible for oxidizing tyramine. Both classes are characterized by a number of toxicities, with the MAO inhibitors being the more lethal of the two. One of the most dangerous properties of the tricyclic antidepressants is a cardiotoxicity that increases the tendency for arrythmias (Mior et al., 1972).

Two other notable characteristics of antidepressant therapy are a delayed onset in response and limited efficacy. A full therapeutic response is seldom noted with less than a week of continuous medication, and, typically, 1–3 weeks of treatment is required before there is a significant improvement in subjective symptoms (Denber, 1975). With regard to efficacy, up to 30% of patients fail to respond to these medications. Side effects, toxicity, long latency to response, and limited efficacy have spurred the continued development of antidepressant drugs.

A number of new antidepressants have been developed since the early 1960s (Fig. 1, Table 1) (Van Dijk et al., 1978). Many of these are referred to as "second-generation" or "atypical" antidepressants.

TABLE 1
Acute Neurochemical Actions of Selected Second-Generation Antidepressants

Compound	Possible mechanism of action	Clinical data
Monoamine uptake inhibitors		
Tandamine	Norepinephrine	Saletu et al., 1977
Nomifensine	Norepinephrine and dopamine	Ananth and van den Steen, 1978
Viloxazine	Norepinephrine	Magnus, 1975
Lofepramine	Norepinephrine	Obermeier and Poldinger, 1977
Maprotiline	Norepinephrine	Amin et al., 1973
Amoxapine	Norepinephrine	Fabre et al., 1977
Pridefine	Norepinephrine and dopamine	Mielke and Gallant, 1978
Danitracen	Dopamine	Kaumeier et al., 1977
Bupropion	Dopamine	Halaris et al., 1981
Fluvoxamine	Serotonin	Wright and Denber, 1978
Zimelidine	Serotonin	Coopen et al., 1979
Fluoxetine	Serotonin	Shopsin et al., 1981
Trazodone	Serotonin	Feighner, 1980
Facilitators of monoamine release		
Nomifensine	Dopamine	Ananth and van den Steen, 1978
Mianserin	Norepinephrine	Itil et al., 1972
Monoamine oxidase inhibitor		
Caroxazone		Cecchini et al., 1978
Activators of GABA/benzodiazepine receptors		
Alprazolam	Benzodiazepine	Hester et al., 1971
Progabide	GABA	Morselli and Lloyd, 1985
Unknown mechanism		
Iprindole		Hicks, 1965
Azepindole		Shopsin et al., 1981
Zometapine		Shopsin et al., 1981

Although lacking in precision, these expressions suggest important differences from earlier substances. The aim of the present chapter is to summarize some of the pharmacological, biochemical, behavioral, and clinical characteristics of second-generation antidepressants in order to assess the current status of this field and to make projections about the future. A second-generation drug is defined as an antidepressant, regardless of structure or date of discovery, which has some distinct pharmacological or biochemical differences from the original (first-generation) tricyclic antidepressants or MAO inhibitors (Fig. 1). These differences normally relate to the selectivity of the biochemical effects, to the side effect profile, and to toxicity. This reflects the ongoing effort to design molecules that maximize the actions on central monoaminergic systems while reducing the ancillary pharmacological effects thought to be unrelated to therapeutic efficacy.

2. GENERAL PROPERTIES OF SECOND-GENERATION ANTIDEPRESSANTS

One of the more difficult tasks in clinical psychopharmacology is establishing antidepressant efficacy. Clinical studies indicate that depression is not a single entity, but rather may be a consequence of a variety of biological disorders. Therefore, it is conceivable that a drug may be effective in only a subgroup of patients, making it difficult to detect efficacy in a limited trial. Conversely, clinical results are complicated by the fact that depression often remits spontaneously and by the finding that there is a significant response to placebos among depressed patients. This makes inclusion of appropriate control groups mandatory. Furthermore, the lack of a definitive biological marker for depression makes it difficult to establish therapeutic utility objectively. It is prudent, therefore, to withhold judgment on a new agent until it is possible to examine the results of a large number of clinical studies that include, if possible, a cross-over design with comparison to standard medications and a placebo (Shopsin *et al.*, 1981). Although dozens of substances have been proposed as second-generation antidepressants, only a handful have met the criteria necessary for establishing therapeutic utility. Although there are data suggesting therapeutic efficacy for the second-generation agents discussed in this chapter, inclusion should not be taken as a sign that the drug is an established antidepressant. Furthermore, some of these compounds have been withdrawn from clinical testing because of toxicities, making it unlikely that they will ever be marketed.

Illustrated are some of the more extensively tested second-generation antidepressants (Fig. 1) (Feighner, 1981; Shopsin *et al.*, 1981; Richelson,

1984). Nomifensine, trazodone, mianserin, and iprindole have all been marketed either in the United States or in Europe. Given their structural diversity, it is not surprising that there are differences in their pharmacological profiles when compared to the original tricyclic antidepressants. A striking example of this is found when the relative affinities for the cholinergic muscarinic receptor are compared; first-generation tricyclics are anywhere from 4 to over 1000 times more potent as anticholinergics than second-generation agents (Richelson, 1984). This typifies one aspect of progress in drug development; elimination of pharmacological properties thought responsible for side effects. As predicted, none of the illustrated second-generation agents has any appreciable anticholinergic activity in humans.

Less success has been achieved in eliminating antihistaminic and α-adrenergic blocking properties (Richelson, 1984). For example, mianserin has a higher affinity for histamine H_1 and α-adrenergic receptors than does imipramine or nortryptyline, and trazodone is a more potent α-adrenergic blocking agent than these first-generation drugs. Although sedation is observed with trazodone and mianserin, it is a beneficial side effect in some patients; it is however, intolerable in others.

Research has indicated the existence of at least two distinct forms of monoamine oxidase, MAO-A and MAO-B (Costa and Sandler, 1972). Selective inhibitors of these enzymes have been developed, and there are data suggesting that these drugs, in particular MAO-A inhibitors, may be antidepressants (Murphy *et al.*,1979). This, too, illustrates the trend to develop more specific agents. By designing compounds that inhibit a particular form of this enzyme, it may be possible to develop drugs having fewer side effects than first-generation agents.

This principle is illustrated further by examining a more extensive list of second-generation antidepressants (Table 1). Whereas first-generation tricyclic antidepressants were relatively potent as inhibitors of both norepinephrine and serotonin uptake, second-generation drugs have been designed to have a greater separation in affinities for the two transport sites. Tandamine, viloxazine, lofepramine, maprotiline, and amoxapine are much more selective as inhibitors of norepinephrine than of serotonin accumulation as compared to imipramine. Although these drugs are not necessarily specific in this regard, the separation is great enough to assume that inhibition of catecholamine uptake predominates over inhibition of indolamine accumulation. Conversely, fluvoxamine, zimelidine, fluoxetine, and trazodone are more selective as inhibitors of serotonin transport than of norepinephrine uptake. It should be borne in mind that these distinctions are based primarily on data obtained from *in vitro* studies, making it conceivable that metabolites may alter selectivity *in vivo*.

There has also been an effort to develop antidepressants that influence dopaminergic transmission (Table 1). In addition to inhibiting norepinephrine accumulation, both nomifensine and pridefine are relatively potent inhibitors of dopamine uptake into brain tissue. Although the relationship between dopamine and depression has not been clearly defined, it is known that manipulation of dopaminergic systems profoundly affects mood and behavior (Creese, 1983). A major biochemical effect of amphetamine is activation of brain dopaminergic systems resulting from an enchancement in the release and inhibition of the reuptake of this monoamine. However, amphetamine is not considered an antidepressant, since it is difficult to establish selective efficacy in depression as opposed to the generalized central stimulation that it provokes. It is notable that side effects associated with nomifensine include psychostimulation, sleep disturbances, restlessness, and paranoia (Shopsin *et al.,* 1981). These symptoms are more severe in individuals with agitated, rather than retarded depression. Such effects may be directly related to dopaminergic activation. It is not surprising that nomifensine may be particularly active in this regard, since, like amphetamine, in addition to inhibiting dopamine reuptake, it also causes a release of this monoamine (Ananth and van den Steen, 1978).

Danitracen and bupropion appear to be highly selective inhibitors of dopamine accumulation. Both have demonstrated clinical efficacy, suggesting that a subtle manipulation of this transmitter may yield a selective antidepressant response. Nevertheless, abuse potential must always be considered a possibility when dealing with drugs of this type.

Another way to activate brain monoaminergic systems is to facilitate transmitter release. As mentioned previously, nomifensine induces the release of dopamine. Mianserin, although having little effect on neurotransmitter uptake or metabolism *in vitro,* has been shown to increase the release of norepinephrine (Fludder and Leonard, 1979). This action is thought to be the result of an inhibition of presynaptic α_2-adrenergic receptors. Blockade of these autoreceptors diminishes a normal feedback inhibition of norepinephrine release.

Caroxazone is a benzoxamine derivative that acts as a reversible inhibitor of monoamine oxidase (Moretti *et al.,* 1974). This drug differs from first-generation agents in that its effect is more transient.

Although most efforts to develop second-generation antidepressants have focused on catecholamines and serotonin, data suggest that manipulations of γ-aminobutyric acid (GABA) may prove beneficial in depression. Alprazolam, a benzodiazepine, is reportedly effective against some forms of depression, especially those associated with anxiety (Feighner, 1981). These data are intriguing inasmuch as classic benzodiazepines, such as diazepam, reportedly have no antidepressant activity (Schatzberg and Cole, 1978). Given the relationship between benzodiazepines and GABA receptors (Enna and Karbon, 1986), this finding suggests that manipulation of GABAergic transmission may be a worthwhile strategy for developing novel antidepressants. However, it could be argued that alprazolam is not a selective antidepressant but rather reduces symptomatology by decreasing the anxiety associated with certain types of affective illness. Such an effect may be more apparent than with other benzodiazepines if there is a greater separation between the anxiolytic and sedative doses of alprazolam. Accordingly, the apparent lack of antidepressant efficacy for diazepam could be the result of its sedation, which obscures other potential clinical effects. It is also possible that alprazolam selectively interacts with a subpopulation of benzodiazepine sites that mediate an antidepressant action. Reports suggesting the existence of multiple benzodiazepine binding sites lend substance to this speculation (Johnson et al., 1983). However, there is no evidence indicating that alprazolam differs from diazepam in regard to binding site selectivity.

Preliminary results indicate that progabide, a GABA receptor agonist, may have antidepressant efficacy (Morselli and Lloyd, 1986). Although the present data are insufficient to establish conclusively that progabide is an antidepressant, initial findings are sufficiently encouraging to warrant further investigation. Given the ubiquitous distribution of GABAergic neurons in the CNS, and the evidence indicating a multiplicity of GABA receptors (Enna and Karbon, 1986), it seems likely that GABA plays a major role in a variety of mental processes.

It has not always been possible to identify a neurochemical effect that may explain the clinical activity of some second-generation drugs (Table 1). This is true for iprindole, azepindole, and zometapine. As their names imply, the former compounds are indole derivatives and therefore related to serotonin (Fig. 1), making it likely that their antidepressant activity is related to an effect on this transmitter system. Neither appears to be an inhibitor of MAO, nor do they influence monoamine uptake or release. Zometapine is structurally related to the benzodiazepines and, therefore, may act in a manner similar to alprazolam.

It should not be assumed that the listed actions are necessarily those most responsible for mediating the antidepressant effects of these drugs. Rather, these neurochemical actions, based on precedent, are assumed to account for efficacy. Many of these drugs and their metabolites interact with a variety of neurotransmitter processes, which may contribute to their mechanism of action. For example, a primary metabolite of trazodone is *m*-chlorophenylpiperazine, a serotonin receptor agonist (Melzacka et al., 1980), which may, in part, contribute to the effectiveness of this agent (Caccia et al., 1981; Kendall et al., 1983).

None of the second-generation antidepressants consistently acts more rapidly than first-generation drugs, nor do they appear to be more efficacious. This suggests that direct manipulation of monoaminergic transmission may not be the best approach for treating depression. Indeed, modifications in monoaminergic transmission may represent only one facet of this disease. Perhaps a rapid-acting, broad-spectrum antidepressant may display a neurochemical profile different from what is presently thought to characterize antidepressant drugs. Thus, although the exquisitely selective compounds that manipulate individual monoaminergic systems are less toxic, they are not effective in a greater proportion of patients nor do they display a more rapid onset of action, which emphasizes the importance, and limitations, of monoamine manipulations in the treatment of depression. Alternatively, regardless of the neurochemical site of action, it may require a fixed period of time for antidepressant-induced changes in brain to compensate for the imbalances responsible for the illness. In this case, an extended lag time may be unavoidable. If second-generation antidepressants can be characterized as safer and neurochemically more selective than first-generation agents, third-generation drugs will be those that influence other transmitter systems and that, it is hoped, will display a more rapid onset of action and a greater range of activity.

3. METHODOLOGICAL APPROACHES

Unlike research on cardiovascular or infectious diseases in which a clinically relevant response can be quantified in the laboratory, tests designed to detect antidepressant activity are based solely on neurochemical and behavioral responses to standard medications. Because the assays may have more to do with the properties of standard drugs than the disease process itself, such tests may not detect antidepressants having novel mechanisms of action. This may explain why the majority of second-generation antidepressants apparently have similar mechanisms to first-generations drugs. Therefore, the best hope of discovering an entirely new class of antidepressants is by behavioral analysis. If an animal model can be shown to be analogous to the human condition, or empirically predictive of antidepressant responses, then a drug that demonstrates activity in this assay but that has no obvious effect on monoaminergic transmission may represent an entirely new type of therapeutic agent. This principle is illustrated in the present section outlining a number of the more common laboratory tests used for predicting antidepressant activity.

3.1. Neurochemical Assays

3.1.1. Acute Tests

Given the relationship between antidepressant efficacy and monoaminergic transmission, the standard battery of acute neurochemical tests measures the effect of a test agent on monoamine metabolism, reuptake, and release. Several different methods can be used to examine these phenomena. Since detailed descriptions of methodology are beyond the scope of this review, this discussion is limited to issues of a more general nature.

Initial *in vitro* tests normally include an assessment of the potency to inhibit norepinephrine, dopamine, and serotonin accumulation into brain synaptosomal fractions (Fuller, 1981). Such experiments also reveal whether the compound is a competitive, noncompetitive, or uncompetitive inhibitor of the transport process and provide data relating to the selectivity of the interaction with a particular uptake system. Negative data prove nothing with respect to clinical activity, whereas positive results indicate antidepressant potential.

Another *in vitro* test measures the potency to inhibit brain MAO (Fuller, 1978). If activity is found, experiments are usually undertaken to establish selectivity on the different forms of this enzyme.

There are numerous *in vitro* methods for studying the effect of a drug on monoamine release (Raiteri *et al.*, 1976). In some cases, brain slices are preloaded with radioactive neurotransmitter and the effect of the drug on spontaneous and evoked release is measured. An enhancement of spontaneous release suggests an amphetaminelike action. If the agent has only a minimal affect on spontaneous release, but facilitates evoked release, this may be indicative of an autoreceptor antagonist.

An initial *in vitro* screen may also include an analysis of receptor interactions using ligand binding assays (Peroutka and Synder, 1981). With this test, the potency to inhibit attachment of neurotransmitter ligands to brain membrane preparations is determined. A potent interaction with receptor binding sites suggests that the compound may be a direct receptor agonist or antagonist, which, in some cases, may be predictive of antidepressant potential (Kendall *et al.*, 1983). Interactions with cholinergic muscarinic, histamine, or α_1-adrenergic receptors are generally considered indicative of side effect potential. An analysis of receptor interactions reveals whether the drug is a competitive or a noncompetitive inhibitor and provides information with regard to relative selectivity and potency.

Specific binding sites have been detected for tricyclic antidepressants in CNS tissue (Langer *et al.*, 1981; Palkovits *et al.*, 1981; Lee *et al.*, 1982). These sites appear to be associated with serotonin and norepinephrine transport systems. Although their biological relevance remains a matter of dispute, the selectivity and affinity of some antidepressants for these sites suggests that they may play a role in the action of these drugs. Because only structurally related antidepressants interact with these binding sites, this assay should not be exclusively relied upon in an antidepressant program unless the aim is to develop tricyclic drugs.

A complete characterization of potential antidepressants requires analysis following drug administration. These assays provide information about the penetrability of the drug into the CNS and may indicate the presence of active metabolites. There are a number of methods for examining inhibition of monoamine transport following drug administration (Fuller, 1981). One approach is to conduct *in vitro* uptake experiments after drug treatment. However, false negatives are possible if the tissue concentration of drug is reduced when the synaptosomal fraction is prepared. This problem is obviated by conducting experiments with animals that were treated with an agent known to be accumulated in the brain by monoaminergic transport systems (Fuller *et al.*, 1979). An uptake inhibitor reduces the accumulation of this substance or decreases its effectiveness.

MAO activity is also examined in brain tissue following systemic administration of the drug. Once again, important information is obtained by analyzing enzyme activity in the presence of various substrates to determine whether the compound is selective for MAO-A or MAO-B (Fuller, 1978).

Analysis of brain monoamine metabolites following systemic administration is another useful measure of activity (Sugrue, 1980*a*). A complete analysis should include measurement of the steady-state levels of monoamines and their metabolites. Qualitative and quantitative changes in metabolite patterns can provide indirect evidence as to whether the agent, or a metabolite, influences the storage, reuptake, or degradation of catecholamines and serotonin. Additional information can be obtained by studying the effect of drug treatment on monoamine turnover (Sugrue, 1980*b*).

3.1.2. Tests following Chronic Administration

Given the finding that the clinical response to most antidepressants requires 1–3 weeks of continuous administration, investigators are now examining neurochemical effects following chronic treatment with test compounds (Enna *et al.*, 1981; Enna, 1986). The rationale for this approach is that any effect resulting from chronic, but not acute, administration may be clinically important, since its occurrence corresponds with the appearance of clinical activity (Sulser, 1978). Studies conducted with both first- and second-generation antidepressants have revealed that the effects on neurotransmitter metabolites vary during the course of treatment (Sugrue, 1981). Moreover, there is no correlation between the appearance or disappearance of a particular metabolite and antidepressant efficacy. In contrast, there appears to be a good correlation between antidepressant activity and the effect of chronic administration on brain noradrenergic receptor function (Vetulani *et al.*, 1976). Chronic, but not acute, administration of most first- and second-generation antidepressants significantly reduces norepinephrine-stimulated cyclic AMP production in rat brain cerebral cortex. Most of these agents significantly decrease β-adrenergic receptor binding as well (Enna, 1986). Because this response is obtained regardless of the acute neurochemical effects, it has been proposed as a method for predicting antidepressant efficacy (Sulser, 1978). However, not all clinically effective antidepressants yield a positive response in this test. For example, neither trazodone nor fluoxetine has yet been shown to have a significant effect on norepinephrine-stimulated cyclic AMP accumulation when administered chronically. In any event, the majority of antidepressants are active in this assay regardless of their chemical structure or acute neurochemical actions, making this a potentially useful neurochemical method for identifying novel antidepressants.

β-Adrenergic receptors are not the only ones influenced by chronic administration of antidepressants (Enna, 1986). Serotonin receptors are reduced in number following administration of some agents, and α-adrenergic receptor binding is also modified in some cases. These responses are not as consistently observed as the alteration in β-adrenergic function.

This brief exposition illustrates the multiplicity of neurochemical tests used for predicting antidepressant activity. However, as virtually all these assays are based on the premise that antidepressants must influence monoaminergic transmission, they are unlikely to detect active agents working through a different mechanism. Nevertheless, these neurochemical approaches are useful for refining antidepressants in regard to selectivity and side effect potential, the primary characteristics that differentiate second- from first-generation agents.

3.2. Behavioral Assays

Animal models are the most likely means for detecting a drug having a totally novel mechanism of action if the model is based on a behavioral effect that can be reversed by antidepressants per se and is not simply a function of their monoaminergic nature. It is unclear whether such an animal model exists. Only clinical trials can absolutely differentiate between an inactive compound and an inappropriate test. Second-generation antidepressants have been useful in identifying the most appropriate animal models for detecting antidepressants of diverse structure and mechanism of action. Three tests that have recently become popular include the "learned-helplessness" model (Maier, 1983), differential reinforcement for low rates of response schedule (DRL) (O'Donnell and Seiden, 1982, 1983), and drug discrimination (Jones et al., 1980) (Table 2).

Learned-helplessness testing assesses the ability of a drug to reverse a learning impairment induced by exposure to inescapable shock. Data interpretation is based on the assumption that animals exposed to inescapable shock learn that nothing can be done to terminate the aversive stimulus. When subjects are reexposed to the shock, but in a situation

TABLE 2
Pharmacological, Physiological, and Behavioral Tests Found Useful for Predicting Antidepressant Activity

Animal mode or test	Reference
Learned helplessness	Maier, 1983
Differential reinforcement for low rates of response schedule	O'Donnell and Seiden, 1983
Drug discrimination	Jones et al., 1980
Potentiation of dopaminergic activity	Cooper et al., 1983
Potentiation or inhibition of serotonergic activity	Hyttel, 1982; Blackwell, 1981
Enhancement of yohimbine lethality	Malick, 1981
Reserpine reversal	Moretti et al., 1981
Blockade of isolation-induced hyperactivity	Garzon et al., 1979
Blockade of apomorphine-induced hypothermia	Meignen et al., 1982
Attenuation of separation-induced depression	Crawley, 1984
Attenuation of stress-induced pathological responses and changes in locomotor activity	Katz and Sibel, 1982
Increase in clonidine-induced aggression	Maj et al., 1982a
Alterations in electroencephalographic profile	Itil, 1983

where escape is now possible, "helpless" animals fail to learn the escape procedure. As the failure to learn a subsequent avoidance task is not manifest in rats never experiencing an inescapable shock, the learning impairment is interpreted as a surrender to aversive environmental conditions, which are perceived to be beyond control. Such active avoidance deficits appear to be sensitive to reversal by a large number of antidepressant treatments, including tricyclic agents (Telner and Singhal, 1981), MAO inhibitors, and electroconvulsive shock (Sherman et al., 1982). Second-generation antidepressants, such as mianserin and nomifensine, are also active in this test (Kametani et al., 1983).

An animal model that is conceptually related to learned helplessness is "behavioral despair" (Porsolt et al., 1978). Rats or mice are placed into a large container of water (25°C) from which they cannot escape. Their initial response to immersion is to search for an exit, but, once these efforts prove futile, a prolonged period of passive inactivity follows. It is conceivable that this immobility is a behavioral reflection of the surrender to uncontrollable environmental pressures (learned helplessness). Upon reimmersion, these animals exhibit immobility for a longer period of time than untrained controls. Many antidepressants reduce the duration of this immobility. Second-generation antidepressants exhibit varying degrees of activity in this test (Cooper et al., 1983). Although nomifensine and danitracen reduce the period of immobility (Herman et al., 1981), fluvoxamine (Fuxe et al., 1981) and citalopram (Hyttel, 1981), serotonin uptake inhibitors, are inactive. Trazodone has been found to be inactive in the behavioral despair model by some investigators (Leonard, 1984), whereas others have found it to be effective. Indeed, the major limitation of the behavioral despair model is its apparent lack of selectivity for antidepressant drugs, with many antihistamines provoking a false positive response (Rogoz et al., 1981).

The DRL procedure is an operant test in which animals are trained to press a lever to obtain either a food or a water reward. The contingency in DRL tests is that the animal must wait a predetermined period of time between successive lever presses to obtain the reward. For example, in the DRL-72-sec test (O'Donnell and Seiden, 1983) animals must wait 72 sec between lever presses to receive rewards; premature presses are penalized by resetting the 72-sec clock. Two variables of interest in the DRL test are the rate of responding and the number of rewards obtained in a test of fixed duration. Antidepressant drugs increase DRL efficiency. Rats treated with antidepressants exhibit reduced response rates and obtain an increased number of rewards per session. First-generation tricyclic antidepressants are active in this test, as are such second-generation compounds as iprindole and mianserin. However, nomifensine is inactive (O'Donnell and Seiden, 1983). MAO inhibitors are also positive in this test, whereas other classes of psychoactive compounds, such as alcohol, chlordiazepoxide, morphine, pentobarbital, chlorpromazine and diphenhydramine, are not (O'Donnell and Seiden, 1982, 1983).

For drug discrimination studies, animals are trained to differentiate between psychoactive agents and control vehicle by being given a reward for pressing a particular lever in a two-lever cage when an active drug has been administered, and by being rewarded only when pressing the other lever following treatment with vehicle. Bupropion is sometimes used as a training drug in this test. When animals are trained with bupropion and nomifensine or viloxazine are subsequently administered, they press the bupropion-appropriate lever. This suggests that these compounds share a similar stimulus cue that, it is hoped, is related to their antidepressant potential (Jones et al., 1980). However, amphetamine elicits a bupropion-appropriate response, and nomifensine is self-administered in rats (Spyraki and Fibiger, 1981). These data suggest that the stimulus properties of these drugs may be more related to abuse potential than to antidepressant activity.

Like bupropion, many antidepressants potentiate dopaminergic responses induced by the administration of amphetamine or L-dopa (Cooper et al., 1983). Among second-generation antidepressants, viloxazine and UP-614-04 potentiate amphetamine-induced stereotypy as well as the ability of L-dopa to reverse reserpine-induced catalepsy (Meignen et al., 1982). Tricyclic antidepressants potentiate the anorexic effects of amphetamine and, indeed, are known to be anorexic themselves (Blavet and DeFeudis, 1982). The anorexic properties of these compounds may also be explained by the fact that amphetamine, amitriptyline, and bupropion induce a taste aversion in animals exposed to a flavor associated with illness (Miller and Miller, 1983).

Another animal model is based on the interaction of antidepressants with adrenergic mechanisms, with many drugs potentiating the pharmacological effects of yohimbine and clonidine. The least ambiguous, and therefore most commonly used, index is yohimbine lethality. Tricyclic antidepressants potently enhance the lethal effects of this drug, although some second-generation compounds, such as fluoxetine, zimelidine, and nisoxetine, exhibit only weak activity in this regard. Bupropion, mianserin, viloxazine, and iprindole are active in this test (Blavet and DeFeudis, 1982; Malick, 1981). Clonidine induces aggressive behavior in mice, an effect that is enhanced by the chronic administration of some second-generation antidepressants. Nisoxetine and pizotifen potentiate this response, but citolopram and fluvoxamine do not. This suggests that the potentiation of clonidine-induced aggression may be useful in identifying α-adrenergic drugs (Maj et al., 1982a).

The induction or potentiation of the behavioral effects associated with serotonergic activation is characteristic of some second-generation compounds. For example, citalopram, a serotonin reuptake inhibitor, induces a serotonin syndrome in mice (Hyttel, 1982). This syndrome is characterized by the overt performance of at least four of the following behaviors: lateral head weaving, forepaw treading, hindlimb abduction, straub tail, tremor, and rigidity (Jacobs, 1976). Citalopram potentiates serotonergic agents in this test and potentiates the head twitch response induced by the serotonin precursor L-5-HTP (Hyttel, 1982). Like fluoxetine, citalopram at high doses causes convulsive seizures, which are blocked by serotonergic antagonists; like femoxetine, it blocks fenfluramine hyperthermia (Hyttel, 1982). Fluvoxamine, a serotonin reuptake inhibitor, does not alter L-5-HTP-induced head twitches in mice but does block the hyperthermic effect of fenfluramine (Maj et al., 1982b). Although fluvoxamine is without effect on tryptaminergic convulsions in rats, the antidepressant candidate BRL-14342 potentiates the anticonvulsant action on L-5-HTP (Clark et al., 1980).

The contribution of serotonin to the action of antidepressants is complicated by the finding that some inhibit, rather than activate, this neurotransmitter system. Serotonin antagonist properties have been described for a number of second-generation antidepressants, including mianserin (Blackwell, 1981) and zimelidine (Cooper et al., 1983). Curiously, although zimelidine acutely depresses the electrophysiological activity of serotonergic cells, chronic administration is without effect on the responsiveness of hippocampal pyramidal cells to serotonin (De Montigny, 1981). Like zimelidine, acute administration of viloxazine, mianserin, or trazodone blocks serotonin-agonist induced head twitches, whereas chronic administration of trazodone or iprindole enhanced the response to these agonists (Friedman et al., 1983). Fluvoxamine and citalopram decrease serotonin histofluorescence in the dorsal raphe nucleus but increase fluorescence in nearby capillary walls (Constantinidis et al., 1981).

One of the oldest, most popular tests for predicting antidepressant activity is reserpine reversal. The constellation of effects observed after reserpine treatment includes hypothermia, ptosis, and hypomotility. Second-generation antidepressants, such as caroxazone and lofepramine, potently reverse many of these effects (Moretti et al., 1981; Sjogren, 1980). The hypothermia is reversed by viloxazine (Blackwell, 1981; Meignen et al., 1982), UP-614-04, and BRL-14342 (Clark et al., 1980). Nomefensine, zimelidine, and trazodone also show activity in this test, but mianserin and iprindole do not (Leonard, 1984). It has been proposed that compounds activating β-adrenergic receptors preferentially block the hypothermic affects, whereas α-adrenergic and serotonergic agonists block the ptosis. Reversal of reserpine hypomotility is thought to be a consequence of dopamine receptor stimulation (Bourin et al., 1983). Thus, antidepressants devoid of monoaminergic activity would presumably be negative in this test.

Antidepressants also influence the responses to chronically administered reserpine. For example, treatment with low doses of reserpine increases locomotion in an open field, an effect that can be blocked by chronic administration of mianserin (Jancsar and Leonard, 1983).

Tetrabenazine induces a syndrome virtually identical to that of reserpine. These effects are reversed by prior administration of bupropion, mianserin, iprindole, and nomefensine (Cooper et al., 1983; Miller and Miller, 1983). Although the mechanism of action of tetrabenazine is thought to be the same as that of reserpine, some antidepressants that are inactive in reserpine reversal are active in the tetrabenazine assay. It is possible that these results are the result of differences in experimental design (dose or time of drug administration).

Upon acute administration, viloxazine and mianserin reduce the effect of reserpine or tetrabenazine on exploratory behavior (Cuomo et al., 1983). Chronic administration of zimelidine, citalopram, mianserin, or iprindole prior to acute treatment with reserpine increases the locomotor response. This effect is opposite to that observed following reserpine administration to untreated animals. However, not all antidepressants are positive in this test, with fluvoxamine being inactive (Maj et al., 1983).

Viloxazine and trazodone block isolation-induced hyperactivity in rats (Garzon et al., 1979). Desipramine, amitriptyline, and MAO inhibitors are also active in this test, but neuroleptics and anxiolytics are not (Garzon et al., 1979). The hyperlocomotion induced by coadministration of LSD and apomorphine has also been shown to be blocked by second-generation antidepressants, in particular, danitracen, mianserin, and pizotifen (Gold et al., 1980).

Reversal of the hypothermic response to apomorphine is also used as a screen for antidepressant potential. In mice, very high doses of apomorphine (16 mg/kg) induce a hypothermia that is blocked by α-adrenergic agonists, as well as by tricyclic antidepressants, nomifensine, viloxazine, and UP-614-04 (Meignen et al., 1982; Puech et al., 1981). Neuroleptics are inactive in this assay.

Some animal models rely on environmental rather than drug-induced manipulations. When male–female pairs of Siberian hamsters are seperated, there is an increase in body weight and a decrease in social interactions and exploratory behavior. Inasmuch as some of these symptoms are attenuated by imipramine, this model could prove to be a useful test for antidepressant activity (Crawley, 1984). Indeed, stress-induced behavioral alterations have proven to be quite popular as models for antidepressant drug screening. Bupropion, iprindole, and mianserin all normalize increases in open-field activity that result from acute noise stress (Katz and Sibel, 1982). Rats subjected to prolonged immobilization stress develop ulcers; nomifensine administration protects against this response (Bickel, 1980).

The effect of antidepressants on brain electrical activity also appears to be a useful measure of therapeutic potential. Electroencephalographic (EEG) seizure activity can be detected in many brain areas following repeated exposure to focal electric currents. When the effects of antidepressants upon kindled seizures at various brain loci were investigated, a preferential action was noted in the amygdala relative to cerebral cortical areas. At high doses, mianserin blocks only amygdala-kindled seizures; imipramine blocks cortical seizures as well. However, the response in the amygdala is not an absolute indicator of antidepressant potential in that iprindole has no effect upon seizure activity in this area (Knobloch et al., 1982).

Drug-induced changes in the normal EEG have been used to identify antidepressants. In fact, alterations in EEG profiles were of key importance in identifying the antidepressant potential of mianserin (Itil, 1983). Two types of EEG profile have been associated with antidepressant activity in humans. The thymeretic response is induced by desipramine and suggests activating properties; a thymoleptic profile identifies antidepressants with sedative properties (Saletu, 1982). Nomifensine and fluoxetine induce thymeretic activity; maprotiline and fluvoxamine, however, induce thymoleptic EEGs. Mianserin and viloxazine induce thymolepticlike changes in the EEG, and VRL-14342 causes an activating EEG (Blackwell, 1981; Clark et al., 1980; Herman et al., 1981).

Although many other tests are used to predict antidepressant activity, these selected models have all had their predictive utility clinically verified. Since no model has yet been proven to unequivocally demonstrate antidepressant activity, a program aimed at discovering new antidepressants must rely upon a battery of tests to generate convergent data that are empirically related to clinical efficacy.

4. SUMMARY AND CONCLUSIONS

A common characteristic of first-generation antidepressants is that they appear to activate monoaminergic transmission. Besides forming the basis for the monoamine theory of depression, this finding made possible laboratory tests for predicting antidepressant potential. These tests have led to the development of a number of structurally diverse compounds which have demonstrated antidepressant activity. The acute mechanism of action of most of these drugs, which are referred to as second-generation antidepressants, appears to be similar to that proposed for first-generation compounds. That is, the majority of second-generation antidepressants are relatively potent inhibitors of monoamine reuptake and, in some cases, facilitate the release of these neurotransmitters. The major differences between first- and second-generation drugs relate to the selectivity of their neurochemical actions and to side effect potential. Although second-generation antidepressants do not appear to be more efficacious or rapid acting than first-generation compounds, these drugs represent a therapeutic advance because the reduction in side effects increases safety and patient compliance.

Second-generation drugs have also contributed to the fundamental understanding of antidepressant drug action. By developing more selective agents, and by reducing ancillary neurochemical effects, work in this area has shown the importance of monoaminergic systems in mediating the symptoms of depression. However, since a significant number of patients still fail to respond to drug therapy, and the onset of action remains delayed, there is still room for improvement. Given the possibility that the underlying biochemical abnormality may not be the same in all forms of affective illness, it is conceivable that no single drug is capable of 100% effectiveness. On the other hand, if all types of depression have a common neurochemical basis, a single medication capable of redressing this imbalance should be more generally effective. The clinical data on second-generation antidepressants indicate that direct manipulation of catecholamine and serotonin neurotransmission is insufficient for this purpose. Therefore, the next generation of drugs will most likely be compounds that interact at nonmonoaminergic sites in brain. Some possibilities include drugs that modify peptide or amino acid neurotransmitters and neuromodulators. Because the present group of laboratory tests is based upon principles related to the actions of first- and second-generation antidepressants, it may be difficult to detect clinical potential in a drug having a novel mechanism of action. Such an agent is most likely to be discovered in a behavioral test or during clinical trials for other indications. Once clinical efficacy has been established, such an agent will be invaluable in defining the biological basis for affective illness and will point the way toward the development of third-generation antidepressants.

ACKNOWLEDGMENTS

Preparation of this manuscript was made possible in part by grants from the National Institute of Mental Health (MH-36945 and MH-00501) and Bristol-Myers, Inc. We thank Mrs. Doris Thornton for her excellent secretarial assistance.

5. REFERENCES

AMIN, M., BRAHM, E., BRONHEIM, L. A., KLINGER, A., BAN, T. A., and LEHMANN, H. E., 1973, A double blind comparative trial with Ludiomil (CIBA 34 276Ba) and amitriptyline in newly admitted depressed patients, *Curr. Ther. Res.* **15**:691–699.

ANANTH, J., and VAN DEN STEEN, N., 1978, A double blind controlled comparative study of nomifensine in depression, *Curr. Ther. Res.* **23**:213–221.

BALDESSARINI, R. J., 1975, The basis for amine hypotheses in affective disorders: A critical evaluation, *Arch. Gen. Psychiatry* **32**:1087–1093.

BICKEL, M., 1980 Antiulcer effects of nomifensine, a new antidepressant, on stress-induced ulcers in the rat, *Arzneim-Forsch. Drug Res.* **30**:69–73.

BLACKWELL, B., 1981, Adverse effects of antidepressant drugs, *Drugs* **21**:273–282.

BLAVET, N., and DEFEUDIS, F. V., 1982, Inhibition of food intake in the rat, *Neurochem. Res.* **7**:339–348.

BOURIN, M., PONCELET, J., CHERMAT, R., and SIMON, P., 1983, The value of the reserpine test in psychopharmacology, *Arzneim-Forsch. Drug Res.* **33**:1173–1176.

CACCIA, S., BALABIO, M., SAMANIN, R., ZANINI, M. G., and GARATTINI, S., 1981, (O)-*m*-Chlorophenylpiperazine, a central 5-hydroxytryptamine agonist, is a metabolite of trazodone, *J. Pharm. Pharmacol.* **33**:477–478.

CECCHINI, S., PETRI, P., ARDITO, R., BAREGGI, S. R., and TOREITI, A., 1978, A comparative double-blind trial of the new antidepressant caroxazone and amitriptyline, *J. Int. Med. Res.* **6**:388–402.

CLARK, M. S. G., JOHNSON, A. M., McCLELLAND, G. R., and NELSON, D. R., 1980, Pharmacological and biochemical properties of BRL 14342, a novel antidepressant drug, *Neuropharmacology* **19**:1207–1208.

CONSTANTINIDIS, J., DICK, P., and TISSOT, R., 1981, Antidepressants and serotonin neurons of the raphe, *Neuropsychobiology* **7**:113–121.

COOPEN, A., RAMMA RAO, V. A., SWADE, C., and WOOD, K., 1979, Zimelidine: A therapeutic and pharmacokinetic study in depression, *Psychopharmacology* **63**:199–202.

COOPER, B. R., HOWARD, J. L., and SOROKO, F. E., 1983, Animal models used in prediction of antidepressant effects in man, *J. Clin. Psychiatry* **44**(5):63–66.
COSTA, E., and SANDLER, M. (eds.), 1972 *Monoamine Oxidases—New Vistas. Advances in Biochemical Psychopharmacology*, Vol. 5, Raven Press, New York.
CRAWLEY, J. N., 1984, Evaluation of a proposed hamster separation model of depression, *Psychiatr. Res.* **11**:35–47.
CREESE, I. (ed.), 1983, *Stimulants: Neurochemical, Behavioral and Clinical Perspectives*, Raven Press, New York.
CUOMO, V., CAGIANO, R., BRUNELLO, N., FUMAGALLI, R., and RACAGNI, G., 1983, Behavioural changes after acute and chronic administration of typical and atypical antidepressants in rats: Interaction with reserpine, *Neurosci. Lett.* **40**:315–319.
DE MONTIGNY, C., 1981, Enchancement of the 5-HT neurotransmission by antidepressant treatments, *J. Psychol. (Paris)* **77**:455–461.
DENBER, H. C. B., 1975, Pharmacotherapy of depression, in: *Psychopharmacological Treatment—Therapy and Practice* (H. C. B. Denber, ed.), Dekker, New York, pp. 121–135.
ENNA, S. J., 1986, *In vitro* receptor modifications as a measure of antidepressant potential, in: *Receptor Binding in Drug Research* (R.A. O'Brien, ed.), Dekker, New York, pp. 409–427.
ENNA, S. J., and KARBON, E. W., 1986, GABA receptors: An overview, in: *Benzodiazepine/GABA Receptors, Chloride Channels* (R. W. Olsen and J. C. Venter, eds.), Liss, New York, pp. 41–56.
ENNA, S. J., and KENDALL, D. A., 1981, Interaction of antidepressants with brain neurotransmitter receptors, *J. Clin. Psychopharmacol.* **1**:12–16.
ENNA, S. J., MANN, E., KENDALL, D. A., and STANCEL, G. M., 1981, Effect of chronic antidepressant administration on brain neurotransmitter receptor binding, in: *Antidepressants: Neurochemical, Behavioral and Clinical Perspectives* (S. J. Enna, J. B. Malick, and E. Richelson, eds.), Raven Press, New York, pp. 91–105.
FABRE, L. F., MCLENDON, G. M., and GAINEY, A., 1977, Double-blind placebo-controlled comparison of Amoxapine and Imipramine in depressed out-patients, *Curr. Ther. Res.* **22**:611–619.
FEIGHNER, J., 1980, Trazodone, a triazolopyridine derivative in primary depression, *J. Clin. Psychiatry* **41**:250–255.
FEIGHNER, J. P., 1981, Clinical efficacy of the newer antidepressants, *J. Clin. Psychopharmacol.* **1**:23–26.
FLUDDER, J. M., and LEONARD, B. E., 1979, The effects of amitriptyline, mianserin, phenoxybenzamine and propranolol on the release of noradrenaline in the rat brain *in vivo*, *Biochem. Pharmacol.* **28**:2333–2336.
FRIEDMAN, E., COOPER, T. B., and DALLOB, A., 1983, Effects of chronic antidepressant treatment on serotonin receptor activity in mice, *Eur. J. Pharmacol.* **89**:69–76.
FULLER, R. W., 1978, Selectivity among monoamine oxidase inhibitors and its possible importance for development of antidepressant drugs, *Prog. Neuro-Psychopharmacol.* **2**:303–311.
FULLER, R. W., 1981, Enhancement of monoaminergic neurotransmission by antidepressant drugs, in: *Antidepressants: Neurochemical, Behavioral and Clinical Perspectives* (S. J. Enna, J. B. Malick, and E. Richelson, eds.), Raven Perss, New York, pp. 1–12.
FULLER, R. W., SNODDY, H. D., and PERRY, K. W., 1979, Nisoxetine antagonism of norepinephrine depletion in brain and heart after α-methyl-*m*-tyrosine administration, *Neuropharmacology* **18**:767–770.
FUXE, K., OREGEN, S. O., AGNATI, L. F., ENEROTH, P., HOLM, A. C., and ANDERSSON, K., 1981, Long-term treatment with zimelidine leads to a reduction in 5-hydroxytryptamine neurotransmission within the central nervous system of the mouse and rat, *Neurosci. Lett.* **21**:57–62.

GARZON, J., FUENTES, J. A., and DEL RIO, J., 1979, Antidepressants selectively antagonize the hyperactivity induced in rats by long-term isolation, *Eur. J. Pharmacol.* **59:**293–296.

GOLD, R., MORGENSTERN, R., and FINK, H., 1980, Effects of atypical antidepressants on LSD potentiated apomorphine hypermotility in rats, *Acta Biol. Med. Germ.* **39:**917–921.

HALARIS, A. E., STERN, W., and HAETO-TRUAX, M. S., 1981, Clinical efficacy of the new antidepressant bupropion (Wellbutrin), *Psychopharmacol. Bull.* **17:**140–142.

HERMAN, Z. S., PLECH, A., BLIEN, E., and JEZ, W. W., 1981, Effects of cholinomimetics, cholinolytics and atypical antidepressants in the behavioral despair test in the rat, *Pol. J. Pharamcol.* **33:**485–489.

HESTER, J. B., RUDZIK, S. D., and KAMDAR, B. V., 1971, 6-Phenyl-4H-s-trizolo (4,3a) (1,4) benzodiazepines which have central nervous system antidepressant activity, *J. Med. Chem.* **14:**1078–1081.

HICKS, J. T., 1965, Iprindole, a new antidepressant for use in general office practice: A double-blind, placebo-controlled study, *Ill. Med. J.* **128:**622–626.

HYTTEL, J., 1982, Citalopram—Pharmacological profile of a specific serotonin uptake inhibitor with antidepressant activity, *Prog. Neuro-Psychopharmacol. Biol. Psychiatry* **6:**277–295.

ITIL, T. M., 1983, The discovery of antidepressant drugs by computer-analyzed human cerebral bio-electrical potentials (CEEG), *Prog. Neurobiol.* **20:**185–249.

ITIL, T. M., POLVAN, N., and HSU, W., 1972, Clinical and EEG effects of GB-94: A tetracyclic antidepressant, *Curr. Ther. Res.* **14:**395–413.

JACOBS, B. L., 1976, An animal behavior model for studying central serotonergic synapses, *Life Sci.* **19:**777–786.

JANCSAR, S. M., and LEONARD, B. E., 1983, Behavioral and neurochemical interactions between chronic reserpine and chronic antidepressants, *Biochem. Pharmacol.* **10:**1569–1571.

JOHNSON, R. W., TALLMAN, J. F., SQUIRES, R., and YAMAMURA, H. I., 1983, Benzodiazepine receptor heterogeneity and regulation, in: *Anxiolytics: Neurochemical, Behavioral and Clinical Perspectives,* Raven Press, New York, pp. 93–112.

JONES, C. N., HOWARD, J. L., and MCBENNETT, S. T., 1980, Stimulus properties of antidepressants in the rat, *Psychopharmacology* **67:**111–118.

KAMETANI, H., NOMURA, S., and SHIMIZU, J., 1983, The reversal effect of antidepressants on the escape deficit induced by inescapable shock in rats, *Psychopharmacology* **80:**206–208.

KATZ, R. J., and SIBEL, M., 1982, Animal models of depression: Tests of three structurally and pharmacologically novel antidepressant compounds, *Pharmacol. Biochem. Behav.* **17:**461–465.

KAUMEIER, S., DOHREN, J., and FLACH, D., 1977, WA 335 (Danitracen): A preliminary evaluation of a potential antidepressant compound. A comparative double-blind study with WA 335 and amitriptyline in the treatment of depressive patients, *Curr. Ther. Res.* **21:**108–113.

KENDALL, D. A., TAYLOR, D. P., and ENNA, S. J., 1983, ^{3}H-Tetrahydrotrazodone binding: Association with serotonin, binding sites, *Mol. Pharmacol.* **23:**594–599.

KNOBLOCH, L. C., GOLDSTEIN, J. M., and MALICK, J. B., 1982, Effects of acute and subacute antidepressant treatment on kindled seizures in rats, *Pharmacol. Biochem. Behav.* **17:**461–465.

LANGER, S. Z., RAISMAN, R., and BRILEY, M., 1981, High-affinity ^{3}H-DMI binding is associated with neuronal noradrenaline uptake in the periphery and the central nervous system, *Eur. J. Pharmacol.* **72:**423–424.

LEE, C., JAVITCH, J. A., and SNYDER, S. H., 1982, Characterization of ^{3}H-desipramine binding associated with neuronal norepinephrine uptake sites in rat brain membranes, *J. Neurosci.* **2:**1515–1525.

LEONARD, B. E., 1984, Pharmacology of new antidepressants, *Prog. Neuro-Psychopharmacol. Biol. Psychiatry* **8**:97–108.

MAGNUS, R. V., 1975, A placebo-controlled trial of Viloxazine with or without tranquillisers in depressive illness, *J. Int. Med. Res.* **3**:207–215.

MAIER, S. F., 1983, Learned helplessness, depression, analgesia, and endogenous opiates, *Psychopharmacol. Bull.* **19**:531–536.

MAJ, J., ROGOZ, Z., SKUZA, G., and SOWINSKA, H., 1982a, Effects of chronic treatment with antidepressants on aggressiveness induced by clonidine in mice, *J. Neural Trans.* **55**:19–25.

MAJ, V., ROGOZ, Z., and SKUZA, G., 1982b, Fluvoxamine, a new antidepressant drug, fails to show antiserotonin activity, *Eur. J. Pharmacol.* **81**:287–292.

MAJ, J., ROGOZ, Z., SKUZA, G., and SOWINSKA, H., 1983, Reserpine-induced locomotor stimulation in mice chronically treated with typical and atypical antidepressants, *Eur. J. Pharmacol.* **87**:469–474.

MALICK, J. B., 1981, Yohimbine potentiation as a predictor of antidepressant action, in: *Antidepressants: Neurochemical, Behavioral, and Clinical Perspectives* (S. J. Enna, J. B. Malick, and E. Richelson eds.), Raven Press, New York, pp. 141–155.

MEIGNEN, J., GROGNET, A., DENIARD, M. J., DALPHRASE, F., ROUX, E., and DeFEUDIS, F. C., 1982, Pharmacological comparison of potential antidepressant UP 614–04 with viloxazine and imipramine; behavioral studies, *Gen. Pharmacol.* **13**:381–391.

MELZACKA, M., RURAK, A., and VETULANI, J., 1980, Preliminary study of the biotransformation of two new drugs, trazodone and etoperidone, *Pol. J. Pharmacol. Pharm.* **32**:551–556.

MIELKE, D. H., and GALLANT, D. M., 1978, A controlled evaluation of a pyrrolidine derivative (AHR-1118) versus imipramine, *Curr. Ther. Res.* **24**:734–737.

MILLER, D. B., and MILLER, L. L., 1983, Buproprion, d-amphetamine, and amitriptyline-induced conditioned taste aversion in rats: Dose effects, *Pharmacol. Biochem. Behav.* **18**:737–740.

MIOR, D. C., CORNWELL, W. B., DINGWALL-FORDYCE, I., CROOKS, J., O'MALLEY, K., TURNBULL, M. J., and WEIR, R. D., 1972, Cardiotoxicity of amitriptyline, *Lancet* **2**:561–564.

MORETTI, A., PEGRASSI, L., GLASSER, A. H., and SUCHOWSKY, G., 1974, Effetto del Caroxazone, nuovo farmaco antidepressivo, sulle mono-amino-cerebrali, *Boll. Chimico Farmaceutico* **113**:36–42.

MORETTI, A., CACCIA, C., CALDERINI, G., MENOZZI, M., and AMICO, A., 1981, Studies on the mechanism of action of caroxazone, a new antidepressant drug, *Biochem. Pharmacol.* **30**:2728–2731.

MORSELLI, P. L., and LLOYD, K. G. (eds.), 1986, *GABA and Mood Disorders*, Raven Press, New York.

MURPHY, D. L., LIPPER, S., CAMPBELL, I. C., MAJOR, L. F., SLATER, S. L., and BUCHSBAUM, M., 1979, Comparative studies of MAO-A and MAO-B inhibitors in man, in: *Monoamine Oxidase: Structure, Function, and Altered Functions* (T. P. Singer, R. W. VanKorff, and D. L. Murphy, eds.), Academic Press, New York, pp. 457–475.

OBERMEIR, W., and POLDINGER, W., 1977, Doppelblindvergleich der Wirkungen eines neuen trizyklischen Antidepressivums (Lofepramin) und eines tetrazyklischen Antidepressivums (Maprotilin), *Int. Pharmacopsychiat.* **12**:65–78.

O'DONNELL, J. M., and SEIDEN, L. S., 1982, Effects of monoamine oxidase inhibitors on performance during differential reinforcement of low response rate, *Psychopharmacology* **78**:214–218.

O'DONNELL, J. M., and SEIDEN, L. S., 1983, Differential reinforcement of low rate 72-second schedule: Selective effects of antidepressant drugs, *J. Pharmacol. Exp. Ther.* **224**:80–88.

PALKOVITS, M., RAISMAN, R., BRILEY, M., and LANGER, S., 1981, Regional distribution of ^{3}H-imipramine binding in rat brain, *Brain Res.* **210**:493–498.

PEROUTKA, S. J., and SNYDER, S. H., 1981, Interactions of antidepressants with neurotransmitter receptor sites, in: *Antidepressants: Neurochemical, Behavioral, and Clinical Perspectives* (S. J. Enna, J. B. Malick, and E. Richelson, eds.), Raven Press, New York, pp. 75–90.

PORSOLT, R. D., ANTON, G., BLAVET, N., and JALFRE, M., 1978, Behavioral despair: A new model sensitive to antidepressant treatments, *Eur. J. Pharmacol.* **47**:379–391.

PUECH, A. J., CHERMAT, R., PONCELET, M., DOARE, L., and SIMON, P., 1981, Antagonism of hypothermia and behavioral response to apomorphine: A simple, rapid, and discriminating test for screening antidepressants and neuroleptics, *Psychopharmacology* **75**:84–91.

RAITERI, M., ANGELINI, F., and BERTOLLINI, A., 1976, Comparative study of the effects of mianserin, a tetracyclic antidepressant, and of imipramine on uptake and release of neurotransmitters in synaptosomes, *J. Pharm. Pharmacol.* **28**:483–488.

RICHELSON, E., 1984, The new antidepressants: Structures, pharmacokinetics, and proposed mechanisms of action, *Psychopharmacol. Bull.* **2**:213–223.

ROGOZ, Z., SKUZA, G., and SOWINSKA, H., 1981, Effects of antihistaminic drugs in tests for antidepressant action, *Pol. J. Pharmacol.* **33**:321–335.

SALETU, B., 1982, Pharmaco-EEG profiles of typical and atypical antidepressants, in: *Typical and Atypical Antidepressants: Clinical Practice* (E. Costa and G. Racagni, eds.), Raven Press, New York, pp. 257–268.

SALETU, B., KREIGER, P., GRUNBERGER, J., SCHANDA, H., and SLETTEN, I., 1977, Tandamine—A new norepinephrine re-uptake inhibitor, *Int. Pharmacopsychiat.* **12**:137–152.

SCHATZBERG, A., and COLE, J., 1978, Benzodiazepines in depressive disorders, *Arch. Gen. Psychiatry* **35**:1359–1365.

SCHILDKRAUT, J. J., 1978, Current studies of the catecholamine hypothesis of the affective disorders, in: *Psychopharmacology: A Generation of Progress* (M. S. Lipton, A. DiMascio, and K. Killam, eds.), Raven Press, New York, pp. 1223–1234.

SHERMAN, A. D., SACQUITNE, J. L., and PETTY, F., 1982, Specificity of the learned helplessness model of depression, *Pharmacol. Biochem. Behav.* **16**:449–454.

SHOPSIN, B., CASSANO, G. B., and CONFI, L., 1981, An overview of new "second generation" antidepressant compounds: Research and treatment implications, in: *Antidepressants: Neurochemical, Behavioral, and Clinical Perspectives* (S. J. Enna, J. B. Malick, and E. Richelson, eds.), Raven Press, New York, pp. 219–251.

SJOGREN, C., 1980, The pharmacological profile of lofepramine, a new antidepressant drug, *Neuropharmacology* **19**:1213–1214.

SPYRAKI, C., and FIBIGER, H. C., 1981, Intravenous self-administration of nomifensine in rats: Implications for abuse potential in humans, *Science* **212**:1167–1168.

SUGRUE, M. F., 1980a, Effects of acutely and chronically administered desipramine and mianserin on the clonidine-induced decrease in rat brain 3-methoxy-4-hydroxyphenylethyleneglycol sulphate content, *Br. J. Pharmacol.* **69**:299.

SUGRUE, M. F., 1980b, Changes in rat brain monoamine turnover following chronic antidepressant administration, *Life Sci.* **26**:423–429.

SUGRUE, M. F., 1981, Chronic antidepressant administration and adaptive changes in central monoaminergic systems, in: *Antidepressants: Neurochemical, Behavioral, and Clinical Perspectives* (S. J. Enna, J. B. Malick, and E. Richelson, eds.), Raven Press, New York, pp. 13–30.

SULSER, F., 1978, Functional aspects of the norepinephrine receptor coupled adenylate cyclase system in the limbic forebrain and its modification by drugs which precipitate or alleviate depression: molecular approaches to our understanding of affective disorder, *Pharmakopsychiatr. Neuropsychopharmakol.* **11**:43–52.

TELNER, J. I., and SINGHAL, R. H., 1981, Effects of nortriptyline treatment on learned helplessness in the rat, *Pharmacol. Biochem. Behav.* **14**:823–826.
USDIN, E., 1978, Classification of psychotropic drugs, in: *Principles of Psychopharmacology*, 2nd ed. (W. G. Clark and J. del Guidice, eds.), Academic Press, New York, pp. 193–246.
VAN DIJK, J., HARTOG, J., and HILLEN, F. C., 1978, Nontricyclic antidepressants, *Prog. Med. Chem.* **15**:262–320.
VETULANI, J., SCHWARTZ, R. J., DINGELL, J. V., and SULSER, F., 1976, A possible common mechanism of action of antidepressant treatments, *Naunyn-Schmiedbergs Arch. Pharmacol.* **293**:109–114.
WRIGHT, J., and DENBER, H., 1978, Clinical trial of fluvoxamine; a new serotonergic antidepressant, *Curr. Ther. Res.* **23**:83–89.

INDEX

ABTX, 426
Acetylcholine
　aggression, 198
　electroconvulsive shock, 386
　hypothalamic, aggression, 187
　morphine withdrawal, 252
　synthesis, electroconvulsive shock, 398–399
ACTH, see Adrenocorticotropic hormone
Adrenergic receptors
　beta, electroconvulsive shock, 391–393
Adrenocorticotropic hormone
　analogs, 545
　memory, 543–546
Affective states, conditioning, 26–36
Aggression
　acetylcholine, 198
　　hypothalamic, 187
　affective, 194
　amphetamine, 263
　autoaggression, 228
　brain lesion-induced, 195
　brain stimulation-evoked, 194–195
　brain tumor, 194
　cannabis, 255–261
　clonidine, 196
　cocaine, 263
　"code," 187
　drug treatment, 204–205
　frustration-induced, 193
　hallucinogens, 196, 252–263
　interspecies, 203
　intraspecies, 203
　isolation-induced, 188–189
　lysergic acid diethylamide, 253–254
　maternal, 202–203
　mescaline, 254–255

Aggression (cont'd)
　methylphenidate, 263
　methylxanthine, 263
　morphine, 196
　morphine withdrawal, 251–252
　pain-induced, 189, 192–193
　pathological, 254
　phencyclidine, 255
　predatory, 203–204, 226
　prevalent aggressive behavior pattern, 267
　psychopharmacology, 183–277
　resident-intruder, 201–202
　seizure, 198–199
　serotonin, 187
　sexual, 233–234
　status-related, 199–201
　tetrahydrocannabinol, 255–261
Alcohol
　aggression, 235–245
　　animal, 235–241
　　determinants, 238
　　dose–effect relationship, 238
　　homicide, 241–245
　　mechanism, 245
　　testosterone, 239
　　violence, 241, 242
Alpha-methyl-p-tyrosine, dextroamphetamine, 339
Alprazolam, mechanism of action, 611
Alzheimer's dementia, 549
　model, 452
Amitriptyline
　assay, 623
　carbohydrate ingestion, 133, 135
　predatory aggression, 226
　structure, 610

Amoxapine, 611
Amphetamine
  aggression, 263
    clinical data, 274–275
    determinants of effect, 266–271
    dose-related response, 267
    drug administration, 271
    drug antagonism, 272
    rage response, 266
  anorexic effect, 21
  antiaggressive effect, 272
    drug antagonism, 272
    efficacy, 275
  conditioned place preference, 33
  conditioned taste aversion, 28
  dopamine release
  feeding behavior, 152
  feeding pattern, 142
  vs. fenfluramine, 152
  food intake, 129
  6-hydroxydopamine, 196
  locomotor activity, 169
  mechanism of action, 74–75
  motor activity, 71
  nicotine blockade, 447
  orexic *and* anorexic effect, 169–171
  quantitative effects, conceptualization, 170
  reverse tolerance, 18
  social status-dependent effect, 269
  stereotypy, 577
  stress response, 8
  substance P blockade, 552
  Tourette's syndrome, 96
Amygdala, 482
Anabasine, 426
  generalization with nicotine, 439
Analgesia (*see also* Pain)
  amygdala, 482
  endogenous systems, 485–495 (*see also* Opioids)
  footshock-induced, 485, 490–493
  opiate, 478–484
  stimulation-produced, 480
  stress-induced, 7, 23
Androgens, 135
Anesthetic hypotension, 502
Angel dust, *see* Phencyclidine
Angiotensin II, 550
Anorexia, 161–168
Anorexia nervosa, 136
Antiandrogenic agents, 233–234

Anticonvulsant drugs
  aggression, 232–233
  tolerance to, 24–26
Antidepressant drugs
  aggression, 223–228
  assay, 623
  binding sites, 617
  vs. electroconvulsive therapy, 376
  food intake, 133
  receptor binding, 619
  second-generation, 609–631
    behavioral assays, 619–625
    mechanism of action, 612–616
    neurological assays, 616–619
    serotonin antagonism, 622
Apomorphine
  A10 neuron activity, 338
  aggression, 269
  attack behavior, 269
  food intake, 130
  morphine withdrawal, 252
  nicotine blockade, 447
  stereotypy, 577
Appetitive behavior, 600–602
Arcuate nucleus, 13
Arecoline, 386
  catalepsy, 386
  discrimination, 447
Arginine vasopressin, 540
Attention deficit disorder
  diagnosis, 68
  differential diagnosis, 69
  with hyperactivity, 64, 68–74
  neurochemistry, 75–84
  phenylethylamine, 83
  Tourette's syndrome, 96
  treatment, 74
Attentional dysfunction, 61, 70
Atropine
  food intake, 129
  tachycardia, 15
Autoreceptor, 337
  nerve terminal, 337
  supersensitivity, 355
Avoidance response, 577
Azepindole, 611

Barbiturates
  aggression, 213–214, 216–217
  food intake, 134
Behavior
  aggression, 183–277

INDEX

Behavior (cont'd)
  feeding, 123–181
  predatory, 197
Benzedrine, 84, 86
Benzodiazepines
  antiaggressive effect, 220
  food intake, 133, 134
  rage reactions associated with, 222
  receptors, 220
  taming action, 213
Beta-adrenergic blockers, 211–213
Beta-funaltrexamine, 500
Bicuculline, 381
Blood pressure, 15
Body temperature, 9–12
Bombesin, 130
Brain tumor, 194
Bulbocapnine
  cardiovascular effects, 15
  mechanism of action, 15
Bupropion
  assay, 624
  mechanism of action, 611
  structure, 610
  as a training drug, 621
Butyrophenones
  aggression, 205, 210
  catalepsy, 578
Bypass surgery, intestinal, 127

Caffeine
  aggression, 275
  food intake, 135
Calcitonin, 130
Calcium, 400–401
Cannabinoids, 196
Cannabis, 255–261; see also
    Tetrahydrocannabinol
Carbachol, 426
Cardiovascular system, 15–16
Caroxazone, 611
Catalepsy, 578
Cathine, see Phenylpropanolamine
Cathinone, 132
Central nervous system
  dopamine receptors, 338
  nicotinic receptor, 454–457
Cerebral vascular disorders, 502
CGS 8216, 132
Chemotherapy, 36–37
Childhood psychiatric disorders, 59–121
Chloralose, 134

Chlordiazepoxide
  aggression, 214–215
  food intake, 133
  nicotine, 442
  satiation, 141
Chlorimipramine, 226
Chlorisondamine, 426
  nicotine blockade, 447
p-Chlorophenylalanine, 379
Chlorpromazine
  aggression, 206–208, 210
  amphetamine aggression, 272
  food intake, 133, 134
Cholecystokinin, 550–551
  food intake, 130, 551
  memory, 551
Cigarette smoking, 451
Circadian rhythm, 8
Clonidine
  aggression, 196
  attention deficit disorder with
      hyperactivity, 74
  dosage, 101, 102
  food intake, 135
  haloperiodol with, 102
  vs. haloperidol, Tourette's syndrome, 101
  onset of action, 101
  side effects, 102
  Tourette's syndrome, 97, 101–102
  withdrawal symptoms, 98
Clothiapine, 211
Clozapine
  aggression, 211
  food intake, 134
Cocaine
  aggression, 263
  food intake, 131
  reverse tolerance, 18
Conditioned drug effects, 2
  cardiovascular, 15–16
  drug self-administration, 37
  paradoxical conditioning, 9
Conditioned place preference, 28
  amphetamine-induced, 33
  cocaine-induced, 33
  development, 33
Conditioned response, 2
Conditioned stimulus, 1
Conditioned taste aversion, 27–29
  loss of, 32
  naloxone, 31
  nicotine, 435–436

Conditioning
  drug effects, 2
  evidence, 4
  optimal conditions, 5–6
  tests, 3–4
Contingent tolerance, 21
Cotinine, 443
Corticosterone, 259
Cyclic AMP, 399–400
Cyproheptadine
  anorexia nervosa, 136
  food intake, 134, 136
Cyproterone acetate, 233, 234
Cytisine, 426
  generalization with nicotine, 439

d-Ala^2-d-Leu^5-enkephalin (DADLE), 501
Danitracen, 611
De Lange syndrome, 266
Depressive illness, 375
Desipramine, 623
Desmethylimipramine, 352
Dextroamphetamine
  A10 neuron activity, 338
  alpha-methyl-p-tyrosine, 339
  vs. fenfluramine, 146
  haloperidol antagonism, 344
  learning disability, 90
  mechanism of action, 70
  rebound effect, 72
Diazepam, 379
Diethylpropion, 146
Dimethyl-phenylpiperazinium, 426
Diphenylhydantoin, 233
L-dopa
  A10 neuron activity, 338
  morphine withdrawal, 252
Dopamine
  A8 neurons, 331
  A9 neurons, 331, 332–334
  A10 neurons, 331
    vs. A9, 332–334
    chronic neuroleptic administration, 352
    effect of agonists, 338–348
    GABA, 351, 355–358
    isoproterenol, 359
    piperoxan, 359
    rauwolscine, 359
    serotonin, 358–359
    substance P, 360
    yohimbine, 359

Dopamine (cont'd)
  agonists, 267
  amphetamine-stimulated, 19
  appetitive behavior, 600–602
  attention disorder deficit with
      hyperactivity, 75
  cerebral cortex, 330
  depletion, 578
  electroconvulsive shock, 380–382
  intracranial self-stimulation, 579
  mesocortical system, 330–332
  mesolimbic system, 330–332
  midbrain systems, 330–332
    A9 vs. A10, 332–334
    electrophysiological identification, 334–337
    neuron regulation, 337–355
  nigrostriatal system, 330
  opiate reward, 498
  reciprocal action with serotonin, 146
  synthesis, 390
Dopamine receptors
  CNS, 338
  D-2 subtype, 338
Drug(s)
  of abuse, 235–277
  aggression, 204–235
  antidepressants, see Antidepressant drugs
  food intake, 126–136
  pediatric medication, 65–67
  tranquilizers, see Tranquilizers
  treatment, 40
Drug effects
  conditioned, 2
  multiple, 6–7
  observed, 2
Drug self-administration, 37–40, 423
  conditioned drug effects, 37
Drug tolerance, 354
  conditioning factors in, 18–26
Dyslexia
  neuropsychological syndromes in, 85
  piracetam, 92

Electroconvulsive shock
  acetylcholine, 386
  vs. antidepressant drugs, 376
  beta-adrenergic receptor, 391–393
  clonidine-induced neuroendocrine response, 401
  dopamine, 380–382

Electroconvulsive shock (cont'd)
  GABA, 383–386
  haloperidol-induced catalepsy, 383
  5-hydroxytryptamine, 377–380, 402
  naloxone, 386–387
  neurotensin, 400
  norepinephrine, 382–383
  opioids, 386–387
  substance P, 400
Electroconvulsive therapy
  calcium levels, serum, 400–401
  depressive illness, 375
  mechanism of action, 375–408
Endorphins, see Opioids
Enkephalin, 480
Enterogastrone, 130
Epinephrine
  blood pressure, 15
  cardiovascular effects, 15
  food intake, 129
Estradiol, 259
Estrogens, 130
Ethanol (see also Alcohol)
  anticonvulsant effects, 24
  hypothermia, 11
  tolerance, 16, 20
Ethyl-β-carboline-3-carboxylate, 220
Euphoria, 579–580
Extinction, 3

Feeding behavior
  amphetamine, 152
  control, models, 171–173
  fenfluramine, 152
  vs. food intake, 137
  serotonin manipulation, 145–155
  structure, 139–142
Feeding patterns, 160–161
Fenfluramine
  vs. amphetamine, 152
  anorexic activity
    context-dependency, 171
    mechanism, 147, 149
  feeding behavior, 152
  feeding patterns, 142
  food intake, 130
  vs. other anorexic agents, 146
  satiation, 142
Fluvoxamine, 611
Fluoxetine
  mechanism of action, 611

Fluoxetine (cont'd)
  predatory aggression, 226
  structure, 610
Flurothyl, 377
Flutamide, 233
Food intake
  alteration, 139
  carbohydrates, 144
  control, 125–126
  drugs, 126–136
  enhancement, 132–136
  fat, 144
  vs. feeding behavior, 137
  naloxone, 155–158
  naltrexone, 159
  nicotine, 450
  protein, 144
  psychopharmacology, 123–182
  satiation, 141
  serotonin, 149–150
  serotonin synthesis, 144–145
  suppression, 128–132, 136–137
  xylamidine, 150
Formamidines, 135

Gamma-aminobutyric acid (GABA), 232
  A10 dopamine neurons, 351, 355–358
  electroconvulsive shock, 383–386
  synthesis, 393–395
Gates Diagnostic Reading Test, 90
Glucose, 129
Glutamic acid, 351
Glutamic acid decarboxylase, 396
Glycerol, 129
Gray Oral Reading Test, 85

Hallucinogens
  aggression, 196, 252–263
Haloperidol
  aggression, 208, 210
  amphetamine aggression, 272
  amphetamine-induced conditioned place
    preference, 33
  clonidine with, 102
  vs. clonidine, 101
  dextroamphetamine, 344
  dosage, 101
  with methylphenidate, 100
  onset of action, 101
  side effects, 100
  tardive dyskinesia, 100–101
  tolerance, 354
  Tourette's syndrome, 95, 99–100

Heart rate
  conditioned, 16
  deceleration, 16
Hexamethonium, 426
Homovanillic acid, 80
Horseradish peroxidase, 331
Hydroxycitrate, 129
6-Hydroxydopamine, 331
  amphetamine, 196
  attack behavior, 268
  irritability, 196
5-Hydroxyindoleacetic acid, 96
5-Hydroxytryptamine
  electroconvulsive shock, 377–380, 402
  head-twitch behavior, 388
  receptor, 388
  synthesis, 387
5-Hydroxytryptophan
  electroconvulsive shock, 378
  feeding pattern, 142
  food intake, 130
Hyperactivity (see also Attention deficit
    disorder, with hyperactivity)
  animal models, 76–79
  diagnosis, 68
  3-methoxy-4-hydroxyphenylethylene
    glycol, 80–82
  prevalence, 68
  vanillylmandelic acid, 83
Hyperkinetic child, 64 (see also
    Hyperactivity)
Hyperphagia, 127
Hypertension, essential, opioids, 502
Hyperthermia, 10
Hypoglycemia, 14
Hypophagia, 127
Hypothalamus, 194
Hypothermia
  ethanol, 11
  impromidine-induced, 387
  pentobarbital, 12

ICI 154, 129, 502
Idazoxan, 352
Imipramine
  antiaggressive effects, 223, 224
  hyperactivity, 228
  increased aggressiveness, 226
  vs. placebo, 91
  structure, 610
Immune response, 16–17
Impromidine, 387

Insulin, 135
Insulin receptor, 13
Insulin secretion, 14
  cephalic phase, 14
  conditioning of changes, 12–15
Intracranial self-stimulation
  dopamine, 579
  nicotine, 448–449
  thresholds, measurement, 586
Iowa Test of Basic Skills, 90
Iprindole
  assay, 621
  mechanism, 611
  structure, 610
Isoproterenol
  A10 dopamine neurons, 359
  food intake, 132

Killer weed, see Phencyclidine
Korsakoff's syndrome, 540

Learned helplessness, 619
Learning; see also Memory
  defined, 533
Learning disability, 64, 84–93 (see also
    Learning disorder)
  dextroamphetamine, 90
  long-term therapy, 91–92
  methylphenidate, 87
Learning disorder
  diagnosis, 84–85
Lesch–Nyhan syndrome, 266, 540
Lipid synthesis, 128
Lisuride, 130
Lithium
  aggression, 228–232
  antiaggressive effect
    clinical evidence, 231
    mechanism, 230
  conditioned taste aversion, 230
  pediatric use, 232
  predatory behavior, 230
Lithium chloride
  anorexic activity, 162–168
  conditioned taste aversion, 28
Lobeline, 426
  nicotine binding, 441
Locomotor activity
  amphetamine, 169
  morphine, 19
Lofepramine, 611
LSD, see Lysergic acid diethylamide

INDEX 639

Lysergic acid diethylamide
    aggression, 196, 253–254, 261
    predatory killing, 254
Lysine vasopressin, 535
    amnesia, 540
    avoidance task, 536

Maprotiline
    mechanism of action, 611
    predatory aggression, 226
Marihuana, see Cannabis,
        Tetrahydrocannabinol
Mazindol
    vs. fenfluramine, 146
    food intake, 129, 130
Mecamyline, 426
    nicotine discriminative effects, 447
    nicotine-induced conditioned taste
        aversion, 436
Medroxyprogesterone acetate, 234
Memory
    defined, 533
    James–Lange theory, 559
    neuropeptides, 531–573
        adrenocorticotropic hormone, 543–546
        neurotensin, 549–550
        opioids, 546–548
        oxytocin, 542–543
        somatostatin, 548–549
        substance P, 552
        vasopressin, 535–542
Meprobamate, 133, 134
Mescaline, 196, 254–255
Metenkephalin, 248
    electroconvulsive shock, 397
3-Methoxy-4-hydroxyphenylethylene glycol
    hyperactivity, 80–82
    Tourette's syndrome, 97
5-Methoxy-N,N-dimethyltryptamine, 254
Methylphenidate
    A10 neuron activity, 338
    aggression, 263, 274, 275
    antiaggressive effect, 275
    controlled trials, 90
    dosage, 87
    efficacy, 90
    half-life, 87
    haloperidol, 100
    learning disability, 87
    mechanism of action, 70
    morphine withdrawal, 252

Methylphenidate (cont'd)
    vs. placebo, 91
    Tourette's syndrome, 96
Methylxanthine, 263
Methysergide
    amphetamine aggression, 272
    discrimination, 447
    food intake, 134
    5-hydroxytryptamine-mediated behavior, 379
Mianserin
    assay, 621
    serotonin antagonism, 622
    structure, 610
Midazolam, 447
Midbrain
    dopamine systems, 330–332
    dopamine-containing neurons, 329, 332–334
        electrophysiological identification, 334–337
        regulation, 337–355
Milenperone, 211
Minimal brain dysfunction, 64
Molindone, 211
Monoamine oxidase inhibitors, 223
    antiaggressive effects, 225
    assay, 623
Morphine
    aggression, 196, 245–253
    body temperature, 10
    cardiovascular effects, 15
    discrimination, 447
    heart rate, 15
    hyperthermia, 10
    locomotor activity, 19
    reverse tolerance, 18
    stress-induced analgesia, 7
    tolerance, 23
    withdrawal, 30, 251
Motivation theory, 168
Muscimol, 131

Nalorphine, 38
Naloxazone, 502
Naloxone
    aggression, 247
    cigarette smoking, 451
    conditioned taste aversion, 31
    electroconvulsive shock, 386
    feeding pattern, 142, 160–161
    food intake, 131, 155–158, 249

Naloxone (cont'd)
  social interaction, 248
  stimulation-produced analgesia, 480
  stress-induced analgesia, 7
Naltrexone
  aggression, 248
  feeding pattern, 142
  food intake, 159, 249
Neimarck Memory Test, 93
Neuroleptic drugs, 575–607
  anhedonia hypothesis, 580
  anticipation-invigoration, 595
  apomorphine stereotypy, 577
  appetitive task performance, 577
  catalepsy, 578
  passive avoidance response, 577
  response-reinforcement matching, 589–592
Neuropeptides
  blood–brain barrier permeability, 556–557
  memory, 531–573
Neurotensin
  electroconvulsive shock, 400
  memory, 549–550
  sites, 549
Nicotine, 421–457 (see also Cigarette smoking)
  analogs, 439, 442
  as an aversive stimulus, 434–437
  as a negative reinforcer, 435
  as a punisher, 434–435
  chlordiazepoxide, 442
  CNS receptor, 454–457
  cocaine generalization, 443
  conditioned taste aversion, 435–436
  cue, origin
  discriminative stimulus effects, 437–448
    blockade, 447
    characteristics, 445
    chlorisondamine, 447
    mecamylamine, 447
  drug generalized with, defined, 439
  food intake, 450
  intracranial self-stimulation, 448–449
  picrotoxin, 442
  as a positive reinforcer, 429–432
  self-administration, 430–433, 452
Nisoxetine, 622
Nomifensine
  food intake, 130
  mechanism of action, 611
  structure, 610

Noradrenaline, see Norepinephrine
Norepinephrine
  attention disorder deficit with hyperactivity syndrome, 75
  electroconvulsive shock, 382–383, 390–393
  food intake, 129
  morphine withdrawal, 252
Nortriptyline, 610
Nucleus raphe magnus, 481
Nucleus reticularis gigantocellularis, 481

Observed drug effects, 2
Obesity, 153–154
Operant behavior, 598–600
Opiates, 467–529
  cardiovascular effects, 499–502
  defined, 467
  mechanism of action, 478, 479
  vs. opioids, 467
  pain transmission, 478–484
  receptors, 500–501
  reward, 495–499
Opioids
  electroconvulsive shock, 386–387
  memory and learning, 546–548
  vs. opiates, 467
ORG 6582, 130
Orthostatic hypotension, 502
Oxazepam, 223
Oxytocin, 542–543

Pain
  opiates, 469–495
  transmission
    afferent pathways, 471–478
    opiates, 478–484
Paradoxical conditioning, 9
Peace pill, see Phencyclidine
Pemoline, 96
Pempidine, 426
Pentobarbital, 12
Pentobarbitone, 447
Phencyclidine
  aggression, 196, 255
  discrimination, 447
Phenelzine, 610
Phenothiazines (see also specific agents)
  aggression, 205, 210
  catalepsy, 578
  weight gain, 133
Phenoxybenzamine, 272
Phenylephrine, 383

Phenylethylamine
    attention disorder deficit with activity, 83
    food intake, 132
Phenylpropanolamine, 132
Picrotoxin, 442
Pimozide
    aggression, 208
    amphetamine aggression, 272
    cardiac effects, 103
    chemical structure, 103
    clinical trials, 103
    dosage, 103
    efficacy, 103
    euphoria, 579–580
    mechanism of action, 103
    pediatric dosage, 103
    vs. placebo, 103
    reinforcement-suppressing effect, 579
    side effects, 103
    Tourette's syndrome, 102–103
Pindolol, 212
Piperoxan, 359
Pipotiazine, 353
Piracetam, 92–93
    dyslexia, 92
    vs. placebo, 92–93
    senile dementia, 92
Piribedil, 130
Pizotifen, 622
Prazosin
    amphetamine aggression, 272
    dopamine neurons, 352
Pridefine, 611
Progabide, 611
Promazine
    aggression, 211
    food intake, 134
Propranolol
    aggression, 211, 212
    amphetamine aggression, 272
Prostaglandins
    food intake, 131
    precursors, 131
Psychotherapy, 99
(3)-Pyridyl-methylpyrrollodine, 439

Quinine, 162–168
Quinuclidinylbenzylate, 399
Quipazine
    discrimination, 447
    food intake, 130
    seizure threshold, 385

Rauwolscine, 359
Reinforcement, 450
Ro 15-1788
    benzodiazepine antagonism, 220
    diazepam antagonism, 220
Rocket fuel, *see* Phencyclidine

Salbutamol, 132
Satietin, 129
Satiation, 141
SCH 12, 679
Scopolamine, 447
Seizure
    aggression, 198–199
    bicuculline, 381
    functional changes following, 377–387
Senile dementia, 92
Serotonin
    A10 dopamine neurons, 358–359
    aggression, 187
    antagonism, 622
    attention disorder deficit with hyperactivity syndrome, 75
    dietary self-selection, 151–152
    drug-induced aggression, 196
    feeding behavior, 145–155
    food intake, 130, 149–150
    morphine withdrawal, 252
    reciprocal action with dopamine, 145
    synthesis, 144–145
Serotonin syndrome, 623
Somatostatin
    Alzheimer's dementia, 549
    food intake, 130
    memory, 548–549
Spinothalamic nociceptive neuron, 473–478
Spiperone, 142
Spiramide, 208
Stereotypy
    amphetamine, 577
    apomorphine, 577
Stimulants
    clinical effects, 70–74
    in pediatrics, 70–74
Stress response, 7
Strychnine, 385
Substance K, 360
Substance P, 551–553
    A10 dopamine neurons, 360–362
    amphetamine blockade, 552

Substance P (*cont'd*)
  electroconvulsive shock, 400, 552
  memory, 552
Sulpiride, 352

Tandamine, 611
Tardive dyskinesia, 100–101
Taste aversion, 27–29
Temperature, body, *see* Body temperature
Tetrabenazine, 623
Tetrahydrocannabinol
  aggression, 255–261
  analgesic effects, 257
  antiaggressive effect
    estradiol treatment, 259
    mechanism, 261
    morphine withdrawal, 259
    temperature, 259
    tryptophan hydroxylase, 259
  corticosterone, 259
  dose-related response, 257
  food intake, 131
Testosterone, 239
Thioridazine, 210
THIP, 131
Threochlorocitrate, 129
Thyrotropin-releasing hormone, 130
Tifluadom, 248
  food intake, 135
Tolerance (*see also* Tolerance under specific drugs)
  contingent, 21
  drug, *see* Drug tolerance
Tourette's syndrome, 93–106, 266
  amphetamine, 96
  attention disorder deficit with hyperactivity, 95
  choice of medication, 104
  clonidine, 97, 101–102
  CSF 5-hydroxyindoleacetic acid, 96
  diagnosis, 99
  EEG abnormality, 94
  etiology, 94
  genetic aspects, 95
  haloperidol, 95, 99–100
  incidence, 95
  3-methoxy-4-hydroxyphenylethylene, 97

Tourette's syndrome (*cont'd*)
  methylphenidate, 96
  motor coordination, 94
  multiple handicaps, 105–106
  neurochemical research, 95–98
  pemoline, 96
  pimozide, 102–103
  psychotherapy, 99
Tranquilizers, 133
Tranylcypromine
  predatory aggression, 226
  structure, 610
Trazodone
  mechanism of action, 611
  serotonin antagonism, 622
  structure, 610
Tryptophan
  feeding pattern, 142
  food intake, 130
Tryptophan hydroxylase, 259
Tubocurarine, 426

Ultradian rhythm, 8
Unconditioned response, 2
Unconditioned stimulus, 1

Vanillylmandelic acid, 83
Vasopressin, 535–542
  learning and memory, 535–542
  physiological action, 535
Viloxazine
  mechanism of action, 611
  serotonin antagonism, 622

WA 355-BS, 134
Wide Range Achievement Test, 85, 89, 91, 93

Xylamidine, 150

Yohimbine
  A10 dopamine neurons, 359
  food intake, 135

Zimelidine
  mechanism of action, 611
  serotonin antagonism, 622
Zometapine, 611

RAYMOND H. FOGLER LIBRARY
DATE DUE